The
New HOLISTIC
HEALTH Handbook

The New HOLISTIC HEALTH Handbook

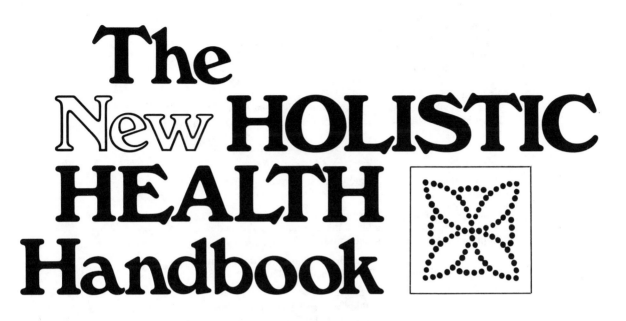

Living Well in a New Age

Berkeley Holistic Health Center

Edited by **SHEPHERD BLISS**, *John F. Kennedy University*

EDWARD BAUMAN □ LORIN PIPER
ARMAND IAN BRINT □ PAMELA AMELIA WRIGHT

A PLUME BOOK

PLUME
Published by the Penguin Group
Penguin Books USA Inc., 375 Hudson Street, New York,
New York 10014, U.S.A.
Penguin Books Ltd, 27 Wrights Lane, London W8 5TZ,
England
Penguin Books Australia Ltd, Ringwood, Victoria, Australia
Penguin Books Canada Ltd, 10 Alcorn Ave., Toronto, Ontario,
Canada M4V 3B2
Penguin Books (N.Z.) Ltd, 182-190 Wairau Road, Auckland 10,
New Zealand

Penguin Books Ltd, Registered Offices: Harmondsworth,
Middlesex, England

Published by Plume, an imprint of New American Library, a
division of Penguin Books USA Inc. Previously published in a
Stephen Greene Press Books edition.

First published in 1985 by The Stephen Greene Press, Inc.
Published simultaneously in Canada by Penguin Books Canada
Limited
Distributed by Viking Penguin Inc.

10 9 8 7 6 5 4 3 2 1

LIBRARY OF CONGRESS CATALOGING IN PUBLICATION DATA
The New holistic health handbook.
    Rev. ed. of: The Holistic health handbook / compiled by the
Berkeley Holistic Health Center; Edward Bauman . . . [et al.].
c1978.
    Bibliography: p.
    Includes index.
    1. Health—Addresses, essays, lectures.   2. Holistic
medicine—Addresses, essays, lectures.   I. Bliss, Shepherd.
II. Berkeley Holistic Health Center. III. Holistic health
handbook.   [DNLM: 1. Holistic Health.   2. Therapeutic
Cults.   W 61 N5315]
RA776.5.N48 1985   613   85-70528

 REGISTERED TRADEMARK—MARCA REGISTRADA

Printed in the United States of America

*The drawings on pages 48, 50, 95, 156, 190, and 291 are by Cata
Carney. Those on pages 63 and 351 are by Amanita Mageau. Those
on pages 54, 122, and 148 are respectively by Phil Gardner, Rainbow
Canyon, and Deborah M. Cotter.*

Contents

V. Bodywork and Movement   323

VI. The Growing Legitimacy of Holism   353

VII. Out Into the Wider World—Beyond the Individual   379

INTRODUCTION   *Shepherd Bliss*   *380*

Acknowledgments

It's always easier to take over a "going concern," so my greatest acknowledgment must be to Eddie Bauman, Lorin Piper, Amelia Wright and Armand Brint who put so much love and care into the first edition of this book. Without their base, the revision would not have been possible.

During the full 12 months that I labored to bring this book into being, many individuals and groups made its growth from the 1970s version to this 1980s version possible. Most of those people live in or around Berkeley, California, though a substantial number of them reside in the Boston area—two key regions where the holistic health movement is growing.

Beginning with my Berkeley support, Naomi Steinfeld and her experienced editorial skills must receive my first and foremost acknowledgment. Her creativity and persistence helped transform many of the book's articles. She joined me soon after the original flush of enthusiasm for the book—that is, when the real work of soliciting articles and working on them was necessary. Naomi was the patient editor who worked with many writers and their writings, helping them (much like a midwife) to bring a written communication into being—to render what they knew as health practitioners in their hands, bodies, and minds onto the page.

Among my San Francisco Bay Area colleagues who were vital was Ellen Freeman. Her positive human energy and commitment was crucial, especially in keeping our publications office running. Support I received from John F. Kennedy University, where I teach, and from one of my deans, Anne Langford, was also most helpful. Two of my other deans, Ron Levinson and Keith McConnell, in Graduate Psychology, have helped indirectly by supporting me through the years by allowing me to explore new areas and subjects to teach, such as holistic health. Other key support groups and individuals were Psychotherapists for Social Responsibility, especially Barbara Green, and Interhelp, especially Fran Peavey, Barbara Hazard and Sara Chapman. Health experts such as Dana Ullman, writers such as Peter Beren of Sierra Club Books and editors such as Michael Castleman of *Medical Self-Care* and Stephan Bodian of *Yoga Journal* were also particularly helpful. Though he was too often off in Tunisia or the Fiji Islands in the

Peace Corps, I also want to appreciate Gordon Murray. And Linda Seymour up in Oregon.

Substantial amounts of work occurred in the Boston area, where I lived during the 1970s and continue to spend many months of each year. My friends—Joseph Pleck, Mark Gerzon, and Sam Osherson among them—came through for me in important ways. I also want to appreciate Frank Collins of Radcliffe Publishing Procedures, Tova Green and Nancy Moorehead of Interhelp, Christina Engels, R.N., and two editors of *Whole Life Times*, Randy Showstack and Shelly Kellman. They each led me to valuable resources which improved this book.

I must reserve a special word of thanks for the poet Robert Bly—whose work has inspired me for over 20 years now, from the time I was in the U.S. Army. He has helped teach me how healing the arts and the expression of deep emotions, such as grief, can be.

In the year that I have been working on this book it has gone from its original publisher, And/Or Press in Berkeley to The Stephen Greene Press in Massachusetts to Viking/Penguin in New York. The stabilizing element in this development has been publisher Tom Begner, whose persistence and patience were most helpful. Managing editor Kathy Shulga has done a marvelous job coordinating all the details necessary to produce such a book.

My deepest appreciation must go to those nearly 100 writers who contributed to this volume, most of whom volunteered their labor. You taught me many things about health and other vital aspects of life. To the dozens of editors whom I have worked under and often struggled with during the last 20 years as a writer, let me also say that I am now much more sympathetic to the problems you face in the classic writer-editor struggles. *Kharma* caught up with me, and I unfortunately found myself doing to my writers many of the same things that I so strongly criticized you for doing to me. Writers, I have appreciated your patience and tolerance with me.

My final acknowledgments are to those brave people everywhere who have suffered at the hands of health-care delivery systems that did not meet their needs. Those individuals have been crucial in the development of the holistic health movement. Three come to mind:

- Chellis Glendinning, a contributor to both the original and to this current edition. She is one of millions of women to suffer a disease caused by a product taken into her body for birth control purposes which damaged her. She continues to speak out actively against such abuse and to work for a healthier planet.

- Deena Metzger, who combatted breast cancer by integrating her "healing stories" into various medical approaches, was finally victorious, and has become a beacon to women everywhere.

- Alice Miller Bliss, my mother, who lost part of herself over 30 years ago to an unnecessary hysterectomy to correct a cancer that did not exist.

These three women are valiant survivors who struggled and each continue to struggle for personal and social health.

Another guiding light for me as I worked on this book was my father in Omaha, Nebraska, recently crippled by a stroke. Holistic health practices can significantly reduce the individual and social forces which produce such diseases, unnecessary operations, many kinds of cancers and illnesses that are caused or worsened by physicians and our current health-care systems. To all those who have taught me through their example or writings about diet, exercise, friendship, love and work, and the other essential ingredients of holistic health, I hereby honor you. Scott and Helen Nearing epitomize such teachers. Scott died on his farm in Maine at the age of 100 just before I began working on this book and Helen continues their life's work, which has surely touched millions of people through their 50 books and open-door hospitality. Long live the healthy, robust spirits of people like Helen and Scott Nearing!

Shepherd Bliss
Berkeley, California
March 1985

Preface

We now live in the 1980s. This book was written for our times and for the people of this age—which some call "the new age."

The Berkeley Holistic Health Center compiled the first *Holistic Health Handbook* in 1978. That book captured the spirit of those times, placed holistic health within an historical context, and even involved the future. This book seeks to do for the 1980s what that book successfully accomplished for the 1970s.

Much has happened in the health field and in the world as a whole in recent years. During the 1960s and 1970s holistic health was an alternative movement associated with the "counter culture"; during the 1980s it has been moving into the mainstream of American life. A growing number of health practitioners and laypersons look to holistic health for healing. No longer relegated to small centers, holistic health is now practiced in major hospitals, taught in universities, and used in businesses and corporations.

This growth was reflected by Lawrence LeShan, Ph.D., president-elect of the Association of Humanistic Psychology (AHP), at a meeting in Boston in August of 1984 when he noted, "The Army Surgeon General is a devotee of holistic health. Consequently, Walter Reed Hospital is becoming one of the most holistic hospitals in the world." Holistic health is truly influencing a variety of environments.

Another speaker at that AHP meeting, Roger Walsh, Ph.D., addressed our age, "The number-one health issue for us at this time is the survival of the human race." Understanding what is happening in the world as a whole helps us see the role of holistic health in the 1980s. Health begins with personal responsibility and includes social responsibility. One's own health is influenced not only by what happens inside at the level of atoms and cells but what happens outside in the general environment.

Dealing with social issues such as environmental pollution and the threat of nuclear annihilation has much to do with individual health. Worldwide movements toward individual, social, and planetary well-being are growing. An increasing number of people see the human species within its larger context. The new articles and sections in this book reveal some of the growing concerns that were barely visible in the mid-1970s when the first version of this book appeared.

As I searched for a clear way to define what holistic health means, I entered a local copy center. "What would you recommend for my asthma?" the woman behind the counter asked. "I'll ask my colleagues at the Berkeley Holistic Health Center," I answered. So I approached our acupuncturist. "Do you treat asthma?" His response: "No, but I do treat people who have asthma." This distinction between treating the whole person and treating the disease helps define holistic health.

The contributors to this book offer various definitions of holistic health. We hope these distinct approaches will stimulate readers to develop their own personal understandings. Let's look at a few definitions:

- Psychologist Kenneth Pelletier, Ph.D., writes, "Fundamental to holistic medicine is the recognition that each state of health and disease requires a consideration of all contributing factors: psychological, psychosocial, environmental and spiritual."

- James Gordon, M.D., asserts that holistic health "encompasses and is at times indistinguishable from humanistic, behavioral, and integral medicine."

- In his introduction to the 1978 *Holistic Health Handbook*, Edward Bauman observes, "Holistic health is a new name for a very old concept of being. It is a reminder of the unity of all life and the essential oneness of all systems." Bauman maintains that holistic healing, "has been especially effective in the areas of psychosomatic illness, chronic pain, and stress, where doctors and drugs have provided only symptomatic relief."

Some of the most prominent figures in holistic health have made contributions to this book, including people well known nationally and even internationally, others who are recognized in the Berkeley, California area, and others whose contributions are beginning to be acknowledged. The book begins with an interview of author and teacher Norman Cousins, whose best-selling *Anatomy of an Illness* (1979) helped popularize holistic health during the 1980s. Physicist Fritjof Capra—whose best-selling books, *The Tao of Physics* and *The Turning Point*, bringing together western science and eastern philosophy—appears here. Philosopher Ivan Illich, whose book *Medical Nemesis* explores "the gravest health hazard we face today: our medical system," joins us. Prominent physicians such as Tom Ferguson of the magazine *Medical Self-Care*, Rick Ingrasci of the *New Age* magazine, Carl Simonton, James Gordon, and Malcolm Todd, former president of the American Medical Association, are also contributors to this volume.

Health practitioners such as Oriental medicine doctor Ted Kaptchuk and death and dying counselors Elisabeth Kübler-Ross and Stephen Levine contribute to this volume. They are joined by an impressive array of psychologists, bodyworkers, homeopaths, hypnotists, writers, musicians, poets, researchers, lawyers, dream workers, and practitioners from diverse fields.

This book was compiled by first carefully studying the original *Holistic Health Handbook*, which inspired other books to bring health education directly to people. That book was successful partly because it was a practical hands-on guide that emerged from the creative Berkeley, California context. Berkeley and the San Francisco Bay Area of which it is a part are centers of experimentation, innovation, and growth. People come here from all over to be nourished—physically, intellectually, politically, emotionally, and spiritually. They come as explorers in search of something. This is the fertile ground within which this book has grown. It retains its creative Berkeley flavor and complements it by deepening its theoretical base and including articles from New England and other areas where holistic health has been growing.

I read hundreds of manuscripts in order to bring this book into being. Some of the best articles from publications such as *Medical Self-Care, Whole Life Times,* and *Yoga Journal* appear here. Excerpts from some of the most important new books on health are included. I also asked prominent health writers and practitioners to write special articles for this book.

A greater number of articles written by M.D.s are included in this book than in the first version. This does not represent a change in attitude toward traditional Western allopathic medicine, with its strengths and weaknesses. It represents an increasing number of M.D.s acknowledging the limitations of purely scientific methods and turning to more subtle and intuitive teachings, and combining them with their traditional training. Respect within the traditional medical community for holistic health practices is growing. Whereas some M.D.s fail to consider wisdom from holistic health, some practitioners who describe themselves as holistic make the equally serious error of dismissing valuable insights from traditional allopathic medicine. The paths to wholeness and health are multiple. A holistic health practitioner is usually strongly rooted in a specific tradition and open to learning from other practices.

Holistic health is many things: a body of knowledge and practices; attitudes and approaches to life; a movement and a community. I've felt all these aspects in the full year I've worked on this book. I've learned a lot—about myself, others, and the world. I've been healed and nourished by holism's practices, attitudes, and approaches. I've felt the movement's momentum, and I've appreciated the community's support. Editing this book has encouraged me to do more running, dancing, and other physical activity, to work in a garden, to eat better and less, and to take more time for relaxation. Editing this book has changed me; I hope that in reading it you will open your heart to discover more of yourself and the world in which we live. Transformation can heal specific dis-eases and the organism as a whole, and individuals and the social fabric of which we are a part.

In the "Intent" which initiates the original *Handbook*, Armand Brint observes, "The intent of this book is to nourish you. The *Holistic Health Handbook* aims to be a living environment." With this revision we seek to continue that intent and the commitment to nurture a living reality. We agree with what Brint wrote seven years ago, "This principle underlies holistic thought: we are all sentient beings who are continually creating our own realities. We are responsible for creating those relationships and situations in which we find ourselves; our choice is whether we create them consciously or unconsciously."

Shepherd Bliss
Berkeley, California
March 1985

I

Holistic Health
in the 1980s

INTRODUCTION *by Shepherd Bliss*

THE FACTORS THAT maintain optimal health and promote healing are many and diverse. They include forces within a person and can be assisted by forces from outside—such as physicians. Yet these same elements can hinder health; an individual can get in the way of his or her own health, as can health professionals. Educating oneself about health and health techniques available is crucial. This introductory section helps orient the reader toward how holistic health can aid in developing and maintaining optimal health.

We begin, appropriately enough, with an interview with Norman Cousins, whose historic *Anatomy of an Illness*, published in 1979, helped popularize holistic health. He describes here how positive emotions such as love, hope, and faith and activities such as laughter, playfulness, and creativity can be curative. Cousins expresses his thoughts in conversation with skillful interviewer Tom Ferguson, M.D., editor of the magazine *Medical Self-Care*.

Our health-care system has been changing in recent years, as has our view of health. Richard Miles charts five basic categories of health care, from traditional Western medicine to the paradigm of holistic health. Miles' systematic thinking helps us differentiate these various systems.

The Clinical Director of the Berkeley Holistic Health Center, David Teegarden, M.D., writes from his own clinical experiences to help define holistic health and place it within various contexts: historical, scientific, philosophical, clinical, and medical. Another prominent physician, James Gordon, M.D., demonstrates how holistic health practices are on the cutting edge of medicine today. Dr. Gordon writes about experimenting on himself and discovering various tools, including acupuncture, meditation, yoga, Tai Chi, bioenergetics, fasting, and physical exercises. Dr. Gordon came to "regard illness . . . as an opportunity for personal growth and change," and "the physician as a catalyst and guide in this process."

In addition to these major contributions, also included are shorter items by: Malcolm Todd, M.D., a past president of the American Medical Association; Lawrence LeShan, Ph.D., President-elect (1985) of the Association of Humanistic Psychology; and eternal iconoclast Ivan Illich.

The eight contributors to this section approach holistic health historically, analytically, scientifically, intuitively, and poetically, with questions and inspiration.

Panic as a Disease

Norman Cousins, in conversation with Tom Ferguson, M.D.

ABOUT A year ago at UCLA I was asked to see a 34-year-old man who thought he was going to die. Larry had gone in for a check-up the previous week. His doctor had taken one look at his electrocardiogram (EKG) and asked him, "When did you have your heart attack?"

Larry gasped. "I've never had a heart attack."

"Oh yes you have," the doctor said. "It's all right here. The EKG doesn't lie. You've had an unmistakable heart attack. You don't remember having any chest pain?"

"No," Larry said. "I've never had any pain."

"Well," the doctor said, "you had a silent coronary, a massive heart attack. Are you sure you don't remember having any pain?"

That night, for the first time in his life, Larry had chest pain. He worried himself into a state of severe panic. Early the next morning he went back to the clinic. They put him on a treadmill. Moments later there was a sharp drop in his blood pressure and an ominous change in his EKG.

They put him in the hospital and gave him an angiogram—ran a catheter up into his heart, injected a dye, and took x-rays. The x-rays showed a substantial blockage of the major arteries of his heart.

They scheduled Larry for coronary bypass surgery. But he was so emotionally devastated that his doctors feared he couldn't withstand the procedure. I'd just recovered from a heart attack myself, so they asked me to see him.

"I Don't Want to Die"

When I came into Larry's hospital room, his first words were, "I don't want to die."

I said, "What makes you think you're going to die?"

"The doctors said I've had a serious heart attack," he said. "I flunked my treadmill test. I flunked my angiogram. My EKG is all screwed up. And now they say I've got to have major heart surgery."

I sat down beside him and put a hand on his shoulder. "You know, Larry," I said, "I've heard and read a good deal about your case, and I think you've got a great heart.

I've got a hunch that if we can get you back into that treadmill room without those doctors scaring you half to death, you'll knock the socks off that thing."

He looked surprised. "Why do you say that?"

"You've never had any symptoms in your life," I said. "I don't think you could have had a serious heart problem without knowing about it. These tests can be wrong, especially in younger men with strong, muscular hearts." And I showed him some papers by the great cardiologist Paul Dudley White to prove it.

I saw him every day for three days, and was finally able to convince him to give the treadmill another try. We went up to the treadmill room an hour and a half early. I told him some funny stories to get him into a good mood. I'd arranged for Larry to operate the controls himself, because one of the flaws of the treadmill is that when you're on it, you don't exercise—*it* exercises *you*—the floor under your feet starts to move and if you don't run, you fall down. If you can control the whole thing yourself, the experience is totally different.

I got on the machine first. We made a game of it—I ran while Larry operated the controls. Gradually he began to lose his fear of the machine. Then he got on, started out slowly, and gradually increased his speed. After five minutes of steady running he was doing fine. We had music playing. He was laughing away, cracking jokes. Finally he said, "Bring the man in."

We invited the cardiologist in. Larry operated the machine. The doctor watched his EKG and followed his blood pressure. Larry gradually increased his speed and increased the upward angle of the treadmill. At three miles an hour with a 15-degree uphill grade, he was still feeling no discomfort of any kind. After 20 minutes of strenuous exercise, he was still perfectly comfortable. He exhibited no symptoms at all. The doctor turned off the machine and cancelled the surgery.

Iatrogenic Disease

The term *iatrogenic* is used to describe doctor-caused injury and disease. But iatrogenic illness and injury is not limited to the surgeon who cuts in the wrong place or to the doctor who overprescribes or prescribes in error. There is such a

Reprinted by permission of the author and *Medical Self-Care*, P.O. Box 1000, Point Reyes, CA 94956.

thing as a psychologically produced iatrogenic problem. Physicians can also create disease by their attitudes, their words, and the ways they communicate.

How many people like Larry go on to have heart surgery? How many people put themselves through the risk, expense, and pain of this and other major operations and procedures *when their disorder is partly or totally the result of the treatment they've received from their physicians*? How many die, unnecessarily, of the complications from these unneeded procedures?

"Everything is Crapped Out"

I was recently sitting with a patient in his hospital room. This man had been through a whole battery of tests. He and his family were waiting for the diagnosis. They were scared.

After some time, the doctor arrived. He didn't sit down. He spread his hands, shook his head, and looked grim. "Well, Charlie," he began. "What can I say? Your kidneys are crapped out. Your liver is crapped out. Everything's crapped out. There's not a hell of a lot we can do. I'm really sorry."

In San Francisco, a woman I know recently went in for a biopsy. She was quite naturally concerned, and telephoned the oncologist the next day to ask what he'd found. She was told that no diagnoses were given over the phone— she would be receiving the results in a letter.

Several anxious days later, the envelope arrived. It was a certified letter. It said: "I regret to say that your biopsy was positive." Can you imagine how devastated and abandoned these two patients must have felt?

The Right Way

Let me give you an example of how a similar situation might be handled by good doctor-patient communication—as demonstrated by a Houston cancer specialist who pays a great deal of attention to his client's attitudes and feelings. He calls it "potentiating the patient."

When he gets patients with new diagnoses of cancer, he sits down with them and tells them he's convinced they are going to make it. He tells them it's nonsense to equate the word "cancer" with death. He tells them he has an excellent treatment for their condition, and that they have an excellent treatment of their own—their body's own natural healing process.

"And you can activate that healing process," he tells them, "by building up your confidence in yourself and your confidence in me. By building up your joy, your appreciation of life, by your urge to go on to do everything you've always wanted to do." He tells them that they're in possession of the most magical system the world has ever known for the treatment of disease.

"Now," he says, "here's the partnership I propose. I'll work with you on the things you'll be doing to build up your confidence, your joy, your hope, your faith. Beginning tomorrow I'm going to introduce you to five other patients who had exactly the same kind of cancer you have and came through it successfully. I will make sure you receive the best treatment medical science has to offer.

We're going to have a lot going for us, and I'm convinced that we can whip this thing and that you can make it." Then he holds out his hand and says, "Now how about a partnership?" They always take his hand.

He doesn't send them away in a mood of emotional devastation. On the contrary—they leave with a growing faith, a renewed sense of hope. And hope is a powerful medication, for no matter what else happens, if the patient does not have hope, the treatment is much less likely to be effective.

A Strong Partnership

I saw another example of good doctor-patient communication when I recently spent a morning with a urologist in Denver. He was seeing a patient who had just been diagnosed as having cancer of the prostate. The CAT scan showed that the cancer had spread throughout his body— they were able to identify 230 separate tumors.

The doctor sat down with the patient and said, "Well, Michael, I can't conceal from you the fact that this is very serious. You have cancer, and it's spreading. But serious as it is, I'm convinced that you can make it through. I've seen many cases, far more serious than your own, which have completely remitted.

"I think those cases have remitted because there's been a strong partnership between doctor and patient. I would like the two of us to join in such a partnership.

"My job will be to knock out the male hormone. I'm going to give you estrogen. We may also have to have some surgery.

"Your job is to have the best time of your life. I want you to exercise your will to live as you've never exercised it before. Vitamin C can help restore adrenal function, and the adrenal glands become depleted in many illnesses, so I think you should begin taking Vitamin C.

"I want you to eat the most highly nutritious diet you can possibly arrange, because I've got a hunch that many cancer patients die as much of malnutrition as they do of the disease itself.

"You've got to become extremely strong—through regular, gentle exercise. Strengthen your body in every possible way. If you do so, the treatments I'll be giving you will have a much better chance.

"I think you have a very good chance. I'm willing to do all I can from my end. Now—how about it?"

I saw that patient's x-rays six months later. Two thirds of his tumors had disappeared—because that doctor not only provided effective treatment, he also potentiated the patient and helped him make the best possible use of the resources at his disposal.

The Dangers of Diagnosis

Over the last five years I've had the chance to meet about 600 people with malignancies. In most cases these people's diseases took a sharp turn for the worse shortly after they received their diagnoses.

How was it, I wondered, that a person brings an accumulation of symptoms to a doctor, receives a diagnosis, and then suddenly experiences a rapid intensification of the illness? I became convinced that there was something about the presentation of the diagnosis that actually intensified the disease. How did that happen?

I got some valuable clues at a recent high school football game in Los Angeles. During the game, four people came to the physician on duty complaining of nausea, vomiting, and abdominal pain—the symptoms of food poisoning. The doctor determined that all four had consumed Coca-Cola from one particular Coke machine under the stands. An announcement was made. The fans were told that there had been some cases of food poisoning, and they were warned not to consume soda from this particular machine.

Within moments, the entire stadium became a sea of fainting, retching bodies. Ambulances from five hospitals raced back and forth, transporting the victims. These people showed all the symptoms of systemic food poisoning, and the symptoms were real. A number of them had to be hospitalized.

A quick analysis of the suspect machine showed that it contained no contaminants. When this was announced, the affected people mysteriously began to improve. They recovered as quickly as they became ill.

Conversion Hysteria

How is it that words passing through the air can be translated into disease? Psychologists have a name for this kind of phenomenon: *conversion hysteria.* Words are converted into hysteria, into panic, and the panic is converted into disease.

If hundreds of healthy football fans can be first made ill and then cured by a few words over a P.A. system, imagine what can happen to people with cancer or heart disease. They bring their collection of symptoms to a physician, and the doctor applies the magic word, "CANCER," or "HEART ATTACK." And those words are processed into hysteria and panic. Panic constricts blood vessels. This reduces blood flow, and makes it difficult for the different systems of the body to function. It makes it especially hard for the brain to do its job.

When I speak of the brain doing its job, I don't mean trying to think oneself into a higher state of consciousness. I'm talking about the human brain as a gland—the most prolific gland in the human body.

Five years ago, when I came to UCLA, I asked my colleagues at the Brain Research Institute for a list of all the secretions produced by the brain. I received a list of 34 substances. Some of these allowed the body to alleviate its pain. Some helped combat infections. Others helped fortify the immune system.

Today they don't even dare count the number of brain secretions. The brain can combine the subunits available to it into an almost infinite number of substances. The brain is a powerful apothecary. In some circumstances it can secrete and "prescribe" substances far more helpful than any drugs. But under circumstances of fear, panic, pain, exasperation, or rage, it is extremely difficult for the brain to produce the appropriate substances.

When a person has deep confidence in a physician, a treatment, and his or her own abilities to help produce a cure, there is an almost irresistible force in the direction of the desired outcome. But when the patient is distressed, fearful, depressed, exasperated, or angry, it is extremely difficult for medical science to do the job it needs to do, and difficult for the body to do the job that it naturally tries to do.

I'm sorry to say that the present state of medical education for laypeople in the United States does not encourage the most positive results. Quite the contrary.

I'm thinking not only of what happens in our schools, though that's bad enough—I'm also thinking of what happens in the general environment in which people talk about health, and of the bombardment of TV ads pushing Tylenol, Anacin, Bufferin, Excedrin, and other drugs. Our upbringing and our education make us all the more likely to panic.

The constant emphasis is on "see your doctor at the first sign of pain or abnormality." As a result, our doctors' offices are clogged with people who have no business being there. Dr. Franz Inglefinger, the late editor of the *New England Journal of Medicine*, estimated that 85 percent of the patients who see doctors could handle the problem on their own. That is to say, 85 percent of the illnesses for which we go to doctors can be handled by the body's own healing powers.

The human body is perfectly capable of taking care of its needs—as long as we don't have to deal with the complications produced by panic and fear.

"Hypochondriacs"

I recently saw a film designed to train doctors to deal with hypochondriacs. I didn't see any hypochondriacs in that film. I saw a series of very frightened people who had pain they didn't understand.

There was a scene in which a doctor told a fearful young woman, "We've done a great number of tests, and there's absolutely nothing wrong with you." And I saw that young woman cringe with shame as she left the office. She clearly felt she'd been accused of imagining her symptoms.

The next scene was some weeks later. The same woman came back again. The doctor put her through the same tests. Again, they were all negative. "There's absolutely nothing wrong with you," she was told. Again she slunk away, looking guilty and discouraged.

The film then asked: "Now, Doctor, what do you do when the same patient comes back a third time?" The suggested answer: "Send her to the new doctor in town."

I found myself imagining a much different scene, a revised version of the one in which that young woman had just completed her first series of tests. The doctor would greet her courteously, make her comfortable, and sit down across from her in his office.

"The first thing I want you to know," he would say, "is that the news is very good. You don't have cancer. You don't have heart disease. You don't have any other organic problem that showed up in the tests. There are no tumors anywhere. You heart is sound as a dollar. There are no cellular abnormalities.

"But you do have this pain. And as long as you do, we're going to take it seriously—very seriously. It may represent the early stages of something our tests can't pick up. Because pain means that your body is trying to tell you something.

"For the next two weeks, I want you to pay very close attention to what your body is trying to tell you. The message could be that you're eating or drinking or smoking too much; that you're having a difficult time at work or at home; or that your life is too crowded and you're overburdened. You'll be the best judge of all that.

"I'd like you to keep a journal, and to write down your thoughts and insights. I'd like you to come back in two weeks and let me know what you've come up with. And I want to assure you that one way or another, we're going to get to the bottom of this."

Instead of sending the patient away shamed and depressed, the doctor would encourage and support her and set the stage to find her own way to recovery.

If You Had a Heart Attack....

This same kind of encouragement and support could help people survive heart attacks. The reason so many people do die—50 percent within the first day—is not the heart attack itself. It is largely because of the panic that almost always accompanies it.

Imagine for a moment that you are a 55-year-old man at home after dinner. Suddenly you feel some sharp pains in your chest.

You become terribly afraid. You stagger into the kitchen and gasp to your wife, "I...I think I'm having a heart attack!"

Somebody calls the neighbors. People begin streaming into the house, running back and forth. Someone has the presence of mind to call the hospital.

The paramedics arrive. They fly at you, stick needles into your arms and put a mask over your face. They pick you up, put you on a stretcher, and rush you out to the ambulance.

Next comes a spine-tingling, high-speed ride to the hospital, with lights flashing and sirens wailing. And if you think that the siren sounds hideous coming down the street, you can hardly imagine what it sounds like from inside the ambulance.

You arrive at the hospital. The first thing you see is a large, bright-red neon sign: EMERGENCY. They wheel you in, do a surgical cut-down on your arm, inject a long catheter into your heart, and rush you up to the intensive care unit.

At the ICU they keep your panic-stricken friends and loved ones outside while they hook you up to an exquisitely accurate and precise battery of meters and gauges which measure and record the decline of half a dozen of your vital functions.

Through this whole ghastly procedure, the most important, most helpful thing anyone could offer you would be a quiet hand on your shoulder, and a few reassuring words: "Look. Don't worry. You'll be fine. You've got a great heart. You're going to be all right."

"Sir, You've Got a Great Heart"

As I mentioned before, I had a heart attack myself not long ago. Just recently, I had a chance to observe the same process again. I was driving past a golf course in Los Angeles when an ambulance drove in. I followed it. The ambulance pulled up beside a man in golfing clothes, lying on a stretcher.

He was in a state of total panic. His skin was ashen. His lips were trembling. His eyes were closed. The paramedics ran up to him and began doing what they had to do. They connected him to an oxygen tank. They hooked him up to an EKG. They stuck several needles into his veins. They were all very busy and efficient. But no one was talking to him.

The EKG monitor showed a tachycarida, a runaway pulse with an irregular heartbeat. I put my hand on his shoulder. "Sir," I said, "you've got a great heart."

He opened his eyes and looked up at me. "Why do you say that?" he asked.

I gestured toward the monitor. I said, "I'm looking at your EKG. It's been pretty hot out here today. You've probably gotten a little dehydrated. It's easy to upset the sodium-potassium exchange that's so vital to the proper functioning of the heart. But I assure you, everything's going to be O.K. In a few minutes you'll be at the best hospital in the world. Take it easy. Believe me, you're going to do just fine."

He opened his eyes, propped up his head, and began looking around. Within 30 seconds, that tachycardia began to recede. Within 90 seconds, he was within the survival range.

Panic and the Heart

That man's panic was constricting his blood vessels, reducing the blood flow to a heart which was already in precarious condition. And yet it seems that almost everything done in response to heart attack seems designed to foster panic. Even in CPR classes, the emphasis is on mouth-to-mouth resuscitation, cardiac massage, and other impersonal, mechanical interventions.

The first thing you have to do with any heart attack victim is to calm the person. Say confidently: "You're going to make it. You're going to make it."

There is nothing more important you can do for someone during a heart attack—or any other serious illness—than to liberate that person from panic. And yet, almost everything we do tends to push them toward panic.

This man was being treated as though he were an automobile. They had attached him to diagnostic equipment and were all set to start installing spare parts. But the human body is much more subtle than that. It has a tendency to fulfill its expectations—positive or negative.

Red Pills and Green Pills

One of the most interesting experiments I know of involved two pills—a super-tranquilizer and a super-stimulant. The subjects were 100 volunteer medical students.

The tranquilizer—a green capsule—was held up before them and all the effects—including side effects—were carefully described. Next a red pill—the super-stimulant—was held up and *its* effects described.

Then half the students got red pills and the other half

got the green ones. What the students didn't know was that the contents of the pills had been switched—the green pills really contained the stimulant. The red pills contained the tranquilizer.

Both groups of students experienced very specific and consistent symptoms—but not the symptoms that should have been produced by the drugs they took. A majority of each group experienced the exact symptoms that had been described to them. The students' bodies created the expected effect—even though to do so, they had to overcome the opposing effects of a very powerful drug.

What does this tell us? It tell us that, in this case, *the human body was more powerful than the medication.*

I suspect that this is often the case. Yet how many physicians respect the ability of the mind to produce such powerful effects? How many of us have confidence in our own ability to deal with illness? How many of us tend to panic at the slightest symptom, to fear the worst about ourselves and our loved ones. How many of us actually make our own conditions, and those of our family members, relatives, and friends, worse by our panic?

The Positive Emotions

If negative emotions like panic can create disease, what is the role of positive emotions—love, hope, faith, laughter, playfulness, creativity? I've come to the conclusion that the function of the positive emotions is to interrupt the negative ones.

The positive emotions protect the body against the bolts of fear, anger, worry, and despair. They are blockers, magnificent blockers. And why not? The role of blockers in medicine is well known. Many of our most widely used medications are blockers: We have the beta blockers and the calcium blockers. Aspirin, our most widely used drug, is a prostaglandin blocker.

The positive emotions may be the greatest blockers of all, blocking, as they can, the disease of panic, which can intensify virtually any underlying illness.

It is not possible to entertain two contrary feelings. The positive emotions drive out the negative. You can't panic and laugh at the same time.

Not long ago a panel of non-Catholic physicians examined some of the so-called miracles at Lourdes. They came to the conclusion that they were miracles indeed. What happened in each of these cases was that the patient's panic dissolved with their love and their faith. You can't entertain contrary emotions.

Voodoo Suicide

Some years ago, the great physiologist Walter Cannon became fascinated by the physiology of the hex. How was it, he asked, that a voodoo doctor, just by pointing a bone at someone, could say, "Two weeks, two days, two hours from now, you will be die"—and the man would die at exactly the appointed time?

After studying a number of cases for some time, he found the answer: The voodoo doctor didn't kill the man. The hex didn't kill him. The victim committed suicide. He believed in the hex. The hex created expectations, and the body followed the path of those expectations. The victim accepted an appointment with death, and kept that appointment. He was programmed to die.

If I had one wish for people with serious diseases, it would be that through their own efforts, through the love and caring of their friends and family, and through the wisdom of the health professionals who care for them, they could be liberated from fear and panic. I would wish they could be programmed to live.

NORMAN COUSINS *is adjunct professor of psychiatry and biobehavioral sciences at UCLA School of Medicine. He is the author of* Anatomy of an Illness.

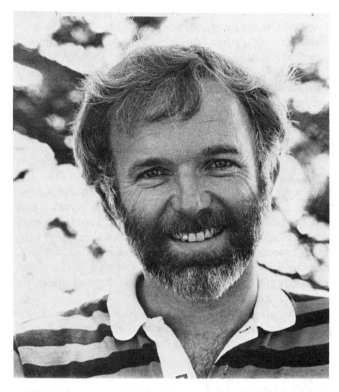

TOM FERGUSON, *M.D. founded the journal* Medical Self-Care.

In addition to serving as Editor of Medical Self-Care, *he is Medical Editor of* The Whole Earth Catalog *and* The CoEvolution Quarterly. *He is also Editor-in-Chief of Medical Self-Care Books. He is the author of* Medical Self-Care: Access to Health Tools *(New York, Summit Books, 1980). His new book,* The People's Book of Medical Tests *(co-authored with David Sobel, M.D.) will be published in 1984 by Medical Self-Care Books/Summit Books.*

Humanistic Medicine and Holistic Health Care

Richard B. Miles

This article deals with the imminent changes in our evolving health-care system. As our views of health and medicine change, we must find ways to understand and deal with the issues raised by these changes. Richard Miles charts for us five basic categories of health care, further defining the difference between alternative methods and a truly holistic approach.

AS ONE of the early participants in and facilitators of what is now called the "Holistic Health Movement," I have spent much time and energy in working out concepts about how the field of holistic health is evolving. I see this movement as being both analogous to and an expression of a much broader shift in values and paradigms that is taking place in Western thought. The Western view of the world is changing; hence our view of life, health, and disease is also changing.

One result of this shift has been great confusion. Since persons who have adopted different value systems will measure events and situations in different ways, communication between them will become difficult, and sometimes impossible.

For centuries our culture has looked upon confusion as incompetence, and upon being "knowledgeable" and in control as competence. The acquiring of objective knowledge and hence of "control" over life and nature has been the principal measure of competence, both individually and societally. Nature has been seen as an enemy to be dominated and mastered (a ubiquitous theme in Western science). But now these assumptions are changing.

It is interesting to look at the root meaning of the word "confusion." It derives from the Latin *confundere*, meaning "to mingle or blend together." This is what appears to be happening in the health field. Many varied and confusing ideas abound in the scene and are in the slow, and sometimes frustrating, process of merging together into a new paradigm called "holistic health."

First, let me state some of the basic issues I have perceived.

The Difference between Modalities and Perspectives

There is a difference between modalities, relationships, and perspectives. The same modalities (systems of techniques) may be used in several different perspectives. How they are used in the provider/patient relationship will depend on that relationship and on the life perspectives of the provider and the client.

There has been a great deal of confusion about this. Since we Westerners identify so strongly with definition and structure, we have quickly labeled practices as "holistic," "humanistic," etc. The practices are simply the techniques and methods. Whether they are humanistic or holistic will depend on how they are employed and the outcome desired, and especially on the relationship between the provider and the client. One can easily practice reductionistic, cookbook acupuncture to relieve symptoms in an allopathic model. One can also practice acupuncture in a systemic/energy-balancing approach in the Chinese model. And one can offer acupuncture as a tool for learning on the part of the client (such learning is not necessarily part of the systemic/energy system). In brief, it is only the entire perspective which can accurately be labeled allopathic or holistic, and not the particular technique being used.

Current Medical Systems

Let me now outline the five categories of medical systems that I see operating, and comment on how their interactions create confusion.

Allopathic Medicine

Based on the reductionist, cellular-structure view of the life process, allopathic medicine has emerged as a science of structural manipulation of the boy intended to "fight," conquer, and destroy disease. This rather aggressive position was tempered in the past by the human relationships between physicians and patients in the local community. As medicine became more scientific and technological, and less based on the physician/client relationship, the impact

T A B L E 1: COMPARISON OF PERSPECTIVES OF SEVERAL SYSTEMS OF HEALTH AND DISEASE

	Allopathic	Alternative	Humanistic	Systemic/Organic	Holistic
View of Nature	As erratic cellular/molecular system needing management	Same as for allopathic	Bio/growth process	Interactive system of energy flow	Consciousness system that supports human creativity
Health	Normalcy/absence of symptoms	Normalcy	Commitment to personal growth	Balance of energy systems	Joy; participation in creativity and fulfillment
Disease	Error in system, enemy to conquer	Same as for allopathic	Blocks to growth/error in system/hills to climb	Imbalance of energy systems	Feedback message to choosing person
Patient	Minimized to set of symptoms	Same as for allopathic	Grower/struggler; locator of blocks	Flow of energies	Learner, chooser, creator
Psychological components	Minimized	Studied, considered	Key to growth	Director of or interferer with energies	Manager of body process, creator of fear and anxiety
Provider	Manipulator of cellular structure	Same as for allopathic	Caring: part guru, part authority	Manipulator of energy flows	Guide, facilitator, teacher
Role of patient	Obeyer of instructions (uninformed)	Obeyer	Part obeyer, part struggler, part chooser	Learn to balance energies	Participator, chooser
Measure of success of treatment	Disappearance of symptoms	Disappearance of symptoms or behavior	Clearing of blocks	Achievement of balance	Lesson learned from it
Measure of quality of system	Conformity/peer review	Not established	Good feelings of client	Not established	Client feedback/interaction
Professional education	Detailed knowledge of reductionist bioscience	Same as for allopathic, plus exploration of wider possibilities	Allopathic science, plus relationship and facilitation skills	Widely varied by discipline; mostly apprentice system	Widely varied and misunderstood
Person responsible for outcome	Provider	Provider	Not always clearly defined/toward client	Provider	Client
Needs of system	Larger view of nature, humanity, life, health, disease; patient outcome—quality control; change of fee-for-service motive	Same as for allopathic, plus more open discussion of efficacy of processes	Clarification of person/system relationship; clarification of dichotomies of humanistic and reductionist perspectives in science	Greater understanding of disciplines; clearer educational processes; patient outcome—quality control	Clearer understanding of new paradigm of thought; development of personal responsibility; clarification of intention; development of educational processes

THE NEED FOR A NEW HEALTH PROGRAM

Malcolm C. Todd, M.D.

IN ORDER to develop a sound basis for the optimum health for our twentieth-century society, it may well be necessary for health professionals and for the general public to become fully aware of the many new approaches to health and disease. Since World War II the technical and scientific advances in medicine have far exceeded the social and cultural advances. We physicians need to reassess the total health of our individual patients, and, in turn, that of our entire society. In this all people may benefit from the cultural, the environmental, the mental, the physical, and the religious advances. Further, it seems not unreasonable that physicians must integrate (and engage sooner or later in) the practice patterns that deal with physical, mental, spiritual, and environmental health in some comprehensive manner.

Since the late fifties and sixties, a goal of the A.M.A. has been a program of integrating body, mind, and spirit in the treatment of the whole patient. This was part of our program of medicine and religion. And considerable progress has taken place. The World Health Organization in its preamble finds health is a state of complete physical, mental, and social well-being, and not merely the absence of disease or infirmity. Now that is quite a laudable goal, and it cannot be accomplished overnight.

Holistic has been defined as a state in which an individual is integrated in all his levels of being: body, mind, and spirit. It has been suggested that all modalities of treatment may be used in holistic healing; that is, surgery, medicine, chemotherapy, radiation, nutrition, rehabilitation, yes, hypnosis, acupuncture, psychics, and, of course, religion. To achieve such a broad goal it will be necessary to tap the resources of our most learned scholars, our most sophisticated researchers, and expert commissions and practitioners. For that ultimate goal is to use these authorities to teach an individual to assume responsibility for himself and to heal himself by modifying any unhealthy attitudes, values, or lifestyles.

Thus far, physicians have shown little objective interest in promoting health and preventive care. We actually have a disease-oriented cure system rather than a health-oriented care system in this country today. Oh, I know my surgical colleagues have excelled in the technical aspects of colon and open-heart surgery. The internist is master at cardiopulmonary dysfunction. Psychiatrists have added much to the treatment of the mental illness of our people. But we have demonstrated little knowledge thus far in utilizing the potentials of genetics and biochemistry.

Menninger states in his writings that the inability of doctors and psychiatrists to practice the medicine that integrates the body, the mind, and the environment is most striking. Resistance by the medical profession to these new approaches may be due to one or two conceptual polarities in medicine; that is, body/mind dualism, and the separation of health from illness. If this be holistic medicine and if it does merit a place in our society, then doctors should give leadership to see that the expansion, the growth of this concept, takes place in a responsible manner. Of course, it will not replace traditional medicine, but it might very well complement and become an integral part of it.

Dan Feldman of the University of California, Irvine, states, "The holistic view of illness postulates that it is a composite phenomenon contributed to and shaped by a number of influences which may or may not bear a direct causal relation to each other. The management of illness requires understanding of as many of these influences as possible."

Such an attitude is particularly important to patients with chronic disabling diseases, since they have not only organic medical problems with their illness, but also social, economic, environmental, and behavioral problems as well. Chronic disabling conditions should be examined within the context of the total human environment. Therefore, holistic medicine may interface basically with patients who have psychiatric and behavioral problems, and secondly with the growing number of chronically disabled citizens in our society.

Perhaps most significant is the concept that each individual is responsible for his own health, which becomes a part of a nation's health. I truly believe that this concept will require changes in the lifestyle of many of us. Disciplining our own lives against self-abuse, evaluating our own moral and ethical standards of living, and the ultimate elimination of poverty will do much to improve the quality of life for all our people. In recent years, more and more attention has been focused on health education. This is as it should be. There has been, of course, interest in preventive care. This interest goes far beyond the scope of traditional immunizations and innoculations, which form

This article is excerpted from a talk given by Dr. Todd. It was first published in the *Journal of the Association for Holistic Health* and is reprinted here by permission of the Association for Holistic Health.

the basis for many preventive-care programs. The primary purpose of health education is to help people establish patterns of living that will discourage disease and enhance health, and in this way improve the quality of life for all of our people.

Since the turn of the century, health-education needs have emerged in this country from four major developments. The first is the emergence of major disease problems that are intimately related to patterns of living learned early in life. Second is the emergence of a health-care delivery system that depends for its successful functioning on informed and motivated consumers. Third is the emergence of the idea that health is a state of total positive functioning, not just the absence of disease. Fourth is the emergence of an ecological view of the world that sees man synergistically and simultaneously related to all of his environment. A view that recognizes attempts to improve human well-being must be viewed within this broad perspective.

The remarkable advances in medicine and public health during the past 75 years, along with growing material affluence and growing freedom from preoccupation with survival activities, have encouraged the idea that health is not the mere absence of disease, but a positive quality of living. Although positive health is a relative and somewhat utopian concept, it clearly calls for a new framework in which new activities in health professions can take place.

This growing new view of man as intimately and synergistically related to his environment is producing a shift from a mechanistic to an organic view of the world that may well be the first fundamental reorientation of human thought since Bacon and Descartes. The goal of positive health viewed from an ecological perspective has profound implications for all who would work to improve human well-being. The A.M.A.'s commitment to positive health as an ecological perspective has been expressed by the holding of three national congresses on the quality of life. I believe it's obvious that the four major developments discussed thus far speak forcefully of the need for coordinated, comprehensive health programs, in our schools, in our colleges, in our communities, and in health-care delivery systems.

Dangerous and apparently illogical health behavior appears as such only from the detached, rational, scientific view that the health professional assumes when he judges the health behavior of others. Such behavior may appear logical and necessary when viewed from inside the consumer's world. In addition, much counterproductive and dangerous health behavior is created and sustained by our society's values. Overwork, overeating, self-medication, cigarette smoking, alcohol abuse, the lack of exercise, all are examples. It is not likely that such ingrained and culturally reinforced behavior patterns can be changed solely by short-term, crisis-oriented health-education programs. Health education needs to be permanently integrated throughout society in a manner that will shape healthful lifestyles in the American people. Health education is a long-term goal, not a short-term panacea.

Many of the nation's future health problems exist now in our school population, and the nature and extent of such problems will be determined largely by how these youngsters manage their lives during the next twenty or thirty years. In like manner, the way in which today's youth use tomorrow's health-care resources will be determined by habits and attitudes developed during their school years. Although some good health education is going on in the schools of this nation, it is apparent that health education has extremely low priority in program development funding and administrative commitment.

The unfortunate fact is that most youths of the nation do not now have an opportunity to participate in comprehensive health-education programs, since health education in many schools is either nonexistent or provided on a fragmented and inadequate basis. Medicine's success in the scientific treatment of illness and injury in the past few decades now makes it possible to turn to preventive care. During the past ten years much has been written and spoken on preventive care. As a matter of fact, the provision of preventive care is one of the requirements by law in the health-maintenance organization, HMO. Yet none of them to my knowledge really offer true preventive services. Oh yes, they give and provide shots and immunizations—some of them have some multiphasic screening—but real preventive medicine involves the individual as well as the provider and it begins, really, with health education.

Let me review with you in a somewhat simplistic form some of the most tragic results that we ourselves create by poor living habits, self-pollution, and individual faulty living. This year Americans will spend ten billion dollars on tobacco, and 10.5 billion dollars on alcohol and wine; 35 million people will be taking stimulants and tranquilizers; and 40 million Americans will spend over one billion dollars trying to control their weight. In other words, a big percentage of the nation's sicknesses and deaths are a fault, at least in part, of the patients themselves. And, yes, don't forget 60,000 Americans died in automobile accidents in 1976.

In the future the well-being of mankind will depend to a large extent on successful education of consumers and professionals alike. Perhaps now there is need for a truly comprehensive system, a new conceptual model of understanding, diagnosis, prevention, and treatment of illness to be achieved by means of education.

MALCOLM C. TODD, *M.D., President of the A.M.A.* *(1975), has studied medical trends in China, Russia, and other parts of the world.*

of this perspective has become more apparent. Although frequently looked upon as a "system," the present practice of allopathic medicine comprises several systems.

It is particularly effective in treatment of traumatic structural damage and burns (accidents) and infectious diseases. It is marginally, if at all, effective in treating chronic degenerative disease and lifestyle problems (alcoholism, obesity, drug addiction, stress), since the facts in these situations do not fit at all well into its model of cellular/structural manipulation. It is iatrogenic (disease-causing) in highly interventive neurosurgery, orthopedic surgery, and obstetrics (areas of highest malpractice activity), because its emphasis on manipulation of nature is completely inappropriate to many of the life situations that are presented in these cases.

Alternative Medicine

Because allopathic medicine is ineffective in dealing with chronic degenerative disease and with lifestyle problems, and also because allopathic practitioners are still attempting to maintain tight control over medical practices, "alternative" providers are emerging in these problem areas. These "alternative" providers are almost always physicians, but are looked on with disdain by most allopathic practitioners. The alternatives they use generally involve manipulation of the body processes bionutritionally or by means of behavior modification, rather than by means of pharmaceutical or surgical treatment, and include such modalities as megavitamin therapies, orthomolecular medicine, chelation, hyperbaric oxygen, and nutritional regimens.

It is unfortunate that many of these alternative providers call themselves "holistic," for they are not. They are simply using alternative methods of symptom manipulation within the allopathic model. Furthermore, because of the reputed success of these alternative modalities, these alternative providers sometimes reap great wealth, simply because these modalities cannot be used freely by their more-conservative colleagues.

Humanistic Medicine

Humanistic medicine is an attempt to temper and soften the cold, scientific, "nature as enemy" perspective of allopathic medical science. It recognizes that the feelings and anxieties of the patient (and of the provider) are significant components in the provider/client relationship. Most of the activity in this area has focused on providing personal-awareness experiences for health professionals that will enable them to have a more sensitive relationship with clients. It is, in a sense, an attempt to return medicine to the "caring" style of the family physician of the past and to clarify the provider/client interaction.

Humanistic medicine is defined not by the set of modalities it uses, but by its shift of focus onto the client's needs (or at least onto *more* of those needs). A humanistic provider would be less likely to offer highly interventive or iatrogenic therapies, and more likely to include psychological alternatives that deal with client attitudes and feelings. The humanistic attitude remains essentially well within the mainstream medical system, albeit with modifications and "humanizing." I see it as one step in the movement away from alienating allopathy and toward interconnecting holism.

Systemic/Organic Medicine

Eastern thought and new philosophies of biological systems have introduced to the Western scene the concept that the interaction between individual and world is a process of life-energy flow. Older Eastern ideas and newer ones—acupuncture, aikido, yoga, meditation, polarity therapies, jin shin jitsu—have joined some new Western ideas—Reichian thought, bioenergetics, rolfing, Feldenkrais, Alexander—in this arena.

These systems seek balance of body/universe energies rather than "normality" as a measure of health. The provider manipulates energy rather than chemistry and structure. The client is seen as a system of interaction rather than in terms of an isolated symptom or cellular/structural error.

Practitioners in this area also call themselves holistic, sometimes rightly, in my view, and sometimes not, since holism is not a question of modality, but of intent and relationship. A client can go to a "balancing" practitioner, get "fixed," learn nothing, and operate in the same disconnected allopathic model as before. Or, with much greater chance of discovering something worthwhile, he could find a "holistic" practitioner of one of these modalities and learn a great deal about the life process.

Holistic Health

Holistic health is significantly different from all the above categories because it focuses on development of the joyful expression of good health, not on the achievement of normalcy or balance. A holistic system may include identification and treatment of disease, as one possible choice among many, but it does not focus on problems and errors, as all the other systems do outright (or tend to do). It focuses, instead, on clarity of intention, development of well-being, and enjoyment of life in a system of self-responsibility.

Holistic health therefore cannot be defined in terms of a set of modalities or licensable practices, since a system transforms to its own ends whatever elements it happens to include. This holistic-health system consists essentially of enabling good health to emerge from within the person who recognizes and acts upon life stresses, and undertakes a commitment to maintain self-expression in an environment of goodwill. Disease is seen as an important feedback message, to be dealt with consciously as part of the life process, not as a victimization by a hostile nature. The holistic assumption is that the body knows how to heal itself, is a natural "healing" system intent on good health, and that we must learn how to get our stresses and misunderstandings out of its way.

Perhaps the clearest analogy to holistic-health education is the biofeedback unit. An individual interacting with a biofeedback unit is gaining more discrete information about body function than his previous experience made available. Acting upon this new information, the "trainee" can learn to modify body habit patterns which have been unproductive, and to create habit patterns with more desirable outcomes. There is no way to impose this learning on someone, nor to explain the process in linear language. (Try to explain to someone the body processes involved in learning how to ride a bicycle.)

This analogy leads us to a basic definition: a "holistic" practitioner is one who offers the client more discrete information about the processes of body, mind, and spirit than the client's previous experience had made available. The client can then choose the course of action, the learning pattern, which will offer more productive and healthy life experience. The fact that he has chosen it makes it uniquely his and places the responsibility in the only place it can truly rest: within the individual.

We have endeavored for centuries to control incompetent practitioners and to maintain a level of "safety" for the public, in health and in other institutions. However, the only completely successful way to do this is to develop the competent "buyer," the well-informed constituent who can tell from his own experience whether or not the practitioner is "real" and working for the client's best interest. Hence I think we should shift our emphasis away from "licensing and control" and toward public information and education. We *must* allow the constituents to make some mistakes, since that is the only way we human beings learn *anything*.

In the words of Thomas Jefferson:

> The only safe depository of power in a democracy is in the people themselves. And, if the people fail to exercise their power with discretion, the answer is not to take the power from them (through control), but to educate their discretion.

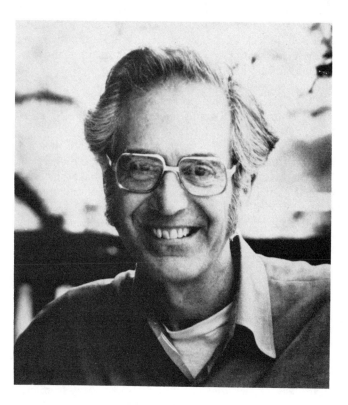

RICHARD B. MILES *is a pioneer in the holistic health field who organized the first major series of innovative conferences in the early '70s* (The New Dimensions of Healing *for the Academy of Parapsychology and Medicine and* Frontiers of the Mind *for AHP). He was the initial co-director of the Holistic Life University in San Francisco, then moved on to join the Health Science faculty at San Jose State University. He has authored* Freedom From Chronic Disease *(J. P. Tarcher, 1979) about the work of Arthur Kaslow, M.D., of Santa Barbara. Richard was the founder and director of the graduate program in Clinical Holistic Health Education at John F. Kennedy University in Orinda, CA, and has served on the boards of the Berkeley Holistic Health Center and the San Andreas Health Council. He is now writing and consulting in the health-care field.*

Holistic Health and Medicine in the 1980s

David Teegarden, M.D.

H OLISTIC health is not merely the absence of disease. It is a state of well-being and vitality that brings about an optimal level of physical, mental, and spiritual functioning. In this state, you experience a sense of joy, wonder, and love toward your self and the world. Holistic health also extends to a wider sphere: It may include a high level of social, ecological, and political awareness, and a commitment to improve not only your own health and well-being but also that of the surrounding world.

What Is Holistic Medicine?

Holistic medicine is a system of medical care that emphasizes the *whole* person. Rather than focusing only on the malfunctioning body part, it also explores the broader dimensions of the patient's life—physical, nutritional, environmental, emotional, spiritual, and lifestyle. In aiming to foster the natural healing process, holistic does not espouse one method over another, but rather encompasses *all* safe methods of diagnosis and treatment—including medication and surgery, when appropriate. Patient and practitioner cooperate to achieve the desired result. Personal responsibility and participation are emphasized.

Holism is more than a medical method—it is a philosophy of life that relates to the whole rather than to the parts. Currently, both medical practitioners and the public are moving toward a holistic view of health and illness. The term *holistic* is itself vague, overused and abused. In the absence of clear standards and definitions, the field of holistic health abounds with controversies and legal questions. Thus, one task of medical and holistic health practitioners in the 1980s is to define their approaches to health and illness, and to ensure that these are cost-effective and safe.

Science and Holism

Contemporary western science dates back to the seventeenth-century philosophy of René Descartes. Descartes assumed that the human mind was the absolute basis for objective reality ("I think, therefore, I am"), and from this established an analytical scientific model for understanding the physical world: The human mind is separate from nature; the universe functions like a machine, with direct cause-and-effect relationships; reality is best understood by reducing matter and energy to their smallest, most elemental forms, and then constructing the physical world out of these discrete entities.

This Cartesian model proved powerful. It was responsible for our space programs, modern conveniences of every kind, and advances in longevity and health.

In earlier centuries, western scientists equated this paradigm with reality and with God's plan for the universe. But discoveries made in atomic physics have since informed us that this paradigm is actually just one approximation of reality.[1]

The concept of *holism* was first presented early in the twentieth century by Jan Smuts, a South African philosopher. This perspective opposes the reductionist tendencies of Cartesian thought, and emphasizes the need to look at the whole rather than its parts.

General systems theory is an emerging scientific paradigm that sees the world and reality as a system of interrelationships. These interrelationships include the influence of the observer and his or her perspective. Systems theory focuses on the interrelated behaviors of entities.

Holism and general systems theory are similar in that their view of the world is distinctly different from the Cartesian paradigm. But while "holistic" is the more popular in current issues, general systems theory provides more rigorous means of scientifically studying issues related to holistic health.

A Holistic and Systems View of Life

In the Cartesian paradigm, humans were superior to nature. The goal of human endeavors was to control and conquer the natural world. This perspective has its limi-

[1]Science, as a discipline or philosophy, must successively refine its models. In a field as basic as physics, the Cartesian model cannot explain the behavior of the most elemental particles. According to one of the most advanced theories in physics, the Heisenberg Uncertainty Principle, it is impossible to "pinpoint" electrons and protons in both time and space. The more precisely we define the location of a subatomic particle, the less we can define the time it will be there, and vice versa.

tations and fallacies, as we have all experienced—ecological disasters, racism, overpopulation, the energy crisis, the threat of nuclear war, the rise of drug addiction, and increasing adverse reactions to pharmacological drugs come from the Cartesian philosophy's tendency to divide, analyze, and control.

In the holistic or systems view, any drastic intervention or action in one system would affect other related systems. Thus, using pesticides in the agricultural system, for example, would cause the organisms that previously were eaten by the "pests" to grow beyond their usual bounds. In a systems perspective, these effects can and must be accounted for. The peace movement, the ecology movement, and the holistic health movement all share the same perspective: that the universe is made up of interdependent systems.

From Orthodox Medicine to Holistic Health

The change from one worldview to another takes place slowly, based on experiences and a shift in values and perspective. Each of us continuously undergoes this process. The sum total of our shared process creates a movement and, ultimately, a change in society.

My own evolution toward the holistic health movement illustrates this process. Brought up in a traditional American community, I went through most of medical school believing that physicians were the heroes of health. We saw lab tests, X-rays, and drugs as the mainstays of our trade. We scorned vitamins as placebos. Interns and residents boasted of their ability to make a diagnosis from test results without ever seeing the patient. When patients died, it was a point of pride if they died with all their lab values "within normal limits." During the 1960s, in the midst of my medical training, my orthodox values were confronted by the blatant discrepancies of our society and by the Vietnam war. I temporarily left school to come to terms with these social upheavals, and later further questioned the validity of orthodox assumptions about other areas of life, as well.

In my first years as a physician, stress and long hours caused me to have severe back pain. When I found myself taking valium and codeine just to get to sleep at night I consulted several orthopedists. They felt that the problem was an early disc hernia, and all of them recommended simple back exercises and walking. The bottom line, they implied, was surgery. Depressed and desperate, I ultimately committed the heretical act (for a physician) of consulting a chiropractor. The chiropractor spent time with

WHAT IS IATROGENESIS?

Ivan Illich

THE medical establishment has become a major threat to health. The disabling impact of professional control over medicine has reached the proportions of an epidemic. *Iatrogenesis*, the name for this new epidemic, comes from *iatros*, the Greek word for "physician," and *genesis*, meaning "origin." Discussion of the disease of medical progress has moved up on the agendas of medical conferences, researchers concentrate on the sick-making powers of diagnosis and therapy, and reports on paradoxical damage caused by cures for sickness take up increasing space in medical dopesheets. The health professions are on the brink of an unprecedented housecleaning campaign. "Clubs of Cos," named after the Greek Island of Doctors, have sprung up here and there, gathering physicians, glorified druggists, and their industrial sponsors as the Club of Rome has gathered "analysts" under the aegis of Ford, Fiat, and Volkswagen. Purveyors of medical services follow the example of their colleagues in other fields in adding the stick of "limits to growth" to the carrot of ever more desirable vehicles and therapies. Limits to professional health care are a rapidly growing political issue. In whose interest these limits will work will depend to a large extent on who takes the initiative in formulating the need for them: people organized for political action that challenges status-quo professional power, or the health professions intent on expanding their monopoly even further....

Thoughtful public discussion of the iatrogenic pandemic, beginning with an insistence upon demystification of all medical matters, will not be dangerous to the commonweal. Indeed, what is dangerous is a passive public that has come to rely on superficial medical housecleanings. The crisis in medicine could allow the layman effectively to reclaim his own control over medical perception, classification, and decision-making....

My argument is that the layman and not the physician has the potential perspective and effective power to stop the current iatrogenic epidemic.*

---

me, taught me about my body, and gently worked on my muscle spasms and misaligned spine. I committed myself to getting *well*, not just to getting *by*. I gradually improved but eventually reached a plateau. Even this treatment was basically passive; therefore, it was limited as an avenue to optimal health.

I turned to aikido, an active martial art. But because I was in poor physical condition, during the first few months I dislocated my shoulder and underwent surgery. I soon learned how to prepare myself, to warm up, to correct my movements, and to bring my mind and body together. I also learned to work within my physical limits.

Awareness of my ups and downs eventually led me to question other factors in my health. What was my potential? What were my real health risks? How did my nutrition and stress affect me? I decided to find out. I monitored my pain and energy daily. I consulted health practitioners, teachers, and friends; I received guidance and support from all of them. Through trial and error, I changed my lifestyle in profound ways. As I had hoped, I became far healther—and happier. This long, painful struggle also gave me a much deeper appreciation of the meaning of life and health.

My work as a health practitioner changed as a result of my own experiences with illness and recovery. I had learned three important principles:

1. Ultimately, *I* was the only one who could change my condition. Certainly, I learned much from many people, but it was my own consistent and enthusiastic application of this learning, as well as an attitude of self-responsibility, that made the difference. Thus, in holistic medicine, the patient must take an active, responsible part to achieve optimal health.

2. The healing process depends greatly on spirit and on interpersonal relationships. Both holism and general systems theory emphasize the underlying interdependence in the universe. It is healing to be in touch with our spirit and the spiritual process in the world. It is healing to acknowledge, through our behavior and values, our interdependence with people, the community, the environment, and the world. It is healing to discover our path in the world and to follow it with faith, sincerity, and dedication. And it is healing to have trusting and supportive relationships with guides, friends, teachers, or healers.

3. In order to be healthy, our perspective must change from *illness orientation* to *health orientation*. The aim of holistic health is to steer patients away from a medical model of health (in which they passively receive treatment or drugs) to a health model (in which they strive to maximize their vitality). The circumstances of each person's life, genes, experiences, and environment are all unique, therefore, everyone's need for health care is unique. Everyone has the potential to move to greater independence and health through application of a holistic philosophy.

Making Choices: Orientation to Holistic Practices and Techniques

Which shall it be—allopathy, homeopathy, psychology, naturopathy? You must decide which health practices and practitioners to choose (keeping in mind the importance of self-responsibility, the role of spirit, healing interpersonal relationships, and a health-oriented philosophy). From my experience in treating clients holistically, an eclectic approach is best. No single system of treatment or self-care will provide the most effective pathway to health over your lifetime. The holistic health field offers an array of approaches that can be confusing, competitive, or contradictory.

General systems theory has a concept called *stratification* that may help to clarify this confusion: *Self-organizing systems*, including human beings, are organized into different dimensions, or strata, of interdependent activity. One example is the stratification of a person into mind, body, and spirit. Each strata represents a different but interrelated level of human life process.

The table below illustrates a more comprehensive conceptual stratification of life process. The strata next to each other are more directly interrelated, but the dysfunctions or imbalances in any strata will ultimately affect all the others. For example, a person who eats poorly may develop biochemical dysfunction, such as a high cholesterol or low blood sugar, or subtle vitamin deficiencies. These in turn may cause dysfunctions of the immune system, with frequent colds or allergies at the cellular level, or poor work-performance at the lifestyle level, which can lead to depression or anxiety at the psychological level, and so on. From another strata, a person may have a learned psychological need to constantly accomplish. People with this psychological imbalance (characterized as the Type A personality) have a distorted sense of how much they can accomplish within a given period of time, and thus fail to get the relaxation necessary for internal health. A current view is that this dysfunction can lead to psychological imbalances that result in increased risk of cardiovascular disease.

The table also illustrates how health practices, naturalistic therapy, and orthodox or radical therapy might be used to intervene in imbalances at various strata. In the holistic model, self-care practices are the most preferable, using naturalistic interventions when necessary, and radical therapeutic techniques for severe dysfunction. The radical interventions, of course, have a much greater risk of adverse effects.

To find health through holistic practices, you must make a commitment to start somewhere. You can seek the most appropriate and effective level to work at, set goals, obtain information and treatment, work on these goals daily, and then evaluate your progress. When you reach a plateau of no progress, it's time to shift to other levels of work. It is valuable to consult with good teachers or practitioners. But be cautious when choosing practitioners and techniques. We live in a consumer-oriented society that promotes largeness and newness, and that rewards entrepreneurial salesmanship. As a holistic "seeker," you must question practitioners about their professional training, and get references from previous clients, if possible. Holistic techniques and products can be costly, and their effectiveness may not be scientifically proven. Again, get references or results of good research. Take the time to learn how various modalities function and what to expect in the course of treatment. Above all, trust your own feel-

DIMENSIONS OF HOLISTIC HEALTH AND HEALTH CARE

Strata of Life Process	Self-care Practices	"Natural" Therapeutic Interventions	Orthodox or Radical Therapeutic Interventions
Spiritual	Medication Spiritual practices Prayer	Spiritual counseling Pastoral counseling Group religious practice	Psychiatric drugs Cults
Environmental	Awareness of toxins Detoxification	Environmental clean-up Allergy presensitization	Chemotherapy
Societal/Cultural	Social/Political involvement Productive work	General political process	Institutionalization
Community/Family	Communication skills Committed relationships	Family or group therapy Community activity	Institutionalization
Psychological	Stress reduction Coping skills	Counseling	Tranquilizers, etc.
Mental (attitudes, values)	Self-awareness Self-responsibility Planning Commitment to goals Learning	Psychotherapy	Cults Institutionalization
Lifestyle	Awareness of negative addictions Learning General health practices	Group therapy Counseling	General illness care
Anatomical	Aerobic exercise Dance Yoga Martial arts	Physical therapy Spinal manipulation Massage Bodywork Metabolic therapies	Surgery
Genetic/Cellular	Detoxification Visualization	Metabolic therapies Meganutrition	Chemotherapy Radiation therapy
Biochemical	Improved nutrition balance	Meganutrition	Chemotherapy
Energetic	Awareness Energy practices	Acupuncture Reflexology Homeopathy	

THE MECHANIC AND THE GARDENER

Lawrence LeShan, Ph.D.

THERE has been a conflict at the heart of medical practice since Roman times at least. This is the question as to whether the physician should concentrate on actively intervening in disease or whether his primary emphasis should be on helping the patient's self-healing systems to work more effectively. The viewpoints both of the public and the profession have swung back and forth on this question in different historical periods. It is this problem which is at the center of the present confusion about "holistic medicine." We are now reaching for a new synthesis of the two viewpoints, an understanding of the strengths and weaknesses of both. We are beginning to learn where each is useful and how best to combine them.

From *The Mechanic And The Gardener*, New York: Holt, Rinehart, and Winston. Reprinted by permission.

In order to understand what is going on in medicine today, it is necessary to examine a basic conflict that has been continually fought in this field for at least 2500 years. This is the problem of what the physician primarily should try to do. Should he actively and forcefully *intervene* when the patient is ill by the use of surgery and strong medicaments to *conquer* the disease? Or should he instead concentrate on finding ways to support the patient's natural healing processes? In effect, should he be primarily a *mechanic* and repair the ill body, or should he be primarily a *gardener* and help the body grow past disease and toward health?

LAWRENCE LeSHAN, *Ph.D., research psychologist and author, is currently the President-elect of the Association of Humanistic Psychology (AHP).*

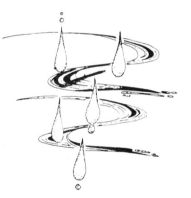

ings and judgment, and your sense of the practitioner's healing and spiritual qualities.

Directions in Holistic Health and Medicine: Moving Toward an Integrated Health-Care System

At this point in history, we can choose from a veritable cornucopia of health-related modalities. These range from CT scans, pharmacology, and surgery to the 2000-year-old Chinese practices of acupuncture and Tai-chi. At the Berkeley Holistic Health Center and other such centers across the country, a team of practitioners (health educators, physicians, psychologists, physical therapists, chiropractors, nutritionists, acupuncturists, and others) combine various modalities into clinical programs for the treatment of illnesses. Clients work with these practitioners in integrated programs to improve their health and vitality, and in the process learn how to maintain their own health.

This, after all, is the goal: to become increasingly independent in one's own health practices.

Presently, we are working to overcome several major obstacles in this integrative process. One involves the need for adequate research. The traditional research methodologies of physical science, which rely on a reductionist conceptual framework, are inadequate for the study of holistic treatment programs. Other methodologies, including those from the behavioral sciences, will be needed to accurately studying the safety and effectiveness of these programs.

Another major problem involves the seeming incompatibility of theoretical frameworks from various healing systems. Different systems see the same problem in different ways. For example, the orthodox medical system may see hypertension in one way, while the Chinese system may see it as an imbalance of different organs, and the homeopathic system may see it as just one of a complex of other symptoms. How to select the optimal treatment modalities from various systems? We are trying to meet this complex and challenging task.

There are also problems of cultural and social bias. Each of us has a cultural and social perspective. The deeply rooted beliefs and value systems held by people of different races or cultures can augment healing, but they can also limit the *inter*cultural integration of healing work. We all need to understand the dynamics of this process and grow beyond its limitations. Finally, we must learn how to make our society and environment as a whole more healthy. There are only a few instances in which holistic health organizations have been able to effectively influence legislative and cultural organizations to implement healthful laws and policies. The holistic health movement must join with other holistically oriented organizations to become an active force in the political process.

It is our collective experience of healing that will ultimately form the basis of an effective program in holistic health and medicine. I invite you to participate with us in this process.

I wish to acknowledge my indebtedness to the works of Fritjof Capra, my friends, and other leaders in the holistic health field in the creation of this article.

Suggested Further Reading

1. Hastings, Fadiman, and Gordon, editors, *Health for the Whole Person.* Bantam Books, 1980.
2. Jeffrey Bland, *Your Health Under Siege.* The Stephen Greene Press, 1982.
3. Fritjof Capra, *The Turning Point, Science, Society, and the Rising Culture.* Simon and Schuster, 1982.
4. Tom Ferguson, editor, *Medical Self-Care.* Summit Books, 1980.
5. Andrew Stanway, *Alternative Medicine.* Pelican Books, 1979.

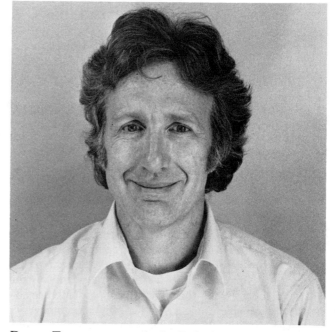

DAVID TEEGARDEN *received a B.S. from Harvard University and an M.D. from Stanford Medical School. He is Board Certified in Family Practice and a member of the American Holistic Medical Association. Serving presently as the Clinical Director of the Berkeley Holistic Health Center, he also has a private practice in Berkeley, California. Dr. Teegarden is a Sho Dan (Black Belt) in Aikido and is interested in a variety of holistic health practices.*

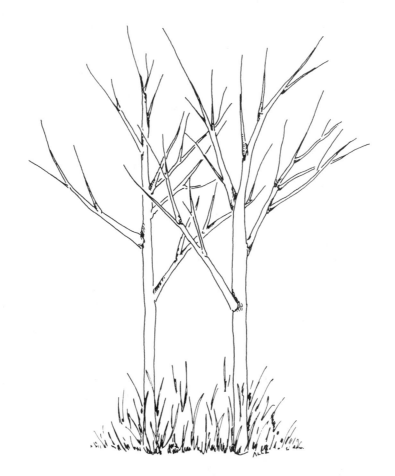

Holistic Medicine: Fringe or Frontier?

EXPLORATIONS BEYOND THE BIOMEDICAL MODEL

James S. Gordon, M.D.

HOLISTIC medicine. To some, the words are offensive: the adjective seems to profane the noun. Others reserve wry derision for its practitioners, for the curious and unconventional therapies they may prescribe. Some embrace holism as if it were messianic, embodying all that is innovative and redemptive. And still others, perhaps the vast majority, are puzzled. What is holism? Is it new or old, revolutionary or redundant? What does it actually contribute to the day-to-day practice of medicine? And why are so many people involved in it, or at least intrigued by it?

The concept was first popularized by South African statesman Jan Christian Smuts (perhaps better known in his military and political capacity) in his 1926 book *Holism and Evolution*. To Smuts, holism was a way of comprehending and describing organisms and systems as entities greater than and different from the sum of their parts, a corrective to the analytic reductionism of the prevailing sciences.

In the last decade, the word "holistic," and its Anglicized cousin, "wholistic," has been revived and applied—and misapplied—to almost every human endeavor, from primary education to jogging to home building. Perhaps its most fertile ground has been in medicine and health care—in part because its principles have always been integral to healing. Hippocrates, for example, emphasized the environmental causes and treatment of illness, and the importance of emotional factors and nutrition.

We are also now realizing, as microbiologist Rene Dubos suggested in *Mirage of Health*, in 1959, that there are inherent limitations to the technological advances which have proved invaluable in treating acute illness, and have helped cure or correct infectious diseases, vitamin deficiencies, and congenital defects. Such advances have been unable to stem the tide of "mental" and environmentally related illnesses—including hypertension, diabetes, obesity, cancer, depression, and alcoholism—which have in the last half-century become the chief agents of our mortality and morbidity. For both patients and providers of care, there are difficult side effects—economic, interpersonal, and biological—of unnecessary diagnostic and surgical procedures, over-medication, and an impersonal, fragmented system of care.

Whatever the present shortcomings of holistic medicine—and I will discuss some of them later—its ideal represents an antidote to the narrowness of specialization, a fresh attempt to understand and treat whole people in their total environment. Without neglecting the treatment of disease, it includes an appreciation of patients as mental and emotional, social and spiritual, as well as biological and psychological beings. It emphasizes approaches—diet, exercise and massage, introspection, biofeedback, and attitudinal change—which respect the patients' capability for healing themselves.

My own journey toward holism, or, more precisely, my discovery of the holistic tradition in medicine, has been quite personal and circuitous.

When I graduated from Harvard Medical School in 1967, most of my classmates and I moved confidently forward into our specialty and subspeciality training, focusing on the latest physiological or pharmacological advances in our particular area of interest. Some kept a hand in basic research, or admired colleagues who did. Even those of us who gave primacy to the "humanistic" aspects of health care suspected the real frontiers of medicine lay with the painstaking explorations of the biomedical scientist.

I was, if not typical, at least on the bell curve for that year's aspiring psychiatrists. I had considered becoming a surgeon like my father, or a general practitioner like my grandfather. I liked the idea of taking care of whole families over many years. But my real pleasure, I discovered, was in talking to people, in exploring their inner worlds, in understanding and helping them to understand the connections between their life histories and illnesses. I had worked on the wards at Massachusetts Mental Health Center, and, in my senior elective, with autistic and schizophrenic children.

By the time graduation came, I was prepared to believe there was an important distinction between physical and mental illness. The former, though influenced by emotions, was basically physiological, appropriate for definition and treatment according to a biomedical model. "Mental" illness (I began to consider this an inappropriate metaphor), with such obvious exceptions as phenylketonurea, pellagra, and perhaps autism, was basically psychological and social.

Over the next 10 years I explored the possibilities of psychosocial treatment in and outside of mental hospitals.

Harvard Medical Alumni Bulletin, Winter 1984. Reprinted by permission.

I grew to believe that medication, particularly in an institutional setting, was often used as a tool for foreclosing, under the aegis of therapy, ideas and behavior which were unconventional and disturbing to the staff. As a chief resident at Albert Einstein College of Medicine, I created with my coworkers a safe setting for psychotic people to re-experience, so they could reintegrate, fragments of early experience and fantasy—a place for what Scots psychiatrist R.D. Laing had called "the natural healing process of madness."

Later, in the community psychiatry laboratory of the National Institute of Mental Health, I worked with non-professionals to create supportive settings—hotlines, runaway houses, and group foster homes—for troubled and troubling young people.

I became fascinated by the way different social and attitudinal settings seemed to affect the very nature of our patients' "mental" illness. "Everywhere else," one chronic schizophrenic young man remarked, "I'm crazy. But here I'm sane."

Our refusal to emphasize psychopathology with these young people, and our insistence on their strengths, seemed to change how they felt about themselves. Parents who came to the runaway houses often marveled that the surly, rebellious, spaced-out kid who had always resisted the therapy they had suggested, was now cleaning his room, hauling out the garbage, and insisting on family counseling.

When I wasn't working with these community-based services, writing about them, or, later, directing NIMH's work with them, I was seeing private patients. My professional life seemed very much in order. There was a satisfying continuum stretching from the dynamic interpersonal psychotherapy I practiced with individuals and families in my private practice, to my attempts to alleviate "mental" illness by changing the settings and attitudes of therapy and therapists, to my concern with larger institutional and social change. People were respectfully reading what I was writing. I was becoming an expert.

Yet something was beginning to nag at me. It was obvious that just as psychological factors could affect physical health, so biological factors could affect psychosocial functioning. What really bothered me, I realized, was the reductionist way we viewed biology itself, and the biological therapies we had developed to treat aspects of "mental" illness. Too often such treatments seemed to violate thoughts and feelings of our patients, or relieved one set of biological problems only to create others.

Perhaps one could view biological symptoms, like psychological symptoms, as clues to the origins of the disturbance, as opportunities for growth and change. Perhaps patients could, with our help, apply an introspective approach to their disturbance and its origins, and could discover and use nontoxic remedies.

I cast about for answers to my questions, and discovered excerpts from Chinese scientific journals, which I found hard to believe, about the successful and widespread use of acupuncture analgesia in major surgery, and the relatively successful treatment by acupuncture of anxiety, schizophrenia, osteoarthritis, and bronchial asthma. There was no apparent anatomical reality to the channels or "meridians" which were presumed to run beneath the skin, no reason I could puzzle out that a needle placed in the foot would improve liver functioning.

At first I thought the successes of acupuncture might be placebo responses: the combination of the patients' positive expectations and their esteem for the practitioners in a supportive social context. But the technique had been used by hundreds of millions of people for several thousand years. There must be more to it.

Then I read that acupuncture was being successfully used in veterinary medicine. Either the Chinese scientists were lying, or.... Something shifted in my mind; my narrowness and chauvinism dropped away, at least for the moment. Here was an apparently effective healing practice based on premises quite different from our own, one which conceptualized the physical and mental as two aspects of an embracing "energy" system, a practice which brought the same, apparently non-toxic, techniques to bear on treating both.

At about the time I was beginning to read about acupuncture, a series of events brought one of its practitioners, an osteopath named Shyam Singha, to my house for a three-day visit. He was unlike any physician I had ever known, as strange and fascinating as the root workers and brujos I had briefly met in ghettos and barrios, or the shamans I had read about in the pages of Eliade, Levi-Strauss, and Castaneda.

Dr. Singha's discussion of Oriental medicine, of the balance between Yin (negative) and Yang (positive) energy and the Law of Five Elements, seemed by turns brilliant and absurdly fanciful, more like religious belief than medical fact. I didn't trust half of what he said, but just when I was about to dismiss him as a charismatic quack, he connected physiological functioning to acupuncture principles, or quoted the relevant articles from the Chinese, and even the British, medical literature. I knew he knew something I didn't.

A year or two after I began to reconsider my attitude toward the biomedical model, six months after I met Dr. Singha, in the middle of my tentative explorations of Chinese medicine, I injured my lower back. I had pains in the lumbosacral area, and numbness and paresthesias in my left leg and foot. I was bent almost double.

I consulted the orthopedic surgeons at Bethesda Naval Hospital (I was in the Public Health Service), who prescribed bed rest, muscle relaxants, and a heating pad, and deferred their diagnosis.

I stayed in bed, bemused and nonfunctional from the muscle relaxants, and arose two weeks later little better. When I returned to Bethesda I was told I might, indeed *should*, have back pain, but couldn't possibly have the symptoms I detailed unless I had a disc problem—and, so far as they were concerned, I only had lumbosacral strain.

I began to think, with, I confess, far greater sympathy than before, about all the patients who had described vague symptoms which fit no known syndrome for whom neither I nor other doctors could do anything.

For about two months I did the prescribed back exercises, and rested when told to. Then, only marginally better and quite impatient, I turned to the highly recommended chief of orthopedics at one of the city's major teaching hospitals. He reviewed my x-rays, expressed concern, mentioned a myelogram, but offered no answers, no help.

Finally I decided, at a friend's urging, to see a local osteopath. The idea made me exceedingly nervous. It was one thing, I realized, to learn the theory of another medical system, or even to talk to a curious, maddening, and perhaps mad, fringe practitioner like Shyam Singha. It was quite another to submit my own body—a body used to the most scientific and sophisticated Western medicine—to one of its adherents.

The osteopath I consulted announced I had a "lesion" in my back, that the lumbar vertebrae were pressing on the nerve roots as they emerged from the spinal cord, and that he could do something about it. He put me on my side, one leg dangling from the examining table, and "manipulated" my back.

The crunch I heard as he leaned hard on my hip conjured dreadful visions—discs extruding, paralysis, and impending impotence.

Within minutes I was standing—not bending over, but actually standing. The numbness and tingling were receding. I was ecstatic, until, five minutes later, the pain and paresthesias returned. Still, I was hopeful: something had happened, even if it had lasted only briefly. I returned a few times, but the results were similar. Finally, close to despair, just before I was to submit to a myelogram, I called Dr. Singha in London.

Stop the medicine, he said. Take hot baths with Epsom salts and then cold showers. Eat three pineapples a day for a week and nothing else.

I thought the trans-Atlantic phone had gone bad. He repeated his prescription. I could hear what sounded like the roar of the ocean in the line while I stood with my mouth open.

"Why?"

"It won't make sense to you."

"Why?"

"Pineapple has malic acid."

"Yes, I understand that." (I am impatient.)

"Malic acid affects the lung and colon." (He is fast losing credibility.) "In Chinese medicine the lung and colon are the mother of kidney and bladder." (The mother?) "The bladder and kidney are connected to the back...."

He was right. It made no sense. But I didn't want the myelogram, and I didn't want surgery, and something about Dr. Singha, an authority I did not understand, moved me. I decided to do it. I was desperate.

I took my baths and showers, and, to my own amazement, and the amusement of my friends, and colleagues, I ate my pineapple. After three days, I called London. "My mouth," I reported, "is full of sores and I have a 103-degree fever. My back hurts as badly and the paresthesias are as prominent as when I first injured it."

"For the sores," he said, "coat your pineapple with honey. So far as the rest goes, it is very good. In Chinese medicine, a chronic disease must be made acute before it can be healed."

At first I assumed that in my feverish delirium I had misunderstood. Then, suddenly, for the first time some piece of the treatment made sense to me. In psychotherapy,

one often has to relive painful traumatic experiences in the process of recovery from a chronic debilitating way of thinking or feeling. Perhaps, I thought, the healing of my body was proceeding in a similar way.

At the end of the week I went back to my osteopath. This time the adjustment held.

My mild curiosity about alternative healing techniques now became a kind of fascination. Perhaps the principle of making the chronic acute could be applied to the biological treatment of "mental" as well as physical illness. Perhaps techniques that had been disparaged or ignored in my training could be of use to me and my patients. It was certainly worth some time.

I read about other approaches to health and illness: osteopathy, chiropractic, homeopathy, nutrition and herbalism, relaxation therapies, autogenics and hypnosis, massage, and Rolfing.

I experimented on myself. Over time, I discovered tools—meditation, yoga, Tai Chi (a Chinese moving meditation)—which helped me experience from the inside organs I had once palpated in surgery, and become aware of physiological processes I had seen recorded on laboratory instruments. I discovered that, by sitting quietly and concentrating on my breathing, I could raise the temperature in my fingers, relax my muscles, still my mind. Bending forward and back, moving from one yoga asana to another, I could feel the individual vertebrae form the curves of my spine.

Each time I had an ache, a pain, or an illness, I tried something new. I began to ask myself what I was anxious about, or why I had been careless: What was in it for me to be sick now? I let the images or the words come: "You don't really feel like going to work but don't feel right about missing a day; Your voice is hoarse because there's something you want to say but are holding back." Unresolved conflicts, it seemed, were often the necessary if not the sufficient cause of my ailments.

For a headache, instead of taking aspirin I now tried to use a relaxation technique or imagery—watching in my mind's eye as the muscles in my neck and scalp softened and lengthened. I used herbal teas for sleeplessness and diarrhea, and acupressure, not antihistamines, for allergies. My treatments were by no means always successful, and rarely was relief as swift as from allopathic medicine. But I was learning from my illnesses—about myself as well as alternative therapies—and I knew I wasn't creating any new problems with my treatment.

I spent several months in England with Dr. Singha learning the fundamentals of acupuncture and osteopathy. In the U.S. I attended lectures and workshops, and consulted the practitioners of different therapies who seemed most knowledgeable and responsible. Sometimes I was sorry: there certainly are a number of incompetent and venal people flourishing at the fringe of medical orthodoxy, feeding on frustration and despair. At other times, I was impressed.

The more I learned, the more curious my previous ignorance seemed. Why had our training omitted musculoskeletal manipulation? It had apparently been part of all the world's healing traditions, and clearly could work to alter peripheral function, perhaps even to modify the feedback loops to the central nervous system.

In my psychiatric training, hypnosis had been dismissed as fraught with authoritarian possibilities, capable only of producing symptom substitution. As I came to understand more about it—and the relaxation techniques to which it was related—I began to see its potential for treating physical as well as psychological problems. I realized that trance states were not unlike those I had entered on the psychoanalyst's couch, that hypnotic suggestions, like the analyst's interpretations, could permit access to memories, thoughts, feelings, and images which might relieve pain, improve functioning, or help resolve psychological dilemmas.

And what about nutrition? I could remember only a few lectures on severe dietary deficiency diseases—scurvy, rickets, pellagra—which we were unlikely to encounter in the United States. Yet it was clear, once I began to pay attention, that how much and what kinds of food I ate affected my mental and physical state.

After awhile, some friends began to ask for help with nagging debilitating problems unrelieved by their primary care physician or specialists, problems such as back pain, sinusitis, vaginitis, arthritis, insomnia, and pre-menstrual tension. I agreed to help, but was apprehensive, partly because I had no formal medical training since internship, partly because there was no body of research, and no articles in refereed journals, to justify my treatments.

I made sure all of my patients had had a thorough, and thoroughly orthodox, medical work-up before they saw me, and comforted myself with the fact that I would in any case be doing them no harm. Finally I decided that I would put all financial incentives on their side—by treating my new patients without charge.

Some of my first patients got better, much better. Some whose physical symptoms didn't disappear still felt better. The success could have been due to specific techniques I used, but I knew it might have been a result of my relationship with my patients and their confidence in me. I couldn't rule out the possibility of a Hawthorn effect—a difference, any difference, making the difference. Still, something useful was happening.

I found that studies on the therapies I was learning were—and still are—not good. There were a few reports from the Soviet Union on fasting, anecdotal accounts on the effects on mood of food, food allergies, and acupuncture, and a few papers on jogging and depression.

I did find much better studies that expanded my view of the interrelationship between physical, psychological, and social well-being—and of the role of the doctor/patient relationship in the treatment of physical as well as "mental" illness. A number of recent works have explored the implications of Hans Selye's decades-old research into the pyscho-physiology of stress, and have provided evidence to substantiate and extend the clinical descriptions of such pioneers in psychosomatic disorders as Franz Alexander, Helen Flanders Dunbar, Willhelm Reich, and George Engel. Studies indicate, for example, that people who have recently experienced significant loss, particularly those who

are not close to their parents, are more likely to develop a variety of chronic diseases than matched controls.

Salvador Minuchin and his coworkers have shown a clear relationship between the free fatty-acid levels of diabetic children and their parents' interactions. Harvey Brenner's epidemiological work has demonstrated a relationship between fluctuations in our national economy and the incidence of a variety of disease conditions. And Arthur Kleinman, Leon Eisenberg, and Byron Good have described how successful treatment of even the most discrete clinical entity can be frustrated by ignorance of the familial and cultural context in which it occurs.

For several years I kept my practices separate: psychotherapy for people with emotional problems, my free clinic and the alternative therapies for those with physical problems that had been refractory to conventional treatment. However, the more patients I saw, and the more I learned about the healing systems of other cultures—all of which I was also investigating at NIMH—the less it made sense to make sharp distinctions between physical and psychological or indeed spiritual, familial, or social problems.

For a few years, I proceeded tentatively, trying first one therapy, then another. Over time I developed a more comprehensive approach, based on my training in psychiatry and psychosomatic medicine, on Chinese conceptions of balance and change, and on my steadily increasing knowledge of the effects of food and exercise, attitude, relaxation, and medication on physical and emotional health.

By the late '70s, the term "psychiatry" didn't cover all I was doing, either in my own practice, or at St. Elizabeths, the federal mental hospital where I had become chief of the Adolescent Service as part of my NIMH work. There I was teaching barely literate, periodically psychotic inner-city teenagers to appreciate the connection between what they ate and how they felt, and helping them shape and control their anger and violence not only by expressing and exploring it verbally, but also with relaxation exercises and Kung Fu practice.

It now seems to me that the most therapeutic attitude for physican and patient alike is one which regards illness, whatever its primary symptoms, as an opportunity for personal growth and change—and the physican as a catalyst and guide in this process. The treatments of choice at any level are therefore those which most effectively promote the individual's capacity for self-awareness and self-care.

My current practice resembles in many ways my grandfather's of 60 years ago. I work with family members of all ages, singly and together, and consult about family problems and decisions as well as about acute and chronic illnesses. I make house calls when someone who needs me is too ill to come to my office. I rarely prescribe the powerful drugs that have been developed since my grandfather's practice—including the neuroleptics, antidepressants, and anxiolytics that are the staples of biological psychiatry—and still more rarely hospitalize my patients.

Many of those who come to me present with the kinds of problems that might bring them to any psychiatrist. But I am perhaps more likely than most to engage them actively

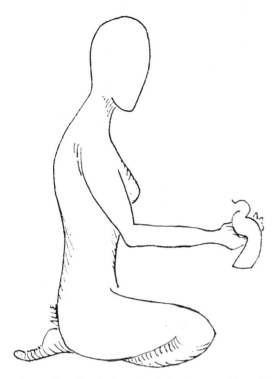

in work on the physical and spiritual, as well as the psychological and interpersonal, aspects of these problems. I tend to see, and help my patients to see, that psychological problems are not simply indicators of underlying pathology. They are, often enough, signs that a new or renewed source of meaning and purpose in life are necessary.

Among the techniques I use—in addition to dynamic psychotherapy, Gestalt, guided imagery, and bioenergetics—I have found that periods of fasting (I must confess I have not resorted to the pineapple fast) can interrupt, or help a patient work through, a depressive or schizophrenic episode. I recommend exercise—everything from jogging and aerobic dancing to Tai Chi and yoga—trying to tailor the technique to the person. And I use acupuncture as well, which seems to relax patients, improve their moods, at least temporarily, and at times help them move through emotional blocks. During the treatment, depressed and affect-less people may dissolve in tears; repressed ones may feel surges of anger. Some rise from the acupuncture table with fresh insights: "I'm only staying sick," one depressed woman announced, "so I can make my husband take care of me."

Others present with longstanding serious physical problems. They come after receiving the most up-to-date and exhaustive work-ups—when they are about to take another plunge into psychotherapy, or undergo yet another series of diagnostic tests, another change in medication, or another surgical procedure. They come—I warn them in advance—prepared to take a fresh look at themselves, their illness, and its treatment.

A middle-aged woman, for example, presents with asthma and emphysema. Chronically dependent on steroids, inhalers, and emergency treatment with epinephrine, she's Cushing-oid, morbidly anxious, and suicidally depressed. Under my supervision, she changes her diet radically, substituting brown rice, vegetables, and fish for coffee and doughnuts, hamburgers, and pizza. She sees some dimi-

nution in her pulmonary symptoms and begins to lose weight, which increases her feeling of self-sufficiency and encourages her to let me gradually reduce her medication. When acupuncture proves capable of aborting an acute asthmatic attack, she is willing to use acupressure at home to relieve attacks that previously might have brought her to the emergency room. The more she is able to take care of herself, the more willing she is to learn techniques she can use on her own. The better she feels, the more confident she becomes, the greater the improvement in her pulmonary functioning.

If holistic medicine has provided its proponents with a rallying point, it also offers us and our critics a challenge. We need to achieve a balance between openness to unconventional healers and regulation of unscrupulous practitioners who capitalize on the despair of prospective patients. There is nothing holistic about allowing poorly trained personnel to practice, condemning more traditional medical care, or claiming that diet, chiropractic, acupuncture, or homeopathy can cure every illness.

The diagnostic and therapeutic techniques that are increasingly widely used cry out for careful and sophisticated research. Even more important, we need to bring new methods, and indeed new attitudes, to the study of the approach to health care—call it holistic or not—that is evolving. Investigators will need to remember that established methods, such as the double-blind study, may be inappropriate for evaluating techniques which depend for their efficacy on the informed and active participation of patients.

The longer I practice, the less I am awed by the techniques themselves. I am increasingly aware of their utility as vehicles for the healing interaction between me and my patients. In the past we have too often factored this "placebo effect" out of our clinical investigations. We now need to take a thorough and critical look at this interaction, its development, and its biological as well as psychological consequences. We need to understand those factors which facilitate or frustrate the development of physicians who are able to establish a healing bond with their patients, and at the environments—emotional and physical, educational and social—in which physicians, other health-care workers, and patients may flourish.

In my own work, I am eager to create a setting for bringing together and putting to use what I have learned in mental health services, and my private "holistic" practice. I want to see if the holistic approach that has been developed among the well-to-do few can be extended to the masses of people, and determine if it offers an efficacious, cost-effective, and satisfying modification of conventional practice.

Whatever the outcome of these studies and efforts, I imagine the name "holistic medicine" will eventually be dropped, as it is ultimately a device of historical utility, not a necessity. Holistic medicine is not a new specialty. The name serves as a reminder of what is best and most enduring in medicine, and an opening into a new synthesis of contemporary biomedicine and the larger healing tradition of which it is but a part.

It is a way of approaching all health care, as useful and exciting for the surgeon and psychiatrist as for the family practitioner, as vital to practice in a tertiary care setting as in a rural retreat. It is, finally, an attitude of thoughtful openness to everything that may be useful in health care— to the healthy techniques we may have ignored or disparaged, as well as those we learned in medical school and specialty training, to the healing power of the therapeutic encounter, to our patients' capacity to understand and care for themselves, and to our ability and need as physicians to grow and change.

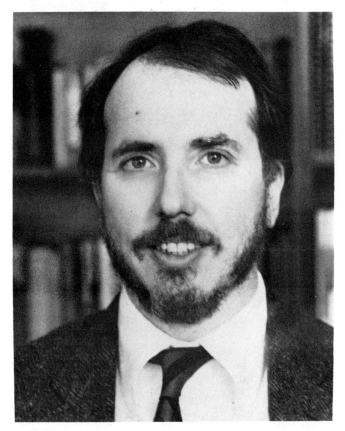

JAMES S. GORDON, *M.D., is Clinical Associate Professor in the Department of Psychiatry and Community and Family Medicine at the Georgetown University School of Medicine in Washington, D.C., and a trustee of the American Holistic Medicine Association. For ten years he was a research psychiatrist at the National Institute of Mental Health. He has written two books on alternative mental health services for adolescents and was the author of the Special Study on Alternative Mental Health Services for President Carter's Commission on Mental Health. He is co-editor of* Health for the Whole Person: The Complete Guide to Holistic Medicine *(Bantam, 1981) and* Mind, Body and Health: Toward an Integral Medicine *(Human Sciences Press, 1984) and co-author of* New Directions in Medicine *(Aurora, 1984).*

II

Healing Systems from Around the World

INTRODUCTION *by Naomi Steinfeld*

IN THIS SECTION you will find three different modalities of healing systems—the Oriental, the Native American, and the Western. Perhaps you are anthropologically curious, or seeking a cure for a particular ill, or in pursuit of the cross-cultural roots of healing. Whatever your ostensible purpose, you are likely to find something of value here.

What is a "system"? Webster gives many definitions, among them:

1. a regularly interacting or interdependent group of items forming a unified whole;
2. an assemblage of substances that is in or tends to equilibrium; and
3. a harmonious arrangement or pattern.

The systems you will encounter here share the basic premise that the old saying, *the whole is greater than the sum of its parts,* is actually true. We are each part of a larger framework (or "fabric," or "network," or "tapestry"—or, "system." Healing, being a nonanalytical dimension, must be alluded to by image or by metaphor). This means that we ourselves are a "system"—an "interacting group of items" such as a heart, lungs, a liver, blood cells, tissue, and so on. And each component of the system is itself a system—our hearts are not massive blocks of matter, but living, highly complex and organized interconnections of parts. And so on, smaller and smaller, and larger and larger. A system is a microcosm (the large within the small), and also a macrocosm (the small within the large). You can start anywhere—it all leads to the same truth: we are not alone.

It is when we cut ourselves off from the awareness of how all the parts are interconnected that we experience illness. Each of these three healing systems speaks to that suturing of the wound, that making whole which constitutes healing. In the 1960s, many young people experienced the wound of analysis—the dividing the whole into parts—and sought to "holistify" the parts. Thus they embraced ancient, other-cultural ways, yoga rather than competitive sports, Oriental massage to learn touching without sexuality, wearing feathers and beads and living in sky-fronted domes in an attempt to reclaim the intimate relationship with nature that the Native American culture never lost. At the same time, Western ways were seen as the antagonist (much as Western medicine saw the body as a vulnerable fortress susceptible to attack from foreign germs and viruses). So in the '60s and '70s, there was a lot of brave new experimenting with nonindigenous healing systems. There was also a lot of flashy behavior and self-righteous rejection of the familiar.

But these are the 1980s, and times, as each of us knows full well, have changed. We have lived through the exultation of the foreign and the diminution of the domestic, and now we are getting back to basics in various ways, redefining and living out the American virtues of work, free enterprise, the democratic system, and so on. So holistic health is going mainstream, and now it's time to assimilate all that is useful from every tradition, including even our own.

This omnivorous investigation helps us develop a sensitivity to our real needs. And when we know what we really need—be it a loving touch, a stretching of the spine, or a knowledgeable practitioner to take us seriously—we know how to locate the source of healing. So here, in this section, are three traditions that you can use to become sensitive to that which will heal that which needs healing.

The Western system is particularly fascinating, because (as so often happens) we have experienced the institutionalized understanding of the followers—which is hardly the same thing as the source. If, when we think of Western medicine, we think back to our first polio shot (when the doctor intoned "Now, this won't hurt a bit," while a needle the size of an elephant's tusk made its way toward our baby-fine skin), then from then on, that becomes the filter through which we view Western medicine. Therefore, it is profoundly eye-opening to read about the *roots* of Western medicine—Hippocrates' careful, respectful words on the nature of the healer-healee relationship, not to mention the working-with-nature ways of naturopathy and homeopathy.

The Native American system, while "foreign" to many of us, is utterly indigenous to this country. In its sacred appreciation for the environment, it views medicine not as a "specialty" but as a way of life: the earth is not a material to support the concrete that leads to the doctor's waiting room, but the healer itself. The round drum beat by a circle of drummers, the prayer circles, the sun, the earth— wholes characterize this way of being, as cubicles and insularity characterize the ills of modern life. In the Native American system, healing is not an action, but a *relationship* of person to environment—of part to whole.

The Oriental system says that we are already whole, and that what causes our ills is the lie that we are not. Our ills first appear in our minds, as thoughts of separation from our larger self. By clearing the mind of the illusion that we are anything other than already whole, we bring our entire beings—body, mind, emotions, and spirit—into harmonious alignment. And one way to clear the mind is to move the body in a particular way, which is the path of yoga.

Which is the "right" system? To answer this question, ask yourself another: "Which is better, your heart or your lungs?" You quickly see that there is a proper place and function for everything. It all depends on what you need and what you are able to accept.

So read on, without preconceptions about what you will find. If you have a hunch about what you are looking for (or if you are *willing* to let that hunch become apparent to your conscious mind) then you can feel your way into discovering a significant piece of information. This information you can then use to make, from the pieces of your life, a "unified whole."

Which will make your life a working system.

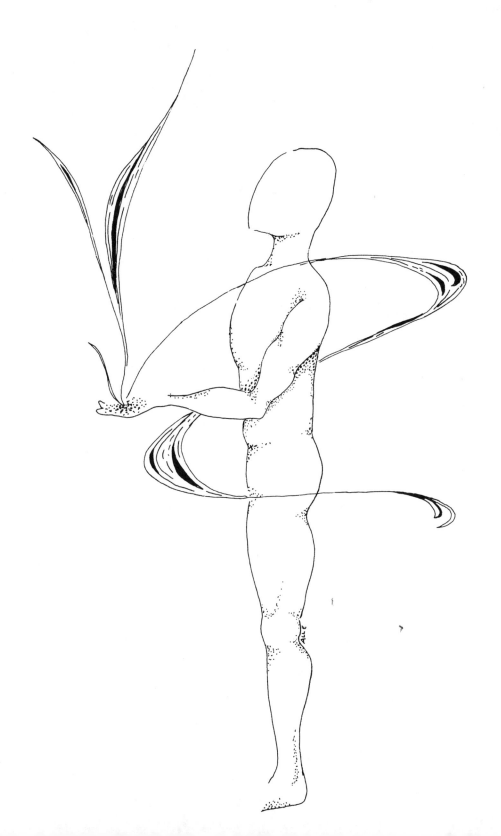

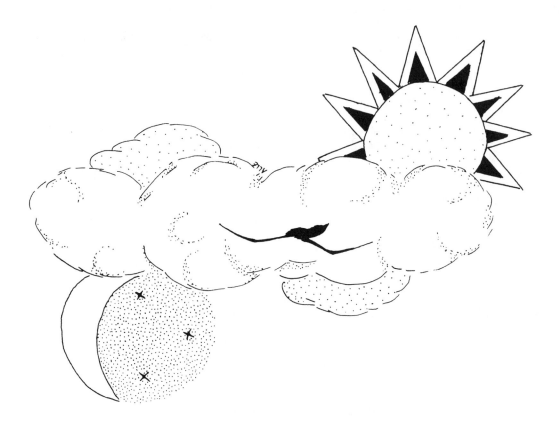

A. ORIENTAL SYSTEMS

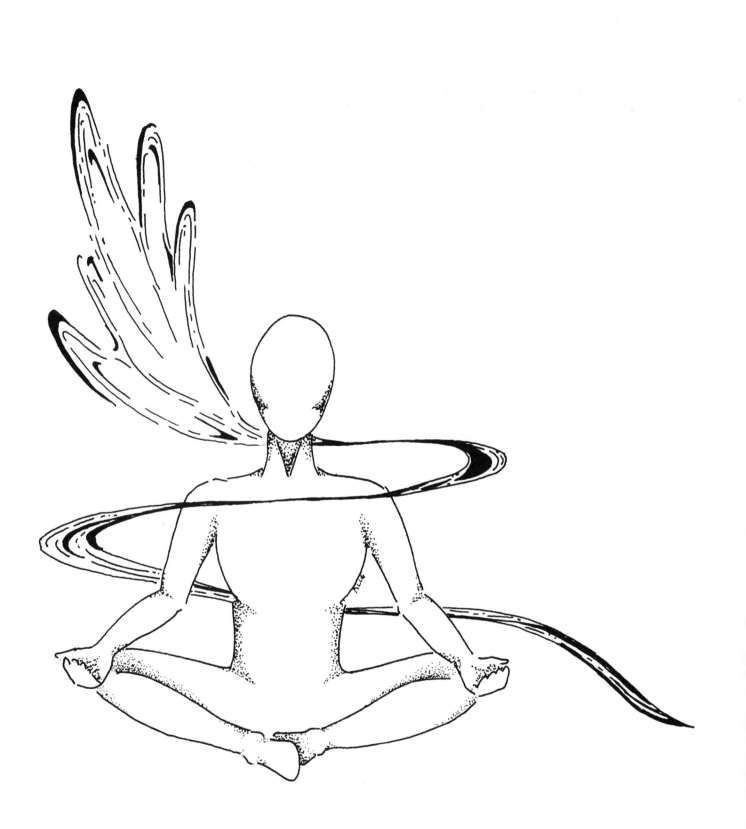

Yoga: An Ancient Technique for Restoring Health

Judith Hanson Lasater, Ph.D.

Yoga is a wonderful way to promote fitness, flexibility, and relaxation. It can be practiced in groups or alone. It has been found to steady the mind, calm the emotions, and tone the body. Basic elements of many yoga systems include asanas, or stretching postures, pranayama, or breathing purifications, and some form of meditation or internal centering. These elements, as well as various individual yoga systems, are elaborated upon in this article, which demonstrates that yoga is of universal appeal, not limited to European culture.

"Having mastered the body by means of the Yogic teachings, so that it becomes a fit habitation for the soul; having the senses, emotions, and mind under control, the wise person discards the worn-out sheaths of desire, fear, and confusion and passes into the state of enlightenment and freedom."

Bhagavad Gita

HEALTH IS just beginning to be studied in the West as a positive state, something to be sought and maintained for its own sake, rather than as the absence of disease. Current students of health are rediscovering some old concepts and philosophies about health, some of them Eastern. One such philosophy is *yoga*.

Actually, yoga is more a technique than a philosophy; it is a practice of the principles of the Indian philosophical system of *Samkhya*, as well as an application of some of its basic premises. In practice, yoga is an applied science of the mind and body. Practice and study of it help to bring about a natural balance of body and mind in which the state of health can manifest itself. Yoga itself does not create health; rather, it creates an internal atmosphere which allows the individual to come to his own state of dynamic balance, or health.

History of Yoga

The term yoga has been bandied about for so many years in Western cultures that it has almost lost its meaning. The word is Sanskrit; it derives from a verbal root, *yuj*, meaning "to yoke or join or fasten or harness, as in horses to a chariot; to concentrate the mind in order to obtain union with the Universal Spirit; to be absorbed in meditation."[1]

The major systematic presentation of yoga was made in the *Yoga Sutras*, or more formally the *Yoga Aphorisms of Patanjali*, in approximately the second century B.C. The literal meaning of "*sutra*" is "thread"; Patanjali's work is a collection of many such threads, short terse sentences which convey the barest minimum of teaching about yoga. The rest was to be learned from a teacher in person.

Little is known about Patanjali; he was supposedly a physician, Sanskrit scholar, yogi (one who practices yoga), and teacher who lived in India. Some authorities believe that he was more of a cataloguer than an author, and that he did not so much originate as collect and edit the teachings, which were already traditional.[2] But it is interesting that a physican was so greatly concerned with philosophy, since this is evidence that he, and perhaps many others at that time, considered one's outlook on life to be related to one's health.

Patanjali is traditionally credited with being the originator of the yoga system. It is relatively unimportant whether he actually did originate it, because, whether he was author or editor, his *Yoga Sutras* are the purest presentation of yoga available, and offer valuable aid to the student.[3]

The Yoga System

One basic assumption of the *Yoga Sutras* is that the body and the mind are part of one continuum of existence, the mind merely being more subtle than the body. This is the foundation of the yogic view of health. The interaction of body and mind is the central concern of the entire science. It is believed that as the body and mind are brought into balance and health, the individual will be able to perceive his true nature; this will allow life to be lived through him more freely and spontaneously.

Yoga first attempts to reach the mind, where health begins, for mental choices strongly affect the health of the body. Choices of food, of types of exercise, of which thoughts to think, all affect the body. Most Westerners live in a state of constant physical tension, which reflects the mental tension within them. Typically, the Westerner tries

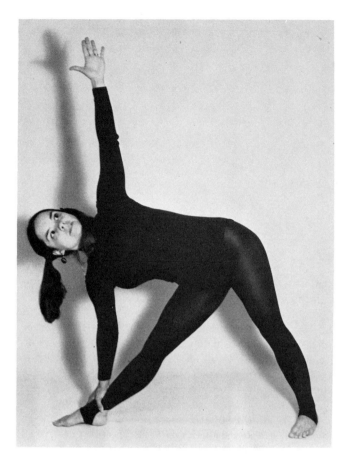

to reduce physical tension without first trying to observe or change the mental patterns from which it arose and will arise again.

In order to still and observe the mind, Patanjali presents a system called *Ashtanga Yoga*, or the Eight-Limbed Yoga. These limbs represent all the aspects of the system. The first two limbs that Patanjali begins with are the fundamental ethical precepts called *yamas* ("rein, curb, or bridle," here used to mean "self-control, forbearance, or any great rule or duty"), and the *niyamas* ("a minor observance"). He continues with the third limb, the basic practices of *asana* ("staying or abiding," here used to mean conscious movements, termed "postures" in the West), and the fourth limb, *pranayama* (*pra* = to bring forth; *na* = the eternal mystical vibation; *ya* = being that; *ma* = to measure). In practice, *pranayama* is the measuring, control, and directing of the breath, and thus of energy within the organism, in order to restore and maintain health and to promote evolution. The fifth limb of the system is *pratyahara* ("drawing back or retreat"), here meaning withdrawal of the senses from attachment to external objects.

These five external, physical yogic practices are followed, in Patanjali's system, by the three internal limbs of yoga: *dharana* ("immovable concentration of the mind"); *dhyana* ("profound and abstract religious meditation"); and *samadhi* ("putting together, joining, or combining with," here referring to the union of the contemplating being with the object of contemplation).

These first definitions indicate a pathway which leads to the attainment of physical, ethical, emotional, and psy-cho-spiritual health. Yoga in no way seeks to change the individual; rather, it allows the natural state of total health and integration in each of us to become a reality.

Physical Health from Yoga

Yoga affects the health of the body in many ways, perhaps most importantly by changing the way we think about our bodies. As we practice the *asanas*, we become more sensitive to our weaknesses and strengths; we become more aware of our areas of tightness, and of our areas of free and easy movement. This increase of awareness can help us make health choices that will affect us profoundly. For example, as the body is stretched and used, the muscles alternately contract and relax, the joints are gently stimulated and begin to move more freely, the muscles cease to restrict the free movements of the joints, the circulation to such areas as the discs between the vertebrae is improved, and the body is generally "tuned up." "Life is movement and movement is life."[4] As we begin to move and use our bodies, we become more aware of our health, and begin consciously to choose better nutrition and more exercise, which are badly needed (most doctors would say) by the average sedentary American.

As another example of how awareness can affect health, let us examine one of the first postures, *Tadasana*, or the Mountain pose. The student is instructed, as he or she stands erect, to become aware of where he places his weight—perhaps too far forward or backward—of how he uses his spine, of the position of his head. As he becomes more aware of the imbalances in his standing posture during class, he becomes more aware of how he stands during the rest of the day. Backache and shoulder tension are often created by unbalanced posture; as we become aware of how we are using our bodies, we are better equipped to change the ingrained habits which may be causing our tension, discomfort, and lack of energy.

The physiological changes caused by the practice of yoga have only recently begun to be documented by Western science. Preliminary findings have reported such data as: reduced blood pressure; lowered pulse rates; beneficial changes in the fat level of the blood, and in stress hormones and thyroid hormones; regulation of menstrual flow; elimination of stress incontinence; reductions of joint dysfunction and pain; increase in the range of normal joints; and a general subjective feeling of increased well-being.[5]

Although yoga is widely used as a palliative for various physical problems—with varying degrees of success[6]—it is much more effective when used to create a basic attitude toward health, namely, that the individual can control his or her own health. Yoga restores a state of balance in the body, in which the body can heal and restore itself; yoga is a tool to create a harmonious *milieu* in which the body, in its infinite wisdom, can attain a health which is radiant and unceasing.

Finally, one of the most important aspects of any health program, especially in the tension-racked West, is relaxation. Yoga classes generally end with 5 to 15 minutes of conscious relaxation. This state differs from sleep in that the mind is aware of the process and is not at all dulled; in this *asana* the student is poised midway between wakefulness and sleep, with the body relaxed and the mind receptively alert. This regular practice teaches the art of relaxation, which, again, may be extended into everyday situations where life demands an intense response and yet an alert, focused mind.

Mental Health from Yoga

Mental health is another specific goal of yogic practice. Many Westerners believe that yoga demands withdrawal from interaction with the world. On the contrary, as the 33rd Sutra of the second chapter of the *Yoga Sutras* states, one who practices yoga must interact fully and lovingly with those around him. It is only in a relationship with another, intimate or casual, that one can learn the nature of one's attachments, needs, and fears. A close relationship, for example, might teach one about jealousy and how it shapes one's view of the world. Much self-knowledge is gained by confronting external situations where impediments to internal peace are manifested.

Another premise of yoga psychology is that emotional stability is the first prerequisite for both mental and physical health. As the constant and disciplined practice of *asana*, *pranayama*, and deliberate relaxation begin to bring the student's organism into balance, the periodic emotional storms that occur in everyone's life will come into clearer perspective; and the student will be better equipped to observe and deal with situations that may be precipitating unnecessary problems. By learning to watch the movements of the body and the breath, the practitioner of yoga is brought directly into the present moment; this continual refocusing on *right now* is supremely necessary if one is to let go of past patterns of rigid and neurotic behavior, which limit the full expression of creativity and the enjoyment of life.

Finally, the student of yoga learns to take things more in stride, to accept the ups and downs of life with a little more detachment, but not with less interest. He will simply accept them more calmly, so that his health is not interrupted by emotional tension or imbalance. As the body's health improves, the undistracted mind becomes a true servant of the creative intelligence which lives in everyone.

Asana and Pranayama: Physical Steps to the Mind

But how can these principles of mental balance be concretely applied to one's life? Yoga stresses the very powerful tools of *asana* and *pranayama* as a way in which the mind and body can become more fully integrated—and this is another definition of health.

Western psychology and medicine are fond of separating the body and mind, and of making of them two different aspects of the individual. Science speaks of psychosomatic and somatopsychic diseases. In an Eastern view this would not be correct; rather, it would seem that the body is merely the concrete manifestation of the mind. This concept holds tremendous potential for the psychologist who is willing to recognize the interconnection of body and mind as being literally true. In the West, it is considered that the human embryo begins life as a physical organism; from this life comes the formation of the brain and, finally, the development of the mind. Eastern views disagree, holding that the consciousness associated with mind manifests through the brain and, from that, to the physical body.

Asana is one way in which the student can experience the unity of body and mind. The second chapter of the *Yoga Sutras*, verse 46, defines *asana* as that which is comfortable and easy, as well as firm. It is a dynamic position, in which the practitioner is perfectly poised between activity and nonactivity, between doing and "being done by" the posture. There is a corresponding mental balance between movement and stillness. Indeed, Patanjali teaches that each posture reflects a mental attitude, whether that attitude be one of surrender, as in a forward-bending *asana*, or the strengthening of the will, through backward-bending postures, or the creation of a physical prayer with the body, as in the practice of *Padmasana*, the well-known lotus posture.

Asana is a two-way street. Once the mental attitude has been created, it can then be spontaneously expressed as an *asana*; if one takes on the external form of an internal attitude, soon that attitude moves through body into mind, thus creating it there. Whichever way one works, the results are the same. *Asana* is thus both a preparation for meditation and a meditation sufficient in and of itself. Those who think that a practice like *asana* is unnecessary or unimportant in a healthy life are making the mistake of dividing the mental and the physical, and are failing to see the beauty of life expressed through the form of the physical body.

Another advantage that *asana* has in helping to restore and maintain total health is that *asana* is direct, nonlinear, nonrational, and nonverbal; hence the compulsive "chattering monkey" of the mind can be temporarily quieted during the practice of *asana*. This quieting encourages the balancing of the mental functions of the individual, since it allows the intuitive aspects of the mind to have free play; it is this aspect of brain functioning that has been indicated in the electroencephalographic biofeedback experiments during meditative states.[7]

From this viewpoint, we can see how *asana* can help overcome the perennial dichotomy of Western psychology,

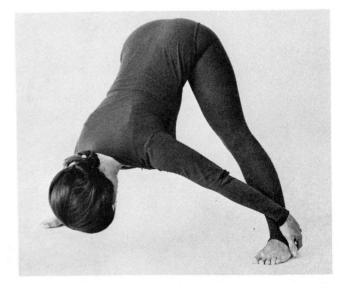

SALUTE TO THE SUN

Lorin Piper

YOGA teachers often say that if you do only one asana a day, it should be the Sun salutation. This is a series of 12 poses linked by a continuous flowing motion, and accompanied by five deep breaths. Do this series at least twice in a row, more if you desire. As always in yoga, do it slowly and consciously.

1. Stand up straight with your feet together and your palms together in front of you. Relax and begin to inhale.
2. Continue inhaling as you raise your arms up and back over your head, arching your back slightly.
3. Exhale as you bend forward and touch your hands to the floor in front of you. Keep your knees straight and let your head hang relaxed.

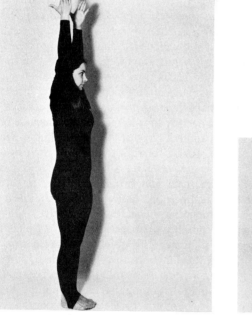
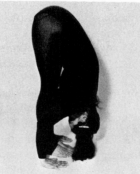
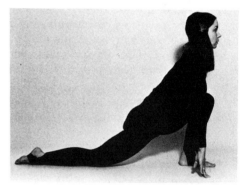

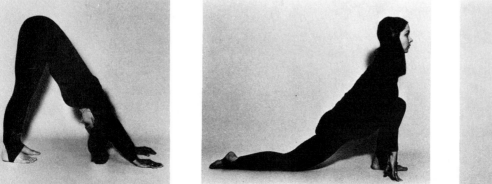
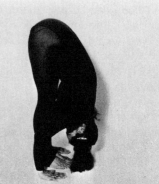

4. Inhale as you move your right leg back, letting the knee touch the floor. Extend this leg back as far as possible. Keep your hands and left leg in place, the left leg bending in the movement. Lean your head back and look up between your eyebrows.

5. Exhale, and place your left leg back next to the right, pushing your buttocks up into a triangle and letting your head hang relaxed. Exhale completely.

6. Holding your breath, lower your body to the floor, touching your chin, chest, knees, feet, and hands to the floor, and keeping your buttocks, thighs, and abdomen lifted.

7. Inhale, relax your lower torso, and bend your upper torso and head backwards until your arms are straight.

8. Exhale as you form the triangle again by pushing your buttocks up.

9. Inhale as you move your right leg forward until it rests on the floor between your hands. Extend the left leg back and lean your head back as in pose 4.

10. Exhale and bend forward until your hands touch the floor.

11. Inhale and stand up, stretching your arms back over your head, arching your back slightly.

12. Exhale as you bring your hands down in front of your chest and relax.

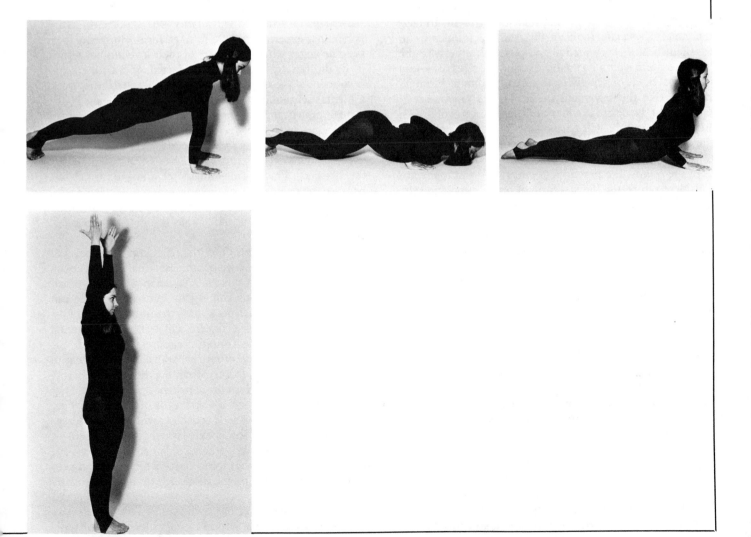

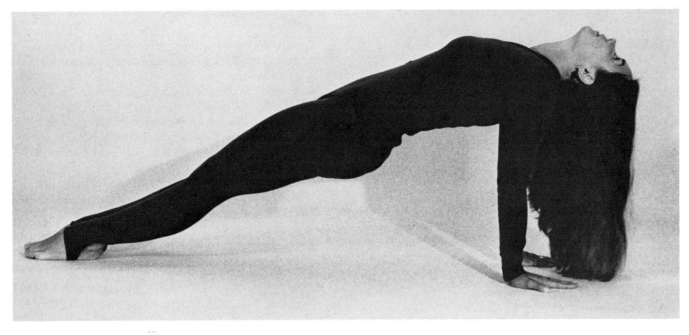

i.e., the seeming difference between the body and the mind. Patanjali does not recognize this split, as can be seen from the way in which he joins the movements of the body and the evolution of the mind in his presentation on yoga. He begins his book with a discussion of the higher states of consciousness that become available to the yogi when body and mind have become perfect vehicles for them. In fact, the state of *samadhi* requires that the practitioner be in excellent health, both mental and physical; otherwise the human system would be unable to stand the stress of losing its normal mode of perceiving reality. In addition, Patanjali suggests that the *asana* and the *pranayama* practices will bring about the desired state of health; the control of breath and bodily posture will harmonize the flow of energy in the organism, thus creating a fertile field for the evolution of the spirit.

In the *Sutras*, the practices of *pranayama* and *asana* are considered to be the highest form of purification and self-discipline for the mind and the body, respectively. The practices produce the actual physical sensation of heat, called *tapas*, or the inner fire of purification. It is taught that this heat is part of the process of purifying the *nadis*, or subtle nerve channels of the body (perhaps akin to the acupuncture meridians), which allows a more healthful state to be experienced and allows the mind to become more calm.

The Remaining Limbs: A Movement Inside

The last four limbs of yoga become increasingly more subtle in their application to the psychology of the individual. The fifth limb, termed *pratyahara*, is the natural outgrowth of the strength gained from the practice of *pranayama*. *Pratyahara* is the conscious and willful withdrawal of energy from involvement with the senses. This does not mean that the individual loses interest in the world, but rather finds himself less attached to the outcomes of various happenings. What *pratyahara* does mean is that the constant disturbances of the mind caused by the senses are no longer so powerful, because the person is less attached to the

sensations as they arrive. These sensations are not only the physical ones, but also the "mental sensations" or emotions, which include love, hate, fear, lust, jealousy, greed, and desire. The yogi does not cease to love; instead, his love becomes more pure, because he expects and asks for less and less in return.

Perhaps an example will clarify this statement. Every person has experienced love in some form. But many have become angry when the object of their love did not return it, or did not act as the lover expected. It was the disappointment of these expectations which produced the anger, a mental sensation which is the opposite of being in the state of *pratyahara*. As one's love is purified by disciplined practice, it can be freely given, because it no longer matters whether the person receiving the love acts "lovable." No expectations are created; so none can be disappointed by the beloved. This is freedom in relationship. Ironically, because the yogi is free of the attachments associated with loving, he can love much more freely and deeply than can one who is bound up in the "What is it going to get me?" attitude toward love.

This concept of *pratyahara* thus has important psychological ramifications. Much of our emotional imbalance can thus be seen to be self-created. A person who is governed by powerful sensations coming in from the outside can never achieve the inner peace and tranquility which most people seek; instead, he or she will waste much mental and physical energy in trying to suppress unwanted sensations and to heighten other sensations, and in trying to manipulate other people into providing desired sensations. The lack of freedom from this constant upheaval in energy will eventually emerge as a physical or mental imbalance, which someone else, usually a doctor, will term a disease.

Patanjali says that the above process is at the root of human unhappiness and uneasiness. When people seek out yoga, hoping to find that inner peace which is so evasive, they find that it was theirs all along. In a sense, yoga is nothing more than a process which enables us to stop and look at the processes of our own minds; only in this way can we understand the nature of happiness and unhappiness, and thus transcend them both. One who has thus overcome this duality will thereby live in the dynamic state of peace and health.

The sixth limb of the system is *dharana*, roughly translated by the word "concentration." This is not the forced concentration of, for example, solving a difficult mathematics problem; rather it is a form of meditation which could be called receptive concentration. When the mind has become purified by the practices detailed above, it becomes able to focus efficiently on one subject or point of experience. If the yogi chooses to focus on a center ("chakra") of the inner energy flow, he or she can directly experience the physical and mental blocks and imbalances that remain in his or her system. This ability to concentrate depends on excellent psychological health and integration and is not an escape from reality, but rather a movement toward perception of its true nature.

The next limb is termed *dhyana*, or meditation. This differs from *dharana* in degree rather than kind. In *dhyana*, the consciousness of the practitioner is in one flow; it is no longer fixed on one subject as in concentration. The distinction can be further made in this way: *dharana* is to *dhyana* as the individual drops of water are to the continuous flow of the whole river.

The final step in Ashtanga Yoga is termed *samadhi*. In this state, it is said, the object of the meditation and the meditator become one. This is like the unity of process; it is like the union of function and structure. The polarity of viewer and viewed, like the polarity of opposites, is no longer relevant; the mind does not distinguish between self and non-self, or between the object contemplated and the process of contemplation.

Importantly, *samadhi* does not mean the "destruction of the ego," as is often thought by the Western psychologist. To the contrary, the perfection of *samadhi* embraces and

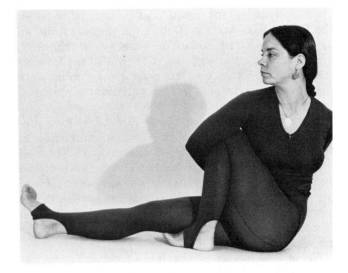

glorifies all aspects of the self by subjecting them to the light of understanding. The person capable of *samadhi* retains his or her individuality and personhood, but is free of the emotional attachment to that personhood which so dominates the consciousness of other people. What could be a more perfect expression of total health than this integration of the physical, mental, and spiritual aspects of the self, with a correspondingly clarified and simplified perception of the world.

Yoga: Unity in Variety

Just as there are many types of people, there are many types of yoga. Besides the Ashtanga Yoga of Patanjali, perhaps the most famous forms of yoga are those described in the *Bhavagad Gita*, the best-known part of the epic *Mahabharata*. The *Gita* mentions *Karma*, *Jnana*, and *Bhakti Yoga*. These are not so much different types of yoga as they are different applications of yoga to daily life. In addition, *Hatha*, *Raja*, *Tantra*, and *Integral Yoga* have been popular, especially in recent times in the U.S. Let us examine the similarities and differences among those various yogas, as well as their applications to health.

Raja Yoga starts with the mind; its goal is a complete stilling of the mind, so that the light of the indwelling spirit may shine out. It makes use of *asana* and *pranayama*, and some consider it merely another name for Ashtanga Yoga.

Tantra, sometimes called *Kundalini Yoga*, is the worship of God as the Divine Mother; it stresses the union of the male and female aspects of the individual, as represented by the archetypal male and female, Shiva and Shakti. The goal of Tantra is the union of dynamic and static aspects of personality; it is quite different from practices which dwell on renunciation and desirelessness, and sees no contradiction between Nature and Spirit.

Jnana Yoga stresses the use of the mind to transcend the mind; it works with that part of the human mind which strives incessantly to know and understand. It trains discrimination; it is eight-limbed, and its other seven limbs are detachment, self-discipline, longing for freedom, hearing the truth, reflection upon that truth, and meditation, which is defined as consolidation and transcendence.

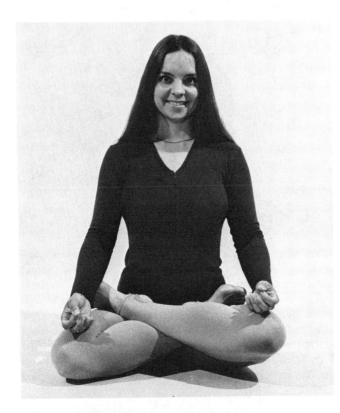

Bhakti Yoga uses the natural desire to love and be loved; the Bhakti Yoga worships God in the personal form, an approach which underlies all the world's great religions.

Karma Yoga is the yoga of action. But all the fruits of the actions are surrendered; the practitioner gives his work freely for the service of others; unconcerned with rewards, he offers them to God.

Integral Yoga, also called *Purna Yoga*, is the form presented by the twentieth-century yogi Sri Aurobindo; it attempts to integrate all aspects of action, wisdom, and peace into one yoga, and is thus nondualistic. Its practices aim at integration on three levels: psychic integration, of the various facets of the self; cosmic integration, of the aspects of the Universe; and existential integration, which comes when one fully realizes that the self and the Universe are one.

Hatha Yoga has several literal translations. The underlying root syllable *hath* means "to oppress," and suggests the use of force or strength; this force comes from the self-discipline of practice. In addition, *ha* has a meaning of "sun," and *tha* of "moon." Thus Hatha Yoga can be understood as the integration of the sunlike and moonlike aspects of the individual; this could mean the left and right sides of the body, and hence the right and left sides of the brain. This integration would be manifested by an even flow through the body's channels of energy, and by a high level of health. Hatha Yoga includes asanas, pranayama, and other purificatory practices, and is sometimes considered to be the same as Patanjali's "tapas."

Summary and Conclusion

It is clear that all the types of yoga which we have explored have common philosophical backgrounds and psychological goals. The most striking common feature is the wholeness of the personality.[9] Western philosophy has constantly been criticized for its inability to reconcile the body and the mind. In yoga, as taught by Patanjali, mind and body are a continuum. Each aspect of self is part of all other aspects. This corresponds with the definition of "holistic" currently in use.

With very few exceptions (among them Carl Jung), Western philosophers have emphasized the rationally approachable aspects of human consciousness. Yoga accepts all of man's consciousness, including the rational, the emotional, the blissful; it excludes none as unimportant or irrelevant. Rather, the integration of all aspects of self results in a higher whole, a vehicle for manifesting health and consciousness. The hallmark of yoga is transformation, not sublimation or elimination; the integrative force which characterizes yoga is manifest in every life form, and the awareness of this evolutionary trend, along with the choice to participate in the process, is just another definition of yoga.

Rather than making the student something that he is not, yoga allows him to become more fully what he already is. Yoga intensifies the individual's consciousness of his perfection and health. Yoga can clearly speak with relevance to the holistic health practitioner. It teaches that to understand health and pathology in others, one must first examine oneself; without self-insight, insight into others is impossible.

Health is the ability to move freely with consciousness from an inner focus to an outer one, to move with consciousness from a rational to a nonrational and motive mode, to move with consciousness from a focus on material values to a oneness with the metaphysical values of the higher self. Centrally, yoga is holistic, integrative, and accepting of the inner nature of man. It is life-affirming and death-accepting. It is a process and a goal. And it is a powerful and versatile tool for creating and understanding health and, therefore, for allowing us to understand, help, and heal one another.

Notes

[1] Monier-Williams, *Sanskrit-English Dictionary*. All definitions in this paper are taken from this work.
[2] Geraldine Coster, *Yoga and Western Psychology*, p. 75.
[3] Two translations of the *Yoga Sutras* available in the United States are those by Rammurti S. Mishra, *The Textbook of Yoga Psychology*, and I.K. Taimni, *The Science of Yoga*.
[4] B.K.S. Iyengar, personal communication, Berkeley, Ca., May 1976.
[5] Paul Copeland, *The Physiology of Yoga*.
[6] ———, "Recent Research of Dr. Bhole," *Yoga Journal*, pp. 31, 33.
[7] Robert Ornstein, *The Psychology of Consciousness*.
[8] Haridas Chaudhuri, *Integral Yoga*, p. 62.
[9] ———, *Integral Psychology*.

Suggestions for Further Reading

Mircea Eliade, *Yoga: Immortality and Freedom*. Translated by Willard R. Trask, Princeton University Press, 1958.
Georg Feuerstein, *The Essence of Yoga*. Grove Press, 1974.
B.K.S. Iyengar, *Light on Yoga*. Schocken Books, 1970.
Swami Rama, Rudolph Ballentine, M.D., and Swami Ajaya, Ph.D., *Yoga and Psychotherapy: The Evolution of Consciousness*. Glenview, Illinois: Himalayan Institute, 1976.
Ernest E. Woods, *Yoga*. Penguin Books, 1968.

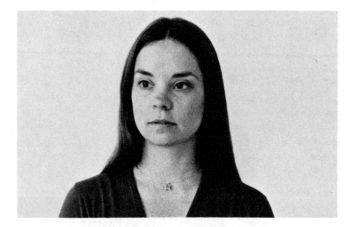

JUDITH HANSON LASATER, *Ph.D, is an instructor in Anatomy and Kinesiology, Institute for Yoga Teacher Education, San Francisco, and has studied yoga with B.K.S. Iyengar both in the United States and India. She has taught yoga nationally for ten years to professional associations, and on radio and television. She is a contributing editor to the* Yoga Journal *and has contributed chapters to* Rediscovery of the Body (Dell, 1977), Yoga Over Fifty (Devin-Adair, 1977), *and* Women's Health Care: A Guide to Alternatives (Reston Publishing, 1984).

The Holistic Logic of Chinese Medicine

Ted Kaptchuk

A STORY is told in China about a peasant who had worked as a maintenance man in a newly established Western missionary hospital. When he retired to his remote village, he took with him some hypodermic needles and lots of antibiotics. He put up a shingle, and whenever someone came to him with a fever he injected him with the wonder drugs. A remarkable percentage of people got well, despite the fact that this practitioner of Western medicine knew next to nothing about what he was doing.

In the West today, much of what passes for Chinese medicine is not very different from the so-called Western medicine practiced by this Chinese peasant. Out of a complete medical system, only the bare essentials of acupuncture technique have reached the West. Patients often get well from such treatment because acupuncture, like Western antibiotics, is strong medicine. But the theoretical depth and full clinical potential of Chinese medicine remain unknown.

As a result, many Westerners have strange notions about Chinese medicine. Some of them see it as hocus-pocus—the product of primitive or magical thinking. If a patient is cured by means of herbs or acupuncture, they see only two possible explanations: either the cure was psychosomatic or it was an accident, the happy result of hit-or-miss pin-sticking that the practitioner did not understand. They assume that current Western science and medicine have a unique handle on truth—all else is superstition.

Other people have an equally erroneous view of Chinese medicine. Deeply and often justifiably disturbed by many of the products of Western science and culture, they assume that the Chinese system, because it is more ancient, more spiritual or more holistic, is somehow also more "true" than Western medicine. This attitude threatens to turn Chinese medicine from a rational body of knowledge into a religious faith system. Both attitudes mystify the subject—one by arrogantly undervaluing it, the other by setting it on a pedestal. Both are barriers to understanding.

Actually, Chinese medicine is a coherent and independent system of thought and practice that has been developed over two millennia. Based on ancient texts, it is the result of a continuous process of critical thinking, as well as extensive clinical observation and testing. It represents a thorough formulation and reformulation of material by respected clinicians and theoreticians. It is also, however, rooted in the philosophy, logic, sensibility, and habits of a civilization entirely foreign to our own. It has therefore developed its own perception of the body and of health and disease.

In order to understand it, we must first accept two principles: that another perspective, though different from our own, can be logical and have predictive validity, and that there can exist another method of healing. In other words, the world can contain two rational and effective medical systems, both describing the same phenomena, but describing them differently. Once we accept these premises, we can begin to understand the Chinese view of physiology.

Chinese medicine considers important certain aspects of the human body that are not significant to Western medicine. At the same time, Western medicine observes and can describe aspects of the human body that are insignificant or not perceptible to Chinese medicine. For instance, Chinese medical theory does not have the concept of a nervous system. Nevertheless, it has been demonstrated that Chinese medicine can be used to treat neurological disorders. Similarly, Chinese medicine does not perceive an endocrine system, yet it is used to treat what Western medicine calls endocrine disorders. Nor does traditional Chinese medicine recognize the bacteria *Streptococcus pneumoniae* as a pathological cause of pneumonia, yet often it effectively treats the disease.

Chinese medicine also uses terminology that is strange to the Western ear. For example, the Chinese refer to certain diseases as being caused by "Dampness," "Heat," or "Spleen." Modern Western medicine does not recognize Dampness, yet can treat what Chinese medicine describes as Dampness of the Spleen. The perceptiveness of the two traditions reflect two different worlds, but both can heal the same body.

The two different logical structures have pointed the two medicines in different directions. Western medicine is concerned mainly with particular categories of agents of disease, which it zeroes in on, isolates and tries to change, control or destroy. The Western physician starts with a symptom, then searches for the underlying mechanism—a precise *cause* for a specific *disease*.

THE AROUND-THE-WORLD MASSAGE

Stephen Chang

I would like to offer you a method of massage that will be absolutely invaluable, in that it will augment the energy within the body, provide for a constant and unimpeded flow of energy along the meridians, and eventually rejuvenate not only an aging body but a fatigued mind as well. I have very appropriately named this invigorating massage the "Around-the-World Massage," for it stimulates the energy along all the main meridians, thereby concurrently affecting the energy in all areas adjacent to those meridians. Applying the following technique will enable you to become acquainted with the paths of the main meridians—an absolute necessity for aspiring practitioners—and to intimately experience the exhilarating effects of such a simple method of massage.

Using the bulb of the thumb or of the index and middle fingers, gently massage the entire length of each of the main meridians in the direction of the flow of energy along the meridian. Massage the meridians in the prescribed sequence shown in Figures 1 through 12, not in any haphazard, random order. The reason for this should be obvious, for the purpose of meridian massage is to stimulate and "build" an unbroken circle of energy circulating within the body, and this can only be accomplished by massaging the meridians in the prescribed sequence. Baby oil, massage lotions, ginger juice, etc., may be used to lubricate the surface of the skin.

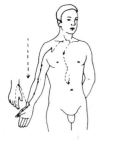

Figure 1. The Lung Meridian, with a descending flow of energy running from the top of the chest, along the inside of the arm to the outside of the thumb, joins a series of 11 bilateral points.

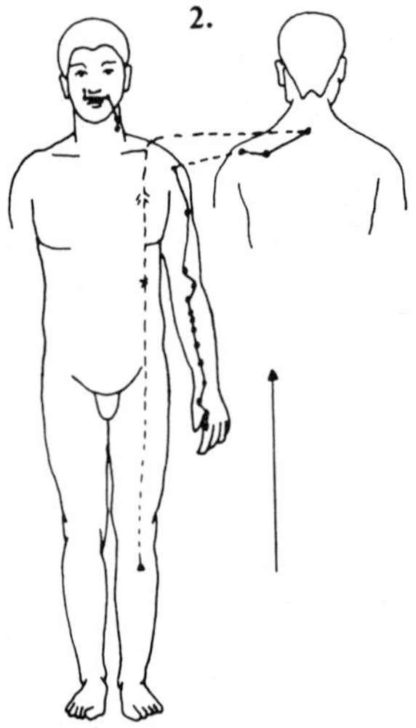

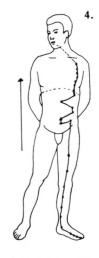

Figure 4. The Spleen-Pancreas Meridian, with an ascending flow of energy running from the foot to the chest, joins a series of 21 bilateral points.

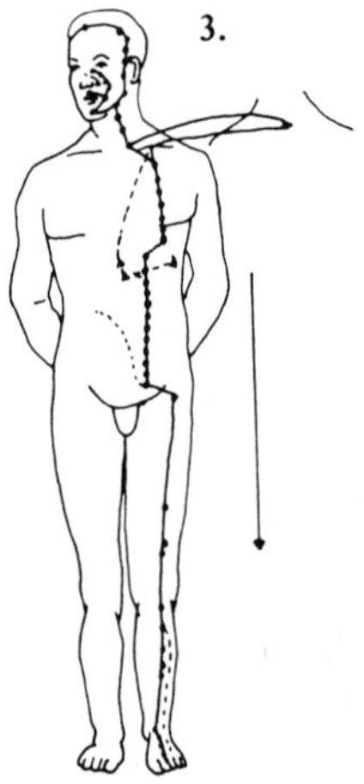

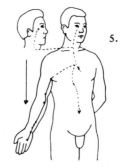

Figure 2. The Large Intestine Meridian, with an ascending flow of energy running from the tip of the index finger of the hand to the base of the eye, joins a series of 20 bilateral points.

Figure 3. The Stomach Meridian, with a descending flow of energy running from the head to the foot, joins a series of 45 bilateral points.

Figure 5. The Heart Meridian, with a descending flow of energy running from the chest to the hand, joins a series of 9 bilateral points.

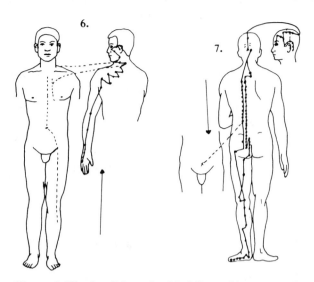

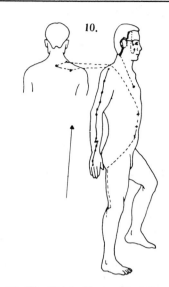

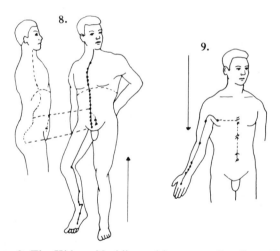

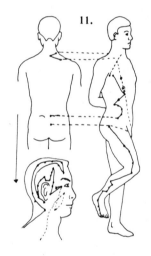

Figure 6. The Small Intestine Meridian, with an ascending flow of energy running from the hand to the head, joins a series of 19 points.

Figure 7. The Bladder Meridian, with a descending flow of energy running from the head to the foot, joins a series of 67 bilateral points.

Figure 8. The Kidney Meridian, with an ascending flow of energy running from the foot to the chest, joins a series of 27 bilateral points.

Figure 9. The Heart Constrictor Meridian, with a descending flow of energy running from the chest to the hand, joins a series of 9 bilateral points.

Figure 10. The Triple Heater Meridian, with an ascending flow of energy running from the hand to the head, joins a series of 23 bilateral points.

Figure 11. The Gallbladder Meridian, with a descending flow of energy running from the chest to the foot, joins a series of 44 bilateral points.

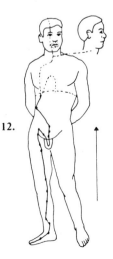

Figure 12. The Liver Meridian, with an ascending flow of energy running from the foot to the chest, joins a series of 14 bilateral points.

Illustrated by Mary Elizabeth Bruno

Patterns of Disharmony

The Chinese physician, on the other hand, directs his attention to the complete individual, including psychological aspects the West often sees as unrelated to health and disease. All relevant information, including the symptom as well as the patient's other general characteristics, is gathered and woven together until it forms what Chinese medicine calls a "pattern of disharmony." This pattern of disharmony describes a situation of distress or "imbalance" in a patient's body. Oriental diagnostic technique does not turn up a specific disease entity or a precise cause, but renders an almost poetic, yet workable, description of a whole person. The therapy then attempts to bring the configuration into balance, to restore harmony to the individual.

This difference between Western and Eastern perception can be illustrated by portions of recent clinical studies done in hospitals in China. In a typical study a Western physician, using upper gastrointestinal X-rays or endoscopy that employs a fiber-optic scope, diagnoses six patients with stomach pain as having peptic ulcer disease. From the Western doctor's perspective, based on the analytic tendency to narrow diagnosis to a single cause, all these patients suffer from the same disorder. The physician then sends the patients to a Chinese doctor for examination.

Upon questioning and examining the first patient, the Chinese physician finds pain that increases at touch (by palpation) but diminishes with the application of cold compresses. The patient has a robust constitution, a reddish complexion and a full, deep voice. He seems assertive and even aggressive. He is constipated and has dark yellow urine. His tongue has a greasy yellow coating; his pulse is "full" and "wiry." The Oriental physician characterizes this patient as having the pattern of disharmony called "Damp Heat affecting the Spleen."

When the Chinese physician examines the second patient, he finds a different set of signs, which make up another overall pattern. The patient is thin. Her complexion is ashen, though her cheeks are ruddy. She is constantly thirsty, her palms are sweaty, and she has a tendency toward constipation, insomnia and night sweats. She seems nervous and fidgety. Her tongue is dry and slightly red, with no "moss"; her pulse is "thin" and also a bit "fast." This patient is said to have the pattern of "Deficient Yin affecting the Stomach," a disharmony very different from that of the first patient. Accordingly, a different treatment would be prescribed for her.

The third patient—with different signs—is diagnosed as having the pattern of "Exhausted Fire of the Middle Burner," sometimes called "Deficient Cold affecting the Spleen." And so on.

Patterns of disharmony in Chinese medicine are real and true in the sense that they provide a way to perceive what the Chinese have called "the web that has no weaver." The web is the macrocosm—the universe—which is considered to be uncreated and to exist through the dictates of its own inner nature; that is, through the constant unfolding of the two polar complements, Yin and Yang. There is no *truth* behind or above the things we see; there is no creator; yet the things we see continue, and their continuing is the eternal process of the universe.

Chief Blind Spot

Can a system of knowledge rooted in such a metaphysics have anything to communicate to Western science? Chinese medicine attempts to locate illness within the unbroken context or field of an individual's total physical and psychological being. It aims to cure through treatments that encompass the whole of the individual as closely as possible. In contrast, the ideal of Western medicine is to probe with laserlike accuracy, penetrating to the microscopic agent of disease in the tissue, in the cell and, ultimately, in the DNA molecule. The chief blind spot of Western medicine, in short, is that it tends not to see the whole.

Chinese medicine also has some notable strengths that Western medicine lacks. Chinese remedies are often more effective than Western ones, and they are always gentler and safer. Chinese prescriptions, for example, do not produce side effects because they are balanced to reflect a patient's entire state of being. Chinese medicine, in addition, is better able than Western medicine to treat illnesses arising from the interrelationships of physical and mental phenomena.

Chinese medicine, because it emphasizes balance and relationship more than measurable quantity, can also frequently discover and treat a disorder before it is perceptible by the most sophisticated Western diagnostic techniques. Chinese medicine is capable of touching those places that evade the microscope and that, after all, constitute human reality.

On the other hand, no honest Chinese physician can fail to be awed by the achievements of Western medicine, by the ease with which a drug such as streptomycin or a technique such as open-heart surgery can penetrate to the core of disorders that Chinese medicine finds complex and intractable.

Because Chinese medicine collects only external signs in order to perceive an overall form, it has blind spots of its own. And one of its greatest strengths—its perception of the body as a whole—can be its greatest weakness. For Chinese medicine can never separate the part from the whole, even when a clinical situation demands that the overall relationships be ignored and a particular part be treated directly. A tumor or a gallstone or an infected appendix must sometimes be identified, isolated and removed. Chinese medicine cannot do this—it lacks both the theory and the technique.

And, because it stresses proportion and sees quantity as secondary, Chinese medicine is weak on prognosis, on predicting the life-threatening quality of a disorder.

Fundamental Matrix

Although Chinese medicine has developed considerably in its history, this progress is a long spiral that moves forever around its point of origin, the ancient texts. Since this point of origin is assumed to contain the seed of everything that can be known, all development is a form of slow exegesis within a broad conceptual framework. Complete and self-contained, traditional Chinese medicine is incapable of assimilating anything that challenges its fundamental assumptions. New ideas and substances can be identified and even incorporated, but they can never expand or transform the fundamental matrix. So, Vitamin B_{12} is very Yang and penicillin is very Yin, but there is nothing beyond Yin and Yang.

At first glance, Western medicine seems equally impervious to alternate modes of perception. Given its current bureaucratic entrenchment, its disposition toward technological solutions, its roots in the profit motive and its arrogant faith in its own destiny, a strong argument can be made that Western medicine will never see anything more in the Chinese system than a bag of tricks.

Yet new ideas in Western science, ideas pointing toward an awareness of the totality of being, have arisen as a direct result of the Western urge to penetrate phenomena and to find the transcendent truth behind them. Western thought, at its most noble and honest, is nourished by the constant tension between unknown and known, imperfect and perfect. This is an idea altogether missing in China, an attitude that contrasts sharply with the Chinese view of truth as inherent in the harmonious arrangement of the given.

Western science can be criticized for insensitivity, for arrogance, for storming Heaven—but the fact remains that it is humble, and humility is integral to the best scientific thought. For all its misuses, the idea of progress implies that not everything has been achieved, that more is yet to come.

In order to remain science, science must believe that what it discovers tomorrow may undermine and revolutionize everything it believes today. Western science, unlike traditional Chinese thought, is necessarily receptive to the new. And there is now a new sense of organism, interconnectedness and unity emerging on the frontiers of modern science. The development of Western thought is creating room for new models and theories.

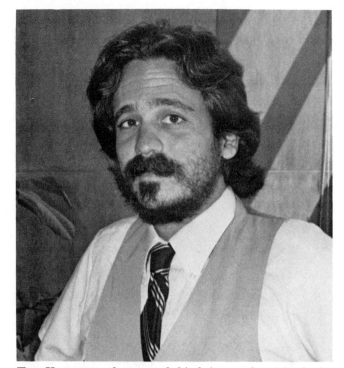

TED KAPTCHUK *has succeeded in being an alternative healer within the established medical institutions. Currently, he is clinical director of the Lemuel Shattuck Hospital's Pain and Stress Relief Clinic in Boston.*

Besides being an adjunct faculty or guest lecturer at most acupuncture schools in the United States, Europe, and Australia, Ted is a thesis reader at Harvard University and a faculty member at Boston University.

He is a collaborator for various research projects sponsored by the National Science Foundation, Harvard Medical School and Boston University School of Medicine. Currently, he is writing a TV documentary on healing for the BBC.

He holds a doctorate in Oriental Medicine from the Macau Institute of Chinese Medicine, China where he spent four years.

B. NATIVE AMERICAN SYSTEMS

Native American Healing

*Sandy R. Newhouse, M.A., and
John Amodeo, Ph.D.*

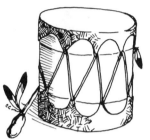

*American Indian healing has its roots in ancient truths
that predate any tribe, nation, or culture. The heritage of
the Native Americans has a message for all of us who are
sharing this land. The present movement toward a more
naturally wholesome and more physically active way of
living results in part from our desire to reconnect with our
roots. Our planet is suffering, and we can help by being
more sensitive to her. This insight is not exclusive to Indian
culture, but a responsibility we all share by being a part
of this stage of our evolution. The Earth is a garden, and
we are its caretakers. Much of the material in this article
is based on lectures by Oh Shinnah.*

THE ART of healing is a way of life to the
Native American people; it is inseparable
from day-to-day existence. Music, dance,
prayer, ceremony, all express relationship to
the Earth and are vital components of Indian healing. They
serve to perpetually renew a sense of harmony within the
community by uniting each individual with the deeper Self,
with others, and with the enveloping cosmos.

Ceremony is the expression of Indian life. Some practices
are shared by all Indian peoples, although many tribes and
traditions are native to this land. Each day begins with a
sunrise ceremony. The Great Spirit's power is welcomed
back to the Earth in a celebration involving prayer, getting
the morning sun, and placing tobacco on the Earth Mother.

A universal practice essential to healthy living is the use
of cedar, sage, or sweetgrass for purification. Burning sacred cedar or sage is a way to center oneself and to unite
the spirit of the community; disharmonious energy is
thought to dissipate, and a neutral situation is created. The
use of the sweat lodge for physical, mental, and spiritual
purification is another common practice. This involves a
highly developed spiritual ceremony of various songs. As
one enters the sweat lodge, one calls upon the spirit of the
ancestors to bring forth messages from the other side.

All healing ceremonies revolve around the drum: its beat
reflects the heartbeat of all peoples on the Earth. They
believe that the beat of the drum will bring Indian people
together again.

Everything is round in the Indian cosmology: the round
dance is performed around the drum; Indians live in round
houses; energy flows in circular movements. Forming circles is an effective way of generating energy and directing
prayer, a sharp contrast to our Western culture's square
cosmology, in which linear communication and square
dwellings prevail.

All healing in the Indian way is closely connected with
the Earth Mother. The relationship to one's environment—the earth, trees, animals, sun, and sky—is intimately involved in healing. Accordingly, whenever possible,
healing is done in a natural setting. The Earth has an
electromagnetic vibration that is able to assist the medicine
man or woman in extracting the imbalanced energy existing
within the person being healed. The healer has his/her
shoes removed for protection, allowing the Earth to draw
the energy through the healer into itself.

Although particular ceremonies, medicines and healing
practices are used, the most essential aspect in the Indian
view is one's relationship to the medicine and environment.
This is radically different from our current Western concept of medicine. To become a medicine man/woman in
the Indian tradition involves 20 to 30 years of study and
taking on a complete way of life. Contrary to Western
medicine, there is no split between a healer's life and one's
healing practice. Medicine people spend as much time
keeping their people healthy through dancing and singing
as they do in healing diseases.

The relationship to the medicine is one of mutual respect
and appreciation for its power. A dynamic relationship
exists between the medicine man or woman and the tools
utilized in the curing rites. For example, when herbs are
used, the plants are gathered and prepared in a definite
way. Prayer is an integral part of all healing. A sacred
relationship must be established in order for the medicine
to surrender its power to the healer for use.

All creation on this Earth contains a spirit, a life force.
This includes rocks, plants, hills, trees, sky, and animals.
The Mother Earth is a living, sensitive, breathing organism. The forces of all creation are dynamically interwoven
into a harmonious whole. Physical and mental illness occurs when this balance is upset. The purpose of all healing

ceremonies is to preserve or restore personal and universal harmony.

Hopi prophecy passed down through history predicts that when the white man's children begin to dress as Indians and return to the ways of the land, the time will have come for Indians to go amongst white people and share their wisdom. In the last few years this prophecy is being fulfilled.

American Indian Spiritual Teachers

Rolling Thunder is a Cherokee Indian Intertribal Medicine Man who has talked to many groups of people throughout the United States and abroad. He is founder and director of the Meta Tantay Indian Foundation,[1] an organization dedicated to traditional life and protection of the Earth Mother. Rolling Thunder's community in Nevada includes people of all races and ages who have come to participate in the traditional Indian way, to learn the natural way of life, and to experience the spiritual way of the Great Spirit. Sunrise Ceremony is shared each day in greeting Father Sun, Mother Earth, and the new day. A day's work includes building dome-shaped homes (called wiki-ups), gardening, tending the animals, cooking, and caring for one another. Crafts such as beadwork, wood carving, leatherwork, jewelry making, and knitting are learned.

Wherever Rolling Thunder travels he shares the music and dance of his people. His central message is clear: Learning the Indian way of life requires living in sensitive and respectful relationship with the Earth and with each other. The Indian teachings are not learned by attending a few talks or workshops or by reading several books. Rolling Thunder stresses the importance of not seeing oneself as a healer or a medicine person. Rather, his emphasis is upon the process of one's own spiritual development. Respect and patience are prerequisites for such growth.

Rolling Thunder teaches the importance of being a spiritual warrior, a man or woman who can stand on his or her own two feet and be in full touch with internal power. He teaches that the greatest pollution exists in the minds of men; all external pollution originates here. Indians describe this as "bad thoughts." It is well known in the native American tradition that whatever thoughts we put out are going to come back upon us, and usually with increased intensity. Rolling Thunder teaches that it is only through good thoughts and energies that we will break down the "buckskin curtain." His main criticism of white people is their obstinate apathy.

Oh Shinnah Fast Wolf is an Apache-Mohawk Servant to the Medicine who represents the Ancient Way. Rather than specifically sharing her Apache or Mohawk traditions, her teachings come from our common source of knowledge and being. It was the prayer of her mother at birth that she would return to this Ancient Way. Most of her healing knowledge comes from her great grandmother, a Mohawk Indian of the Turtle Clan. Her great grandmother taught her how to use touch, massage, and crystals and plants in healing. At the age of nine, she was initiated as a Servant to the Medicine by a medicine man in a ceremony which tested her ability to heal with crystals. She is founder and director of the Four Directions Foundation,[2] a nonprofit

spiritual and educational organization dedicated to the Ancient Ways and protection of the Earth Mother.

Wherever Oh Shinnah speaks, she burns cedar for purification. In the traditional Indian way she offers cornmeal to the four directions, to the Earth Mother, and to the Creator for all of the people present. With her right hand she cuts a hole in the air above for Spirit to come through. She explains that she carriers an "eagle feather which is the symbol of truth. In the way of the Indian peoples, this eagle is the one that flies closest to the Great Spirit; the energy it carries is carried higher than any of the other ones. It becomes a symbol of truth and is a kind of messenger between human kind and spirit." Her eagle feather has been doctored by medicine elders through special ceremony. She describes the feather as "becoming my symbol to you so that the words I carry to you are the truth from the perspective and understanding of my own individual heart."

Oh Shinnah carries a natural quartz crystal as her symbol of the Healing Way. This crystal calls in the spirits of healers. She says, "Everything I talk about is related to healing." Turtle Island was the name the Indians gave to what we call the United States. The turtle represents feminine, healing energies. Her message is that the spirit and energy of this country is Indian. She wants the people in the United States to tune into the ancient teachings of the American Indians and become sensitive to the spirit of this land.[3]

Oh Shinnah teaches many techniques of healing, although she constantly reminds her students that there is no rigid formula to learn. Rather, healing is a relationship; it is an act of putting oneself in touch with our brother or sister. It is necessary to feel the pain and suffering of another person in order to heal.

Crystals and Color Healing

Crystals and color healing are two of the main teachings. Crystals are known to have electromagnetic energy, as does the human body. When a natural quartz crystal is brought into contact with a person's etheric body,[4] the electromagnetic attraction is capable of drawing imbalanced energy out of the human body. According to the nature of the illness, the crystal will become hot or cold as it is passed over the person's aura. The crystal is absorbing the bad energy out of the body, according to these teachings. It is important to remember that "the crystals are your teachers. Hold one in your hand. Be open to its power. It will teach you." Oh Shinnah comments that it is time to heal with crystals when one is given to you. Indian medicine cannot be bought. The reader is cautioned never to attempt using crystals without receiving training, since if used improperly, they can be extremely dangerous.

Color healing dates back to ancient Egypt and other premodern societies. An essential aspect of color healing involves the aura. Particular colors effect a vibrational increase in the physical and etheric bodies. Color healing is based on the law of attraction; the vibration of the color attracts a similar vibration in the human body.

The seven color rays of the rainbow or visible light spectrum are used for healing purposes. There are three hot

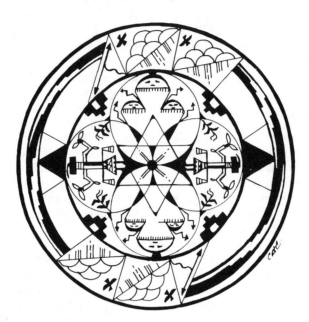

ALL of my life is a dance.
When I was young and feeling the earth
My steps were quick and easy.
The beat of the earth was so loud
That my drum was silent beside it.
All of my life rolled out from my feet
Like my land which had no end as far as I could see.
The rhythm of my life was pure and free.
As I grew older my feet kept dancing so hard
That I wore a spot in the earth
At the same time I made a hole in the sky.
I danced to the sun and the rain
And the moon lifted me up
So that I could dance to the stars.
My head touched the clouds sometimes
And my feet danced deep in the earth
So that I became the music I danced to everywhere.
It was the music of life.
Now my steps are slow and hard
And my body fails my spirit.
Yet my dance is still within me and
My song is the air I breathe.
My song insists that I keep dancing forever.
My song insists that I keep rhythm
With all of the earth and the sky.
My song insists that I will never die.

From Nancy Wood, *Many Winters* (Doubleday, 1974), p. 29.

colors (red, orange, yellow) and three cool colors (blue, indigo, violet); green exists as a balancing, harmonious color at the center. Each color corresponds to each of the seven chakras or body centers (as called by American Indians). Each color ray is used for a specific kind of healing. For example, the red ray corresponds with the body center at the base of the spine. Yellow, which corresponds to the solar plexus, is known as the "mind principle." Green expresses color balance; it is the color of the heart center. One final example is the violet ray, the highest vibration in the visible light spectrum. It may be used by healers to ease birth and death transitions.

Oh Shinnah says, "The power is in the consciousness. Know what is going on with you—predetermine before you cross over that you will come back with that level of consciousness." She also notes that color healing must only be applied by people whose consciousness has been prepared by many years of exposure to the teaching.

Plants

Central to Indian healing is the ceremonial gathering and preparation of plants. Oh Shinnah was 18 years old before her great grandmother allowed her to cut a plant. She was taught that "if you are not in harmony with the plants, you will hurt them. And instead of giving you a song and a healing way, they will scream when you cut them, if you are not in harmony with them, if you do not make an exchange." Our predominant cultural attitude is one of appropriation and exploitation of nature, rather than harmonious interaction. Plants and other living things have feelings, too—a fact currently being recognized through research at Stanford and elsewhere.

The Indian way emphasizes the importance of bringing oneself into harmony with a plant before uprooting it. One is instructed to sit with the plants and intuitively sense the oldest one with the strongest energy, known as the grandmother or grandfather plant. The next step involves talking with the eldest plant regarding the need for this medicine. A prayer is made to effect an essential exchange of energy. Oh Shinnah gives the example, "Creator, let this plant release its energy. Allow my sister to be healed." The grandparent plant itself is never picked, as it communicates with the other plants. After an offering of blessed cornmeal or pure tobacco, a smaller plant nearby is gathered. If the offering is not grown with one's own hands, then relationship must be established in some other way. This can ensue through prayer, by placing it under a small pyramid, or by sending color vibration through the offering.

When picking plants one must become sensitive to their growth cycles. Flowers are gathered while in bloom. Green leafy plants are cut just before the bloom, while the power is still in the leaves. The basic rule is to gather the plant just before it reaches its prime, after which its energy descends into the roots. A careful preparation procedure follows in order to extract the full healing essence of the plant.

The Four Corners Area

"The white man,[5] through his insensitivity to the way of Nature, has desecrated the face of Mother Earth. The white man's advanced technological capacity has occurred as a result of his lack of regard for the spiritual path and for the way of all living things. The white man's desire for material possessions and power has blinded him to the pain he has caused Mother Earth by his quest for what he calls natural resources. All over the country, the waters have been tainted, the soil broken and defiled, and the air polluted. Living creatures die from poisons left because of industry, and the path of the Great Spirit has become difficult to see by almost all men, even by many Indians, who have chosen instead to follow the path of the white man.

"We have accepted the responsibility designated by our prophecy to tell you that almost all life will stop unless men come to know that everyone must live in Peace and Harmony with Nature. Only those people who know the secrets of Nature, the Mother of us all, can overcome the possible destruction of all land and life.... Your government has almost destroyed our basic religion, which actually is a way of life for all our people in this land of the Great Spirit. We feel that to survive the coming Purification Day, we must return to the basic religious principle and to meet together on this basis as leaders of the people."[6]

The Hopi Traditional Village leaders delivered this message to the President of the United States in 1970. Their teaching for all of us is the same today; our time is running out to re-establish a relationship with the Earth Mother and our environment.

A serious problem currently threatens the traditional Hopi way of life at the Four Corners area (where Arizona, New Mexico, Colorado, and Utah meet) in the southwestern United States. The Hopis—meaning peaceful ones—are considered by many to be the oldest known self-sufficient community in existence on the North American continent. The Hopis live a natural, simple lifestyle in the desert, fully in touch with their spiritual teachings.

Public Law 95–531, a Congressional act to divide the "Joint Use Area" of the Hopi and Navajo tribes, and the Land Claims Settlement Docket 196 (described by the Four Directions Foundation as "an attempt to 'pay off' the Hopi with $5,000,000") are two current political issues threatening the Hopis' native land base. The public law calls for the petition of one million acres of the joint use land shared by the Hopi and Navajo, which will clear the way for oil company and uranium development leases. This land, used primarily by the Hopi for agriculture and for grazing by the Navajo, was relatively closed to energy development until Public Law 93–521 was passed; 4,000 to 8,000 Navajos currently living in this area will be displaced as a result. As reported in the Friends of the Hopi first newsletter, "The National Academy of Sciences recently said they believe we may have to declare Indian lands in the Southwest a 'National Sacrifice Area.'"[7]

At the request of his Hopi elders, Richard Kastl, an Osage-Creek Indian, has been speaking to groups throughout the country on Hopi prophecy and the serious exploitation problems at the Four Corners area. At the First Native American Healing Arts Conference in San Francisco, Richard began his presentation by saying, "The Hopi people maintain that through their ceremonies and their songs they maintain a balance in the Western hemisphere. It is necessary for them to be able to grow their corn and to live their lives the way the Great Spirit laid out for them to live." Hopi, Zuni, Apache, and many other Indian peoples say that the Four Corners area is the "heart of Mother Earth," and as such would be a dangerous area for extensive oil-well digging to occur.

Peabody Coal Company is strip-mining the sacred mesas for coal deposits and selling the coal to several large power plants. The coal is transported through pipes to power plants in Las Vegas and Los Angeles; 2,700 gallons per minute of water from the unrechargeable water table is pumped out to push the coal through the pipes. Native Indians, depending on the moisture level in the desert for their survival, are facing a severe agricultural and ecological crisis. Hopi elders report that the corn has grown considerably smaller this past season. Pollution is another problem, with one power plant alone producing three and a half tons of particulate matter a day. There are numerous other coal-burning plants in various construction phases all along the Colorado River, and all through Indian land.

Many of the Hopi prophecies predicting the end of life as we now know it unless we return to a spiritual way of life have already come to pass. Richard Kastl emphasizes that we are coming to a very critical point in time. Concerning the strip-mining situation, it was written in prophecy, "Do not let them take what is under your houses; it is there for your children's children." It was also passed down that "if a gourd of ashes is allowed to drop upon the earth, that many men (will) die" and that "the end of this way of life is near at hand." The traditional Indian leaders view this as the dropping of the atomic bombs on Hiroshima and Nagasaki. Richard says, "These were all signs that we were nearing a point where we must regard our situation in this country; it is time to realize where the imbalance is coming from."

Perhaps the most startling fact about all of this is that so few people in the United States even know about this current struggle of the American Indians. It is known that the U.S. government has broken hundreds of treaties in the past, but not that this is still happening before our very eyes. As Richard says, "People do not even know the struggle we have just to maintain the reservations that they set aside for us. Everything else they took away, and now they come back and want to take away our last lands. But we are standing on our feet and appealing to people's consciousness."

The sacred lands of the Four Corners area is indeed unique. The most intense, magnificent phenomenon of lightning in the world is reported there. Oh Shinnah notes that the strata is primarily quartz crystal, producing tremendous electromagnetic vibration. From air studies, she says, it is known that this area is one of only four places on earth that are radiation and pollution free. (Mount Shasta, Lake Titicaca, Machu Picchu are the three others.) These are sacred lands; we will all suffer from their destruction.

In September 1977, over 100 Indian delegates from North, South, and Central America attended a four-day international United Nations Conference in Geneva on discrimination against American Indians. During this unprecedented meeting, sponsored by the United Nations Committee on Human Rights, requests were made for U.N. protection of Indian rights.

The United States government is receiving international criticism for its continuing policy of cultural genocide of indigenous peoples. Sympathetic supporters and friends are encouraged to write letters and send telegrams to Staff Director Ernest Stevens of the Select Committee of Indian affairs, Room 5331, Dirksen Senate Office Building, Washington, DC 20510, (202) 224-2251, and to President Reagan.

Personal Power

The development of personal power is accentuated in the Native American tradition. Our current time period is a unique one. We are experiencing the transition from the 2,000-year-old Piscean Age to the Aquarian Age. In Hopi Indian cosmology, we are moving from the fourth to the fifth world.

Experiencing our creative energies opens the doorway for the development of personal power. The words creative and creator are derived from the same root. It is through the process of surrendering to Creator that we are able to more fully open ourselves to creative power. Once surrender is accomplished, trust is automatic. In surrendering, we discover that our life is guided by a force greater than ourselves. Oh Shinnah emphasizes that "surrender is accomplished only through free will. To surrender is to give over, rather than to give up." Music, dance, art, and imagination are keys for returning to our creative power.

During this time in history it is essential that people own their personal power and communicate their convictions. It is a time for personal growth consciousness and political awareness to be fully united. Oh Shinnah appeals for action in the following way: "We have a chance at this point in history, right now, to change everything. Not only have we developed intelligent consciousness, there is a very small segment of that intelligence that can actively see and pursue its own spiritual evolution. We can see our evolution. That has never happened before. . . . As we continue to be apathetic about what goes on in our lives, we will not understand surrender. We will not see the future. . . . Yet in two generations, through the children, we can change everything."

Indian People emphasize that they are not a vanished race; they were not all killed off. "We are a reborn people who are coming to form circles with one another once again."

Notes

1. A quarterly newsletter is available from the Meta Tantay Foundation, P.O. Box 707, Carlin, Nevada 89822, for $3 a year. Those interested in visiting the community are requested to write first.
2. For more information of Oh Shinnah's workshop and future tapes and books, write to the Four Directions Foundation, P.O. Box 188, Corte Madera, CA 94925. She frequently lectures on the West Coast and has plans to start a community school in the Southwest teaching the Native American way of life.

3. Gurdjieff also teaches us to look to the spirit of the land in which we live.

4. Oh Shinnah describes the etheric body as wavy lines of energy, emanating about 12 inches out from the body. It is here that physical illness can be recognized.

5. When Indian spiritual leaders speak of white people, they are not referring to skin color or blood, but rather to an insensitive state of mind. Oh Shinnah says "I do not recognize racial difference. I am an Indian because my heart is Indian, because I have a relationship with the Earth Mother, because I care for people, because I am a warrior woman, because I believe in the balance of nature, not because my father and mother had Indian blood."

6. Dan Katchongva, *Hopi: A Message for All People* (New York: Akwesasne Notes, 1973), pp. i–ii. This publication and *Akwesasne Notes* (a quarterly newspaper for native and natural peoples) are available upon donation from *Akwesasne Notes*, Mohawk Nation, via Rooseveltown, New York 13683.

7. Friends of the Hopi, P.O. Box 1852, Flagstaff, AR 86002, issues an excellent periodical newsletter on the current political situation at the Four Corners. More information and petitions to repeal the Public Law are available from the resource communication center.

SANDY R. NEWHOUSE, *M.A., M.F.C.C., is working on her Ph.D. in Clinical Psychology at the University of Virginia, Charlottesville, and works as a therapist at the local community mental health center. She has published articles on cross-cultural medicine, psychosomatic medicine and Tibetan Buddhism in the* Yoga Journal, Tibet Journal, *and* Women's Health Care: A Guide to Alternatives.

JOHN AMODEO, *Ph.D., practices psychotherapy in San Francisco and Mill Valley, California. He is a faculty member of John F. Kennedy University and Sonoma State University and lectures widely. He is a contributing editor to the* Yoga Journal.

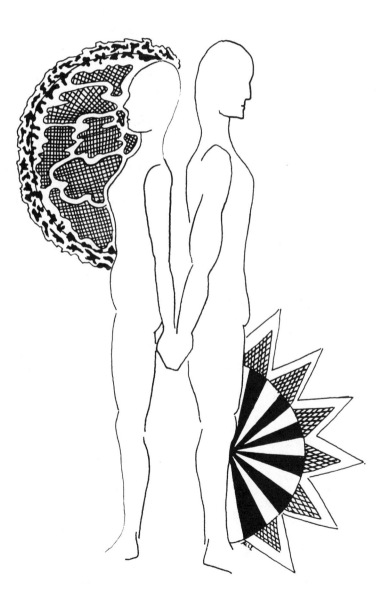

Turtle Island Speaks

NATIVE AMERICAN CONSCIOUSNESS AS MODERN SURVIVAL PARADIGM

Thomas I. Pinkson, Ph.D.

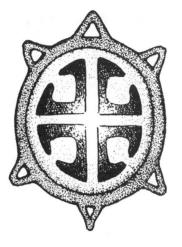

This article describes the use of Native American rituals, particularly the Vision Quest, as part of a therapeutic process. Dr. Pinkson uses traditional Native American rituals, ceremonies, and myths to stimulate the creative process. The programs, classes, and workshops he has developed have been used in several Bay Area colleges and in seminars around the country.

"There are two ways to be fooled: one is to believe what isn't so, the other is to refuse to believe what is so."

—Kierkegaard

"Not obeying the rules handed down from the beginning of time by the ancestors can bring sickness."

—*The Sacred*, p. 129

LONG BEFORE there was a United States there was Turtle Island. It was perceived as feminine by the diverse groups of indigenous people occupying her territory. These first inhabitants of Turtle Island treated her with respect, attuning their lives to the rhythms of her being. Daily interactions with the natural world were made sacred in appreciation of Turtle Island's gifts of food, shelter, clothing, medicine, and beauty.

Today, many years later, the majority of the land's current inhabitants no longer walk with respect upon her body. Modern Americans are not attuned to the natural forces dwelling within their own bodies, nor with those beneath them in the larger body they live upon. Increasing mechanization and stress characterize 20th-century society. Prevailing attitudes emphasizing the supremacy of material reality and of human life over animal life and non-material realities perpetuate alienation from the world of nature within and around us. Increasing incidence of stress-related illness and environmental pollution are manifestation of disharmony between our bodies, minds, feelings, spirit, and physical world. We suffer from a perspective lacking effective methodologies, with which to bring these seemingly disparate realities into a balanced whole. We

focus well on separate bits and pieces of life, but too often miss the synergistic workings of the "whole show."

Yet the "whole show of evolution" moves on, whether we attune to it or not. Advances in physics, genetics, and medical technology bring new perspectives at an accelerated rate. The proliferating nuclear threat and its extension into outer space necessitates attitudinal and geopolitical change to counterbalance the threat of misused technology. One harbinger of hope is the increasing clinical and research data in the fields of psychosomatic medicine, biofeedback work, psychoimmunotherapy and scientific explorations in consciousness studies which indicate cultural acceptance of a radical underestimation of our power to impact our inner physiological being, as well as the physical world around us. We desperately need survival paradigms that teach us to work wisely and harmoniously with the issues of power facing us at this time in history. Thomas W. Wilson, in his paper "Changing Perceptions of National Security" presents the challenge clearly: "... in the real world today the national interests of the separate states converge in the need to defend and sustain the living systems of planet earth—and that includes us."

One model for defending and sustaining the "living systems of planet earth" can be found in the "old ways" of the first inhabitants of Turtle Island. "Rules for living" were passed on by the elders of Native American tribal groups throughout the Americas. They affirmed that all the manifestations and forces of creation are interdependent with one another in an integrated whole. There was a "recognition of life as power, as a mysterious, ubiquitous, concentrated form of non-material energy, of something loose about the world and contained in a more or less condensed degree by every object." Native American beliefs emphasized pragmatic knowledge with which to live in harmony and balance with this "non-material energy, and with the great mystery underlying it all. Wakan Tanka, translated from the Oglala Sioux language, literally means sacred, or Great Mystery.

The shaman and medicine man/woman helped tribal members maintain, or restore when needed, this sacred balance through their healing rituals, rites, and ceremonies. Vital to this process was the relationship to the land they lived on. For Native people there was no concept of ownership or possession of land. They believed their role was caretaker: they were to live on Turtle Island with love, respect, and appreciation for her generous gifts without which they could not survive. This perception of their role as caretakers produced behavioral patterns congruent with this belief. They were to care for their "mother," who in turn was the bearer of life itself. There was no word for religion; there was simply living out their beliefs in their daily lives. A primary dynamic of their caring role was reciprocal interaction with the land and all her creatures. Reciprocity was sacred because it maintained the balance between giving and taking, the "good medicine" responsible for health and well-being. Failure to act within the dictates of reciprocity could lead to illness, misfortune, and even death.

Vision Quest, the seeking of direct contact with the Great Mystery to obtain guidance and medicine power for one's life, was a dynamic rite of passage for many Native American people. The quest consisted of time spent alone in nature praying for a vision. The questor would neither eat nor drink and in some cases would stay awake at night as well. It might go on longer, but two to four days and nights was a frequent duration. The fasting, isolation, and solitude, sleep deprivation and emotionally charged prayer rituals accompanying the sacred quest acted in synergistic fashion to produce an alteration of consciousness.

Similar to psychedelic experience precipitated by psychoactive drugs, psychological set and setting were important determinants in the results of this altered state. The setting for the quest was constant; a wilderness environment, usually atop a mountain or high butte. The set, or cognitive repertoire of attitudes, beliefs, feelings, and philosophy, inculcated into the Native youth since early childhood, emphasized the presence of the Great Mystery in all of creation. If the questors sufficiently prepared themselves through the rites of fasting and purification, and if they truly humbled themselves before the Mystery and waited in patience, their prayers would usually be answered. This was the expectation, and, in a self-fullfilling manner, frequently resulted in a peak experience of mystical union and oneness between creator, creation and perceiving self. The quest experience encouraged and empowered what philosopher Jacob Needleman refers to as a "firsthand sense of identity." The expansion of awareness shifted the identity focus from ego to the transpersonal. The quest experientially validated the cultural belief in the interconnectedness and interdependence of all life, thereby reinforcing the importance of reciprocal interactions with every manifestation of the Great Mystery.

The returning youth was typically welcomed back into the tribe with elaborate rites of incorporation. Often a new name was bestowed, based on his visions, which in turn reinforced the spiritual nature of their identify. His clothing, dwelling, personal belongings, songs, and prayers from this point on, and for the duration of his life, was physical embodiment of his guiding vision from adolescence, the foundation for his medicine power. A strong sense of purpose and commitment to act as a "warrior" and integrate his vision into his life characterized the post-quest experience.

In my doctoral dissertation, published by Free Person Press as "A Quest for Vision," I describe my own quest for vision and subsequent development of a successful adaptation for treating heroin addiction in the early 1970s. Since that time I have offered this program through workshops and classes to people in all walks of life throughout the country. Participants discover helpful guidance, insight, and empowerment to challenge unresolved difficulties impairing their current existence. Might there be a linkage of some sort between the "old ways" of the aboriginals of Turtle Island, ways that helped them obtain the survival wisdom necessary for their times, and our need today for "survival wisdom" on the same land? Rupert Sheldrake speculates that there might be "a subtle but pervasive propert' of nature which organizes and stores information just as the gravitational field organizes matter and stores energy." "Morphic resonance" is the flow of information between elements of the field. Does Turtle Island still speak to modern questors through this "morphic resonance," as it has for millennia to those who would listen?

The model I use in teaching the quest for vision consists of four stages. The initial one is *preparation*. Native youths had the entire web of their culture preparing them for their outings. Ongoing validation for the importance of vision motivated them to seek their own when the timing was right and to do so in a sacred way with the helpful guidance of knowledgeable elders. Today's prevailing paradigm of reality emphasizing the material world, and rationality and logic as the dominant means to "know the world," lacks positive models of encouragement and instruction for those seeking vision on different levels of awareness. Thus modern questors need supportive preparation to develop both a conceptual framework and physical and self-regulatory awareness skills with which to capitalize on the potential of the quest experience. Preparation focuses on exploring the dynamics of sacredness in reciprocity, the meaning and source of medicine power, and how to open and attune to "mystery" within and around us for guidance and direction. We work with dreams, myth, and symbols using guided fantasy, movement, sound, and music. We attune the feelings and intuition and utilize centering exercises, meditation, and prayer to quiet our rational ego-centered minds. We strive to enhance awareness and sensitivity to the deeper psyche and to the animals, trees, rocks, weather, and so forth, of the natural world around us. Dreams are an especially important focus, bridging the personal unconscious with the collective unconscious, the waking state to the altered state during sleep, and the rational to the "wilderness" of the deeper mind. Attunement to intuition and feelings in addressing problematic situations that come up in preparation helps balance overdependence on rational modes of problem-solving which western education teaches us to rely on. Emphasis is on introspection, entering the "looks-within place" to listen for guidance from the "mystery" within.

The intent of these exercises is not to have participants try to become Indians. I myself am not of Native American descent. I have, however, spent the past fifteen years exploring Native American and shamanistic belief systems, rituals, and ceremonies through direct experience with shamans and medicine people; through seeking my own visions and through attempting to integrate the findings of these explorations into my clinical work as a psychologist, a consultant, and teacher. My intent is to use these "old wisdom ways" as a vehicle to expand perceptual models on the nature of reality. The "old ways" open the doors of perception to a larger vista of awareness in which the wisdom of relationships based on reciprocity, harmony, and balance become self-evident as survival necessities.

The second stage, *purification*, begins as we ready ourselves for time on the land. We seek cleansing of our physical bodies, our minds and our spirits so as to "empty" ourselves for our quest. Each questor begins to fast. This helps clean out the body and open awareness and communicative capacities previously unavailable due to digestive and food-related activities. Fasting also helps the individuals to clarify and focus on their goals for the quest. A sweatlodge ceremony deepens this process.

The sweatlodge is a dome-shaped structure of branches with tarps and blankets thrown over it to completely seal out all light. Rocks are heated in an open fire-pit and then brought into the lodge when red-hot and placed in a hole at the center. Participants enter the lodge and form a circle, seated on the ground around the glowing rocks. Water is poured onto the rocks, and hot steam blasts throughout the lodge, cleansing all within.

Native American people view the sweatlodge ceremony as a healing process, complete in itself, as well as part and parcel of other sacred rites such as the Vision Quest. They view the lodge as Jews and Christians would revere their synagogue or church. The sweatlodge ceremony was a symbolic return to the womb of creation. Every act within this sacred setting of earth, air, fire, and water held significance. Prayers were offered as bodies and spirits, minds, and emotions opened and were cleansed. Many healings took place in the lodge. It is one of the most ancient of the old ways and considered very sacred and powerful. Disrespect or misuse can result in serious difficulty.

Modern questors find the sweatlodge to be a powerful experience for them as well, expanding their understanding of purification to a psychospiritual, as well as physical, level. A "Giveaway Ceremony" takes place after the sweat, with each member sharing with the group something of import to his quest. Afterwards we sleep next to one another in a circle, which symbolizes wholeness and the spiritual knowledge we seek from the teaching wheels of the universe.

We rise at dawn to greet the birthing new day in a Sunrise Ceremony, and to review dreams from the previous night. Then we say our goodbyes and each person walks off to an already designated "place of Power" to spend one to three days alone (depending on the length of the outing.)

This period of *solitude and isolation* in the natural world comprises the third stage of the quest. Modern seekers also experience an alteration of consciousness induced by the fasting, ceremony, and ritual. Dissociation from their normal reality structure enhances this alteration as they explore their own nature in the midst of nature. Openness, attentiveness, appreciation, and humility, attitudes stressed in the earlier preparation sessions, enable participants to go deeper into their experience. Solitude, especially in the darkness of a wilderness setting, activates fears and anx-

ieties that ego defenses have successfully held in check in one's normal environment. Questions of: Who am I? Where did I come from? Why am I here? Where am I going? are also activated and explored as each person enacts his/her quest. The cyclic, rhythmic forces of nature pulse in and around them, offering their wisdom-teachings to the perceptive and attentive student.

The group reunites at a central location upon completion of the agreed-upon time of solitude. A celebration of survival and togetherness initiates the fourth stage of the quest—*incorporation*. We reassemble our circle to hear each member's experience. Each person is recognized as both teacher and student, a sacred Medicine Wheel or mirror, as they relate their story. This sharing serves as a rite of integration back into the social world from which we have ventured forth and to which we now return. A prayer of thanksgiving concludes our time in the wilderness. A final meeting one week later focuses on the significance of our quest discoveries for our post-quest lives.

Since 1972, when I first took out a group of questors, over 300 people, ranging in age from 13 to 67 have gone on such outings with me. Almost all reported gaining insight, a sense of purpose, and self-confidence. They discover inner strength and survival capacities that enable them to successfully cope with fear, anxiety, and the stress of the unknown. Their physical survival, which some were not sure of during their time alone, intensifies their appreciation of life, of others, and of themselves. They speak with more assurance and trust of who and what they are, and their sense of connectedness with nature.

"I found what I was looking for and it was me," reports John B., a 44-year-old administrative executive from San Francisco. "I had no great mystery opened to me—no spiritual visitor. My vision is that I've found my own spirit, the real me, beneath my physical and psychological being. I see now that the rules I've lived by have kept me from the natural spirit that is within me. I've been an active churchgoer since college. I know the Christian concept of the soul, but I've always associated it with life after death, not as part of my present existence. The concept of spirit as a part of me never really fell into place. To me, my being was made up of my body and my mind. The idea of a third part of my being, a spirit, never really occurred to me. The rules of society and logic have kept me blinded. My search for my spot was a part of my vision. I learned to trust my feelings even though logic said otherwise.

"The sweatbath continued the vision. My rules said nudity was bad. But when it came time to decide whether to go into the bath or not it felt right to do it. So, I ignored the rule.

"Our giveaway was a part of my vision. I learned that simple giving from the heart, not the size or the fineness of the gift, was what mattered. Joe's gift was the greatest for me. My rules said it was not right for one man to embrace another. I found that Joe's embrace was good and right.

"As I thought of these things this morning, I realized these same rules were keeping me from Nature. Nature was willing and open but I kept myself out. My reasoning said I must fear Nature, that I must protect myself from it. So I kept up the shield that separated me from it.

"I know that I can't cast aside all my rules, but I know now that they're there for me to cast aside when the time is right. I think I can hug my son when I feel it is right and not be guilty—thanks to Joe. I think I can be nude and not be ashamed when the time is right. Finally, I can go to the land and be a part of it, accepting its beauty, its signs, its being.

"After I thought of these things I began to cry. It felt good to cry so I let the tears flow. I cried, I think, in happiness and thankfulness for my vision. Now that I've found my spirit, now that I know it is there, I can seek it out. I know the way."

John's account reflects a broader understanding of himself and greater flexibility in the options he now chooses for his life.

For Native people, as with John and other modern questors, lack of awareness in understanding the consequences of their actions can lead to disharmony and imbalance. Illness and accidents can be a manifestation of this disharmony which might be internal, or interactional, with their social, natural, or spiritual environment. Illness or misfortune were perceived by Native Americans as signs of disharmony. Intervention through physical means was one component of treatment. The more significant intervention was the realignment of the patient back into harmonious relationships with themselves and their environment, the basis of a true and lasting healing.

Modern questors return from the wilderness more perceptive of the disharmony and imbalance in their lives, and with a clearer sense of the role they play in bringing this about. In touch with enhanced personal power, they can now act constructively on their insights to initiate positive transformation in their areas of distress. By spending time alone in the natural world, questors directly and intimately experience the cyclic energy forces of nature and their interconnectedness to them. The medicine power of the shaman was directly related to their own intimate relationships with these forces. Anthropologist Michael Harner points out that the shamanistic system is in fact a "system of consciousness alteration with which to enter alternative realities which modern physics describe as existing all around us." The absence of medicine as we know it today, with its dependence on physical intervention, forced people to "develop the utmost potential of their minds in order to deal with critical matters that cannot be dealt with on a material basis." The shaman, Harner continues, "utilized intentional altered states of consciousness to accomplish a specific mission. Their voyages into altered states helped them to explore and develop mind potentials not usually addressed in current educational models." Quest participants utilize expanded vision to explore their own deeper mind states and potentials for being.

Numerous modern quest participants report transcendence of ordinary ego boundaries while in their altered states. Native American beliefs emphasize that Turtle Island and all who dwell upon her are conscious, living beings. For them, transpersonal relationships with non-human entities is an accepted part of life. It is assumed that all two-legged persons have a specific totem animal/spirit that can help them in their lives and the Vision Quest is an opportunity to initiate this relationship if it has not already begun. Modern questors have powerful learning experiences both with physically present animals as well as with archetypal ones through dreams and visions. New perceptions and avenues of discovery not available in ordinary states of awareness serve as rites of passage into deeper knowledge of self, which in turn provides information with which to walk in balance on the life path. This is the ancient empowerment heritage so badly needed today, passed on by generations of Turtle Island elders.

Ancient Hopi prophecy accurately predicts current conditions of pollution and nuclear threat. They state that we are at an important crossroads. Our actions now determine the severity of purification needed to heal our earth's wounded body. Perhaps we already experience this purification in the dramatic changes in weather patterns around the world and the havoc they have wrought. Solutions must begin within, for pollution begins in our pathological misperceptions of identity and relationship emphasizing myopic vision of separateness and short-term gain. There is, as ecologist Barry Commoner tells us, "no free lunch."

"Modern society critically needs to strengthen its understanding of human, ecological, and spiritual values to balance its runaway technological prowess," declared Willis Harmon of the Institute for Noetic Science. Fred Polack, in *Image of the Future*, further asserts that "bold visionary thinking is . . . prerequisite for effective social change." We have much to learn in seeking vision for effective social change from the old ways of Turtle Island. If the Turtle Island concepts appear alien to our Judeo-Christian background, listen to another elder, also part of the "old ways" as he encourages us to "Speak to the earth and it shall teach thee!" It is Job—in the Bible—12:7–10. . . . The job of seeking survival-based vision beckons us all. Our children's children await our response.

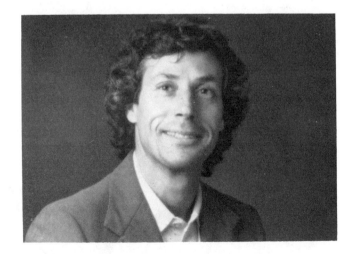

DR. TOM PINKSON *is a transpersonal psychologist in private practice in Mill Valley, California. He is the author of* A Quest For Vision *and numerous articles on his innovative work with cancer patients, rites of passage, death and dying, and attitudinal healing. His consulting and workshops on health promotion, personal empowerment and psychospiritual growth have been utilized by business and corporate groups, hospitals, Hospice programs, mental health, and educational institutions throughout the country.*

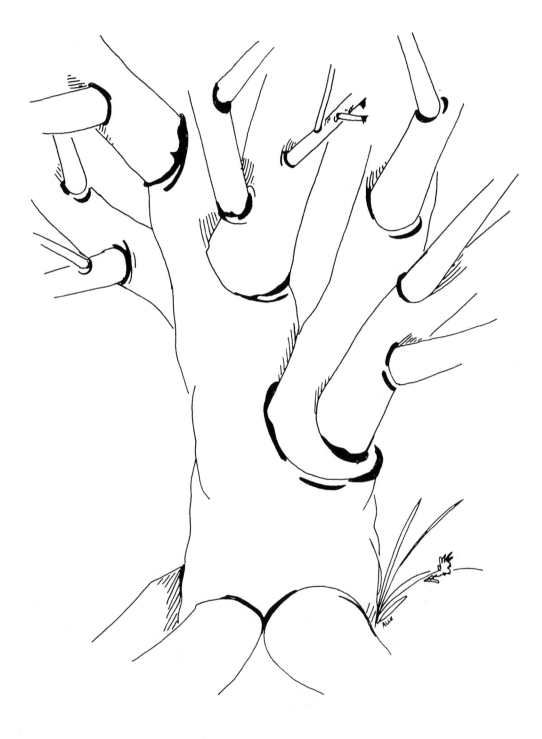

C. WESTERN SYSTEMS

Hippocrates of Cos:
The Founder of Western Medicine

Aidan A. Kelly, Ph.D.c.

Hippocrates was born on the island of Cos in 460 B.C., and was said to have been at least 85, or perhaps 100, when he died. He was an Asklepiade, according to tradition, but the tradition is not clear about just who the Asklepiadai were. They may have been the priests of Asklepios, the god of healing; or a guild of physicians, somewhat like the guild of Homeric poets; or a clan of hereditary physicians who claimed descent from Asklepios; or perhaps some combination of these.

Certainly Hippocrates did not invent the science of medicine out of wholecloth. Instead he built on the work of preceding generations, just as all philosophers of his time did. What he did, apparently, was pull all available knowledge together into a unified system, on which he and others could then build. The extant collection of writings known as the Hippocratic corpus *(easily available in the Loeb Classical Library series) probably contains relatively little that is by Hippocrates himself, and much that was written by his students and followers. Precisely the same is true—although to a lesser degree—of the writings attributed to Plato, Aristotle, Plutarch, or any other Classical author. People then were not as concerned as we are about publishing under their own names, especially since their work had a much better chance for survival if it were attributed to the illustrious founder whose work they were continuing.*

Most of the Hippocratic corpus is technical and, as such, quite outmoded. But I offer here some selections, from the Oath *and from the aphoristic works (largely the* Precepts*), that are as relevant now as they were in the Age of Pericles, and that can remind us again how much we owe to those familiar but alien ancestors of ours, the Greeks.*

HE HIPPOCRATIC OATH
I swear by Healing Apollo, by Asklepios, . . . and by all the gods and goddesses . . .:
To honor my teacher like my own parents, . . . and his sons like my brothers . . .;

To help the sick as best I can, and never to injure or do wrong, never to give poison or allow it to be given, never to give an abortifacient to a woman;

To live my life and practice my art in holiness and righteousness; . . .

To enter any house only to help the sick, abstaining from any intent to harm or do wrong to anyone there, and especially from sexual entanglements with anyone there, whether man or woman, bound or free;

To hold whatever I hear or see, whether in my profession or in my private life, to be holy secrets, not to be divulged or published abroad;

And may my enjoyment of my life and my art, and my reputation among all men, depend on whether I keep this oath or break it.

Sayings of Hippocrates

Life is short, art is long, opportunity fleeting, experiment deceptive, and judgment difficult. Hence not only the physician, but also the patient, and everyone else who is involved in the situation, must cooperate.

Healing is a matter of time, but sometimes also a matter of opportunity. Hence medical practice must not depend primarily on plausible theories, but instead on experience combined with reason.

Do not hesitate to ask the opinion of laymen, if any improvement in treatment may result from doing so.

Care for the sick to make them well, care for the healthy to keep them well, and care for yourself.

It is never a mistake to call in a consultant; for all the help you can get is never enough.

Sometimes give your services for nothing, remembering what gifts you have received, or for the pleasure of the work. And if you have a chance to help an impoverished stranger, give your best. For where there is love of people, there is love of the art. Some patients, even knowing their condition is serious, will recover simply because of their confidence in the goodness of the physician.

Do not adopt an outrageous mode of dress in order to attract patients. Being a little unusual may be in good taste, but too much will harm your reputation. Being pleasant and fashionable is not beneath the physician's dignity.

Eating properly will not by itself keep well a person who does not exercise; for food and exercise, being opposite in effect, work together to produce health.

A wise person should consider health to be the greatest of human blessings, and should learn how to benefit from illness by thinking.

AIDAN KELLY *is a doctoral candidate in Classics and Religion at the Graduate Theological Union, Berkeley, California.*

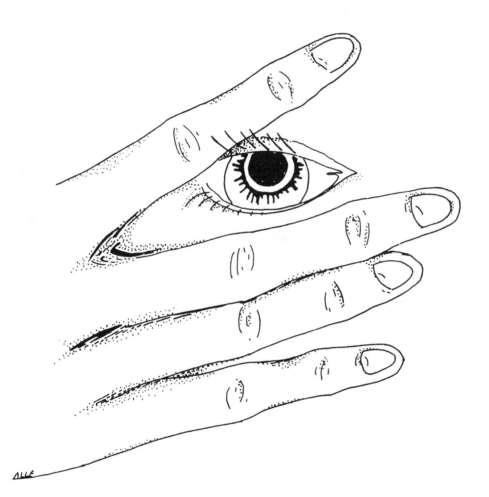

Naturopathy and Disease

Marti Benedict

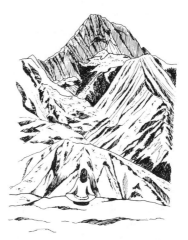

THE PHRASE, "identify the cause of the disease," commonly used in conventional medicine is directly rooted in the cause-effect assumptions of Western philosophy. Naturopathy, in contrast, seeks the *relationship* between the mind/body/spirit of the individual and his environment, in nature. It assumes, in fact, that all the elements which affect a situation coexist simultaneously and interact. The dynamic way in which they affect one another cannot be dissected analytically for observation, but must be construed holistically.

Naturopathy looks to the original state of nature, in which man was formed, as a tool in the treatment of disease. Naturopathy deals with two parameters which influence disease. The first is the virulence of the disease agent; the second, the resistance of the body to disease. The stronger the shield of the individual, the less susceptible he is to attack from the forces which disrupt harmony. In order to change a disease pattern, we alter both of these states: we reduce the virulence of the agent and increase the resistance of the person.

The naturopath views disease as sharing a common origin with lowered vitality of the system. Therefore it uses two fundamental methods to restore health. First, *nourish* the depleted system with pure food, water, thought, movement, and peace of mind. Second, *cleanse* the toxin-ridden body with an internal "housecleaning." These two practices are complementary, and are always used together.

Countless individual variations have been formulated by naturopaths over the years, as they adjusted their own views to the needs of their patients. It is written that Hippocrates practiced naturally, and that he cured the island of Cos of all diseases using a small number of herbs, fresh air, sunshine, exercise, and massage. One may well argue that in simpler times there were fewer diseases, affecting smaller percentages of the population. Yet in the past few thousand years the genetic makeup of the human being has altered little.

Naturopathy and the Disease Process

When working with a patient, we notice a phenomenon known as the "law of cure," which describes the regression of the disease process. Stated simply, as the body becomes better nourished and internally cleansed, the symptoms of old illnesses will begin to appear, in reverse chronological order, that is, the most recent first. Thus if a patient of 45 has arthritis as his chief complaint, but has a history of sciatica, migraines, eczema, poor digestion, teenage acne, headaches, or stomach problems as a child, he might reexperience some of the problems of his past. As the healing process continues and he begins feeling generally better, he may go through various "healing crises" for short periods of time. The naturopath can distinguish "healing-crisis symptoms" from the same symptoms within a current disease process, but the methods are beyond the scope of this article.

The very core of naturopathy lies in sunlight, air, water, and earth. Although many modalities employed by naturopathy have been discussed, nutrition of the mind/body/spirit unity is the fundamental building block of this particular branch of natural healing.

Here is an example of the healing process as performed by naturopathy. A patient complains of a painful hemorrhoid. The practicing naturopath could give him some astringent herbs to shrink the hermorrhoid. The symptom would be relieved, and the patient might leave satisfied that the practitioner had discharged his responsibility.

This may be all the patient wants. However, to comply with the principle of bringing this individual's body/mind/spirit into greater harmony with nature, the conscientious naturopath would have to discover what long-term conditions have interacted to produce this symptom. He may find that the patient has poor nutritional habits, does not exercise enough, shows evidence of poor circulation, liver and gall bladder congestion, lymphatic-waste accumulation, kidney insufficiency, or heart weakness—or that he has been suffering from some job-related tension for the past six months.

The options are many; however, they will all have to deal with some deficiency, whether it is physical, spiritual, or emotional. An optimum course for dealing with it will find the patient and the practitioner working together in a re-education program to improve the patient's diet and his ability assimilate foods, to incorporate daily exercise into his life, to help detoxify the body and improve circulation, to tone up internal organs, and to increase spiritual harmony by means of meditation, breathing exercises, prayer, or progressive relaxation.

With this kind of examination and treatment the patient can walk out of the office feeling comfortable, not only because of the direct intervention, but also because he is assured that the real problems will begin to correct themselves in time. If he accepts the challenge offered him, he may find a new lease on life; the role of his original symptoms (remember the hemorrhoid?) will be seen in its proper perspective, i.e., as an opportunity to get in balance.

Naturopathic treatment, unlike traditional medicine, requires the patient to take a very active role in his healing process. If he is to do his part, he needs patience, great effort, and a willingness to overcome old habits. Some people, of course, will prefer to go to the allopathic physician, have the hemorrhoid removed surgically, and "get it over with." This too will give relief—of a kind. But it has its drawbacks as well: the cost of surgery, the trauma of surgical intervention, the inconvenience and lost time during recovery and, of course, the prospect of another hemorrhoid later on. There is a choice; one man's medicine is, quite literally, another man's poison.

Some Precautions to be Observed

There are two aspects of naturopathy which require careful consideration. First in the cleansing of the body as a means to good health, as advocated in many currently popular books. This is not a universally appropriate method. Some people need a building and repairing process because their systems are depleted. For a person who has a frail, overextended system, cleansing may create an additional stress. On the other hand, a cleansing process may make a relatively well-nourished person feel better and increase his emotional stamina. The better-nourished patient will be able to cooperate with the healing process; his healthier body will be able to discharge toxins more efficiently. But the undernourished patient must be built up in other ways first. It takes energy to have a healing crisis. Judgment must be exercised to choose the course of treatment for each individual, not to fit the patient to the method.

Second, it is important to understand natural nutrition. There are health-food stores which stock protein powders, vitamin and mineral supplements, and so on; but they exclude fresh vegetables, fruits, grains, fish, meat, poultry, and dairy products. There is nothing wrong with supplements in their place, but they cannot be used as substitutes for food. A proper nutritional education will include where and how to shop for food, how to prepare it, as well as when and how to consume particular foods. Again, it's more expedient to pop a pill than to work with a naturopath. Re-education of this sort is time-consuming and expensive. It also costs more effort. Yet, in the course of a

lifetime, it's worth the effort to achieve a basic philosophical involvement with health.

Thirdly, there is the issue of food for the emotions and the spirit, a subject frequently passed over lightly, given lip service, and ignored. These things are most difficult for the average person to talk about, and also the most difficult to put into practice. For example, many people believe they are stuck with their sickness. A common complaint is that someone is "married to his ulcer." It takes great effort to understand that the ulcer is a *chosen* response to a life situation. The person must regain power over his own body and give himself permission to be healthy; he must disown the ulcer that he created in response to interpersonal irritations. Moreover, this change in consciousness may depend on or lead to initiating communication about the very issues that provoked the original irritations. Facing such issues usually means having to go through more pain, anger, and hostility before the problem is resolved.

Then, too, resolution doesn't alway mean winning. It may mean growing by admitting, loving, and giving more space and honest concern to irritations and difficulties. Many prefer not to work on this uncomfortable, psychologically naked level. Yet this is the work of a more evolved consciousness than the one which merely attacks symptoms and balances vitamins.

Finding adequate spiritual food also raises some difficult choices for the young and the consciously searching. In some circles, it is accepted behavior to follow a spiritual leader as part of the process of growth and self-education. The pitfall here is that of "guru-hopping." The seeker who repeatedly moves from one leader or discipline to another, always on the spiritual quest or road, but never really choosing, is actually going nowhere, and may never reach the point of assuming responsibility for himself. The inability to choose a spiritual discipline and stick with it is merely another form of the procrastination and self-delusion which create disease. Therefore the patient must be encouraged to feed his spiritual body actively, not only by searching, but also by participation and choice.

MARTI BENEDICT *has a M.A. from Stanford Medical School. She has studied Chinese medicine and other natural methods for 10 years, in both the United States and the Orient. She is currently in private practice, where her aim is to integrate the appropriate natural techniques for each of her individual clients.*

Homeopathy

George Vithoulkas

Homeopathy is based on the premise that a remedy can cure a disease if it produces symptoms similar to those of the disease in a healthy organism.

Samuel Hahnemann, the founder of homeopathy, found that a dilute remedy could induce healing without creating toxic side effects.

The system of homeopathy is geared toward treating the person, not the disease. By means of exacting study, the homeopath learns to pinpoint the specific remedy, in the voluminous materia medica, *which matches one's particular constitution and the stage of the dynamic disease process. Often this remedy is enough to rectify the imbalance.*

In this article George Vithoulkas, one of the world's leading homeopathic practitioners, shares his knowledge of this rediscovered system of healing.

N 1810 a book called *Organon of the Art of Healing* was published in Toragou, a small town of Germany. Its author, Samuel Hahnemann, was a physician, and in it he stated the laws and principles of a new system of healing which he called homeopathy. This medical system met with bitter opposition, especially when it started, but soon spread all over Europe, and today it is practiced in most of the civilized countries of the world.

What Hahnemann had to say about medicine was at the time most revolutionary, and in the light of current medical practices it is equally revolutionary today.

Briefly stated, he claimed and proved that medical cure is brought about in accordance with certain laws of healing that are in nature; that nobody can cure outside these laws; that there are no diseases as such, but only diseased individuals; that an illness is always dynamic in nature, and that therefore the remedy, too, must be in a dynamic state if it is to cure; that the patient needs only one particular remedy for any given stage of his illness, and no other, so that he is not cured unless that remedy is found, but at the best only temporarily relieved.

Hahnemann never ceased to examine and inquire. He

This article is adapted from *Homeopathy: Medicine for the New Man*, Avon, 1972, by George Vithoulkas; portions of the book were serialized in *Alternatives Magazine* during 1977. Reprinted by permission of the author.

came upon an idea which was to be the germ of this completely new system which we know today as homeopathy. A professor of medicine at London University named Cullen had devoted twenty pages of his *Materia Medica* to the therapeutic indications of Peruvian Bark; and he attributed its success in the treatment of intermittent fevers to the fact that it was bitter. Hahnemann was dissatisfied with this explanation—so much so, that he did something quite extraordinary; he took the medicine himself! This was an action entirely out of keeping with every process of medical research that had hitherto existed. One can only speculate what prompted Hahnemann to do something so unorthodox: but as a result the world was to enter into an entirely new era of medicine. He describes the result as follows:

"I took by way of experiment, twice a day four drachms of good China. My feet, finger ends, etc., at first became cold; I grew languid and drowsy; then my heart began to palpitate, and my pulse grew hard and small; intolerable anxiety, trembling, prostration throughout my limbs; then pulsation in the head, redness of my cheeks, thirst, and, in short, all these symptoms, which are ordinarily characteristics of intermittent fever, made their appearance, one after the other, yet without the peculiar chilly, shivering rigor.

"This paroxysm lasted two or three hours each time, and recurred if I repeated this dose, not otherwise; I discontinued it, and was in good health."

It was through his experiment that Hahnemann came upon his understanding of how all medicine cures: a remedy cures a disease only because it produces similar symptoms in a healthy organism! The whole of homeopathy derives from this law; in it resides the revolutionary breakthrough to a wholly new dimension in the understanding of medicine.

This discovery, and the fact that he was already very well known, attracted around Hahnemann a number of physicians who, like himself, were looking for the truth. They all starting experimenting on themselves by taking different drugs. They continued for six years, and kept scrupulously detailed accounts of the symptoms produced upon each of them by every drug they had taken. And during that time Hahnemann compiled an exhaustive list of poisonings recorded by different doctors in different countries during centuries of medical history. Now, in the symptoms produced upon them by these drugs, Hahnemann and his associates recognized the symptoms of many illnesses for which they had in vain been seeking cures; and, much more important, they discovered that the drugs actually cured those illnesses!

Although he had so clearly grasped and formulated this principal law of homeopathy, Hahnemann did not feel that he had discovered it. He quotes a number of people who, he thought, either stated it or hinted at it long before he came upon it. Hippocrates, for instance, stated this law several times in his teachings; Boulduc wrote that rhubarb's purgative quality was the reason why it cured diarrhea; Detharding said that senna cures colic because it produces a similar effect on the healthy; and Stahl wrote that "the rule accepted in medicine to cure by contraries is entirely wrong; on the contrary diseases vanish and are cured by means of medicines capable of producing a similar affection."[1]

Preparation of Homeopathic Medicines

When he had proved enough remedies, he started prescribing them in the accepted dosages of the time; but although the patient was invariably cured, the drug often caused such an aggravation of the symptoms that any repetition of the dose was a hazardous prospect. Such aggravation was to be expected, since the drug itself was producing symptoms similar to those of the patient. So Hahnemann reduced the dose to one-tenth of its original amount. The patient was still cured, but the aggravation, though lighter, was still there too; this was not good enough. Hahnemann diluted the medicine still further, each time prescribing only one-tenth of the previous dose, and presently reached a dilution that was completely ineffective, because there was essentially no remedy left in it! So the advantages of simple dilution were very limited. It seemed, then, that one had to choose between two evils: either the medicine was strong enough, in which case the symptoms were aggravated, or it was too diluted to bring about a cure. Now it was precisely at this most critical junction that Hahnemann discovered an amazing process which reduced the toxic effects of the remedy and actually increased its healing power proportionately! He simply submitted each dilution to a series of vigorous shakes or succussions, and discovered that progressive dilutions were now not only less toxic but also more potent!

Hahnemann says that the efficacy of a remedy thus processed is increased because "the powers, which are, as it were, hidden and dormant in the crude drug, are developed and roused into activity to an incredible degree." This is how he made all the dilutions of his remedies.

First of all, he considered that distilled water, alcohol, and *sacharum lactis* (lactose) were medicinally inert, so he diluted the drugs in these substances. If the remedy was soluble in water or alcohol, he mixed one part of the substance with 99 parts of the liquid, and submitted the mixture to 100 vigorous succussions. This dynamized mixture he called "the first centesimal potency." Then he mixed one part of this potency with 99 parts of water or alcohol, and again succussed the dilution 100 times to produce the

second centesimal potency of the drug. The third step in the process, of course, diluted the original substance to one part in a million, and the fourth step to one part in a hundred million. He repeated this process up to thirty times and apparently did not go beyond that, although his successors did.

Hahnemann had discovered that there lies hidden in every substance in nature some inner life, and that we can mobilize and use this force if we know how to process the substance. In homeopathy the repeated dilutions and succussions of a remedy release a great curative energy which is inherent in the drug; and in homeopathy we witness the amazing cures that the energized remedy can bring about.

In this connection we are struck by something which Paracelsus wrote: "The Quintessence is that which is extracted from a substance.... After it has been cleansed of all impurities and its perishable parts, and refined to the highest degree, it attains extraordinary powers and perfections.... In it there is great purity, and it is because of this purity that it has the virtue to cleanse the body."

The Concept of the Vital Force

It was this particular insight which, in time, led Hahnemann to the true understanding of the nature of disease. He had the kind of mind that proceeded only from facts obtained from research, inquiry, and experiment. He never accepted any concept that was incompatible with the results of experiment and observation. Now there were two facts that struck him: first, that remedies greatly diluted could only cure if they were homeopathically potentized, that is, dynamized through succussion; and, second, that once they were potentized, they contained no detectable material trace of the original substance. It followed, therefore, that their curative effect was not material, but involved some other factor—energy. He concluded that the succussions must transmit some of the energy of the original substance to the neutral matter in which it was diluted, rather as amber transmits static electricity to paper if rubbed against it, or as electricity, an invisible force, can be stored in batteries which are themselves material. He probably realized that he had gone beyond matter and was working in the domain of energy.

From all this, a chain of logical conclusions necessarily followed. Since the remedy was in fact dynamic and not material, the disorder upon which it worked must belong to the same order of being: so the illness was a derangement primarily on a dynamic plane. But what exactly did that mean? Hahnemann concluded that it was nothing other than a derangement in the life force in man.

Revolutionary Concept

Hahnemann went far beyond his time, and was even in advance of us today in stating that not only the disease but also its cause is dynamic. In other words, it is not the microbes or the virus or the bacteria, nor even their virulent poisons on the biochemical level, that cause disease, but rather their intimate nature, their very "soul," if one may use this expression. And this is something dynamic. Furthermore, this vibrating, pulsating, living inner malevolence of the morbific agents can affect only organisms that are susceptible to them, and can affect them only on a dynamic plane.

If illness were a question of bacteria and their numbers, those most exposed would be the first to be affected. But we all know that this is not the case. There are people everywhere who are exposed to contagious diseases and do not catch them; there are people who sleep in the same bed with patients suffering from tuberculosis or severe staphylococcal infection and are never affected; and then there are others who live in the most healthy environment and contract all kinds of contagious infections. Disease comes about only when two conditions are fulfilled: the presence of an external morbific agent and the patient's own susceptibility. It is not merely the result of exposure to a number of microbic invaders. That is why an epidemic never hits everybody in the area; there are people living in the most intimate relationship to its victims who are not in the least affected.

A homeopath is not concerned with killing bacteria, but with bringing the whole human organism into a state where it is impossible for bacteria to thrive on it.

Let us summarize what we have said so far:

1. A patient is cured only if he is given that medicine that can produce in a healthy organism symptoms most similar to his own.
2. A disease is not just the malfunction of some organ, but, first of all, a disturbance of the vital force that is responsible for the functioning of the whole organism.
3. Medicines cannot penetrate the physical organism to reach and act upon the vital force unless they are in a dynamic, energized state.
4. The cause of disease must be sought on a dynamic plane and not on a physical, chemical plane.

It is interesting to note that today every patient knows the name which orthodox medicine has given to the prominent symptoms of his trouble. But no conscientious homeopath ever prescribes according to the name of a disease: for him every case is completely new, with its own particular symptoms, both mental and physical. Any homeopath who bases his prescription on the name of disease instead of on the patient is not a true homeopath and should not be trusted. Each individual case should be noted down to its last detail. In aphorisms 84 and 86, Hahnemann tells us how this should be done:

84. The patient narrates the history of his complaints; his attendants communicate what they have heard him complain of, and describe his behavior, and other circumstances they have observed. The physician observes, by means of sight, hearing, and touch, what is changed and abnormal about the patient, and writes down everything in precisely the same expressions used by the patient and his attendants. He quietly allows them to finish their story, if possible without interruption.

86. When the patient and attendants have ended their statements of their own accord, the physician

supplies each symptom with more precise definition, to be obtained by reading over the single symptoms communicated to him, and here and there instituting particular inquiry; for instance: at what time did this attack occur? Was it some time before the present medicine? Was it during its use? Or was it some days before discontinuing the medicine? Describe exactly what kind of pain or sensation occurred, and where was the exact place? Did the pain come in single paroxysms, at different times? Or was it lasting and uninterrupted? How long did it last? At what time of the day or night, and in what position of the body was the pain most violent? In this manner every attack or circumstance alluded to by the patient should be made the subject of careful inquiry and description.

Hahnemann knew the complexities of human nature and the difficulties confronting the homeopath in trying to question a patient about his symptoms. In aphorisms 96 and 97, he writes:

It is worthy of remark that the temperament of patients is often abnormally affected; so that some, particularly hypochondriacs and other sensitive and intolerant persons, are apt to represent their complaints in too strong a light, and to define them by exaggerated expressions, hoping thereby to induce the physician to redouble his efforts.

But there are persons of another kind of temperament, who withhold many complaints from the physician, partly from false modesty, timidity, or bashfulness; and who state their case in obscure terms; and who consider many of their symptoms as too insignificant to mention.

Taking the case is only the first part of the picture, for the doctor must then set about finding the remedy. To do so he must go through his books and study the provings of different drugs until he has found the one whose symptoms are the most similar to those of the patient. It often takes hours before the doctor can say that he has found the right remedy for a chronic condition. In homeopathy there are no ready-made formulas. Each case requires its own particular medicine, and no other potentized remedy will have any effect at all.

In homeopathy, diagnosis is nothing more than the recognition of the drug which can cause—and therefore will cure—a certain totality of symptoms. That is why homeopaths all over the world talk about their patients as being a "Sulphur case" or a "Pulsatilla case," and so on. They call the patient and the totality of his symptoms by the name of the remedy they indicate.

Quite apart from the fact that homeopathy definitely works, homeopathic diagnosis has great advantages over the tedious clinical examinations of allopathic diagnosis, since it concerns itself excusively with the patient's symptoms, and discovers from these, only, the cure. For the allopath, the pathological state requiring treatment exists only when he can observe some pathological tissue change in the body—a duodenal ulcer, say, or a tumor somewhere—but for the homeopath the disturbance starts with the patient's own symptoms, which are at the same time the indication to the remedy that will cure him. For him the malady is already far advanced when it qualifies for allopathic recognition. For the homeopath the patient is ill when and because he feels ill. For the allopath the patient is ill only if his doctor can see it in the laboratory. The point is that the patient is right; those very disturbances which are in the beginning his symptoms can, and do, ultimately, result in the tissue changes recognized by allopathy. But the homeopath comes on the scene at the beginning and, by curing the functional disorders, aborts the possibility of a subsequent pathological tissue change. It follows from all this that if the patient has to wait for an allopathic diagnosis before he can be cured, he pays for it dearly. In aphorism 7, Hahnemann states it very aptly:

Symptoms alone must constitute the medium through which the disease demands and points out its curative agent. Hence the totality of these symptoms, this outwardly reflected image of the inner disease, must be the chief or only means for the disease to make known the remedy necessary for its cure, the only means of determining the selection of the appropriate remedial agent.

During the short history of homeopathy, it has survived many bitter attacks from high places. The attacks have always come from those who would be most discredited by recognizing its success; they are the defense mechanism of vested interest, and therefore subject to the greatest caution. In these attacks on homeopathy it is equally significant that the chief complaint against it has not been that it does not work—because it does—but only that accepted medical practice cannot understand how it works. No wonder!

For us homeopathy must be judged by its results; then, and only then, may we ask how it works. And the following is our brief effort to answer this question.

First, what do the symptoms of a disease mean; what do they show; what do they say? A little thinking will reveal that they are the means by which nature tries to get rid of disease. As Hippocrates aptly puts it: "Through vomiting nausea is cured." It seems that each organism is possessed of a defense mechanism which is set in operation as soon as this organism is invaded by a morbific agent. We know that all infectious diseases have an incubation period during which the patient is unaware that he is ill; actual symptoms appear only after this period of incubation, which may last hours or days. A little thinking will help us to understand more clearly the dynamic concept of disease.

In the phenomenon of illness, we see the appearance of certain symptoms; we are confronted with certain symptoms that have been created in the human organisms. But what is the process of creation—any creation? As we know very well, when something is created by man, it is first conceived in his mind. That concept is the birth of the creation at a dynamic level. When a new machine is made, its inventor first conceives it and works it out in his mind.

Mozart often said of his composition, "I have already composed it, and now I have only to write it down."

This rule of the dynamic origin of creation holds for all creation, whether it be for the creation of the universe, or of man, or of man's works. "As above, so beneath." Nature works this way, and disease is created this way, too. When a morbific agent comes in contact with a susceptible organism—and here we have, clearly, the positive and the negative, the male and female, those two eternal factors present in all creation—then the disease is conceived on a dynamic level. Only later do we feel and see its results in the organism.

This dynamic disturbance which shakes the whole organism, starting from its center, sets in motion in that organism millions of inimical changes intending to kill it. But the organism is unaware of these processes until they are violent enough to really endanger its life. It is only then that the organism sets in motion a reactive defense mechanism which, quite wrongly, we call disease. The symptoms of a disease are nothing but this reactive mechanism which is trying to get rid of the toxicosis. The toxicosis is, as we have explained, the material manifestation of an earlier disturbance on a dynamic level.

Perhaps it will be proved in the not too distant future that our organisms fight different morbific agents which attack them every day, but that most of these attacks are counteracted and neutralized on the dynamic level, like ideas which are not forceful or purposeful enough to make their appearance in the material world. Man is unaware of these attacks, and it is only seldom that these dynamic changes manage to reach a materialization—a toxicosis, in medical terms—that is poisonous to the body. When this happens, we have a general alarm of the organism, and it brings forth all its defensive resources which we feel and see as signs and symptoms of disease. Homeopathy does nothing else but strengthen this natural defense of the organism by adding to its resources and energy. It works in the same direction as the vital force and not against it. This direction, this natural intelligence of the vital defense, is precisely that set of symptoms that allopathy would so diligently suppress!

As we have said, illness and health is an affair which involves the vital force of man. This is neither material nor visible. To make an image, we would suggest that it lies in the domain of something akin to vibrations. To bring about a cure, the remedy must be similar to the disorder in its vibrations, as it were—or similar in pitch, if one prefers. A remedy which does not quite cover all the patient's symptoms cannot have any effect on them; nor should it be supposed that two or three drugs taken together will collectively do the work that one is supposed to do. Logic may find it perfectly reasonable that if one drug can produce 80 percent of a patient's symptoms and another can produce the remaining 20 percent, both can be safely administered together, and jointly remove the disease. But it does not work that way, alas! It is not a matter of quantity—adding up the required number of symptoms in a variety of drugs—but rather one of quality. These remedies are all dissimilar in quality, in nature—in vibrational frequency, if one will. Every drug has its own nature, and in order to work, it must be similar to the nature of the disorder. In cases where a number of remedies prescribed together have brought a result, it simply means that one of them has matched the disorder, and acted.

Some More Laws of Cure

A temporary aggravation of the symptoms is to be expected after the right remedy has been taken, and before the cure is completed. This aggravation is hardly noticeable in acute disorders, but very noticeable in chronic disorders. It sometimes attains an intensity which one could well describe as a curative crisis. During such a crisis one can expect such things as a sudden diarrhea, increased menstrual flow, excessive perspiration, profuse expectoration, and of course the reappearance of any suppressed skin eruption. The duration and intensity of the crisis are in direct proportion to the intensity of the case. Two conditions are necessary for such a reaction: first, the right remedy; second, a vital force strong enough to produce such a reaction. This explains why true homeopaths delight in such aggravations.

It often happens that in individuals of weak vitality, this curative crisis comes about only when the organism has been sufficiently strengthened, both by continuous and careful prescribing, and by the right kind of life.

J. T. Kent has described twelve different reactions which might take place after the first prescription. We cannot here go into the minute details exhaustively, but we can say that after the first prescription the symptoms may disappear in one of these four directions:

(1) they may go from the center to the circumference of the body;
(2) they may go from above downward;
(3) they may go from more vital to less vital organs; and
(4) they may disappear in the reverse order of their onset—those that appeared first will be the last to disappear.

Some examples of each of these categories will illustrate what we mean.

First of all, what is meant by the statement that the symptoms may go from the center to the circumference? Which is the center in man? It is the brain, the seat of thinking and all higher functions of the body. If the organism is considered as a whole, the brain is automatically recognized to be its center and its most vital part. Next in importance comes the heart, and then the liver, the lungs, the kidneys, etc., down to the muscles and the skin, which constitute the circumference of the organism and man's least important organs. A scratch, or the rupture of a blood vessel on the skin can safely be neglected; the same thing in the brain could be fatal. We also know that if the center is disturbed, the whole organism suffers profoundly. Now, to give an example, a mental case is treated homeopathically, and in the course of treatment the mental symptoms disappear and are followed by violent symptoms in the stomach. By this phenomenon the homeopath knows that a complete cure will eventually come about, because the direction followed by the symptoms is right: from the cen-

ter to the circumference. Likewise in the case of asthma: if a skin eruption appears during the treatment, it shows that the disease is moving toward the circumference, thus guaranteeing that the patient will finally be cured. But of course only a master homeopath will understand the symptoms of a patient, evaluate them rightly, and treat them accordingly. Alas, it not infrequently happens that after such a favorable reaction the ignorant patient is anxious to have his skin condition immediately removed, and if the homeopath does not explain to him what this skin trouble means in the process of his cure, he will find some obliging allopath to restore him to his previous condition quite swiftly! One of those who have most clearly described the direction followed, if a cure is to take place, is Hippocrates himself!

In the 49th of his aphorisms he writes: "In a person suffering from *angina pectoris*, the appearance of swelling and erythema on the chest is a good sign, for it shows that the disease is moving toward the circumference."

And in section 7, aphorism 5: "In a mental disorder of a maniacal type, dysentery or anasarca is a good sign."

Again in section 6, aphorism 11: "In those suffering from depression of spirits and kidney diseases, the appearance of haemorrhoids is a good sign."

Section 6, aphorism 21: "The appearance of varicose veins or haemorrhoids in those suffering from mania shows that the mania is cured."

And in aphorism 26 of the same section: "If the erysipelas moves from the outside to the inside, it is a bad sign, but if the opposite happens it is a good sign."[2]

In all these examples we can see how correctly this great physician understood and described the law of direction.

The direction from above downward appears mainly in skin eruptions where the trouble moves from the head and the upper part of the extremities toward the fingers and the nails. Likewise, if the symptoms move from the brain to the lungs, this is a movement from above downward, and at the same time from a more vital to a less vital organ.

Finally, the symptoms disappearing in the reverse order from that in which they appeared means, for example, that if a patient suffered from chronic headaches ten years ago, then from vertigo, and after that from depression or epilepsy, the depression or the epilepsy would be the first to disappear; next vertigo would reappear; when this too had gone, the headaches would return and finally they also would disappear. This gives an idea of what detailed and careful work is required from a homeopath in each individual case, if he is to restore his patients to health. It also shows the difficulties he encounters when, in the course of treatment, old symptoms reappear and the patient is in a hurry to get rid of them. That is why it is of the utmost importance for the patient thoroughly to know the theory of homeopathy; otherwise he will perhaps discontinue treatment just when he is improving.

Before concluding, we should like to discuss some of the disturbances and diseases that homeopathy can cure. The following is from a speech by Dr. W. H. Schwartz during an international homeopathic congress in America.

Until now, applied medicine has considered man exclusively as a physio-electrochemical organism. In theory it might admit that there is something beyond his material body, something called the psyche, or the mind. But what do physicians really know about these matters? In their everyday practice, they are called upon to treat skin eruptions that come on after deep distress, Bell's palsy after anxiety, diabetes after disappointment, doudenal ulcers after irritability or tension, insomnia caused by ambition or fear, chorea after mortification or vexation, and so on: the list is without end. So they know in their practice the effects that disturbed thoughts and feelings have upon the body. Yet they have neither the knowledge nor the means to go to the root of these disorders, nor do they ever stop to think that some other treatment may be adequate.

So it is indispensable to teach the practicing physician about the mind and the emotional sphere of man. The homeophatic materia medica deals exhaustively with all these, and therefore the homeopathic physician has the means to detect all disturbances, trace their origin, and treat them radically.

Homeopathy can attune, correct, and purify the human organism so that it functions with efficiency and sensitivity. This is absolutely essential. But true health is much more than this, and comes about when man has harmonized the whole of his being with his Creator.

Notes

[1] Quoted in S. Hahnemann, *Organon of the Art of Healing*, p. 46.
[2] Hippocrates, *Aphorisms*, author's translation from the Greek.

Suggestions for Further Reading

Harris Coulter, *The Divided Legacy*, vol. III, Wehawken Books,
——, *Homeophatic Medicine*.
James Kent, M.D., *Lectures on the Homeopathic Philosophy*.
C. H. Sharma, *A Manual of Homeopathy and Natural Medicine*.
Dorothy Shepherd, M.D., *Homeopathy for the First Aider*.
George Vithoulkas and Bill Gray, M.D., *The Science of Homeopathy: A Modern Textbook*.

These books are available by mail order from Homeopathic Educational Services, 2133 Derby Street, Berkeley, CA 94705, and from Yes! Books, 1035 31st, Washington, DC 20007. Send a self-addressed stamped envelope for price lists and lists of other available books.

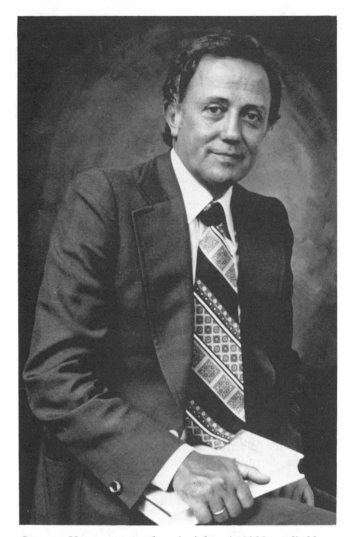

GEORGE VITHOULKAS, *born in Athens in 1932, studied homeopathy in South Africa and India, and introduced it into Greece in 1967. In 1971 he founded the Athenian School of Homeopathic Medicine and the Centre of Homeopathic Medicine. A member of several leading homeopathic societies, he has published articles in scientific journals, including "W.H.O.", and also two books,* Homeopathy Medicine of the New Man *and* The Science of Homeopathy, *now translated into many languages.*

Homeopathy: An Old Medical Science Re-emerges

Dana Ullman, M.P.H.

IT MAY be hard to believe, but it's true: at the turn of the century, 20–25 percent of urban physicians in the United States were homeopathic physicians. At this time there were also 22 homeopathic medical schools, over 100 homeopathic hospitals and more than 1000 pharmacies selling homeopathic medicine. These impressive statistics alone, however, do not give us the sense of the truly significant degree of influence that homeopathy had in the 1800s and early 1900s. Many of the country's professional, cultural, and business elite were patrons of homeopathy, including William James, John D. Rockefeller, Harriet Beecher Stowe, Henry Wadsworth Longfellow, Samuel F.B. Morse, Louisa May Alcott, Daniel Webster and numerous others.

Homeopathic medicine was growing so rapidly in the United States that in 1844 its practitioners formed the first national medical association, the American Institute of Homeopathy. In response to homeopathy's growing popularity, orthodox medicine took the offense. In 1847 they developed their own organization whose goal was, in part, to stop the growth of homeopathy. They called their organization the American Medical Association (AMA).

Shortly after the formation of the AMA, they established a "consultation clause" in their code of ethics that prohibited consultation with homeopaths or other "irregular" practitioners. Historians have noted that the AMA's ethical codes were very rarely enforced against orthodox medical doctors, except for the consultation clause. Astonishingly enough, an orthodox physician was expelled from his local medical society for consulting with a homeopath, even though this consultation was in reference to the treatment of Schuyler Colfax, the Vice President under Andrew Jackson. Another physician was expelled for consulting with a homeopath—his wife.

This consultation clause was finally rescinded in the early 1900s but not for any benevolent reasons. The AMA's new tactic was to give their full support to the Flexnor Report, sponsored by the Carnegie Foundation, on the status of medical education. The Flexnor Report recommended that public and private monies for medical schools should only be given to those institutions that emphasized the strict reductionistic biomedical model as epitomized at

Whole Life Times, 18 Shepard St., Brighton, MA 02135, November 1982. Reprinted by permission.

the time by the Johns Hopkins Medical School. Despite the popularity of homeopathy, other natural therapeutics, and the growing interest in psychology, the Flexnor Report considered these practices as unscientific and unworthy of further study.

(For further information on the history of homeopathy in the United States, see the bibliography for Dr. Harris L. Coulter's *Divided Legacy: The Conflict Between Homeopathy and the American Medical Association*.)

What Is Homeopathic Medicine?

The word "homeopathy" (also spelled "homoeopathy") is derived from two Greek words: "homoios" which means *similar* and "pathos" which means *disease* or *suffering*. Homeopathy is the medical science of using extremely small, non-toxic doses of plant, mineral, animal, or chemical substances which in overdose would have a similar effect of *causing* such a disease in a well person. The theory about how these substances work is that through potentization— or dilution to but a trace of its molecular form—all that remains of the substance is its template, its genetic information, its unique resonance. To call this resonance that remains an "energy" may be confusing; it is perhaps better called a "vibration." There is as yet no concrete evidence to define this resonance, but it has indeed been shown to be there in both laboratory and clinical experiments. This science of microdoses lines up homeopathy with other healing arts in what has come to be called the field of "energy medicine."

Both ancient and futuristic energy medicine deals with fields and forces. Included in this family of healing are acupuncture, therapeutic touch, and other bodywork practices, Reichian psychotherapy, and the use of electrical current to stimulate bone growth and wound healing (as used in the orthodox practice of orthopedic medicine). Homeopaths have done much research to discover the specific physical, emotional, and mental symptoms that various substances cause in overdose. Clinically, homeopaths extensively interview their patients to note their unique physical, emotional, and mental symptoms in detail. The homeopaths then look for the substance in nature which has the toxicology that matches the person's total symptoms.

Homeopathy in First Aid

Dana Ullman, M.P.H.

THE practice of classical homeopathy is a deep and exciting study with a lengthy history. It requires comprehension of an elaborate philosophy of health and disease, along with the systematic study of hundreds of homeopathic remedies and their psychophysiological personality.

The use of homeopathic remedies in first aid, however, doesn't require as in-depth a study as does classical homeopathy. In fact, any health practitioner or consumer can readily learn practical applications of homeopathic remedies in simple first-aid situations. Whereas a classical homeopath's treatment of a person with an acute or chronic syndrome requires strict individualization of the person's total body-mind symptoms, treatment for accidents and injuries tends to require less strict individualization. When different people cut themselves, get burned, or break a leg, they all need a similar metabolism to heal their injury. While people in diseased states require individualized treatment, homeopathic remedies in first-aid conditions are generally effective for specific conditions for people *or* animals.

It should be recognized that there will be times in first-aid conditions that individualization is needed and that greater knowledge of the homeopathic remedies is vital for the benefit of the injured person. Still, it is useful to know what remedies are most commonly given in specific conditions. Hopefully, your success with the remedies will stimulate you to study homeopathic philosophy and *materia medica* more deeply.

But why should a practitioner consider homeopathic remedies in first aid? The answers are simple:

1) There are few things a person can do for injuries other than resting and letting time pass.

2) The homeopathic remedies work very well, and sometimes rapidly, in building the person's ability to repair him/herself.

The use of other deep-acting therapies is not usually recommended when a person is receiving classical homeopathy for a chronic condition. Such therapies can, however, complement homeopathy in first-aid treatment (except for the use of herb teas, which sometimes can neutralize the remedies). It is also important to know that use of the remedies does not replace the standard practices of first aid or appropriate medical care.

Reprinted by permission from the monthly magazine *Let's Live*, March 1981, Copyright© Oxford Industries, 1981.

Care and Handling of Homeopathic Remedies

Most homepathic remedies are in pill or globule form after they have been "potentized" (a pharmaceutical process where one part of the remedy and nine parts solution are mixed and vigorously shaken; then they are diluted 1:9 and shaken again). The number of times the remedy is potentized is signified by an "x" (as in 6x, 30x). Homeopaths have empirically found that the more a substance is potentized, the deeper it can act within a person; and fewer doses are generally needed. *It is extremely important to remember that even though the remedies are very small in crude substance, they still are powerful in an energetic way and must be used with caution.*

Homeopathic remedies require special handling and storage so that they do not lose their power and become inert as the result of deterioration or contamination. If the remedies are handled correctly, they have been known to maintain potency for several generations. Since determination of a remedy's continued potency is only possible by frequently monitoring the extent of its clinical failure, the following precautions should be taken to ensure proper care of the remedies:

• *They* should be kept away from strong light, from temperatures higher than 100 degrees, and from exposure to strong odors like camphor, menthol, mothballs, or perfumes.

• *They* should always be kept in the container in which they were supplied and never transferred to any other bottle which has contained other subtances.

• *They* should be opened for administration of the remedy for the minimum time possible. One should be careful not to contaminate the cap or cork before replacement.

• *It* is important never to open more than one bottle at a time in a room. Failure to take this precaution can result in cross-potentization and spoiling of the remedies.

• *If,* by accident, more pills than the number specified in the prescribed dose are shaken out of the bottle, do not return them to the container; throw the excess away to avoid possible contamination.

Administration of the Remedy

Since homeopathic remedies first came into use, homeopaths have noted that certain substances could also neutralize a particular remedy's action. Much controversy swirls around which substances should and shouldn't be avoided. At the least, as a precaution, I believe clients should avoid the following substances for a minimum of 48 hours after taking their final dose: coffee, camphorated products (including tiger's balm, anti-chap lip balm, counter-irritant muscle relaxing creme), teas (including herb teas), mentholated products, cough drops, and mouthwash. It is generally recommended that coffee and camphor be avoided for longer periods in chronic cases.

The dose should be put into a "clean mouth." Food, drink, tobacco, toothpaste, and other substances should not be put into the mouth 15 minutes before or after the remedy. Allow the remedy to dissolve underneath the tongue before swallowing.

Homeopathic Pharmacies

To ensure that the remedies have been made correctly, always obtain them from a reliable homeopathic pharmacy. Following is a list of some of the leading homeopathic pharmacies in the United States:

Standard Homeopathic Pharmacy, P.O. Box 61067, Los Angeles, CA 90061.

John A. Bornemann & Sons, 1208 Amosland Rd., Norwood, PA 19074.

Boericke & Tafel, 1011 Arch St., Philadelphia, PA 19107.

Luyties Pharmacal Co., 4200 Laclede Avenue, St. Louis, MO 63108.

Humphreys Pharmacal Co., 63 Meadow Rd., Rutherford, NY 07070.

General Rules for Determining Dosage

Beginners in homeopathy can effectively use 6x or 30x remedies. The higher potencies (200x, 1000x, etc.) *should only be used by practitioners deeply knowledgeable about homeopathy.*

If a person is under homeopathic care, it is recommended that the person contact the homeopath to determine if another remedy at this time is appropriate.

An injured individual will tend to need more frequent doses shortly after the injury. In very severe cases this may mean every 30 to 60 minutes. After a couple of hours, the frequency of doses can spread to every other hour or every fourth hour, depending upon the severity of pain. In non-severe injuries, doses every four hours or four times a day are common. The most important rule for determining dosage, however, is severity of pain. Generally, a person will not need to take a remedy for more than two or three days, except in the case of a fracture or severe sprain, where the person may take one to three doses daily for five to seven days.

A remedy should be taken only for as long as the pain persists. Do NOT continue doses unless there are still symptoms (pain, swelling, etc.). If a person continues to take doses, he or she risks the possibility of experiencing a proving (overdose) of the remedy. **The basic idea is to take as little of the remedy as possible and yet enough to lessen pain and stimulate one's healing powers.** Generally, the more severe the condition, the more often will its repetition be necessary.

Following is a partial list specifying the characteristics and attributes of remedies recommended by homeopathic physicians for the conditions indicated or type of relief for which the remedy is traditionally used:

Arnica (Mountain Daisy)

—any shock or trauma from any injury! Arnica should be given in most first-aid injuries, either by itself or a few hours before another remedy is given;
—relieves pain, shock and swelling;
—before and after surgery (dental surgery, too!);
—before and after childbirth for the mother and for the infant (the remedies are very small and dissolve easily—no choking);
—for old injuries which still bother (especially head injuries);
—some toothaches!
—bruised or tired muscles from overwork (external application).

Internally: Arnica should be repeated as needed—anywhere from every 15 minutes to three times a day (*it depends upon severity*). 6x or 30x are most commonly used by beginners.

Externally: Available in mineral oil solution called "Arnica Oil." Put directly over bruised or tired muscle, but DO NOT USE EXTERNALLY IF SKIN IS BROKEN OR RAW, NOR IN THE EYES OR ANY MUCOUS MEMBRANES. It can be used in massage oils!

Calendula (Marigold)

—an anti-bacterial agent (prevents infection *and* promotes healing);
—*wounds with broken skin*; especially clean cuts, knife wounds, scratches, and abrasions;
—stops hemorrhage;
—good for sunburns and for *first-degree burns*;
—dilute the tincture or oil and use for a mouthwash in dental hemorrhages;
—for diaper rash in infants;
—tincture diluted, useful as an eyewash, especially for cuts on the cornea.

Externally only: Available in mineral oil (Calendula Oil) in tincture or in ointment. If you have the oil or ointment, you can put it directly on cut. If you have the tincture, it is better to dilute it.

Hypericum (St. John's Wort)

—a natural antiseptic;
—lacerated wounds, *septic (infected) wounds*;
—*injuries to nerves* or to parts of the body richly supplied with nerves, especially if wound is *sensitive to touch*, (examples: crushed fingers or toes, or falls on the spine);
—good for any shooting pain which was the result of injury;
—closes up open wounds;
—snake bites or any bite with shooting pains.

Internally: Take doses depending upon severity (same as Arnica as well as all the remedies in first aid).
Externally: Available in tincture only. Dilute tincture approximately 1:10 and put directly on wound.

Ledium (Marsh Tea)

—*puncture wounds* (rusty nails, needles, septic scratches);
—*bites and stings* (from animals, dogs, cats, wasps, mosquitoes, bees, and insect stings);
—severe bruising (black eyes, blows from firm objects);
—if affected part *feels cold* and feels *relieved by cold applications*, this is a good indication for Ledium's use (the part is not sensitive to touch and non-inflammatory—unlike Hypericum).

Internally only: Number of doses depending on severity.

Urtica Urens (Stinging Nettle)

—first-degree burns.

Internally: Whenever there is pain with a burn.
Externally: Dilute 10 drops tincture per ½ cup water (soak gauze pad, apply to burn, cover with cotton and bandage; renew when dry). Soaking burned part in lukewarm water directly after burning acts homeopathically.)
Second-degree burns: Causticum (internally); Hypericum (externally). Third-degree burns: Cantharis (internally and externally).
DO NOT FORGET ARNICA FOR THE SHOCK OF THE INJURY!
After initial healing, Calendula externally will prevent scarring.

Rhus Tox (Poison Ivy)

—ruptured ligaments and tendons near joints (*Sprains* and *Strains*);
—especially the type of sprain that is *worse upon initial motion, but better upon continued motion*;
—dislocation of lower jaw—use four hourly (not longer than two days);
—if injury is more severe where it wrenches tendons, splits ligaments, or bruises the bone or bone covering, RUTA is preferred. If this injury is not tolerable to any movement without pain, BRYONIA is recommended. If it is a muscle injury, ARNICA is advised. ARNICA can be applied externally in concomitance with internal medicine, except *not* in open or raw wounds.

Internally only: Number of doses dependent upon severity.

Ruta (Rue)

—acts upon torn and wrenched tendons, split ligaments of joints, and *bruised covering of bones* (periosteum);
—bruises to the kneecap, shin bone or elbow;
—synovities, inflammation of the ligaments, inflammation of the knee joints and wrist joints.

Internally only: Number of doses dependent on severity.

The logic of this pharmaceutical approach is that homeopaths (as well as most others who are involved in natural healing methods) recognize that symptoms are the organism's efforts to re-establish homeostasis and to heal itself. A person's defense system, however, is not always strong enough to heal itself fully, so symptoms tend to recur. Since the homeopathic medicine is prescribed specifically for its ability to create the similar symptoms that the person is experiencing, the medicine works *with* rather than *against* the person's efforts to heal him or herself.

This use of "similars" in medicine is both ancient and modern. Physicians and healers have used it and made reference to it throughout history and throughout the world.

In the 4the century B.C. Hippocrates wrote, "Through the like, disease is produced, and through the application of the like it is cured." There is also record of the use of the law of similars in ancient Egypt and China as well as in the Mayan civilization.

Conventional medicine today commonly uses the law of similars in its application of immunizations and allergy treatments. It also uses radiation to treat cancer (radiation causes cancer), digitalis for heart conditions (digitalis creates heart conditions), and ritalin for hyperactive children (ritalin is an amphetamine-like drug which normally causes hyperactivity). It is, however, important to note that homeopaths *very* rarely utilize any of the above treatments.

Aconite (Monkshood)

—acts similarly to Arnica which means that it is good for shock. However, it is good for people who are very anxious and fearful after their injury (Arnica's shock has more confusion and dullness).

Internally only: Number of doses dependent upon severity.

Symphytum (Comfrey)

—*fractures*;
—injuries to the periosteum (bone covering)—like Ruta;
—injuries to the eyeball, the bones around the eye, and the cheekbones.

Internally only: Three times a day for a few days and then perhaps once daily for no more than five to seven days (depending upon the severity of the fracture and the pain).

The following abbreviated list of eight homeopathic books is offered in the hope that it may help your understanding of homeopathy and aid you in the correct prescription of the homeopathic remedies:

Introductory and Self-Help Books

1) *Homeopathy: Medicine For The New Man*. George Vithoulkas. This book is the best introduction to homeopathy. It is written by one of the world's foremost contemporary homeopaths.
2) *Homeopathic Medicine*. Harris Coulter, Ph.D. This book is a good introduction to homeopathy, especially for health professionals.

3) *Homeopathic Medicine At Home*. Maeismund Panos, M.D., and Jane Heimlich. This book is the most comprehensive self-help book on homeopathy available today. The use of 28 homeopathic remedies are discussed for their use in injuries and acute conditions.

Books for the Serious Student or Practitioner of Healing

4) *The Science of Homeopathy: A Modern Textbook*. George Vithoulkas. This book is the most comprehensive up-to-date book on homeopathic principles and methodology.
5) *A Brief Study Course In Homeopathy*. Elizabeth Hubbard-Wright, M.D. This concisely written book clearly discusses the methodology of the homeopathic science.

Books for the Serious Student or Practitioner of Homeopathy

6) *Lectures On Homeopathic Materia Medica*. James Tyler Kent, M.D.
7) *Drug Pictures*. Margaret Tyler, M.D. This materia medica summarizes what some of the greatest homeopaths said about the most commonly prescribed remedies.
8) *Introduction To Homeotherapeutics*. Drs. Neiswander, Baker, and Young. This is a good materia medica to study in conjunction with others.

Most of these books can be obtained through Homeopathic Educational Services, 5916 Chabot Crest, Oakland, CA 94618. For a full booklist, prices, and additional homeopathy reference sources send self-addressed stamped envelope.

Although these therapies are in part based on the law of similars, they do not follow other important principles of homeopathy such as the use of the infinitesimal non-toxic doses, the strict individualization of a medicine to each person, and the use of only one medicine at a time. As a result of these differences, conventional medicine's treatments are often toxic and only temporarily relieve symptoms rather than deeply cure the person. These conventional treatments are not even considered homeopathic.

Homeopathy is as much an art as it is a science. The best homeopaths are those who are rationally oriented and can also draw ideas from intuition. Through interviewing a patient, the homeopath must amass a lot of information in a systematic way while intuiting the subtle emotional and mental characteristics of the person. The homeopath deals with a synergy of characteristics of an individual as well as a variety of toxicological symptoms.

SOME CONTROVERSY:
The Homeopathic Pharmaceutical Process

Whereas homeopathy's law of similars can be readily understood and accepted, homeopathy's special pharmaceutical process is its most controversial procedure. This process is called "potentization" and refers to a specific procedure of serial dilution. One part of a medicinal substance is diluted with nine parts distilled water or ethyl alcohol and then this solution is vigorously shaken. One part of this solution is diluted further with nine more parts distilled water or ethyl alcohol and then shaken. This process of dilution with shaking is continued 6 times, 30 times, 200 times, 1,000 times, 10,000 times or more (when a homeopathic medicine is labeled as 30x, this means that the dilution with shaking has been completed 30 times.) Homeopaths have not only found that the medicines work deeply to re-establish a person's health, they have generally found that the more a substance in potentized, the deeper it acts, and the less doses are needed.

There have been elaborate and eloquent writings in the scientific literature about how the homeopathic medicines work. Most homeopaths, however, are more interested in learning how to find the correct medicine for a person than why the medicines work. Despite the provocative theories about how the medicines work, this answer may, like the workings of most orthodox drugs today, remain a mystery.

Since a person's symptoms are their efforts to heal themselves, the homeopathic medicine provides an added informational message or stimulating resonance to the organism's defense system. In the same way that immunizations stimulate the person's defense system against a specific pathogen, the homeopathic medicine which is prescribed based on the *totality* of the person's symptoms is able to stimulate the person's *total* defense system.

Some argue that homeopathy has not been scientifically explained. But initial inaccurate explanations of gravity didn't disprove gravity's existence.

The wealth of experience of homeopathic physicians for almost 200 years in this country and throughout the world lends some evidence that there is something about their medicine that works. The historical fact that homeopathy gained its greatest popularity here and in Europe during the epidemics of the 1800s is further evidence that the medicines have a definite effect on people who are ill.

Hering's Law of Cure

But the homeopath does not just offer a therapeutic medicine and end the process there. If you just treat the symptom you only provide temporary relief. A holistic perspective to evaluating a person's progress toward health requires an analysis of all mind and body symptoms, which must be observed and compared over a period of time. Constantine Hering (1800–1880), the father of American homeopathy, recognized the importance of this perspective and noted through careful observation that there were three postulates of cure that described how one can determine if a person's health is improving or deteriorating. These postulates are called "*Hering's Law of Cure*" and are as follows:

1) Healing moves from the deepest part of the organism (the mental and emotional states as well as the vital organs) to the more superficial parts (the skin, muscles, ligaments, and extremities).
2) Healing flows from the upper part of the body to the lower parts.
3) Healing progresses in reverse chronological order of the appearance of symptoms.

A basic assumption behind these postulates is a definition of health that recognizes three different levels of a person's experience—the physical level, the emotional level, and the mental level. Health is defined as a state of freedom from limitation on any of these levels. The person thus experiences physical well-being, emotional centeredness, mental clarity and creativity. A person's overall state of health according to a homeopath is defined primarily by his mental state, secondarily by his physical state. Thus, a person with schizophrenic delusions with few chronic physical symptoms is generally considered by a homeopath to be more sick than a person who has chronic arthritic pain but who is relatively clear mentally and emotionally. There are of course exceptions to this general rule, for the major determinant is the degree to which a person's symptoms limit his/her freedom to live and act within the world.

Homeopaths are not the only practitioners who have postulated the existence of Hering's Law. Acupuncturists have witnessed aspects of this law for thousands of years. Naturopaths who guide their clients in long fasts and psychotherapists who lead their clients into deep psychotherapy have occasionally noted this phenomenon, too.

Classical Homeopathy

In my own practice I follow the path of the classical school of homeopathy which was developed by Dr. Samuel Hahnemann. James Kent took the science further and today George Vithoulkas of Greece is expanding it even further as president of the International Foundation of Homeopathy, an organization which trains professionals. Hahnemann emphasized that only one medicine at a time should be given to initiate a cure, even if the person had numerous and varied symptoms. He asserted that all the symptoms of a person are a part of a single diseased state. The one correctly chosen medicine stimulates the person's overall immune response system which begins the curative process of the person's various symptoms.

Finding the correct medicine for each individual is not always easy. The classical homeopath takes a lengthy interview of the person in order to obtain physical, emotional and mental symptoms. Notes are made of the various subtle symptoms of body language, human values, and idiosyncratic behavior. Sometimes a couple of visits and even a couple of different prescriptions are necessary before the right deep-acting medicine can be found.

Combinations

Recently, some American companies have begun massmarketing mixtures of homeopathic medicine. Distinct from the classical homeopathic approach which recommends taking only one medicine at a time, these "combination medicines" include three to six low-potency (usually 3x to 6x) remedies that are commonly given to treat a specific condition. Although many people are only recently learning about these combination medicines, these mixtures have been sold throughout this country and throughout the world since the beginning of homeopathy. In fact, at present, the combination medicines are more popular in Europe than the classical approach. In this country most homeopaths recommend only one medicine at a time, while consumers who are new to homeopathy and who don't know how to individualize the choice of a medicine to themselves tend to purchase combination medicines.

An example of a combination medicine would be to take four commonly used substances that a homeopath would use to treat the symptoms of a cold, and mixing these together in a single solution to create a new mixture which can treat a broad number of people. Such a combination might include weak potencies of *arsenicum* (arsenic) *allium cepa* (onion), *acontium* (monk's hood) and *kali bic* (potassium bichromate).

Classical homeopaths consider this is a shotgun approach to treat people who have individually different symptoms of a cold. The new mixtures create a different substance from the original components and have not yet been proven by homeopathic research.

Classical homeopaths assert that manufacturers of combination medicines should complete experimental "provings" of their medicines. (Provings are experiments where human subjects are given continual doses of a substance until toxic symptoms are developed. Whatever symptoms a substance creates in overdoses, it cures in potentized doses. All homeopathic medicines are "proven" in this way to determine their individual application.) When substances are mixed together, the mixture causes (and cures) some symptoms similar to its component parts, but most of its symptoms are unique to its new combination. Classical homeopaths therefore are concerned that consumers cannot know what a medicine is really effective for, without provings.

Despite this seemingly logical critique, people throughout the world have used the combination medicines with success in treating numerous types of acute conditions. The low potency combination medicines may sometimes effectively relieve pain and even stimulate a curative response; however, there is general recognition that they do not act as deeply in promoting cure as the single dose of the correctly chosen (often higher potency) medicine. Also, in some cases, the frequent use of combination medicines may make it more difficult for a classical homeopath to find the one best singular medicine for the person.

Some words of warning about homeopathy in general are that one should never take any medicine for prolonged periods of time. Nor should one frequently take different homeopathic medicines. Frequent dosages of homeopathic medicines can cause the person's present symptoms to get worse or new symptoms to develop.

The Status of Homeopathy Today

Homeopathic medicine is not well known today in the United States, but it is known and respected throughout the world. Virtually every country has its homeopaths. Homeopathy is particularly popular in India, where there are over 70,000 registered practitioners. It is also widely practiced in France, where approximately 6,000 M.D.s use homeopathy and 16 percent of the French public have tried the medicine. The Royal Family of England has been under homeopathic care since the mid-1800s, and homeopathy has begun to grow quite rapidly there. A recent survey published in the *British Medical Journal* (July 30, 1983) found that 80 percent of a random group of young physicians expressed interest in being trained in either homeopathy, acupuncture, or hypnosis.

Other countries where homeopathy is relatively popular include The Netherlands (where a recent government report noted that at least 20 percent of the Dutch people have gone to alternative practitioners and that homeopaths and acupuncturists were the most popular practitioners), Greece, Argentina, Brazil, Mexico, Pakistan, and the USSR.

There are no official statistics about homeopathic medicine in the United States. There are approximately 1,000 M.D.s involved in homeopathic practice and an equal number of other licensed professionals (dentists, veterinarians, nurses, physician assistants, naturopaths, chiropractors, acupuncturists, psychologists, etc.) practicing with homeopathic medicines. There are an uncertain number of lay practitioners.

Homeopathy can provide dramatic and lasting results in many people. However, it's unrealistic to expect impressive cures always. Chronic conditions tend to improve gradually, and between 20 to 50 percent of chronically ill people may get worse for a short period of time and then follow Hering's Law of Cure. For those whose lives have been effectively and permanently improved through homeopathy, it's well worth the wait.

Suggested Further Reading

Stephen Cummings, F.N.P. and Dana Ullman, M.P.H., *Everybody's Guide to Homeopathic Medicines*. Los Angeles: J. P. Tarcher, 1984.

George Vithoulkas, *The Science of Homeopathy*. New York: Grove, 1979.

Harris Coulter, Ph.D., *Homoeopathic Science and Modern Medicine: The Physics of Healing with Microdoses*. Berkeley: North Atlantic, 1981.

Harris Coulter, Ph.D., *Divided Legacy: The Conflict Between Homoeopathy and the American Medical Association*. Berkeley: North Atlantic, 1973.

Edward C. Whitmont, M.D., *Psyche and Substance: Essays on Homeopathy in Light of Jungian Psychology*. Berkeley: North Atlantic, 1980.

Source of Homeopathic Books, Tapes, & Medicine Kits

Homeopathic Educational Services
2124 Kittredge St.
Berkeley, CA 94704

Homeopathic Organizations

National Center for Homoeopathy
1500 Massachusetts, N.W. #41
Washington, DC 20005

International Foundation for Homeopathy
1141 NW Market St.
Seattle, WA 98107

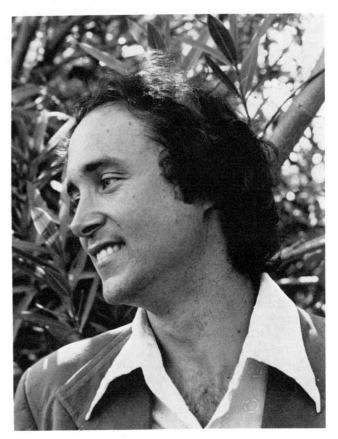

DANA ULLMAN, M.P.H., *co-authored* Everybody's Guide to Homeopathic Medicines *(Tarcher, 1984) and is one of the pioneers of the resurgence of homeopathy. He directs Homeopathic Educational Services, a comprehensive mail order service of homeopathic books, tapes, medicines, medicine kits, and general information on homeopathy. He has also organized conferences on alternative health care for U.C. Berkeley, federal health agencies, and other institutions and community organizations. Dana is also known for his work on legal issues of alternative health care. In 1976 he was arrested for practicing medicine without a license. He won an important court settlement in 1977 and then was almost successful in getting the California medical board to consider changing the law based on proposals by him and some colleagues.*

III

Tools for Keeping Healthy

INTRODUCTION *by Naomi Steinfeld*

WHAT IS HEALTH, and how can the tools in this section help you find and maintain it?

We suffer from an excess of fragmentation and specialization. We develop one aspect of ourselves—one area of personality, one area of knowledge—and then we come to identify with that one aspect as "all there is." But somewhere, in some deep, unrecognized place within us, we remember that there is more—other parts of ourself, other, radically different perspectives from which to know our worlds (those worlds that range from inner-subjective to physical body to social body to cosmic). And that place which recalls that something more—that place from which we recall (though dimly) the wholeness—calls out again and again, like a loving, all-forgiving parent to a lost, bewildered, angry child. That place re-calls: "Come back; all is well; come home."

Thus, this section could just as well be titled, "A Call to Wholeness" as "Tools for Keeping Healthy." These articles *are* tools, of course—in the sense that anything that helps you turn individual components (fragments) into something new, distinct, and usable is a tool. A hammer is a tool, and a computer is a tool, and writing an article is a tool, and reading (i.e., receiving) that writing is a tool. So this is an energetic, dynamic process, this giving and using of tools.

The material contained in the pages of this section represents the two levels of communication:

• *The exhale.* This itself has three levels:

—The accumulated seekings and findings of many dedicated people;

—Their self-posed questions, and the research they have done in the course of attempting to answer these questions; and

—The traffic signs they have posted along the way for those who come after them: "SLOW DOWN—BUMPY ROAD AHEAD"; "BE CAREFUL IN THE FAST LANE—THERE ARE DEEP, HARD-TO-SEE POTHOLES"; "IF YOU'RE SLEEPY, PULL OVER AND REST—DON'T JUST DRINK COFFEE, POP UPPERS, AND LISTEN TO LOUD MUSIC TO KEEP AWAKE"; and so on.

• *The inhale.* To the extent that you can receive it, the material in this section (and in the entire book, for that matter) represents the opportunity for you to take *in*—to grapple with these questions in a way that is personally meaningful to you, and thus to make the questions (and perhaps the authors' answers) your own.

The particular aspects addressed in this section are not all-inclusive; admittedly, they are aspects, parts, pieces. But they span a multileveled range, from physiological to sensorial to emotional to intellectual to intuitional to spiritual; they speak (if you will listen) to different levels of yourself. Some levels you may be quite intimately and expertly familiar with. Perhaps you have devoted many years to eating well, or to meditating, or to reducing stress, or to alternative medicine. Other levels may be brand-new to you—for example, have you ever considered the human-relations consequences of the computer revolution? Have you ever considered the possibility of surgery as a collaborative, healing experience? Have you ever considered the possibility of using the mind's capacity for seeing inner images—the ability to visualize—to dispense with the need for surgery altogether? What about music—is it more than supermarket jingles and Top 40 entertainment? Does it have any innate properties that relate to healing? Can we be "tuned" like instruments? And are our dreams and nightmares only products of indigestion (as Dickens' Ebenzer Scrooge suggests), or are they messages to our waking minds that have the same energizing, dynamic, healing capabilities as the words in these pages?

You can begin reading anywhere—with what you already know, or with what you don't know. There is no wrong place to start; there is no wrong place to go from there. Whatever in you calls out for wholeness will help you call forth exactly that which you need in order to become your fuller self. To become whole.

So here are the tools. By opening up this book, you have called them forth. Use them well; build what you need built.

A. AWARENESS

Biofeedback:
A Mind-Over-Body Matter

John E. Alle

CAN YOU train your mind to control your health? Leading physicians and scientific researchers around the world say you can—through biofeedback.

Biofeedback, a relaxation technique less than 20 years old, enables people to gain control over some bodily functions previously thought to be "involuntary." Biofeedback can help alleviate many ailments, including: high blood pressure, migraine headaches, muscle spasms, back and neck pain, asthma, general tension, cerebral palsy, epilepsy, some heart problems, rheumatoid and osteoarthritis, drug and alcohol withdrawal, and some psychosomatic illnesses.

What Is It?

Biofeedback is basically the conscious monitoring of internal body states. By watching and/or listening to sensitive recording machines—or amazingly simple home devices—you can learn to control many internal body processes. For most of Western medical history, these functions, for example, blood pressure, were regarded as completely involuntary and beyond conscious control. But now, with the advent of biofeedback, researchers—and an increasing number of health consumers—are discovering that our ability to control our own bodies has been greatly underestimated.

Even if you have never heard of biofeedback, chances are you've used it sometime in your life. When you stand on a bathroom scale, for example, you receive immediate "feedback" about your weight. Thermometers, blood pressure cuffs, stethoscopes and other instruments that display information about the body are also biofeedback devices. None of these instruments does anything *to* you. Each relays information about some aspect of your body's functioning. Some kinds of biofeedback are available without any instruments at all; you can take your pulse by simply placing a finger on your wrist.

In biofeedback training, you use the information about the body process you're monitoring to learn how to change that process voluntarily. With a little instruction and daily practice, almost anyone can learn to regulate pulse rate, body temperature, muscle tension or other internal processes.

Kansas State University Professor David Danskin, Ph.D., a psychologist who heads the Applied Biofeedback Laboratory there, said that in biofeedback, people take "a more active role in their treatment of their health problems by learning how to regulate voluntarily the body functions that may be causing them. The biofeedback user is, to a degree, both patient and doctor."

Some of the most widely publicized results of biofeedback have been achieved by psychologist Elmer Green, Ph.D., head of the Voluntary Controls Program at the Meninger Foundation in Topeka, Kansas. Green has taught migraine headache sufferers to eliminate their headaches and to prevent new ones by altering their skin temperatures, one measure of relative physical tension.

How to Begin

Ultimately, our goal may be to rely solely on one of the inexpensive, do-it-yourself home biofeedback devices now available (see Resources), but people experienced with biofeedback advise the novice to begin with the assistance of a trained professional instructor. Learning the correct technique is essential for long-lasting results, and for most people, the training takes only a few 45-minute sessions a week for two to four weeks. In addition, most biofeedback trainers assign home exercises between sessions: practicing various breathing techniques, listening to recorded instructions, or practicing on small home biofeedback machines.

Suppose you've been diagnosed as having migraine headaches. If your physician tells you you're too tense and need to relax more, biofeedback may help. If you cannot obtain a referral to a biofeedback training clinic from friends or a local holistic health practitioner, The Biofeedback Society of America or the American Association for Biofeedback (see Resources) should be able to provide a referral in your area.

At the clinic, you will probably be asked to lie down and shut your eyes while the trainer attaches several surface electrodes, coated with conducting fluid, to your forehead. The electrodes are connected to an electromyograph (EMG) machine, which monitors muscle tension. First, you can expect to hear a high-pitched tone that indicates that the

From *Medical Self-Care*, P.O. Box 1000, Point Reyes, CA 94956, Fall 1982, and reprinted by permission.

muscles in your forehead are tense. Then the trainer will probably begin describing a series of pleasant images to help you relax. As you relax, the tension should begin to flow out of the muscles in your forehead and the pitch of the tone should drop. Greater relaxation drops the pitch further, until finally, it becomes a low hum, which signals that your forehead muscles are relaxed. At first, the process usually takes 30 to 45 minutes, but when it's over, you may well notice that your headache has improved or disappeared.

After several training sessions where you turn those high-pitched tones into low hums, you'll probably be able to repeat the process successfully almost anywhere to reduce headache pain or eliminate it entirely.

Machines similar to EMGs may inform you of relaxation progress by beeps, blinking lights or a fluctuating needle on a dial. Most inexpensive home devices measure skin temperature.

No matter which biofeedback machine you learn on, once you have mastered the technique to control stress or other nervous reactions, there is no longer any need for the more complex machines.

The Importance of a Good "Coach"

The role of the biofeedback trainer—the physician, nurse, psychologist, or other therapist—is crucial to learning the skill properly.

"Biofeedback takes time, effort, practice and a good coach," Dr. Melvyn Werbach, M.D., director of the Biofeedback Medical Clinics in Beverly Hills and Tarzana, California, explained. "Biofeedback trainers give support, manage training exercises, and have to be psychologically sensitive to their trainees."

Dr. Lee Baumel, M.D., director of the Brotman Medical Center's biofeedback department in Culver City, California, said, "If people can eliminate their symptoms in the biofeedback room, but not outside it, we haven't accomplished our goal."

Most authorities suggest that beginners arrange at least one 45-minute training session per week, with practice sessions at home for 20 minutes twice a day.

Biofeedback for Rehabilitation

Some victims of stroke and paralysis have used biofeedback to help them regain muscle function. To move a partially paralyzed arm or leg, there has to be sensory input to the brain as well as motor output. For example, a football place-kicker who loses his sight cannot kick field goals consistently. But if different buzzers sound depending on where he places his kicks, he can relearn place-kicking by substituting sound for sight. Biofeedback instruments can make similar sensory substitutions for stroke and paralysis victims. The person learns to monitor muscle activity through a different sense. Eventually most patients regain at least partial reuse of "paralyzed" muscles or limbs.

Dr. John V Basmajian, M.D., professor of Medicine and director of rehabilitation services at Emory University in Atlanta, has used biofeedback with more than 500 rehabilitation patients. "We never succeed in restoring full function," he said, "but we can restore some useful function."

At the Casa Colina Hospital Rehabilitative Medicine Center in Pomona, California, a man who had worn a leg brace for two and a half years because of a stroke explained how he used biofeedback for rehabilitation: "I would practice every day, one hour in the morning and one hour at night. I'd practice starting and stopping the noise from the machine about 600 times an hour. In three or four weeks, I was able to control my ankle and strengthen it to the point where I got rid of the brace."

Does Biofeedback Work for Everyone?

Probably not. Success in biofeedback depends mostly on the type of ailment and on the degree of concentration the person invests in the training. Doctors explain that biofeedback may not work if a person has serious psychological problems or if severe pain prevents adequate concentration. Personal motivation also plays a key role. According to Werbach, two-thirds of the people in his clinics who attend the basic series of 10 sessions show clear improvement by the end.

With proper training, biofeedback researcher Dr. Elmer Green said, biofeedback clients have "approximately an 80 percent success rate in reducing or eliminating their ailments. But some patients are so used to thinking that there must be drugs or other cures for them they can't believe they can control their disorders themselves."

The Future: What Are the Limits?

The future of biofeedback is uncertain because currently no one knows the limits of mind over body. Proponents of biofeedback hope for the day when it may be used to alleviate and prevent more stress-related ailments, from ulcers to skin problems. There is even the possibility that biofeedback might be applied to ovulation control and be used for contraception in the future.

Dr. Werbach said he thought the next five years would see dramatic new uses for biofeedback: "There are many other symptoms we hope to treat very soon." New biofeedback equipment is beginning to help people who from birth have been unable to control their bowels. It has also helped insomniacs learn to sleep and people suffering from hyperdrosis, excessive sweat production, learn to control that problem.

As with any new and unconventional therapy, however, some doctors have expressed fears that seriously ill people may fall victim to unscrupulous practitioners who advertise biofeedback as a cure-all. That's why it's important to check your trainer's credentials. Several times during the last 10 years, the federal Food and Drug Administration has acted against manufacturers who have made unsubstantiated claims that their biofeedback devices "cured" ulcers or high blood pressure. Biofeedback is not a cure; it's a relaxation technique that has medical applications.

"Exaggerated claims have been made from time to time," biofeedback researcher David Danskin said. "It's still new and we're still experimenting with it."

For now, biofeedback should be considered a useful adjunct to conventional medical treatment. But in the future, it may possibly change the way physicians practice medicine. Instead of treating people after they become ill, doctors may spend more of their time teaching biofeedback—and other stress-reduction skills—to help people stay healthy.

How to Select a Home Biofeedback Machine

If you want to learn to relax more effectively, you need not wait until a biofeedback training center opens near you. Home biofeedback devices are now a big business, and several are amazingly simple and inexpensive.

There are two types of biofeedback devices: home trainers that are quite accurate and cost as little as $25, and sophisticated clinical machines that can provide several different types of biofeedback as well as research-oriented, data-gathering capabilities and may cost up to $20,000.

If you simply wish to gain better control over nervous tension, one of the many home devices should be sufficient. Usually you need to use the device for only three or four weeks to master the skill and learn to control your target body process. After that, you should be able to do it without the aid of the device.

Several home biofeedback devices are based on the observed correlation between skin temperature and internal tension. Stress cools the skin; relaxation warms it. Dr. Tim Lowenstein offers an inexpensive temperature gauge as a biofeedback instrument (see Resources). A tiny sensor, usually placed on one finger, detects minute changes of less than one-tenth of a degree. Lowenstein also sells relaxation tapes.

Bob Kall has developed a home biofeedback device similar to Lowenstein's. It's an attractive finger ring thermometer with a liquid crystal display mounted in the center (see *Futurehealth* in Resources).

If you decide to spend more money for a sophisticated biofeedback machine, comparison shop. Match the machine with your needs. Check the machine's detection capabilities and make sure the feedback is delivered in a form that suits you. Verify all the advertising claims before you purchase and, if possible, consult with a professional trainer. Also, select a machine that offers a warranty.

Many organizations now produce relaxation tapes for use in conjunction with biofeedback (see Resources). Also, you might find them at your local public library. More and more libraries buy and lend relaxation cassettes.

Resources

For more information about biofeedback, contact:

The Biofeedback Society of America
4301 Owens Street
Wheat Ridge, CO 80030
(303) 422-8436

American Association of Biofeedback
2424 Dempster Street
Des Plaines, IL 60016
(312) 827-0440

New Mind, New Body
Barbara Brown, Ph.D.
  1974; 464 pages
  $9.95 from
  Harper and Row
  10 East 53rd Street
  New York, NY 10022
  A useful, valuable, accessible book on the development of biofeedback.

Biofeedback: An Introduction and Guide
David Danskin, Ph.D., and M. Crow, Ph.D.
  1981; 150 pages
  $9.95 from
  Mayfield Publishing, Co.
  285 Hamilton Avenue
  Palo Alto, CA 94301
  A concise, readable overview of biofeedback.

Beyond Biofeedback
Dr. Elmer Green and Alyce Green
  1977; 369 pages
  $10.95 from
  Dell Publishing
  1 Dag Hammarskjold Plaza
  New York, NY 10017
  Two prominent biofeedback researchers discuss their work in the field and speculate on how and why biofeedback works.

Conscious Living Foundation
P.O. Box 513
Manhattan, KS 66502
(913) 539-2449
  Distributes a free catalog that contains the small hand-held biofeedback thermometer and relaxation tapes of Tim Lowenstein, Ph.D.

Emmett Miller Tapes
P.O. Box W
Stanford, CA 94305
(415) 328-7171
  Another good source of relaxation tapes. Catalog free; sample cassette with selections from 10 different tapes, $2.00.

Self-Health Institute
Route 2, Welsh Coulee
La Crosse, WI 54601
  Also sells relaxation tapes.

Echo, Inc.
P.O. Box 87
Springfield, OH 45501
(513) 322-4972
  Another source of small handheld biofeedback thermometers. Best price for orders of 500 or more.

Futurehealth, Inc.
Dept. P-100
P.O. Box 947
Bensalem, PA 19020
(215) 752-7665
  Sells Bob Kall's liquid crystal display thermometer rings and relaxation tapes.

William S. Kroger, M.D.
BK Enterprises
P.O. Box 6248
9478 Olympic Boulevard
Beverly Hills, CA 90212
  Excellent source of relaxation tapes.

JOHN E. ALLE *is a freelance health and science writer based in Los Angeles.*

Psychotherapy for a Crowd of One

Gita Elguin-Bödy, Ph.D., and Bart Bödy, Ph.D.

To be made whole we must learn how to integrate the multifaced nature of our being. If different aspects of our personality are in conflict, we cannot expect to find harmony in our environment. This internal battle will be constantly projected onto the external world.

This article gives methods for expressing our many parts without overidentifying with them. By using these techniques we can gain a fuller knowledge of self and a greater ability to live in the world.

 URKING WITHIN each of us is a vast and varied assortment of "subpersonalities." Each of these subpersonalities represents a complex of tendencies which, in its drive to be expressed, has developed an identity and character of its own. In other words, it was born out of some physical or psychological need. But then, as it gained autonomy, it may well have developed its own axe to grind—often at the expense of other subpersonalities; as well as of the individual whose needs were the original reason for its existence.

The cast of characters is not fixed or static. As with any group, the members are constantly changing, interacting, developing, regressing. One character may strut on center stage for a time, then retire to the wings. New members appear; old ones fade out. Subpersonalities, like people, have their own life cycles: they are born, develop and grow, take on new features, fuse with ("marry") other subpersonalities, and also die.

Few individuals ever suspect that they are hosting a whole crowd of subpersonalities within them. Most people may be dimly aware of perhaps one or two. We do not readily recognize what is going on, because we are continually identifying with one or another of these subpersonalities, and are not able to view the scene as a whole. Just as in sleep we may dream ourselves to be a child, a general, or a circus performer, so in our waking life we may act the part of "The Boss," "Flirt," "Doubter," "Adventurer," or "Lonely Child" according to the pull of circumstances. Asleep or awake, we are tricked into believing that we *are* the role we happen to be playing at the moment.

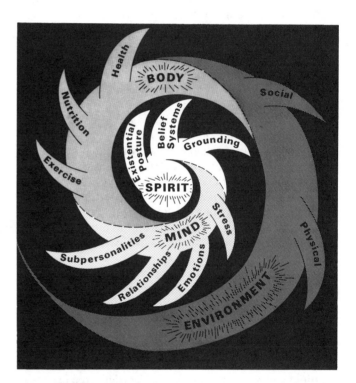

Losing sight of the overall picture, we confine our expression in a given situation to the repertoire of just the one subpersonality that "pops up" from force of habit. However, by identifying with just one subpersonality, we limit ourselves. Allowing the press of circumstances to make these choices for us dampens our spontaneity and reduces our effectiveness.

As we make the acquaintance of our various subpersonalities and work with them, we begin to see ourselves as separate and distinct from each of them, as well as from the sum total of the cast of characters. Thus we learn to dis-identify from any and all subpersonalities, to gain conscious control over them, and to get in touch with who we really are. Understanding the various components of our personality in relation to our own real self, we are able to grow and find fulfillment at a higher level. By attaining command over these disparate components, we become far more effective in dealing with internal conflicts as well as the outside world.

Making the Acquaintance of the Inner Crowd

As we first try to get in touch with our inner cast of characters, our position is akin to that of a myopic director faced with a group of actors fighting for the director's chair instead of the spotlight. The first step in getting the act together is to coax each of them, one after another, up to front stage center, into the spotlight of consciousness, and have them practice their lines at the same time, we must enforce the off-limits sign on the director's chair. Any problem that is unresolved or incompletely worked through will serve as the psychological "stage."

Suppose the problem has to do with your boss, who has been riding you to be more efficient, more punctual, more dedicated, etc., etc. You see his point, you would like to be all this, but you feel that there is more to life than just following a routine. You dream of faraway places, of all the things you would have liked to do, but have had to put off. So part of you wants to rebel, to cut loose. But another part says, "Wait a minute, you can't just throw your security overboard. Joe Blow would give his eyeteeth to have your job."

Once you have identified the problem that you want to work with in this way, you explore both sides of it. Psychological phenomena are always shadowed by their opposites. When a particular quality or tendency is overdeveloped or given free rein for a time, the pendulum will eventually begin to swing back and reveal the existence of the exact opposite quality or tendency. Let us say you begin by focusing on the part of you that wants security. You identify with it and try to feel its essence. Then you let the feelings that come up coalesce into the image of a person that would exemplify it for you, and you give this "person" an appropriate name. Let us suppose that the image which comes to you when you feel this part of yourself is a business type called "Secure." You proceed to explore this aspect of yourself until you know just how it feels about the situation.

Then you let go of "Secure" and turn to the complementary aspect. Perhaps the image which comes to you this time is that of a carefree, adventuresome adolescent. He has long hair, wears jeans, and is smiling and unencumbered. You baptize him "Adventurer."

You have now assisted in the "birth" of two of your subpersonalities. Actually, they were there before, but now you have deliberately and consciously made their acquaintance. Of course, you still have a problem. One subpersonality wants the security of his job; the other one wants to drop out and go wandering off. Since they have just one vehicle through which to express their desires—your body—they cannot both do what they want at the same time. In short, their conflict is your conflict.

To find out why each of these characters wants what he wants, you may start a dialogue between them. To give them voice, you alternately identify with one and then the other. Probably to your surprise, you will soon discover that what they originally said they *wanted* is not what they *really need*. Yet they are stuck with these wants because they know of no better way to satisfy their real needs.

Very likely, as you prod "Secure" to tell you why he wants to hang onto the job, he will first say that he wants it for the money and power it brings him; and he wants these in order to feel secure; and he wants the security in order to have respect, admiration, and love. So it turns out that what "Secure" really needs is love, but he does not know how to go about getting it directly and seeks it in this roundabout way.

A similar clarification develops when you explore "Adventurer's" motives. Why does he want to be footloose? To escape an oppressive situation. And why escape? Because he cannot handle it. Why not? Because he is too weak. What does he really need then? Strength.

Apparently "Secure" is after money and power, but really needs love; and "Adventurer" is out to travel, but really needs strength. But why does one need love, and the other strength? Going one step deeper, you may find that these two subpersonalities share an even more basic need: to feel good. But they have approached this common need from opposite directions. One has tried to compensate for lack of love by striving for money and power. The other feels too weak to cope and wants to run away from it all. Neither has confronted the problem squarely, and therefore neither has succeeded and neither is satisfied. In the process, "Secure" has become overdeveloped, at the expense of "Adventurer," in whom possibilities for creativity and self-realization lie untapped.

As you continue to work with "Secure" and "Adventurer," other subpersonalities will begin to emerge, and to define and redefine themselves. The appearance and feelings of specific subpersonalities change from one session to the next, depending on their experiences in the interim: who has been in control, who has been inactive, how they felt about themselves and others, how they related to the world, etc. Moreover, a subpersonality may suddenly shrink, expand, change features, or split in two.

The theater of guided fantasy is the basic mechanism for allowing the cast of characters to present themselves and play their parts. They are brought together as a group, where they learn to recognize each other, to interact with greater awareness, to tolerate, accommodate, and even appreciate one another. This procedure is exactly analogous to conventional group therapy, but with one major difference: all members of the group reside in and express themselves through one body.

Resolving the Internal Conflict

Perhaps you are wondering what happened to "Adventurer" and "Secure." Left to their own devices, they would probably continue struggling and bickering. Possibly they might alternate in satisfying their respective wants, by taking ten days in Hawaii and working hard the rest of the year. Or "Adventurer" may break out with a six-month beachcomber tour and then again be submerged for a year or two. Some people even go for years, working hard during the day and drinking hard at night, or going on a bender every other weekend. But this sort of alternation (or time-sharing) is not a solution, because when "Secure" is in control, you feel encaged, and when "Adventurer" is having his fling, you feel guilty. In either case, you wind up with neither love nor strength, much less a sense of fulfillment. Of course, the real issue is not which subpersonality gets its way, but rather whether their/your real needs are met. And meeting these real needs may well require a fuller integration involving other subpersonalities, not just "Adventurer" and "Secure."

The overall goal is for each subpersonality to work in harmony with all the rest, and for you, acting from your center, to be fully aware and directing the show at all times. The process for reaching this goal is a dialectic dance with no prescribed rules or steps. However, there are some common patterns that may be summarized in the following six stages.

1. *Accepting each subpersonality.* It is important to realize that, no matter how negative a given subpersonality may appear, there is a good reason for its existence; it has something to contribute to the total personality.

2. *Developing the subpersonalities that have been suppressed or held back.* This may initially threaten other subpersonalities that have been holding center stage. Such problems can be resolved by increased communication among them. They may require special attention and nurturing.

3. *Harmonizing all subpersonalities.* As they learn to cooperate with each other, their negative traits tend to cancel out and the positive ones to complement one another.

4. *Integrating all subpersonalities around a unifying center of awareness and volition.* As you dis-identify yourself from specific subpersonalities, you begin to experience the center of your being—the "I"—as free and independent of the cast of internal characters, but fully in control of their behavior.

5. *Expanding the "I" into transpersonal and transcendental dimensions.* The "I" is experienced as a reflection of a universal principle of consciousness, the "Higher Self."

6. *Facilitating concrete behavioral changes which reflect the expanding awareness and integration within, as well as greater harmony with relation to family, society, and cosmos.* As you experience yourself more freely and completely, you will find your possibilities in the external world enhanced and potentiated.

Basic Techniques

These stages are attained by creative use of a variety of techniques and procedures, carried out with the help of a knowledgeable guide. Some of the more basic ones are described below.

Guided fantasy.

An essential preliminary is to relax deeply, both physically and mentally (often in a comfortable, prone position) with the mental set: "I am taking a recess from life's problems. I dedicate these moments exclusively to myself." The next step is to conjure up a structured fantasy or guided daydream, usually starting out with a peaceful, relaxing scene, such as lying on a beach or a meadow. Third, specific, subpersonalities are explored, generally by identifying their attitudes toward a current problem or situation.

Intraindividual group process.

Relaxed and aware, you visualize your subpersonalities sitting in a circle, and report on how they look and what they feel at that moment. The subpersonalities are then encouraged to interact with one another. As longstanding or short-range conflicts emerge, they may experience feelings of hurt, fear, anxiety, anger, or possibly ambivalence or some form of positive feelings. They are encouraged to express these feelings directly, in a straightforward manner. Generally, one overriding theme develops, and all the subpersonalities focus on working it through. Toward the end, the group usually arrives at some form of resolution.

Identification and disidentification.

You identify with a specific subpersonality by imagining that you are one with it, that you *are* it. This gets you in touch with its history, its needs, its conditions and ways of behaving. The best way to achieve identification is through guided fantasy, though in some situations "acting" or "role-playing" may be more appropriate. In either case, it is easy to tell when a person has "gotten into" a subpersonality because the whole countenance and bearing change accordingly.

Dis-identification is the opposite: taking an attitude of detached witnessing. This technique enables you to distance your self and achieve a broader, more objective perspective. It is especially useful when you feel trapped inside a given role, feeling, or attitude, and cannot let it go.

The "Independent Observer."

This technique is a process of dis-identification from *all* subpersonalities. You take the position of an outside spectator, impartially observing all aspects of the situation. This is often quite useful for resolving an impasse. The "Independent Observer" usually proves to be a very insightful personage, and using it will make you realize how much common sense and wisdom you possess within yourself.

Role playing

You enact a conflict, alternately taking the part of one subpersonality and then the other, in a developing dialogue. When an impasse occurs, you may need to call in— act out—the "Independent Observer."

All these techniques can be applied not just to subpersonalities, but to any feelings, thoughts, states of consciousness, habits, ideal models, or bodily processes. They may be practiced as part of the guided fantasy, in the normal waking state, during the sessions or as part of your homework between sessions.

Cross-Individual Interactions

The game gets more complicated when several people interact, each bringing his or her own set of subpersonalities that have already been identified and have interacted with one another within their own (intraindividual) groups. Although each set shares many elements with every other, the possible combinations and variations are endless.

The individuals in the group begin by introducing themselves, both as distinct individuals and as a group of subpersonalities. This may be extended into a discussion of the development of each subpersonality, the emergence of new subpersonalities, the resulting balance of forces, and the problems they are currently working on: people are very happily surprised to find counterparts to many of their own subpersonalities, and their dynamics, among the cast of characters that others bring.

Whether you work individually or in a group, the basic task is the same: individuation of specific parts of the personality and their harmonious reintegration, around an aware center. Because there is only one person involved, individual work can be more direct and "clean": the areas of conflict can be dealt with one at a time, and the pace adjusted to each individual. Also, the guided fantasy is more flexible in this context. But the group procedure has its advantages, too. By sharing discoveries and experiences, individuals can increase their own growth. The group process is more complex, more fast-moving; incongruities are more vividly exposed, and group members share and compare perceptions among themselves. Since this process is essentially an exponential version of the individual work already described, the techniques used are basically the same, only expanded and adapted to the group context.

Collectively guided fantasy.

In a collective guided fantasy, group members are asked to focus on any two subpersonalities, have them perform some task together, and be aware of how they interact: who takes the lead, how they share responsibilities, whether they can accomplish the task, etc. Later all members can simultaneously role-play—preferably nonverbally—first one subpersonality, and then the other. In this way subpersonalities of different members come in direct contact.

Feedback.

During group interaction, members learn to become more aware of how their subpersonalities affect other members of the group and how they, in turn, are affected by the subpersonalities of others. They exchange this information, and express their perceptions and reactions to others' subpersonalities.

Dramatization.

Conflicts between your own subpersonalities, or between your own and others' subpersonalities are acted out, with group members playing specific roles in the conflict and identifying with them. To help confront a specific situation, members may be asked to act through only the one subpersonality which is being kept hidden. The rest of the group members pay attention to the reactions of their own subpersonalities, and later relay this information back to the individual.

"Independent Observer."

This can be acted out by the same individual whose conflicts are being dealt with, or by another member of the group.

Group meditation.

Meditation techniques can be used to further group integration as well as personal synthesis.

A System for Physical, Psychological, and Spiritual Growth

There is no definite list of techniques for this work, because new ones continue to evolve and old ones are adapted in novel ways. As therapists and patients learn from each other, they are constantly devising new techniques to fit the needs and dynamics of specific individuals and their subpersonalities: some only to be used on the spot and then forgotten; others to be added to the repertoire and used again and again.

Some techniques have been adapted from sources as diverse as Gestalt therapy and Behavior Modification. For example, you may find that a given situation triggers undesirable reactions that you try in vain to control: perhaps the subpersonalities that tend to react constructively are overshadowed by others that are inappropriate to the situation but are too well-entrenched. To reinforce the operation of the constructive subpersonalities, some directive techniques can be profitably employed, such as progressive desensitization or cognitive behavior therapy.

To keep such efforts from being sabotaged by a recalcitrant subpersonality, it is important to start off by getting a general consensus of the entire group, to let them express their feelings about the proposed changes, and to solicit their commitment to cooperate or at least not to interfere.

But identification and dis-identification are the most fundamental tools in the development and harmonization of the subpersonalities. These two techniques can also be used to gain control over bodily processes, to change specific habit patterns, and to aid in transpersonal and transcendental unfoldment.

For example, any physical illness will generally involve one or more of the subpersonalities as well as the host individual. If the illness is acute, some or all subpersonalities will be temporarily affected. In a chronic illness, on the other hand, it is often just one subpersonality that "owns" the illness—usually the one that the individual tends to identify with the most—whereas the rest enjoy good health. A basic strategy in combating such illness is to make this subpersonality take responsiblity for its state of health. One tactic is to uncover that subpersonality's investment in the illness and find a way to meet its needs in a more constructive fashion. Another ploy might be to identify with one of the subpersonalities that remains healthy. Pain may be dealt with by dis-identifying from it and taking the "Independent Observer" position.

Identification/dis-identification may also be helpful in acquiring a good habit. For example, you may visualize a subpersonality that typifies the desired quality, and then invite it to join the rest of the subpersonalities in the intraindividual group. There may well be some initial resistance from the "older members," but this can be dealt with in the same way as any other conflict within the group. To overcome qualities and habits that are not desired, it is generally best to dis-identify from them and identify with their desirable counterparts; this is much more effective than simply opposing them.

Identification/dis-identification is the basic mechanism

underlying various techniques of meditation. For instance, one way to overcome restlessness is to focus the awareness fully on the restlessness and then to shift the consciousness to the center, adopting the attitude of witness, one totally detached from the restlessness and its causes. Meditating Buddhists and yogis practice a technique of "watching the breath," for breathing is considered a major source of restlessness. The effect of this simple "watching" is to make the breath slow down or even be suspended for an indefinite period. Other bodily processes are likewise stilled, the consciousness expands, and the meditator achieves a transcendental unity with all things.

Individuation and Integration

Synthesis on the psychological plane is achieved by first detaching the disparate elements of the personality into separate dynamics, or subpersonalities, and then harmonizing them and integrating them around the center of awareness and volition. As we attain this sense of unity within ourselves, we are better able to appreciate others as unique individuals who yet share with us a fundamental unity through a higher self. These same techniques are then used in the search for transcendent meaning, leading to transpersonal unfoldment and unity. An ancient Vedic text speaks of it thus:

> "I was one, I became many,
> and now I am One again."

Suggestions for Further Reading

Assagioli, R. *Psychosynthesis: A Manual of Principles and Techniques.* New York: Psychosynthesis Research Foundation, 1965.

Desoille, R. *Théorie et Pratique du Reve Eveillé Dirigé.* Geneva: Editions du Mont Blanc, 1961.

Vargiu, J., *et al.*, eds. *Synthesis*, vol. 1, no. 1 (1974); and no. 2 (1975). Redwood City, Calif.: Psychosynthesis Press.

GITA ELGUIN-BÖDY *(Psy.D., Ph.D.) is a licensed clinical psychologist who specializes in the treatment of people with general health problems and chronic disease, as well as weight reduction and eating disorders. She received her Ph.D. from the University of California, Berkeley, and her Psy.D. from the University of Chile. Since 1979 she has been co-founder and executive director of Holistic Health Associates, a multidisciplinary health clinic in Oakland, California, that promotes well-being through physical, mental, and spiritual development. In 1983–84 she also served as founding director and first president of the Montclair Health Professionals Association, a community-based educational and service organization working to eliminate barriers among health professionals of different disciplines, as well as to draw health providers closer to the community. She has published several articles in professional journals and lay periodicals and also sought to disseminate holistic concepts through her program "Holistic Perspective" on KLW National Public Radio.*

BART BÖDY *(Ph.D.) received his doctorate from the University of California, Berkeley. He is a clinical psychologist specializing in the holistic treatment of people with chronic disease, as well as the enhancement of wellness. He is co-founder and administrative director of Holistic Health Associates, a multidisciplinary health clinic in Oakland, California. He is currently organizing a health education network to make holistic health concepts and techniques better known and utilized throughout the community. He is the editor of "Holos," a newsletter on holistic health and holistic psychology.*

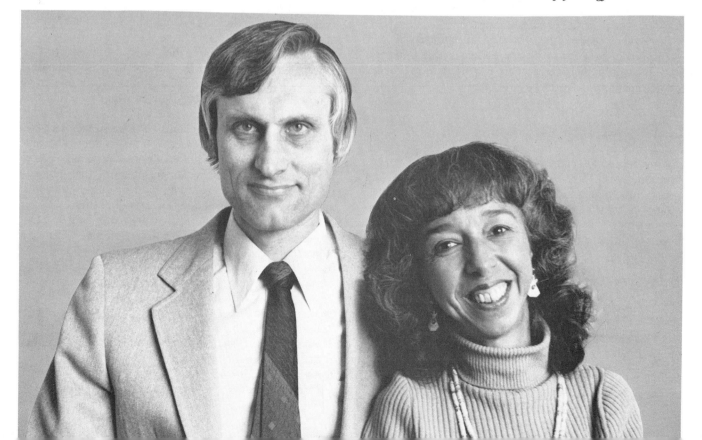

Some Positive Words About Negativity

Naomi Steinfeld

THE NEED for light, and for lightening, is clear, especially at this time in our collective human history. As countries brag, threaten, and joust, today's children doubt whether they will survive to become grandparents. We worry for our children's psyches and their ability to hope; we worry for ourselves; we see overwhelming evidence of darkness around us. Swimming in a milieu of petty-mindedness that affects "innocent bystanders" as well as the jousters, we may find despair within arm's reach. What can we do?

Helplessness is perhaps the hardest to bear. It closes off all doors, saps the strength, dilutes the will. Before we give in to helplessness, we will try something else.

One of the "something elses" tried, particularly within the holistic health movement, is the light touch—surrounding difficulties with white light, affirming the positive, beaming radiance at whatever threatens or ails us. Much of this work has borne rich, nutritious fruit—it is quite empowering to realize that we are not the hapless victims of circumstance but rather, in some sense, the co-creator of our experiences. That perhaps we, because of subconscious beliefs, "ask for" unpleasant experiences—to be hurt, abandoned, exploited, and so on. And that becoming aware of these subconscious feelings and expectations then empowers us to replace our negative expectations with positive ones, thus leading to more positive—more spiritual—experiences. As a friend of mine happily declared, "Before we started doing affirmations my husband and I fought all the time. Now we never fight at all."

But I have watched them, and I have noticed a bright metallic quality, a brittleness, between them. They are always "perfect." And they are rarely really in contact with each other.

I believe that there indeed *is* a deep correlation between one's inner self-concept and one's experiences in the world. And I further believe that there is a connection between an individual's inner conflicts and a larger community's way of projecting fears onto bigger-than-life "bad guys"; between how the individual sees and attempts to resolve those inner, contradictory "pieces" and how a larger community attempts to find, or impose, this resolution. Therefore, to begin to heal the larger community by attempting to heal oneself makes sense to me. There is no other arena in which we have the possibility of so much knowledge, and ultimately so much control.

But I seriously question the ultimate effectiveness of an exclusively positive approach. I wonder whether "affirming the truth" (i.e., the desired outcome) helps people become more powerful, really. I'm not denying that the magic show works—I've had my thoughts read too, and even occasionally done it to others. And I've chanted and felt better; and I've taken vitamins and felt righteous; and I've forgiven my enemies with sweet words forced out from behind grinded teeth, and lo and behold sometimes those enemies would stop bugging me, or even do something nice. I've even done physical healings for people—not just with my hands, but sometimes simply with my thoughts. And that seemed to have an effect, sometimes. So I'm not denying that this stuff works; that it's possible (as I did) to go from a schlemiel to a savior in a couple of New Age workshops.

But what is the cost?

Seemingly, nothing. We gain better health, more radiant beauty, "no more fights"—a kind of ethereal, floaty serenity. We drink our herbal teas and commune with the infinite. And leave the earth-level scrapping to the unenlightened.

What *is* the cost of being addicted to positivity? The cost is that we don't know who we are. We may be "an expression of the infinite"—but we don't know who we are. And we can't know until we know what we are composed of. Every baby learns to name its nose, its toes, it bellybutton. But right now, can you name your grief? Your longings? Your shame? Do you know what drives you, forces you to repeat actions and thoughts that your deepest self abhors? Do you know why you feel false after a party, or reluctant to ask for favors, or decimated by the disappearance of a lover? Until you know your makeup, how can you possibly heal yourself? What are you healing? Who is the healer? Who is the healee?

I speak from experience. I didn't start off all full of light—actually, I felt full of dark. I grew up with two parents who taunted, wheedled, and needled each other to death. This I saw, helplessly, not as "psychopathology" but as real life—the best we could expect. I knew no other way. I did my best to want to survive, in a world that promised such a payoff, but there didn't really seem much worth surviving for.

Then I found The Light! What a shock, what a change!

So there *was* another way. Immediately, my walls were papered with affirmations for everything I might ever want: love, money, beauty, peace, nicer clothes, better jobs, self-forgiveness. I read books on how to remove wrinkles by bathing them in specific colors. I overpowered my terrors with positive litanies: "I am calm, I am clear, all is perfect now." I "forgave my enemies" and thereby felt nobler. (But I had to *reforgive* and *reforgive*—I somehow needed continuous booster shots.) My voice became more mellifluous and soothing; I opened my heart chakra through meditation, prayer, and affirmation. People who had never before noticed me rushed up to tell me their troubles; to be healed; to tell me I was wonderful.

I had never been wonderful before. I would not have given it up willingly.

Except that I finally crashed—fell hard from my perch of wonderfulness into a despair that seemed to have no bottom. And no word of affirmation would reach down that far.

So I had to give it up. Like all addictions, it was ultimately bad for me. The gap between the wonderful, healing person (what I presented to others and to myself) and the bug-sized monster inside me (what I truly felt about myself) was too big to bridge. I let go of my tight-fisted grasp on the positive, on being so wonderful. And to survive (my only wish, then—I didn't know that later would come the will to grow, the will to see clearly, the longing for truth)—to survive, I went back to square one: my own inner darkness.

But this time I was willing to look.

The Mask of Goodness

Why is it so important to be good, to be seen as loving and kind and all that? Why would we rather imprint our minds with "I am loving" than confess "I hate that son-of-a-bitch"?

I think it is because we believe, at base, that we are really bad—that our very *being* is bad—that it is so bad that we must be on 24-hour guard duty to make sure this badness doesn't leak out.

Because if it did, we would be lost, doomed. Annihilated. Nobody must know how bad we *really* are. No one else must know. Certainly, *we* must not know. (Although we know, we know.) Unknown terrors await, should this truth leak out—psychosis? homicide? catatonia? What kind of nuclear holocaust lies latent within our buried psyches, needing excessive fortifications and protection systems? And might we not, by carelessness or accident or in a moment of enraged passion, knock the red phone off the hook, dial the fateful number? We don't admit this. But we fear it.

How did we come to be so bad that we have to cover by being so good?

Early Childhood Heartbreak and a Desperate Child's Decision

If you did not have your heart broken as a child, then you are one of the rare few, and were born to highly enlightened beings. But for the rest of us, we have survived a rough time.

Out parents broke our hearts. Not because they were bad—because they themselves were love-starved, in one way or another. We tend to make light of our childhood traumas, of how much we hurt from them. But from our adult, over-5-foot-tall vantage point, we conveniently forget that when we were little, these events were big. In fact, catastrophic.

For example, here's a story from my childhood that's actually kind of funny now. When I was six, I was in the bathroom and saw a wadded-up pile of toilet paper on the toilet tank. Taking it for garbage, I flushed it down the toilet, thinking my mother would be proud of me for cleaning up. Then I ran to tell her, pleased with myself.

But mommy wasn't pleased at all. I had flushed my father's false teeth down the toilet. Mommy hit and daddy glowered, and I ran off to first grade in suppressed tears. Everything the teacher said seemed silly and distant, as if she were talking underwater. My misery seemed too big to rein in; I could not bear being so cast out from my parents' love. The hours from nine to twelve lasted forever.

But at noon my mother arrived, bearing my lunchbox (in my flight, I had forgotten it). Surprisingly, she was smiling. She told me that the superintendent of our apartment building had managed to find the teeth before they got flushed out into the sewer. (In my mind, I saw the super lying in the middle of the street, cars veering from him right and left, while he poked his right arm down the sewer manhole and managed to sightlessly grab just the right wet clump as it cascaded by.)

She smiled at me. She apologized. She said she loved me.

I beamed at her and kissed her and told her I loved her. And when she left I was able to make sense of the teacher's words, and to practice writing my alphabet as usual.

But the thought—too dangerous to voice, too dangerous to think—came up and up and up: What if the teeth hadn't been found? What would have happened to me then? Would I have been let back in, or not?

This illustrates only *my* version of the childhood heartbreak, but we all have our own stories. We fall in love with our parents, and they don't really fall in love with us back. We wish to do anything at all to please these gods, and they want us to be how they want us to be—strong or weak, a doctor or a carpenter, a thinker or a feeler—but what they don't want us to be is ourselves, following our own inner promptings. This isn't because they are bad or evil—it's because they were once in our same situation: offering up the best of themselves to their parents, who then ignored abused distorted, or manipulated those offerings to match their own needs. Our parents, then, grew up terribly estranged from their own inner selves. Then they had us—and, like their parents, they couldn't see us, either.

A child can stand offering his or her treasures and seeing them get stomped on only so often. At some point must come the decision, "I will not get hurt again in this way." The treasures, the offerings of the true self, get buried, repressed; in their place comes something false, whether this involves conforming to the parents' wishes or rebelling against them. In both cases, there is a hidden sense of grief and outrage, that who we really are should be so unacceptable to the people we love most in the world. Yet this is not the worst of the damage; the worst is that we end up hiding our true selves from *ourselves*. We don't know about it any more. We don't believe we have anything worth knowing. We contort ourselves into a conforming, brittle "goodness"—or even into a rebellious, seemingly spontaneous "badness"—to get the kind of love we never end up getting. (Even getting approval for being "good" can't fill the hole in our heart, because this "goodness" is only a behavior rather than an essential, from-the-self act.)

So we forsake ourselves to survive, and we get no real satisfaction from the rewards reaped by our false, behaving selves. And we don't recall that once we were some way else; that we loved full strength, without fear or reservation.

How Affirming May Get in the Way of Self-Discovery

To affirm the positive when you believe it is one thing, and it is truly empowering. But to substitute positive words for negative feelings can often end up doing more damage than just complaining about how bad things are. It's true that complaining doesn't change much. But at least you're right there where the hurt is—you can point to it and wince if the air hits it wrong. But if on top of this hurt you apply a rainbow-colored bandaid and brightly intone, "There is no hurt!" there is no chance of healing that which "does not exist."

What really hurts us most—grieves us most, betrays us most—is being estranged from ourselves. Of course we want not to get *stuck* in the hurt, to get past it. But first we have to get *through* it. We have to know who hurt us, how they hurt us, what we did with that hurt, what we keep on doing with that hurt—in relationships, on the job, in terms of inner experience and outer activity. To deny the existence of the hurt is to keep ourselves irretrievably distanced from our true selves. And there is no peace, no contentment, no real self-acceptance, no real self-empowerment, if we are ignorant of our true selves.

So we put bandaids on our sores when we rely only on positive thinking. And we do this because we *must* appear good—we must *not* look like the bad, worthless creatures we suspect ourselves to be. (We *must* be that bad! Why else would our beloved parents have turned away our gifts—our love—and tried to change us into something different?) Recognizing the negative feelings inside us seems to strip us of all pretense to human worthiness, seems to expose to the world our secret "truth": "I have no right to be. I deserve worse than I get. I gave my parents my best, and they rejected it. That best was *me*. My essence is no good."

Who can admit that this is their secret feeling? And yet if you allow this in, it may resonate inside and lead you to some truth about yourself. It is quite terrifying to really, experientially acknowledge that under all your activity and efforts to do well and be good is the underlying conviction, "I have no right to be." This is a realization that, seemingly, leads to total destruction. No wonder we avoid it. "Here awaits the unspeakable...."

And yet only be getting to that underlying conviction can we get through to the other side.

What *is* the other side?

Self-Acceptance

Why are some people so willing to undergo the intense psychic struggles that are part of getting to know one's true self? Partly because they are aware of the suffering that living from the false self repeatedly brings. But also, if they have had even a brief experience of thier true self, because they find themselves in a different reality—one in which they are free to do that which can humanly be done. No longer constrained by caring about how they appear to others, they are free to discover what they really want and how they might get it. When they have their own inner approval, they don't need to be seen as good by others. The inner binds and lawyeristic debates that once sapped most of their energy are gone. In their place is a spaciousness, a stillness, in which priorities sort themselves out in terms of what serves the true self and what does not; in which the spontaneous action of one's being gives as much delight as babies get from finding and playing with their toes; in which activities are done for their inner purposefulness, and not for show or to temporarily escape the omnipresent inner critic (the one that perches on your shoulder and says, "You should have run another mile," or "You should get a better job"). Self-acceptance doesn't mean not being flawed; it means compassionately accepting yourself for your perfections *and* your flaws, your strengths *and* your weaknesses. To be self-accepting means to risk doing things your own way—not to be different, or to get attention. But just to be true.

So to become empowered has little to do with telling yourself that you are as wonderful as you wish you were, and has a lot to do with looking at how you actually are—your flaws, your hurts, your secret pain, your hidden shameful longings. These buried feelings are not ends in themselves; rather, they are means toward developing a knowledge of yourself. And when you know who you are, you are powerful. When it comes from within, it radiates outward, and there is no need to "affirm" it methodically and mechanically. When you *are*, then you are powerful.

I want to end with a story from the Sufi literature, about a man who tried very hard to be good.

The Man Who Was Easily Angered

A man who was easily angered realized after many years that all his life he had been in difficulties because of this tendency.

One day he heard of a dervish deep of knowledge, whom he went to see, asking for advice.

The dervish said, 'Go to such-and-such a crossroads. There you will find a withered tree. Stand under it and offer water to every traveller who passes that place.'

The man did as he was told. Many days passed, and he became well known as one who was following a certain discipline of charity and self-control, under the instructions of a man of real knowledge.

One day a man in a hurry turned his head away when he was offered the water, and went on walking along the road. The man who was easily angered called out to him several times: 'Come, return my salutation! Have some of this water, which I provide for all travellers!'

But there was no reply.

Overcome by this behavior, the first man forgot his discipline completely. He reached for his gun, which was hooked in the withered tree, took aim at the heedless traveller, and fired. The man fell dead.

At the very moment that the bullet entered his body, the withered tree, as if by a miracle, burst joyfully into blossom.

The man who had been killed was a murderer, on his way to commit the worst crime of a long career.

There are, you see, two kinds of advisers. The first kind is the one who tells what should be done according to certain fixed principles, repeated mechanically. The other kind is the Man of Knowledge. Those who meet the Man of Knowledge will ask him for moralistic advice, and will treat him as a moralist. But what he serves is Truth, not pious hopes.[1]

References

1. Idries Shah, *Tales of the Dervishes* (New York: E. P. Dutton, 1970), 79–80.

Suggestions for Further Reading

Each of the following books can be read separately. Together, however, they form a totality. For the most incremental benefit, read them in the order in which they appear.

Ballantyne, Sheila. *Imaginary Crimes.* New York: Viking, 1982. This unsparing, exquisitely written novel offers an inside look at what it's like to be the child of love-starved parents who don't know who you are. Gives no solution, but details the dilemma quite poignantly.

Miller, Alice. *The Drama of the Gifted Child: How Narcissistic Parents Form and Deform the Emotional Lives of their Talented Children.* New York: Basic Books, 1981. A psychologist's brilliant exploration of how children learn to give up their own sense of themselves and serve their parents' needs instead. (It is in this ability to divine their parents' unspoken needs that the children are "gifted.") A wonderful companion piece to *Imaginary Crimes.*

Peck, M. Scott. *The Road Less Traveled: A New Psychology of Love, Traditional Values and Spiritual Growth.* New York: Simon and Schuster/Touchstone, 1978. A psychiatrist's penetrating and deeply compassionate look at the trials and joys of the search for love and self-love as a spiritual process. Food for the heart as well as the mind.

Speeth, Kathleen Riordan. *The Gurdjieff Work.* New York: Pocket Books, 1976. Speaking in the language of the teachings of Gurdjieff, psychologist/teacher/writer Kathleen Speeth gives precise information about distinguishing the real self from the false self. A good companion piece with Sufi stories.

Shah, Idries. Various collections of Sufi tales—for instance, *Tales of the Dervishes*; *The Way of the Sufi*; *Wisdom of the Idiots*; *The Dermis Probe* (all published by E. P. Dutton); *Seeker After Truth* (Harper & Row); and more. These collections of ancient Sufi lore and teaching stories appeal in many ways. They can be read as the entertainments they certainly are. But they also can help you become aware of new ways of seeing and of knowing. In fact, if they are read without preconceptions, they can actually be a tool for recontacting your real self. A useful way to read them is not to puzzle them out with your intellect but to identify with each character and to find the equivalent aspect of yourself.

NAOMI STEINFELD, *a professional writer and editor since 1970, has contributed to this edition of the* Holistic Health Handbook *in both capacities. A former coordinator of* editcetera, *a Berkeley, California-based professional editorial association, Naomi has worked as a freelancer for hundreds of publishers and authors across the U.S. In the process, she has learned something about many subjects. She is now moving away from this to explore and promote holistic, growth-enhancing alternatives in her capacities as writer, editor, and future clinician. Recent projects include* Writing, *2nd ed., by Elizabeth Cowan Neeld (Scott Foresman, 1985), for which she was a major contributing writer, and* Ending Hunger: An Idea Whose Time Has Come (*The Hunger Project, 1985*), *for which she was the copyeditor. In addition, she is working toward her M.A., M.F.C.C. in Transpersonal Psychology Counseling at John F. Kennedy University in Orinda, California.*

Dreams: The Mystery That Heals

Alan Bryan Siegel, Ph.D.

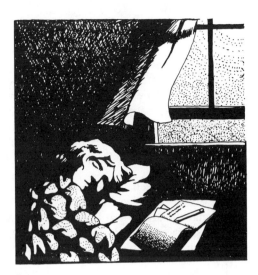

"To be concerned with dreams is a form of self-realization."

Jung

 EMEMBERING your dreams and learning to appreciate their symbolic language will increase their ability to heal. Cooperating with your dreams by the use of imagination and dream elaboration will lead you through the dream gates and on a journey of self-discovery.

Throughout history people have regarded their dreams reverently, and have sensed a meaningful relationship between the inner world of their dreams and the outer world of waking life. The ancient Greek physician Hippocrates practiced dream therapy and encouraged the ritual of dream incubation. This ritual began in Egypt and was extensively practiced for more than a thousand years in ancient Greece. Dream incubation required a pilgrimage to a sacred temple, in which one went to sleep in hopes of having a curative or prophetic dream.

Dreams have been used in many ways in different cultures and eras. Dreams have been used for creative inspiration by poets, artists, and scientists; for psychic and prophetic powers by Native American tribes in their vision quests; for personal problem solving and self-actualization in modern psychotherapy; and for spiritual guidance and enlightenment in religious and meditative traditions. As you begin to explore your dreams, it is important to ask yourself what you want to learn from them. The answer will begin to shape *your* way of working with dreams. Carl Jung (in Jacobi, p. 56) stated that "the interpretation of the dream is to a great extent dependent on the purpose of the interpreter or his expectation about the meaning."

Modern medicine has retained the Hippocratic oath, but has forgotten his teachings about the remarkable therapeutic powers of dreams. Freud reawakened popular interest in the importance of the dreaming mind, and stressed the healing power of interpretation by an expert psychoanalyst. Many people have benefited immensely from the insight and guidance of dream therapists and teachers. Yet a shortcoming of this model is that the dreamer is limited to a passive patient role, and is not always encouraged to discover the dream therapist within.

"The dreaming mind, I suggest, in addition to all its other functions, is the instrument of liberation, capable of breaking up the conventional patterns of human perception and releasing new forms of awareness."

Alan McGlashan,
Savage and Beautiful Country

There are, in fact, many ways to work with your dreams that do not require years of training. The way described in this article is a personal exploration of dreams by means of what Jung called active imagination and by sharing dreams in a supportive atmosphere with family, friends, and other interested dreamers. The emphasis is on an imaginative and nonanalytic approach that relies on experiential understanding, and that encourages the discovery of new perspectives on your life by the use of creative dream elaboration.

"A dream not understood is like a letter unopened."
The Talmud

Remembering Dreams

"I sleep and my heart wakes."

Richard Rolle

Dream research shows that you need to dream, and that, in fact, you dream several times each night. Even if you rarely remember your dreams, they are working to restore the equilibrium that waking life seems to disrupt.

In the dream groups I lead, a frequent topic is how to improve dream recall. Some people are motivated to improve their dream recall because they are troubled by recurring dreams; others have had dreams that have profoundly inspired them. Most people sense that improved dream recall will bring them important insights about their lives.

The *right* way to remember and document your dreams is the way that works best for you and is the most meaningful. The following suggestions may help you to develop a personal ritual for remembering dreams.

In the evening before sleep, make a written or mental review of the day's events, and of your inner feelings about them. As you drift to sleep, progressively relax each part of your body, and suggest to yourself that you will remember that night's dreams. Keep pen and paper by your bedside. All these steps reinforce the suggestion to your dreaming mind that you are sincere. A special journal that is aesthetically pleasing can become a treasure chest of your inner life. The best book on dreams is usually the one that you write yourself.

> "Reveal Thyself to me, and let me behold a favorable dream. May the dream that I dream be favorable, and may the dream that I dream be true. May Mahkir, the goddess of dreams, stand at my head. Let me enter Esaggila, the temple of the gods, the house of life."
>
> Babylonian Dream Prayer
> to the Goddess Mahkir

In the morning, dreams may fade out of awareness without a trace if you immediately jump and begin your waking day. Instead, reserve a few quiet minutes in the morning, and lie still with your eyes closed. You can linger in a half-dream state, and your dreams will often stay with you as you make a gentle transition from sleeping to waking. In this half-dream state, you can sometimes observe beautiful and revealing hypnogogic imagery, which is similar to dreams, but can be observed with greater conscious awareness.

One of the most common reasons for apparent nonremembering of dreams is the belief that a dream is not good enough. Some say that their dreams are too mundane, just repeats of daily events; others complain that their dreams are too fragmentary, or feel bewildered and embarrassed by their shocking dream behavior, and prefer to leave their dreams behind in sleep.

At a dream group I attended, a man claimed to never remember any dreams, except one fragment which he considered too trivial to qualify as a dream. Reluctantly, he described a blurred image of a knife. With encouragement and playful imagining in the group, he was able to derive rich meaning from the dream. The knife was related to his waking fascination with knives. He also saw the blurred image as his uncertainty about his masculinity and sense of assertion. The cutting-through power of a knife symbolized a type of acute perception that he valued and struggled to cultivate. Through this, he realized that he had had many similar brief dreams. Once he believed that his brief dreams were worthy of being called dreams, he began to report other, longer dreams at later group meetings.

> "Sleep offers itself to all; it is an oracle always ready to be our infallible and silent counselor."
>
> Synessius of Cyrene

Always record a dream immediately, no matter how fragmentary, frightening, or seemingly unimportant it may be. During the night, make a few key notes if you awaken with a dream; or else it is likely to fade by morning. Prompt recording of dreams prevents distortion of them by the conscious mind. Because it is difficult to accept what dreams reveal, Wilson Van Dusen, (p. 14) suggests: "Do most of the work on your dream while half asleep, when you can

feel back into it and halfway understand the symbolic language of your inner self." If you awaken with only a fragment of a feeling that you have dreamed, review the dream and let its details fill in by quietly rehearsing and redreaming it. You can aid this process by assuming the sleeping posture that you awoke in.

Henry Reed suggests a strategy of vigilance towards dreams. Dream vigilance can continue throughout the day. You may remember dreams at unexpected times; a dream of water remembered when turning on the shower, or a dream of a jaguar remembered while watching a house cat prowl in the grass. The important task of carrying your dreams with you while you are awake will frequently shed light on their meanings, and bring subsequent dreams that elucidate and further develop the meaning of the first dream.

> "Hunt half a day for a forgotten dream"
>
> Wordsworth

You need not remember every dream, or even remember a dream every day. What is important is not the quantity of dream recall, but the quality of how you integrate the messages of your dreams into your life.

The art of remembering dreams is more an attitude than a technique. It involves sincere desire for self-knowledge, trust in the healing power of dreams, vigilant receptivity to dream images, prompt documentation of dreams, and appreciation of their images and story quality.

Working With Your Dreams

Dreamwork can add to your total program of health maintenance by teaching you how to activate important inner resources. Jung stated (in Jacobi, p. 59) that "Every dream is a source of information and a means of self-regulation," and that "dreams are our most effective aids in the task of building up the personality." The time and energy you devote to the dreamwork will help you clarify important values and resolve emotional conflicts, and will contribute to greater self-sufficiency and responsibility for your life.

> "It is best to treat a dream as one would treat a totally unknown object: one looks at it from all sides, takes it in one's hand, carries it about, has all sorts of ideas and fantasies about it, and talks of it to other people. During this process all sorts of things occur to one about the dream and bring one nearer its meaning."
>
> C. G. Jung

Dreams symbolically reveal how you face central conflicts in your life. They unceasingly dramatize these conflicts until you act to take care of your needs more fully. Dreams frequently portray a variety of creative solutions to your problems. After a long series of dreams about airplane crashes, I had a dream in which I saw a plane, about to crash, that turned into a feather and floated gently to the Earth. As a result of the "Feather-Down" dream, I began the study and practice of progressive relaxation and autogenic training, which gives me the feeling of a gentle landing when I feel that my plane is about to crash.

In my airplane-crash series, I would helplessly watch a

plane lose altitude and crash. A literal interpretation would have been that I should give up flying. Instead I view these dreams as an allegory of an emotional pattern in my life. I get too high flying, too far off the ground, racing away with frantic thoughts. Suddenly I run out of gas and crash emotionally back to Earth. I become a wreck. When I witness this painful process, I know that the wisdom of my dreaming mind is telling me to slow down and feel, or risk a fiery crash.

As a preliminary to dreamwork, begin to reflect on your whole life. What have been the most formative events? Consider life crises and your style of facing anxious and uprooting events. Consider your most important relationships. Ask yourself: Who am I?

Jung (in Jacobi, p. 59) wrote that, "if we wish to interpret a dream correctly, we need a thorough knowledge of the conscious situation at that moment, for the dream contains its unconscious completion." It is always helpful to connect a dream to important events and changes in your life. Ask yourself: What is this dream saying about my life?

A daily ritual of tuning in to deeper feelings is an invaluable aid to understanding your dreams. Even ten minutes set aside for reflection in the evening can help digest the day's events. Writing your daily reflections in a private journal is even more helpful. Keeping a journal can help you to develop an inner sanctuary from which to view the rapidly changing circumstances of your waking and dreaming life. Whether in writing, drawing, or other art forms, the regular expression of your inner reflections will clarify your dream images, and you will find your dreams responding more directly to the concerns of your waking life.

The dreaming mind may be seen as a remarkable oracle. Just as the ancient Greeks consulted their oracles and journeyed to the temples of dream incubation, you can consult your dreams about specific problems, such as difficult relationships, disturbing fears, physical illness, creative blocks, or recurring nightmares. Dreams respond amazingly if you request guidance on a specific question. Dream request requires a thorough conscious examination of a vital issue in your life. When you have exhausted all possibilities, turn to your dreams. Open yourself, and form a very simple question about your issue. Some may wish to form a prayer. The answer might take a few days to appear, or you might wake up in an hour with a revelation. Occasionally a dream may deliver the answer to a totally different (though vital) question.

I have used this dream-request technique many times, and find it useful when I am writing. A dream helped me to begin this article. I read, made notes, and collected my ideas, but found it hard to begin. I relaxed before sleep and asked my dreams to guide me. That night I had the following dream:

I am working on my dream article and remember three counselors I have worked with, who suggest truly confronting barriers and fears that arise in dreams. I write: "You should take your dreams and the changes suggested by your dreams seriously but not overly seriously," implying a serious commitment but not losing humor.

Working with a dream isn't all stern and analytical. Looking at the humor in a dream dilemma can relax the tension momentarily, and open the door for new responses to old problems. Dreamwork can be an enjoyable game; like trying on the costumes of different characters in a play. "Not losing humor" is not losing an enjoyment of the unexpected. In dreams the joke is often on you.

Dreaming the Dream Onward

"We must reawaken the images."
                                                Mircea Eliade

Once you have retrieved a dream, allow your imagination to elaborate it. Soon the dream will begin to work with *you*, guiding you to important growth choices. You can create a relaxed and receptive space for yourself in which outside distractions are reduced. This will bring you close to a dream state, and will activate the intuitive image-making power. Relaxation techniques, meditation, or simply closing your eyes and stretching your imagination awakens an essential emotional participation in the drama of the dream. The nonverbal, imaginative nature of art forms, such as painting, dancing, writing, sculpting, and photography also help recreate the dreamspace necessary for direct experiential understanding of dreams.

"One night I dreamt I was a butterfly fluttering hither and thither, content with my lot. Suddenly I awoke, and I was Chuang Tzu again. Who am I in reality? A butterfly dreaming I am Chuang Tzu, or Chuang Tzu imagining he was a butterfly?"
                                                Chuang Tzu

A simple way to dream the dream onward is to vividly pretend to reenter and redream a dream sequence. You can write a narration of your dream in the first person, or tell it to a friend, or tape-record a dramatization. If you feel inspired, create nonverbal movements to express your feelings as you dream your dream onward. When you reach the end of what you remember, let the story spontaneously continue itself for as long as feels comfortable. The results are surprising. These playful exercises allow you to both participate in and observe a reliving of your dream.

Here is a brief example of dream elaboration. Upon returning from backpacking in an area very close to a large forest fire, I dreamt:

Packing up late at night before a nuclear attack or a natural disaster. Getting all my things arranged. It is cold. Need food and utensils. May be camping for a long time.

Upon waking, I remembered eerie smoke-filled skies, with the sun turning red. I felt the presence of impending danger. I wanted to rise and carefully prepare survival gear. I wrote a short poem based on the dream.

PREPARING

It is time.
In darkness I prepare.
Smoke and thunder fill the air.

Bats and birds are nervous omens
of the Change that is soon coming.

I will wander in the chilly night,
Never losing hope for dawn's light,
But first I gather tools to me
To be ready for Earth's cruelty.

Although the atmosphere of the dream is ominous, the careful preparations reflect increasing feelings of self-sufficiency. Besides the objective meaning of having been close to a disastrous forest fire, I can see other levels of meaning. Many people dream of natural and environmental disasters, including nuclear war, riots, and earthquakes. The fear of such uncontrollably powerful events is real; yet we are not helpless. We can survive and even grow in the face of life's inevitable crises and disasters by learning to care for our needs more fully.

If you have such a dream and are puzzled how to begin, you might choose an element which is the most charged with energy. Without worrying about being right, play with the image or feeling, and make associations to the image, always relating back to the image, as if circling around it. In this dream I chose the feeling of impending disaster. With that in mind, my associations took me back to other near-disasters I had experienced. I remembered preparing for major hurricanes while growing up in Florida, and being lost at night on a cliff near the Pacific in an isolated area of Mexico. Letting my imagination circle around the central feeling led me on an interesting journey through my life, and helped me relate the metaphor of "preparing" to how I am facing major changes in an important relationship and in my living situation.

At first the dream seemed like a rerun of having been near the forest fire. As I dreamed the dream onward, I discovered deeper meanings that touched both my personal life and the roots of our common human experience. Dreaming the dream onward seeks to understand the dream by learning to speak the language of dreams. The language of dreams is not easily translated into everyday words and sentences, nor is it fully explained by interpretations. It must be experienced to be comprehended.

"I believe in the future resolution of the two states of dreams and reality into a sort of absolute reality or surreality."

Andre Breton
The Surrealist Manifesto

Facing Your Shadow

The "shadow," as formulated by Jung, embodies all the unknown and unrealized parts of yourself. The shadow is our unknown other side: our Steppenwolf, our Mr. Hyde. It can be unthinkably impulsive, violent, or blasphemous. Occasionally the shadow may embody higher potential that a person won't allow himself to accept.

"Each night our dreams allow us to be quietly and safely insane."

William Dement

Shadow figures tend to exaggerate emerging parts of oneself. A person who is soft-spoken may have loud screaming animals in his or her dreams, suggesting more aggressive, assertive expression. A person who is fashion-conscious may appear in dirty old rags, indicating the need for a less finicky, more relaxed look.

Your shadow may startle you with nightmares. You may find yourself attacked by a wild animal or committing an act that you consider immoral. Nightmares are like an urgent telegram from your inner Self. Their power demands that you pay attention and work to resolve the inner conflict they point to. Although you will naturally be tempted to forget a nightmare, you must write it down and begin to work with it imaginatively. Try to create alternative endings in fantasy. When falling, imagine landing on a bed of feathers. If imprisoned, let yourself escape through a tunnel into a meadow of spring wildflowers.

There are many common nightmare themes, including disasters, wild-animal attack, being chased, imprisonment, paralysis, visits from the dead, violence, and revisiting events, such as repeated war memories.

Sharing your nightmare with a friend and fellow dreamer will often relieve enough anxiety to let you dream the dream onward and find out what it is trying to tell you. In one dream group I was leading in a psychiatric setting, a woman who was very religious dreamed that the devil was chasing her. As she shakily told the dream, two other group members nodded and stated that they had had similar dreams of diabolical figures. With a sigh of relief, she was able to explore her guilt feelings about actions she had committed which went against her religious beliefs.

Having an imaginary dialogue with the threatening person, animal, or thing is a good way to continue. A dialogue can be done in writing, where you create both voices; in dramatization, where you assume one role and others play the other roles; or in a Gestalt dialogue, where you act out each part in the dream. The purpose for doing the dialogue is to drive home the difficult realization that each character and part of your dream is an aspect of your own personality. You can use the dialogue form to develop important parts of your higher self, as well as to cope with difficult and threatening tendencies. I have had dialogues with my inner wise old man, my wounded child, my inner judge, my nurturing mother, and many other voices within me. Dream dialogues help you to become whole by personifying unknown and potentially useful parts of yourself.

Personification, or giving voices to the characters and objects of dreams, helps you to gain entrance to their sometimes confusing world. This may seem artificial at first. If you place skepticism aside, the dream voices will begin to speak in a lifelike fashion. As you personify, accentuate the emotional state of each character. Always switch roles; but not only the helpless victim, but also the powerful attacking monster.

The following nightmare illustrates personification.

I am on an island that is being attacked by a huge, terrifying Female Bigfoot creature who is killing people by the scores as if they were insects. I hide on the other side of the island and plan with others how to fight it.

Alan: Who are you?

Bigfoot Mama: I am a wild grizzly bear. I'll rip and chew you and sink your island. You will suffer my tortures.

Alan: You terrify me, I must hide. I must fight you or I will die. You are a monster.

Bigfoot Mama: I am pure hate. I will get you with no warning. I will scare you to death. For now you must live in terror of me.

Alan: I will fight you. Your shadow darkens our island. I will gather allies and defeat you. I won't be crippled by fear.

Bigfoot Mama: You are puny. Your fear will choke you. You don't have a chance.

Alan: I will watch and learn your ways. I will find your weakness.

There is a feeling of primitive destructive power from Bigfoot Mama. The dream suggests to me that one way to confront such evil power is to regroup with other friends and work together. In the dialogue I am beginning to confront her and learning to use my powers of observation.

I found it easy to identify with myself as the underdog gathering strength to fight a mighty oppressor. It was more difficult to imagine that Bigfoot Mama is also a part of me. When dialoguing with this dream, I was embarrassed to admit that I became excited by her horrible powers when I assumed her role. The effect of this dream continues. Among other things, it has helped me to observe and be more conscious of my own aggressive and destructive nature, rather than repressing it and letting it build up. If you let your dreams familiarize you with your own evil, you will be less possessed by it and less inclined to act it out.

Dialogue, dramatization, or any other technique for dreaming the dream onward will help you relax and gain an essential new perspective on your dream dilemma. Working with troubling images can help you learn to accept your fears. Always be alert for painful and embarrassing messages. They are your shadow calling to you.

"As Jung said, the shadow side of the personality, which we normally try to keep down in the interests of some (higher) good, is 90 percent pure gold."

Ann Faraday,
The Dream Game

Dreaming Together

Sharing dreams with your friends, family members, or the people you dream about will make your dreams come alive. Sharing dreams enhances your understanding and your dream recall. If you are more curious, you may want to form a dream-sharing group or join an existing one. Telling a dream in a dream group often reveals the universality of the emotional and spiritual dilemmas that we all face. A supportive atmosphere in a dream group can help the dreamer to overcome resistances and to creatively resolve inner conflicts and fears that are difficult to face alone. Asking for help on a dream can be a way of asserting yourself to more fully meet your needs.

Dr. Montague Ullman has pioneered invaluable techniques for a dream sharing process he calls the "Experiential Dream Group." Ullman's dream group principles are outlined in his book, *Working With Dreams*, which he co-authored with Nan Zimmerman. The two key factors in dream groups, according to Ullman, are the *safety factor* and the *discovery factor*. A safe climate is created by giving the dreamer control over any discussion of his/her dream. Each person in the group is encouraged to rely on his/her own intuitive feeling about when a comment about the dream "fits." Encounter techniques are avoided, and questioning or analysis of the dreamer is discouraged. Too much interpretation may stifle further exploration of a dream's meaning and often reveals more about the interpreter's reality than about the dreamer's reality.

In the discovery phase, the dreamer lends his/her dream to the group, and a wide-ranging exploration of images, fantasies, and ideas is encouraged for all group members. Each member empathizes with the dream by imagining that the dreamer's dream is his/her own. Each person then shares his/her emotional reactions and associations to the dream, as if he or she were the dreamer. In this way, the dream group encourages each person to discover as much meaning in the dreams as he or she can accept and use. The varied life experiences and wisdom of group members is enormously helpful in approaching and understanding the dreams. However, it is always the dreamer's intuitive feeling that determines whether a dream meaning "fits."

Mutual dreaming is common in ongoing dream groups. Close relatives, spouses, or dream-group members often have dreams with extremely similar dream content or themes. What at first seems mysterious and coincidental later becomes a clearly observable process of unconscious communication. The dreams in the group seem to respond to common themes as if they were linked together and communicating with each other. In one group, every member had an animal dream on one evening, with no prior discussion of animal symbolism. In another group, a dream about a pet who had died was followed by a revelation that other members had also dreamed about the death of close family members during the prior week. Subsequently, many themes of death, separation, and loss emerged in many of the group members' dreams in response to the original dream about the pet dying. Discussion of these dreams helped to resolve lingering conflicts about important losses in members' lives. I encourage group members to share dreams about the dream group or about their fellow dream-group members, as they lead to insights about important issues in the group process.

Innovations in Community Dream Work

In my ten years of experience leading dream workshops, I have developed three unique applications of the experiential dream-group technique. The first, which I call Dream Quest, is a wilderness backpacking retreat based upon a contemporary dream-incubation ritual developed by Dr. Henry Reed. I have used the Dream Quest retreat in working with inner-city teenagers, adult psychiatric patients, and community college students. As we journey into pristine wilderness areas, I encourage participants to imagine that they are entering a "Dream Time" wherein imagery and dreams have a heightened reality. In the manner of the ancient Greek dream-incubation temples and the Plains Indian Vision Quests, each group member seeks to obtain a dream or image that will help him/her to understand and resolve a pressing personal growth issue. The following elements of the Dream Quest experience combine to enhance the problem-solving aspect of the dreamwork: the feeling of physical well-being generated by being in harmony with the forces of nature; the heightened awareness of the wilderness "Dream Time;" and the supportive feeling of community that develops around the ritual of sharing dreams.

The second approach grew out of my doctoral research in psychology, in which I studied the dreams of first-time expectant fathers. The "pregnant fathers" in my study had many recurrent and similar dream themes. Their dreams revealed a profound process of change in their identity and their relationship with their spouse. Their dreams also suggested that a prenatal attachment to their child begins for some men early in the first trimester of their wives' pregnancy, and continues to evolve throughout the pregnancy. Extremely common in many of the men's dreams were: themes of pregnancy; birth and parenting; sexuality; masculinity and femininity; and many vivid birthing images, such as emerging from caves, animals popping out of bubbles, and scuba divers with umbilical-like air hoses.

Despite the seemingly obvious connection to pregnancy and birth, many men were not aware of how profoundly involved in the pregnancy they were until they actually discussed their dreams with me. Based on these results and my previous work with expectant mothers and couples' dreams, I began using experiential dreamwork techniques with groups of expectant fathers, mothers, and couples. Each dream that was shared in the expectant-parent support group stimulated discussion of important emotional issues, such as anxieties about labor and delivery, changes in sexuality during pregnancy, parenting roles, marital communication, and identity changes.

Dream sharing can be a valuable vehicle for promoting emotional growth in support groups of people undergoing similar life-transitions, physical illnesses, or disabilities. A dream group I led for three years in a psychiatric halfway house was a popular part of the program. In a work setting, I led a year-long staff dream-sharing group, which was designed to facilitate communication. There are many variations of group dreamwork that have been effectively implemented in educational settings, hospitals and clinics, prisons, churches and synagogues, and for arts groups.

A third approach, which I use for dreamers of all ages and in many different settings, is a dream-drawing technique. It involves having all the group members pretend they are dreaming as the dreamer tells his/her dream. Relaxation exercises may help set the mood for the waking-dream experience. Before discussing the dream, all group members make a drawing of the dream, pretending that it is their own. Simple crayon drawings are very effective and allow all the group members to emphathize with the dreamer's experience in ways that are relevant to their own lives. Members all discuss their drawings and their experience of the dream as if it were their own. Often, another group member will have a more dramatic experience of the dream than the dreamer.

Living Your Dreams

You can begin to live your dreams in simple ways. If you dream of being near the ocean, honor your dream by going there if you can. If you are far from the sea, you might draw an ocean scene or read a novel that takes place in a seashore town. I once dreamed of a very peaceful scene of a water lily in shiny water, and a few days later, while out with my camera, I came across the exact image from my dream. I later hung the photo on my wall as a mandala of tranquility. I dreamed of a young boy triumphantly riding a horse. I drew a picture of it, and practiced assuming the balanced and powerful position of the boy riding. The physical enactment of a dream will encourage your whole organism to discover and embody deeper meaning in a dream. Other forms of dream embodiment are dancing the part of one of your dream characters, and pretending to be one character or element in your dream for an hour or a day.

Dreams are not always literal in what they tell you; yet sometimes they suggest specific health practices and ideas. The works of Edgar Cayce document his use of dreams for medical counseling and for the discovery of preventive health practices tailored to the individual's needs. My dreams have suggested specific vitamins and herbs to take during stressful periods. Once when I was contemplating a long trip, my dreams specifically told me that it would be too exhausting, and that instead I should practice relaxation exercises and spend time in nature. Dreams have also encouraged me to take up jogging by showing me graceful gazelle-like movements. In dreams I find I can jog away from tense situations.

Dreams offer models to reach a healthier, more balanced lifestyle. To integrate the wisdom of your inner dreamer, you must test these models in everyday life. Ask yourself not only what a dream is telling you about your life, but also what you will do about it.

Dreamwork is not a panacea. It is up to you to choose which dreams to act upon. Acting upon dreams can avert both physical and psychological distress. The crucial choice you face is how to give form to emerging parts of yourself and to integrate them into your life. As you work with your dreams, you will intuitively sense which dreams to dream on. The most important dream meanings are the ones that both feel right to you and activate you to change your life.

You can honor your dreams by remembering and sharing them, and by dreaming them onward in imaginative ways. Dreaming your dreams onward celebrates the natural healing power of the dreaming mind by inviting the images and voices of your inner Self to guide you.

"If a man could pass through Paradise in a dream, and have a flower presented to him as a pledge that his soul had really been there, and if he found that flower in his hand when he awoke—Ay! and what then?"

Samuel Taylor Coleridge

References

Jolande Jacobi, *C. G. Jung: Psychological Reflections*. Harper, 1953.
Wilson Van Dusen, *The Natural Depth in Man*. Perennial, 1972.

Suggestions for Further Reading

The Dream Network Bulletin. 487 Fourth Street, Brooklyn, NY, 11215. A newsletter that chronicles current developments in dreamwork techniques, including national listings of workshops.

Ann Faraday. *The Dream Game*. New York: Harper & Row, 1974. Emphasis on the Gestalt Therapy approach. Dream diaries, dream themes, nightmares, dream groups, and dreams and altered states.

Dianne Hales. *The Complete Book of Sleep*. Belmont, CA: Addison Wesley, 1981. An excellent summary of research on sleep and dream cycles, clear discussion of insomnia and many varied sleep disorders of both adults and children.

C. G. Jung et al. *Man and His Symbols*. New York: Dell, 1968. a very popular introduction to Jung's psychology written by him just prior to his death. Profusely illustrated.

Henry Reed. *Dream Realizations Workbook*. Available from Dr. Henry Reed, 503 Lake Drive, Virginia Beach, VA, 23451 for $10. A detailed manual for enhancing the creative problem-solving powers of dreams using inspirational writing in a dream journal.

Montague Ullman and Nan Zimmerman. *Working with Dreams*. A highly recommended introduction. Emphasis is given to dream groups by Ullman, who is the pioneer of the experiential dream group.

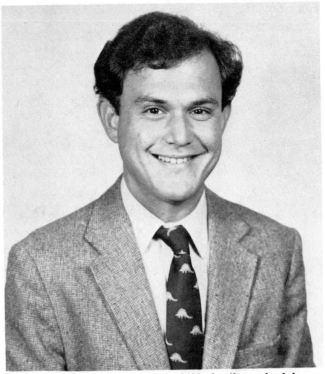

ALAN B. SIEGEL, *Ph.D., is a child, family, and adult psychologist in private practice in Berkeley and San Francisco. He has been leading dream groups and seminars for over 10 years throughout the San Francisco Bay Area. He conducted original research on the dreams of expectant fathers and specializes in working with expectant parents. Dr. Siegel is on the Graduate Psychology Faculty at John F. Kennedy University and is the Coordinator of Continuing Education for the City of Berkeley's Mental Health Clinics.*

WHAT I MISS ABOUT BEING SICK

Lying motionless under the heavy comforter.
Wild cherry cough drops, tamed down to my need by
    two serious, bearded men who stare concernedly
    from their white box.
A bier of crushed kleenexes—white roses calling to
    mind the year I was a tissue-costumed fairy in Miss
    Marhoffer's class play. (She was the one who led us
    each day, in public school, in "The Lord is my
    shepherd." It has dogged me for decades. I mutter
    it now feverishly: "I shall not want.")
All the books I had "no time" to read, now dog-eared
    and landsliding on the night table.
The door truly closed.
    (Unless I call out or cough quite loud—in which
    case a face pops through, tired but somewhat
    willing; shortly after comes a hand bearing not
    grandma's homemade chicken soup with matzoh
    balls (grandma is dead) but Lipton's chicken
    noodle, the kind with real diced-chicken bits. And
    a ragged, stalwart smile that says I am, for at least
    one more day, not indispensable.)
Not answering the telephone.
Stashing my calendar in the other room. Forgetting I
    own it.

The cat nesting on my belly, breathing warmly and
    evenly, purring,
the sweet shock of cool air on my hot face,
the comfort of the weighty air lying on top of me,
the slow, sensual ache of my muscles,
dreams with closed—and open—eyes:
    blue water thickly falling through my fingers,
    landscapes of such dark/bright wonder as to pale
    any date on any calendar,
    all the mysteries clear and now and wordlessly
    comprehensible, unrecordable, untranslatable into
    "life" until I begin to
Remember my hidden treasures, those still places that
    come into focus with my regular breathing

(following the cat, following
    not my will but—all that my body can manage—
    just breathing),
The pulse of me, the pulse of cat, the pulse of leaves
    outside the window, newspaper on sidewalk, worm
    on leaf, leaf on tree, tree in sky, sky in blue ease,
    infinitude;
all boxes, all calendars silly and gone—

That time of great gratitude,
recuperation:
thoughts are still
air has feel
walking to the window is a miracle,
all passersby are beautiful, even those with ghetto
    blasters.
Why had I worried so?
When clearly
the world has ease,
birds glide on invisible strings,
flapping as I inhale, coasting as I exhale.
    (Or is it me, adjusting my breathing to match the
    bird?)
Only one of us
    (the air full of light, a pitch in the wind to sing by)
Only one of us
    (the fullness is all, is enough; I will never complain
    again
      about *any*thing! Oh,
      let me stay in this still moment of blessed gratitude
      for the simple, real things—
      breathing through my nose! Keep me
      from caring about my calendar)
Only one of us, I or the bird,
is trying.

To have this much inner life without the excuse of a
    fever!

NAOMI STEINFELD

Dreams and Holistic Health

Jeremy Taylor

We All Dream

Some people say, "I never dream," but a person who actually does not dream simply does not exist. Rapid eye motion [REM] studies show that everyone dreams, regardless of age, sex, race, and so on. To say "I don't dream" is actually to say "I habitually ignore and forget my dream experiences." All warm-blooded creatures dream regularly—REMs have been observed throughout the animal world.

Prolonged dream deprivation tends to cause severe mental disorientation and emotional upset. Apparently, if the unconscious is deprived of its normal outlets in REM sleep, it demands "its due" and causes people to hallucinate and "dream while awake." Clearly, the dream is a natural phenomenon. It is part of and necessary for the maintenance of natural physical, mental, and emotional health and balance within the organism.

Just as there is no such thing as a person who doesn't dream, there is also no such thing as a dream with only one meaning—all dreams have multiple meanings, much like puns. At one level, all our dreams are always about who we are in the process of becoming as we grow and change. At another level, we are also always dreaming about the physical condition of our bodies at the moment of the dream. At yet other levels, our dreams are invariably concerned with recent memories ("day residue"), childhood and adolescent reminiscences, sexual desires and fears, religious intuitions, the complexities of emotional relationship (or the lack of it), desires for power and competence, synchronous intuitions, other subtle perceptions, and more.

The Healing Dimension of Dreams

Dreams always come in the service of wholeness. They come to correct imbalances in waking attitudes, emotions, habits, and behaviors, and to bring to light the energies for growth and change that have not yet reached conscious self-awareness by other means. Even when our conscious awareness—the ego—is hostile to and fearful of the corrections brought by dreams, the dreams themselves will continue to bring their healing messages of wholeness, and the possibilities for increasing wholeness in waking life.

Indeed, if they are thwarted by forgetfulness, inattention, or even conscious repression, they will tend to take on increasingly horrific and "nightmarish" forms until the ego is forced to at least remember them upon awakening. In this way, nightmarish dreams will at least impress ego consciousness with their seriousness and get past the repression that often makes us forget dreams whose messages we are not ready to heed.

What Do Dreams Mean? (And Why Are They So Hard to Understand?)

The only reliable way to determine what a dream may mean is to seek your own "aha's" or "tingles" about its meaning and significance. Usually, when you hear or think something that may be true about the meaning of your dream, a spontaneous, confirmatory, wordless "aha" wells up into consciousness. *This "aha" of the dreamer is the only reliable touchstone of dreamwork.*

What is this "aha"? It has to do with previously unconscious *memory* coming to the surface of conscious self-awareness. At the unconscious depth from which the dream springs naturally, we already "understand" all our dreams—their meanings are *already* inherent in the dream experience, and come to conscious self-awareness when they rise and break the surface of consciousness, sending ripples through our awareness. The point of all dreamwork—whether solitary, one-to-one, or in groups—is to bring the dreamer's previously unconscious knowledge of the dream's multiple meanings to consciousness.

The dream does not mask or hide, but does its best to reveal—why, then, are most dreams so opaque? *It is because every dream has multiple meanings and multiple levels of meaning, joined into a single narrative or dream experience. It is this multiple, layered quality of dreams that often makes them so obscure to waking consciousness.*

However, when we make the effort to remember and work with our dreams, they regularly reveal startling insights, creative ideas, and conscious understanding of confusing emotions.

Six Basic Hints For Dream Recall

1. Simply deciding that you want to recall your dreams— that you care about your dreams and desire to remem-

---

This section is excerpted from Jeremy Taylor, *Basic Hints for Dream Work* (Sausalito, CA: Dream Tree Press).

ber them—is the single most important step in dream recall.

2. Make it as easy for yourself as possible to record your dreams. Put the tape recorder, or the light-pen and dream journal, or pencil and paper, or what-have-you right next to your sleeping place so that you can use them without having to wake up or move around too much.

3. When you awaken during the course of the night with a dream memory, jot down a few key words or images; most often, this will be sufficient to stimulate a much fuller recollection of the dream upon awakening.

4. Check your diet for B-vitamins. They appear to be important in the chemistry of dream memory for some people (as well as being useful in dealing with stress).

5. If you awaken and do not recall any dreams, try to return to the same physical position you were in when you first awoke. Often, this simple action will trigger a dream memory. If you know what your habitual body postures are over the course of a night's sleep, try them all, one by one.

6. If you still do not recall anything, try imagining the faces of those people you have the strongest emotional response to in waking life (positive or negative). As you visualize these faces, you may notice a background or scene in which one of them appears. This is often a dream memory, and can serve to bring more of the dream to consciousness.

14 Basic Hints For Working With Your Dreams By Yourself

1. Make a written record of your dreams, even if you use a tape recorder to collect them. Note the date and day of the week you awoke with the dream(s). Write them in the *present tense*.

2. Give your dreams *titles* when you write them down. Not only is this crucial for going back and reviewing your dreams over the months and years, but the moment of picking a title is often a doorway to insight.

3. Remember, you are the only person who can know what meanings and significance your dream(s) may hold. The "tingle," or "aha," or "flash," or "bell ringing," or whatever you feel like calling it—*the inner knowledge that something is true and on-the-case—is the only reliable touchstone of dreamwork.*

4. However, the "tingle test" is only a positive test—the absence of a "tingle" does not necessarily mean that an idea of piece of work is wrong; it may be wrong, but it may also be that for some reason you are not prepared to acknowledge some truth about yourself at that moment. In this case, continued attention to your dreams will invariably bring the ignored truth back to your attention. The homeostatic, self-correcting quality of the dreams themselves can be relied upon.

5. Do not put any habitual limitations on the ways in which you record and interact with your dreams. Prose narrative is only one alternative. *Draw pictures* of your dreams. Experiment with different ways of recording and exploring your dreams. Try recording them as *poems.*

6. *Give expression* to the images, ideas, and energies of your dreams in as many different ways as you can. The more expressive work that is done with a dream, the more likely it is that the dream will reveal more of its meanings and insights and gifts for living. Cultivate whatever expressive methods you find satisfying.

7. Do not ignore dream fragments. *The structure of the memory of a dream is often as meaningful as the dream itself.* Most often, the "fragment" is an image carefully edited by memory to make it as simple, subtle, and clear a symbolic statement as possible.

8. Read, think, pay attention to as much of the *full range* of your experience as possible, and try to make sense of it as a whole, in pieces, any way you can.

9. Remember that every dream has many meanings and many levels of meaning, so don't be too dazzled by the first or second set of tingles you have.

10. Remember, everyone is in the same boat.

11. (Which is one of the best reasons I can think of to love your enemies—we are *all* in the same boat—we share one planet on the outside, and one archetypal drama on the inside, and *we must learn to love our enemies because it is the only thing that works.*)

12. Re-experience your dreams in as vivid imagination as possible. Re-experience the dream from the points of view of different characters and figures. Write these imaginings down and reread them. Imagine different ways your dreams might have continued if you had not awakened when you did. (Exercises like these are usually called "Gestalt work" or "active imagination" in the literature.)

13. Go back and look over all your dreams periodically. Be open to seeing new patterns and directions of development. Look over your expressive work at the same time.

14. Share your dreams with people you care about. Ask them about their dreams.

Some Elements That Are Always Present In Dreams

It is the nature of dreams to convey multiple meanings and layers of meaning with a single narrative. To use the metaphor of weaving, there are always certain kinds of threads woven into the fabric of every dream. Sometimes one color or texture will dominate the overall design, sometimes another, but all dreams are woven of essentially the same warps and cross threads, no matter what the design. Here is a partial list of some of those threads of meaning and significance that seem to be woven into every dream:

1. Every dream has an element of sexual desire. Freud is right to this extent (but he is clearly in error when he attempts to reduce *all* dream activity to repressed sexuality).

2. Every dream depicts elements of the dreamer's personality and vital energies in its imagery. This is the basic insight of the Gestalt school of dreamwork. The people and things and situations in your dreams all represent aspects of yourself, but they also often rep-

resent waking-life people, situations, and things *at the same time.*

3. Every dream has an element of reflection of physical health and condition of the body at the moment of the dream. (For a long time, this "plum pudding hypothesis" dominated scientific thought and experiment, and dreams were considered to be only a function of disordered metabolism.)

4. Every dream has a thread of immediate memory drawn from the last day or so, known technically as "day residue." The important question to ask regarding day residue is not so much what particular incident is being recalled, but rather *why* that particular incident and not some other has been woven into the experience of the dream.

5. Every dream has an element representing power and dominance relationships in waking life. Alfred Adler emphasized this aspect of dreamwork.

6. Every dream has an element of childhood and adolescent reminiscence, often associated with the question, "When in my life did I first feel the way I am feeling now?"

7. Every dream has an element of speculation about the future, often associated with the question, "What might happen if I did so-and-so?"

8. Every dream renders feelings and emotions into metaphoric images. Corriere and Hart are right when they say "a dream is a picture of a feeling" (but they are in error when they claim that is all a dream can ever be).

9. Every dream has an element of archetypal drama. Even when dreams are terribly personal and seemingly mundane, there is always some way in which the universality of all human experience is hinted at.

10. Every dream is constructed out of the seeming opposition between polarities (light and dark, good and evil, life and death, possible and impossible, etc.). There is also always a complementary element present, which hints at the ultimate unity of such polarities in a single, unitary, all-embracing reality.

11. Every dream has an element of "synchronicity" (telepathy, precognition, and the like).

12. Every dream has a balancing or compensatory element relative to waking consciousness. Even the worst nightmare or recurring dream has as a major part of its purpose or reason for being the correction of some imbalance in waking attitude or behavior.

13. Every dream has an element of constructive self-criticism.

14. Every dream has an element of creative inspiration or problem-solving.

15. Every dream has an element of religious concern and intuition about the inevitability of death. Religious beliefs from around the world can be seen reflected in common dream experiences (such as leaving the body, dreaming of someone who has died, dreaming of "heaven" and "hell," etc.).

16. Every dream has an element of "return to the womb" and "return to the crucible for melting and recasting." Each dream is a step in the evolution and development of personality, and every awakening is a rebirth into a potentially new life.

17. The dreams of a single night are almost always related to each other thematically. (The failure to detect a theme or thread of meaning in the dreams of a single night is probably a result of our inability to unravel the multiple levels of meaning, rather than an indication that the dreams are actually unrelated.)

18. Every dream reflects a concern for waking-life emotional relationships or the lack of them.

There is no theoretical end to this list. Some elements will predominate and obscure others at various times, but my experience is that these elements are always present to some degree or another in all dreams. It is always worthwhile to ask if one of these elements is a major determinate in the dream experience, and how it may interweave with other universal dream themes.

Suggestions for Further Reading

Faraday, Dr. Ann, *Dream Power*, New York: Berkeley, 1972

Garfield, Dr. Patricia, *Creative Dreaming*, New York: Simon & Shuster, 1974.

Hillman, James, *The Dream and the Underworld*, New York: Harper and Row, 1979.

Jung, Dr. Carl, *et al*, *Man and His Symbols*, Garden City: Doubleday, 1964.

Taylor, Jeremy, *Dream Work—Techniques for Discovering the Creative Power in Dreams*, Ramsey: Paulist Press, 1983.

Ullman, Dr. Montague, and Nan Zimmerman, *Working with Dreams*, New York: Delacorte, 1979.

JEREMY TAYLOR *is a Unitarian Universalist Minister and dreamworker residing in the San Francisco Bay Area. He has taught dreamwork for many years at the Starr King School for the Ministry in Berkeley, and has done dreamwork in a wide variety of settings including schools, churches, hospitals, residential treatment facilities, and prisons. He has worked in the United States, England, and Greece, and has led ongoing dream groups in San Quentin Prison and the Federal Correction Facility at Pleasanton. He is the author of* Dream Work—Techniques for Discovering the Creative Power in Dreams *(Paulist Press, 1983), as well as numerous shorter works.*

Autogenic Training

Vera Fryling, M.D.

Autosuggestion is not new. We suggest ourselves into experiences all the time, only we are rarely aware of the process. Auto (self) genics (produced) is a methodical system of meditative exercises designed to bring about greater personal response-ability. It consciously focuses the creative power of the mind on relaxation and awareness. Dr. Fryling points out the tremendous physiological benefits of this system and outlines exercises that will allow you to achieve this unique self-healing experience for yourself.

 UTOGENIC Training (AT) is a method of self-regulation, deep relaxation, greater awareness, and self-discovery. It was developed by a physician, Johannes Schultz, in Berlin, Germany, around 1930. In developing it, he combined his knowledge of the physiological changes occurring in deep relaxation and hypnosis with the meditative processes he had learned from Eastern practices, such as Zen and yoga.

Schultz developed a series of six standard phrases based on the physiological process of deep relaxation. These are repeated while the attention is held on the corresponding body area, thus combining the advantages of focused meditation and autosuggestion.

The first of the six standard phrases, "My right arm is heavy," initiates the autogenic state with muscular relaxation, which is often subjectively experienced as a sensation of heaviness. The second phrase, "My right arm is warm," affirms the process of vasodilation (relaxation of the muscles around the blood vessels which open or constrict the vessels), which is regulated by the autonomic nervous system.

We quickly learn with this procedure to influence the autonomic functions, which were formerly believed to be outside our ability to control. They cannot be controlled at will; only in a passive, concentrated state with an attitude of receptivity can we allow the desired functions to happen and thereby learn the control of internal states. In this passive "carte blanche" state, we tap the inherent wisdom of the body to achieve optimum balance or homeostasis. This balance is upset for most of us by anxiety, resentment, competitive striving—all components of that tension which must be overcome.

AT is unique as a relaxation method in that it was developed by a physician, within the medical model. Consequently, its effectiveness has been documented in detailed medical case studies of peptic ulcers, constipation, sinus problems, blood pressure, migraines, asthma, diabetes, arthritis, sexual problems, and many others. Twenty-four hundred case studies have been cited by Schultz and Wolfgang Luthe. AT is used for psychosomatic disorders and sleep disturbances, to improve academic and athletic performance, and for stress reduction in industry.

A key principle of the theory of AT is that the body will naturally balance itself when directed into a relaxed state. Homeostatic balancing is a central concept discussed throughout biology; AT is a method for bringing it about by intentional practice.

How to Practice AT

Begin the exercise in a sitting or reclining position with your eyes closed. Distractions from without should be minimized; the phrase, "External sounds do not matter," may be used. This makes it possible to practice in the office, in waiting rooms, even on public transportation.

AT may be practiced lying flat on a comfortable surface, in a reclining chair, or in a straight chair in a "rag-doll" position, with feet flat on the floor, spine relaxed, and hands or arms resting on the thighs. Remember that these exercises involve *passive concentration*. This means that we bring our awareness to a particular part of the body, say the appropriate phrase to ourselves a few times, then simply observe what sensations or emotions we become aware of. Here everyone's experience is unique and valid. AT is to be practiced for two twenty-minute periods each day; it can also be used for a few minutes during the day whenever one needs it to raise energy, calm down, or regain perspective.

The basic mood phrase is, "I am at peace with myself and fully relaxed." Then go through the following steps.

1. Concentrate on the part of the body to which the phrase is directed. Begin with, "*My right arm is heavy.*" Proceed to the left arm, right leg, left leg, neck, and shoulders. (For example, "My neck and shoulders are heavy.")
2. Concentrate again on the part of the body to which the phrase is directed. This time, the phrase is, "*My right arm is warm.*" Proceed to the rest of the body as above.

This exercise increases peripheral blood flow, relaxes the blood vessels, and promotes self-healing physiological changes.

3. Repeat the phrase, "*My heartbeat is calm and regular.*" Make contact with the heartbeat or pulse. If you experience any discomfort, eliminate this phrase and go on to the next one.

4. Repeat the phrase, "*My breathing is calm and regular.*" (Or "*It breathes me.*") This exercise prompts slow, deep, regular breathing.

5. The fifth standard phrase is, "*My solar plexus is warm.*" (This fifth exercise should be done *only* under medical guidance.) Your solar plexus is in your abdominal area, where you feel your center to be. Dr. Schultz reports that this exercise calms the central nervous system, improves muscle relaxation, helps sleep, and increases blood flow to the abdomen. (*Omit this exercise if you have had any severe stomach or abdominal condition, diabetes, or any condition that creates a chance of bleeding from any abdominal organs.*)

6. Mentally repeat, "*My forehead is cool.*" This exercise is performed primarily for its psychological effect, which is to combine deep relaxation with alertness.

7. The exercises are ended with the Return Phrase: "*I am refreshed and alert.*" Take a deep breath and stretch.

You may want to keep a journal in which you record your experiences after going through these exercises each day. It is usual for the effects to increase with time as you keep using the phrases. You may want to use one or two of the phrases for short exercise periods, and run through all of them for longer times.

Autogenic Discharge

Although the structure and process are simple, the effects are often powerful. Frequently the student experiences sudden startling sensations as suppressed affect is released, such as fear or pain from a previous incident that has been retained in the memory of our "biocomputer." This is called "autogenic discharge."

For instance, a woman in our seminar experienced an uneasy feeling on her left side; on investigation she recalled that she had once suffered a burn on her left upper arm when her nightgown caught fire. A young man experienced sudden pain in his knees, then recalled a football injury. A therapist experienced some strange feelings in his bones. He later recalled having arthritis pains twenty years earlier. Most of these incidents are not immediately available to memory, but the trainee may be assisted to bring the event and the associated feelings to awareness.

Autogenic Modification

Another aspect of AT, known as "autogenic modification," consists of the organ-specific formulae (OSF) and the intentional formulae (IF). OSF are physiologically oriented phrases that are used to reinforce the effects induced by the standard exercises. They have been developed for specific disorders, and are used to strengthen the body's own self-healing forces. It is important for these to be developed with the guidance of a medically trained person. Some examples of OSF are: "My sinuses are cool" (which can reduce congestion by constricting blood vessels in that area); "My throat is cool, and my chest is warm" (which could reduce a cough or asthma). For glaucoma, the OSF, "My eyes are soft and relaxed, and drain perfectly" might be used to reduce intraocular pressure.

The intentional formulae (IF) consists of brief, clear, positive self-suggestions which direct attitudinal changes, increase accuracy and speed in sports, and create behavioral modifications. For example, "I move with ease and accuracy; my opponent is quite unimportant," takes the element of strife out of the picture and therefore reduces stress and adrenalin output. After three weeks of AT, a physician in one of our groups found himself joyously moving toward a tennis championship.

Another IF might be: "I am calm and safe, relaxed and free, and my creative thoughts flow easily." On a quite different theme, one member of our group used the IF, "My solitude is replenishing me," as a positive reprogramming of his attitude toward being alone.

Meditative Exercises

Advanced meditative exercises involve visualizing colors and objects; contemplating concepts, such as peace, happiness, freedom; evoking specific feelings; and asking questions of the unconscious and the inner self. These exercises overlap with the methods used in Psychosynthesis, a system developed by the Italian psychiatrist Roberto Assagioli at about the same time as Schultz originated Autogenic Training.

The meditative exercises given here are originally taught to the trainee by the leader, but are eventually practiced and developed by the individual alone.

Exercises to reduce pain in joints or muscles may be used as an adjunct to the six standard formulae. Here is an example.

Imagine yourself at a beach, hearing the sound of the ocean, smelling the fresh breeze (this also works well for smoking control), expanding your lungs and allowing the energy of oxygen to enter all of your body, and feeling the light and warmth of the sun shining upon you. Imagine lying down on the warm sand and letting it run through your fingers; then covering your knees with warm sand (another way to reduce pain in the knees). Seek some shade if you are too warm and need cooling (this is important if the trainee overreacts to heat).

Imagine a color that is soothing to you, and let it flow through your body. Observe what occurs to you when you meditate on the concept of *beauty*. You might wish to evoke a feeling of serenity as you experience nature.

You will notice that this brief meditation includes color, objects, feelings, and concepts, as listed in the outline which opens this section.

Questions about the unconscious may be further explored in exercises such as the following.

Imagine you come to a body of water, an ocean, to explore its life sources. You may take anything you need for your journey—from a snorkel to a submarine. Experience what you see as you travel through the water. You come to the bottom of the ocean: experience what you see there.

There is a word on the bottom of the ocean that is keeping you from what you want. It expresses the root cause of what is holding you back from whatever or wherever you want to be. See that word; remember it. See what you can do with it.

Physiological Visualization

Visualizations can lead to optimal physiological functioning. One can visualize the glucose metabolism bringing energy to each cell. Or you might focus on the circulation:

Get in touch with your heart. Get in touch with your blood vessels, the heart chambers. Feel your heartbeat. Experience how the blood flows through an artery. Just follow it: into the lungs, filling with oxygen, back to the heart, out to the arteries. Follow it through the arteries, branching out into all the smaller blood vessels,...smaller and smaller. The blood vessels are elastic and supportive. The blood gives up oxygen and nutrients to the cells; and it flows on, into the veins, back to the heart. Get in touch with the cycle, with the circulatory system. Picture each part of the cycle of circulation going all through the body. Imagine yourself refreshed as this circulation brings the energy of oxygen and nutrients to the cells of the body.

Psychological Integration Exercise

Imagine that you are going on a journey, on a magic carpet, floating through space. Imagine yourself looking down on your home town, seeing some of the people who are important to you. See their environment, the setting in which they act. Now imagine that you hold thin strings connected with the people and objects below, and that by pulling those strings, you can make things move as you wish them to. You might want to change the scene in this magic theatre.

Now imagine that you are down there too, included in the scene, at the same time as you hold the strings up above. Have people talk together. Give yourself another minute or so to complete the scene. Take in the feeling of it; when you are ready to move on, just let go of the strings and float along. Float up higher; so you can see a larger area below you. See the different kinds of areas on the Earth.

Let yourself float through space now, seeing the sun, moon, and stars. Look down at the variety of people passing under you on the Earth. Watch them from sunrise to sunset, as the moon and stars pass in their 24-hour cycle...sunrise to sunset, a circle.

Imagine what comes to you when you think of *eternity*.

Now gradually float down on your magic carpet; gradually come back to the room you started from.

Sensuality Enhancement

You can use imagery to enhance sensuous and sexual expression.

Imagine a color you associate with excitement. Imagine it flowing into the area of your body where you would like to feel excitement. Then let it spread throughout the body, becoming total excitement. Imagine yourself walking in a meadow, and seeing in the distance a person who is dear to you. See this person coming closer to you. Make contact in a nonverbal way. Imagine yourself to be radiating a color, and your partner radiating a color; let them blend if you wish. Let the new color flow out of your body: give birth to the creation fostered by that merging.

Non-threatening fantasies such as this are used effectively in current sex therapy.

Gestalt Meditation

Gestalt meditation explores the polarities within the self and brings them to completion.

Imagine yourself in a scene that is comfortable and enjoyable to you. Walk through this scene, perhaps a natural one. Look around you and select an object that your attention is drawn to. Now imagine yourself as that object, and express its essence for you. Mentally describe *yourself* as that object; list its qualities in your mind, as your own. Get in touch with its environment: where it stands, or sits, or lies. Allow the environment, with all its qualities, to speak to the object which is you within it. Let it describe to the object how the environment supports it.

Let your imagination carry on a conversation between the object and its environment. Have each say to the other, "What we have in common is...!"

Let go of this image whenever you feel ready.

Transpersonal Imagery

Use the first four standard exercises; then imagine cool, clear water. Imagine seeing your reflection in it. As you look into the water, see a drop on a nearby rock, gently falling into the pond, giving its energy. See and feel the energy that each drop creates.

Now use the phrase, "I am calm and serene." Pay attention to your breathing. As you inhale, take in a sense of love; as you exhale, breathe out caring for self and for others. And use the phrase, "I experience joy and love."

Results

With regular practice, certain psychological shifts occur, such as an increase in production of alpha brain waves, as well as of theta states, which are similar to those dreamlike states experienced between sleep and waking, in which intuition is enhanced and creative ideas are born and flourish. Several trainees have begun writing poetry, which they had not done in years. Painting, as one form of nonverbal expression, in conjunction with AT, can help open up many other creative functions. One of our women, a high-powered executive, found herself writing poetry and, to her surprise, doing gourmet cooking, when she had had little interest in either before.

We can use Autogenic Training to regulate habits, such as smoking, alcohol, or overeating. One internalizes the idea that these things are no longer important. The imagery we can use to direct our unconscious mind, as well as our internal body states, includes endless variations within its basic scheme, and is limited only by our desire for self-exploration and self-direction. Our mind and body play a powerful and fascinating symphony; the tools with which to conduct it have been placed in our hands.

Suggestions for Further Reading

Roberto Assagioli, *Psychosynthesis*. Hobbs & Dunn, 1965.

Hannes Lindermann, *How to Overcome Stress the Autogenic Way*. Germany: Berpelsmann, 1973.

Wolfgang Luthe, *Creativity Mobilization Technique*. Grune and Stratton, 1976.

Wolfgang Luthe and Johannes Schultz, *Autogenic Therapy*. Grune and Stratton, 6 vols. 1959–73.

Karl Rosa, *You and A.T. Autogenic Training*. Dutton, 1976.

VERA FRYLING, *M.D., Assistant Clinical Professor at the University of California Medical School, San Francisco, was trained in Autogenic Training in Germany and has studied at the Gestalt and Psychosynthesis Institutes. She is currently in private practice in Berkeley, and is a consultant to the Biofeedback Institutes, San Francisco and Los Angeles.*

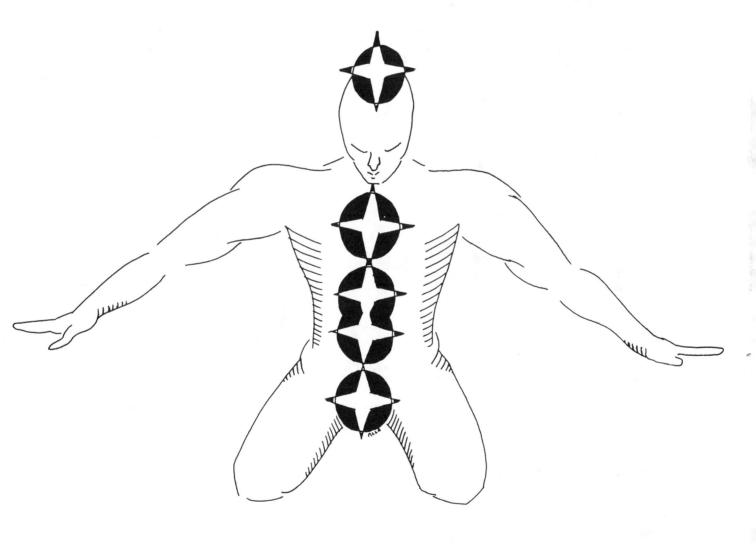

The Healing Potential of Meditation

Kathleen Riordan Speeth, Ph.D.

The healing benefits of meditation are well known. Each aspect of meditation has specific uses and drawbacks, depending on the individual and the circumstances. Kathy Speeth shows how to classify the techniques according to their placement on the body-mind continuum and the degrees of control or letting go that they require. This will help in the sometimes difficult task of choosing the appropriate meditation.

THE power of mind to alleviate suffering, and to contribute to psychological and physiological well-being, has been known in the sacred traditions since before the dawn of history, and was probably first recognized by early shamans. This power has given rise to meditative techniques that are at least as various as the problems which have been, throughout history, attributed to the human condition. Given this variety, to ask, "Can meditation heal?" as many in the human potential movement and the healing professions are now asking, is about as precise as musing, "Can carpentry help?" without a knowledge of the trade or a look into the toolshed.

Meditation is not a single practice, easily defined. It encompasses such diverse methods as formal sitting (as Zazen or Vipassana), in which the body is held immobile and the attention controlled; expressive practices (such as Siddha Yoga, the Latihan, or the chaotic meditation of Rajneesh), in which the body is let free and anything can happen; and even the practice of going about one's daily round of activities mindfully (as in Mahamudra, Shikan Taza, or Gurdjieff's "self-remembering"). All of these are meditation; yet to speak of them all as if they were interchangeable is to obscure the nature of meditation, and makes it difficult to ask meaningful questions.

The question we started with—"Can meditation heal?"—can be more usefully answered if we restate it as, "*Which* meditation techniques can heal *which* human conditions?" In this way, we can "look into the toolshed" and try to match the tool to the job.

One way to analyze meditation practices is to differentiate them along a continuum ranging from control to letting-go: the degree to which one directs or surrenders to what is. If we take this as a useful dimension of meditation to study, we can add a second dimension, which

might be termed the body/mind continuum. We can then visualize a matrix (as in Figure 1) with four quadrants, one concerned primarily with controlling the body, another with controlling the mind, the third with letting go in the body, and the fourth with letting go in the mind. Now we can look at various practices and aspects of meditation in terms of where they fall in these quadrants, and observe their healing potential for body or mind.

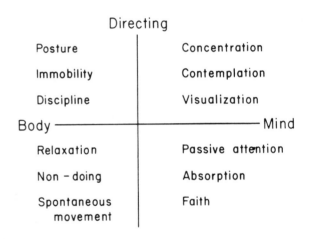

Figure 1.

These aspects of meditation do not ordinarily exist in isolation. In the meditative techniques found in the world's great sacred technologies, they are found in combination, like atoms in a molecule. Inspection of a separate component can give us a lot of information (but not all) about the potential of a combination which includes it.

Let us consider each quadrant of the chart in turn, taking the aspects within the quadrants in order.

Posture

Assuming a certain posture has been central to many meditation techniques, from pre-Aryan Mohenjo Daro (where archaeologists unearthed a statue of a person seated in the Lotus position, dated about 4,000 years ago) to the present. Classic postures, integral to Hatha Yoga, are given in the *Yoga Sutras* of Patanjali, which codify ancient yogic healing practices. Other postures appear in the Kum Nye holistic healing system of Tibet (Tulku, 1976), in Islamic prayer (Shah, 1971), and in Gurdjieff movements (Speeth, 1976). Posture is considered so important in Zen Buddhist practice that Suzuki Roshi (1970, p. 21), former abbot of Tassajara Monastery in Big Sur, said about it, "These forms are not the means of obtaining the right state of mind. To take this posture is itself to have the right state of mind."

A major characteristic of prescribed meditation postures in many traditions is that the spine is kept straight. This is true in Hindu and Buddhist yogas, in the Christian attitude of kneeling prayer, in the Egyptian sitting position, and in the Taoist standing meditation, "embracing the pillar." Any of these postures may challenge personal misalignments which may have come to feel "normal" to the individual. The spine is put back into a structurally sound line, and the weight of the body distributed around it in a balanced pattern in which gravity, not muscular tension, is the primary influence. It is possible, although it has not been conclusively proven, that this postural realignment affects the body's muscular armoring and thus the state of mind.

Reich, Alexander, Feldenkrais and others have shown that bodily posture both reflects and influences the inner posture of the mind. Gurdjieff even asserted that no new thought or feeling can appear without modifying the physical configuration of the body in some way. "No new postures: no new attitudes," he taught, giving as an example the "Stop!" exercise of certain Sufi orders, in which students must freeze in position when they hear the command.

"Feeling himself in this state, that is, in an unaccustomed posture, a man involuntarily looks at himself from a new point of view, sees and observes himself in a new way. In this way the circle of old automatism is broken. The body tries in vain to assume an ordinary comfortable posture. But the man's will, brought into action by the will of the teacher, prevents it."
Ouspensky, 1949, p. 334

It looks as though postural realignment, and the expansion of the repertoire of postures, can bring about not only physiological benefits, but a widening of emotional and intellectual horizons. Posture has other intriguing potentials in the realm of healing; we will look at only one more, the symbolic value of posture.

To take the position which has been used by seekers of enlightenment in many ages, the very position in which the Buddha sat under the famous Bodhi tree, may evoke an archetypal process, in which the individual and the particular encounter the transpersonal in a "peak experience," the effects of which may include a life-saving reorientation of values and habits, reversing, for example, the progress of addiction or disease.

The prescription of certain postures, to be assumed for specific lengths of time in specially designed spaces, within meditative therapeutic communities, is currently being used by a Tibetan lama, Chogyam Trungpa, to treat psychological disorders (Caspar, 1974). Although it is still too early to evaluate the effectiveness of this new process, its very existence shows the importance of posture as a healing agent in the elaborate Tibetan system of holistic healing.

Immobility

Committing the body to absolute stillness has its own physiological and psychological benefits. A mounting body of experimental evidence shows that even inexperienced meditators soon undergo measurable physiological changes: lowered blood pressure, slowed heart rate, decreased oxygen consumption, increased skin resistance, and an increase in the regularity and amplitude of alpha rhythms recorded from the brain. These effects of slowing and quieting are termed a hypometabolic state. At least some of them are probably due not to any esoteric inner changes, but to the physiological effects of immobility (probably in combination with relaxation and posture). However, the mere lowering of the metabolic levels of the body can reduce stress, producing an effect exactly opposite to those of normal life stresses, which lead to hypertension, coronary problems, and so on.

Psychologically, refraining from movement can have important strengthening effects, especially on self-confidence and on what is sometimes called "will." One Zen master recommended that every meditation room have at least one fly. Not scratching an itch, not brushing away a fly—to find the capacity to suppress these movements can have an extraordinarily liberating effect on the mind. Similarly, to remain entirely still as pain mounts in the legs, and the psyche whispers every sort of rationalization for shifting just a bit, can evoke real courage and self-respect; qualities which contemporary life gives us little opportunity to develop or test in ourselves, and for lack of which we fall prey to *anomie*, the sickness of soul in which one can experience no meaning in life. The manna of the hero may be the elixir of health.

Recent research suggests a relationship between immobility and the classic yogic awakening of *kundalini*, in which the meditator feels a serpentine force rising up the spine into the crown of the head, culminating in a rapturous experience. Itzhak Bentov has recorded physiological data which seem to indicate that meditative stillness produces an aortic rhythm of a certain frequency. This beat travels throughout the body, reverberating in the third ventricle of the brain. This third-ventricle rhythm sets off a wave which travels along the sensorimotor projection areas of the cortex, ending in the pleasure centers of the hypothalamus. If this effect proves to be genuine, it would be evidence for the value of immobility to body and mind (Sannella, 1976; Bentov, 1977).

Discipline

The last of the aspects of meditation which have to do with control of the body is discipline. At this point in the evolution of healing methods, there is a strong inclination to value spontaneity and freedom, to look at discipline as "out of date" and "life-denying." Yet there is something inherently healthy in a disciplined existence, the kind of life which can include a regular meditation practice or even commit itself to joining an ashram, a monastery, or a group of like-minded people pursuing the meditative life.

Discipline involves organizing one's day around activities that have meaning and value to oneself, and that therefore support a sense of personal worth. Because many of the basic day-to-day decisions have been made once and for all—when to get up, when to eat, when and how long to meditate, and which practice—attention is freed for inner work during other periods of the day. Moreover, if the meditator has joined a community with a charismatic leader, there may be a great surge of feelings of security and well-being that come with finding a satisfying way of life and an effective guide who can really help. Freud described similar phenomena as "transference cures." Religious people may find the same feeling in certain conversion experiences. Whatever the form in which it is found, this new energy and hope can power major life changes, such as abandoning self-destructive habits and attitudes— which are often put aside forever, even after the "honeymoon" period is over.

Discipline can also benefit the body even if it is not regulated by transcendent values—as, for example, in the armed forces. Regularizing food intake, rest, and activity can reduce tensions and synchronize body clocks to improve physical functioning and minimize stress.

Concentration

What are probably the oldest forms of meditation involve focusing the mind on a single object. Patanjali, who codified the oral tradition of Hindu meditation, considers concentration to be the primary meditative form, whether the focus is on a physical object, on the guru in one's heart, or on a sound, such as OM. Patanjali says (1953, p. 44):

"Sickness, mental laziness, doubt, lack of enthusiasm, sloth, craving for sense pleasure, false perception, despair caused by failure to concentrate, and unsteadiness in concentration; these distractions are obstacles to knowledge. These distractions are accompanied by grief, despondency, trembling of the body, and irregular breathing. They can be removed by the practice of concentration."

The human mind is essentially the same as it was in Patanjali's time, and Patanjali describes the state of *samadhi*, or trance, to be the effect of concentrative meditation. The meditative methods which emphasize concentration are still the ecstatogenic forms. It is fairly easy to achieve altered states of consciousness with such practices—states which can lead to life-giving contact with archetypal innerspace, to movement beyond the realm of the senses, or, unfortunately, to distraction and excitement.

In more concrete terms, the focusing of the mind may disrupt harmful psychosomatic patterns that have taken control of the body. It may support relaxation, thereby reducing stress. It can dissipate anxiety merely by providing an object for the attention, much as happens when, for example, someone with a fear of flying listens to announcements and reads information about the airplane during preparations for takeoff.

Concentration is typically central to psychic healing; this can be true of self-healing as well. One of the most striking example of concentrative meditation is the Hindu practice

of *tratak*. Here the attention is concentrated on the light of a flame of burning *ghee*, or clarified butter. Here is a partial description of the process (cf. Johari, 1974, pp. 73– 74):

"Hold the breath in the lungs and, with a smile, gaze into the midpoint of the flame of a *ghee* lamp which has been placed at eye level, eleven inches from the face. Breathe if necessary, but always deeply, slowly, inaudibly ... When tears flow, empty the lungs and close the eyes. ... Bring eyes to the third eye and concentrate on the afterimage until it vanishes, breathing slowly and deeply."

It has recently been discovered that this age-old practice may have an actual physiological effect on central-nervous-system neurotransmitters. The pineal gland has been shown to be light-sensitive, and its activation seems to change the melatonin-serotonin balance in certain brain areas, producing profound effects on mood and perception.

Contemplation

To extend concentration for a long time can have its own effects. We will refer to such meditative practices as contemplative. Contemplations are often focused on an idea, such as love or truth or God. To sustain these ideas may bring contact with the healing forces associated with them, just as the idea of munching a juicy fruit may cause salivation. We are symbolic creatures; our bodies react to ideas.

Another form of contemplation, widely practiced in Hindu tradition, is having the *darshan* of the *guru* or spiritual teacher, either in actual fact (physical presence), or by experiencing the *guru* as within oneself. Again, if the *guru* represents an ultimate state of well-being, to sustain focus on him is to affirm the value of that state in oneself, and to assert the relative unimportance of various kinds of suffering.

A widespread form of contemplative meditation involves repeating words in the mind. The Hindu term for the practice is *mantra japa*. The practitioner repeats the syllable, word, or phrase continually, sometimes for weeks, months, or years on end. This practice may be done within formal sitting meditation, during life activities, or all the time; a special "rosary" may be used to register each repetition. Each sacred tradition has a rosary, and each has special words to recite: "Guru Om"; "Om mani padme hum"; "La illah ha illa la"; "Hail Mary, full of grace, the Lord is with thee." Is this mere superstition and magical thinking, or is there healing potential in such a practice?

Some traditions claim that certain syllables have healing power for specific purposes. Here is a contemporary account (Davidson, 1966, p. 16) of a healing conducted in a "Temple of Sleep" in Afghanistan by Sufi practitioners:

"After the patient had been assigned a bed, he lay on his back, his eyes fixed upon one of a number of octagonal mouldings. Set in the ceiling, these mouldings were embellished with a nine-pointed diagram. The chief practitioner and his assistants now visited each bed in turn. While the rest of the group maintained a chant of the syllables, "Ya HOO, Ya HUKK!" the chief passed his hands, held together with the palms downward, horizontally over the patient. His hands were held about six inches over the patient's body and passed with a rhythmic movement from the eyes to the toes.... An integral part of the proceedings was that the chief blew upon the patient at about two breaths a second.... The subjects appeared to enter a hypnotic state in about six minutes."

This is a mixed practice, which includes concentration and mantra repetition, as well as another element, evoked by the mantras: these Sufis said that the healing took place because of the transmission of the *baraka*, or grace, of their spiritual forefather, Bahuddin Naqshband.

Even if the reader considers the channeling of power through a spiritual lineage to be only wishful thinking, the repetition of words in the mind may be observed to have healing powers much closer to home. The mantric words, whatever tradition they come from, replace the usual chatter that runs on incessantly in the mind, extending the regretted history and the neurotic self-images forward in time. To disrupt these patterns changes the individual's view of himself and his world; such change can even be permanent. In general, anything is better than these stereotyped, destructive ideas which normally fill our minds; even, as Krishnamurti wryly suggested, chanting, "Coca-Cola, Coca-Cola."

Visualization

Visualization is also used in all religious traditions, but the Tibetan Buddhists are the specialists in this field. Here is a typical Tibetan practice to visualize one deity:

"In the space before us we visualize a pure white cloud, on which rests a golden throne surmounted by a lotus seat and moon-disc. Maitreya Buddha in a position which indicates he is about to rise. His feet rest on a lotus footstool. His body is radiant and golden. His hands are in the *Dharmaçakra* mudra at his heart and from them come two flower stems. The flower on his right supports a Dharmaçakra, the flower on his left a flask of nectar. His ornaments are rich and brilliant. At the center of his chest, at his heart, is a small moon-disc, on which stands the golden syllable *Mai*. Around this letter in a clockwise direction is the Guru mantra; surrounding this is the short mantra of Maitreya, and around this is the extended mantra of Maitreya." (Dreissens, 1974, p. 58).

Clearly this visualization is complicated enough to require much effort by the meditator. Constructing such a scene in the mind takes the utmost attention and focus, leaving hardly any room for ordinary concerns. While the usual activities of "little mind" are absent, it may be possible to "fine tune" the mind toward specific beneficial energies or influences, each of which may alleviate a certain kind of mental and physical suffering.

A specifically Western practice involving visualization has recently emerged in the foreground of the holistic health movement. Carl Simonton, an oncologist working first in the Air Force and then in his own center in Houston, Texas, developed a method of visualizing the disease process, for use with malignancies (Simonton, 1975). The cancer patient is taught to relax and is then guided through a meditation in which the tumor is visualized. The treatment (chemotherapy, surgery, radiation, etc.) is then visualized, and the tumor is seen to slowly weaken, shrink, and finally disappear altogether. The meditation instructions may be taped for home use, four times a day. This technique may prove useful in the treatment of other diseases as well, even where there is no suspected psychogenic component as there is in cancer.

Relaxation

As noted above, many meditation practices involve the deliberate letting-go of muscular tension: relaxation. One of the basic *asanas* (postures) of Hatha Yoga, the *shavasana*, or "corpse posture," involves the profound relaxation of all the muscles of the body. This is done systematically, from feet to head, while lying supine. Other meditation postures work from a seated position, with the weight of the body distributed evenly so that only the large muscles near the spine must work, and the rest of the body can be relieved of tension.

The general effects of relaxation on health are well-known: reduction of habitual muscular tensions; improvement of circulation; restoration of natural rhythms and homeostatic levels; alleviation of stress. The range and depth of possible psychological experiences are increased, especially as the loosening of character amoring produces memory flashes and emotional discharges that had been locked up in bodily tensions—a phenomenon well-known to practitioners of autogenic training and Rolfing.

Nondoing

As we know, formal sitting meditation is typically conducted in a state of immobility. Manipulation of the outside world has to cease for the duration of the practice: coping comes to a temporary halt. Nondoing is a kind of action in inaction. "Just to sit may be the most difficult thing. To work on something is not difficult; but not to work on anything is rather difficult" (Suzuki, 1970, p. 83). Just sitting, not coping, not doing anything, is the greatest challenge we can make against our delusion that the world cannot get along without us—a belief that fosters the familiar list of stress-related diseases. The temporary renunciation of culturally determined goals, strivings, and ambitions frees the meditator from the postures and stance of the social *persona* he or she has developed for the world, allowing room for creativity and new values to come into being.

Spontaneous Movement

By no means do all meditation practices emphasize immobility. Some practices encourage paying close attention to, and honoring, any urge to move spontaneously and freely. The chaotic meditation of Rajneesh is one such method, designed especially for the release of mental, emotional, and bodily tensions before deep practice is attempted (Rajneesh, 1976). The *Latihan* of Subud is also a practice of spontaneous movement, of surrender to whatever inner impulses emerge during the period of practice (Bennett, 1959). Siddha Yoga often involves *kriyas*, spontaneous facial grimaces, gesturing, posturing, rapid and deep breathing, and anything else that may well up in the meditator during his practice (Muktananda, 1973).

All these meditative forms may be particularly useful for those with a tendency toward rigidity of depression. They may make possible the cathartic expression of emotion, with its ability to finish "unfinished businesses." Moreover, some remarkable recoveries of physical health have been reported, such as that of Eva Bartok, who used the Latihan (Bennett, 1959, p. 329).

Passive Attention

Turning now to the fourth and last quadrant of our schema, we come to aspects of meditation that involve "letting go" in the mental domain. All meditation may be said to involve passive awareness: the mind is open to whatever enters it, here and now. The meditative forms which emphasize this attitude most strongly are the great contribution of Gautama Buddha, and complement the concentrative forms in the Buddhist canon. Taken all together, these passive forms are called Vipassana meditation, or insight meditation, and quite aptly so. The meditator simply sits, observing the rising and falling of the abdominal wall. When the mind wanders, the meditator takes note of it, then gently, without exerting any opposing force, returns to contemplation of the abdominal movements. This is the beginning of a state in which the "evenly hovering attention" (as Freud puts it) of the meditator begins to bring to light all sorts of previously repressed thoughts and feelings.

"As you progress in mindfulness, you may experience sensations of intense pain: stifling or choking sensations, . . . pain from the slash of a knife, the thrust of a sharp-pointed instrument, unpleasant sensations of being pricked by sharp needles, or small insects crawling over the body . . . sensations of itching, biting, intense cold. As soon as you discontinue your contemplation, you may also feel that these painful sensations cease. When you resume contemplation, you will have them again as soon as you gain in mindfulness. These painful sensations are not . . . serious. They are . . . common factors always present in the body and are usually obscured when the mind is normally occupied with more conspicuous objects. When the mental faculties become keener, you are more aware of these sensations. With the continued development of contemplation, the time will come when you can overcome them and they cease altogether" (Sayadaw, 1972, p. 16).

This natural biofeedback—in which the attention is made finer, instead of being given a power assist with electronic sensors—can be used to repair, regulate, and heal the body. In a territory hitherto explored mostly by Western psychotherapists, Vipassana can probably offer its own similar long-term benefits to psychological health, depending on how much the meditator can look inward with unconditional positive regard and lack of bias. Contemporary Western procedures analogous to Vipassana can be found in the "continuum of awareness" of Gestalt theory (Perls *et al*, 1951, p. 88) and Gurdjieff's "self-remembering" (Speeth, 1976).

When passive attention is combined with relaxation, there may be a natural waning of learned anxieties and fears. Goleman (1971) called this process "global desensitization." When the body is deeply relaxed (a state which is incompatible with fear) various unconscious and semiconscious memories, images, and thoughts rise to awareness. Each time this happens, there will be some reduction in the negative emotional charge associated with them. Repeated scannings of these disturbing thoughts and feelings while one is in a relaxed and watchful meditative state may cause their negative connotations to disappear entirely.

Absorption

At the deeper levels of meditation, there is a state in which the practitioner gives up the mindful witness, forgets the self, and seems to dissolve into the object of contemplation or even into nothingness. Here is Muktananda's description (1972, p. 55) of such an experience.

"I took the all-pervading consciousness to be Nityananda, firmly regarding the five elements, rivers, oceans, caves and mountains as his different forms. Considering the sky to be his head, the earth his feet, the directions his ears, the sun and moon his eyes, I began to meditate on the all-pervasive Nityananda. My mind became increasingly more absorbed in this contemplation. Thus I meditated, considering the entire outer universe to be his embodiment. Whatever awareness was left, I turned it to contemplate Nityananda within. First I touched my head with my hand, thinking of my beloved Gurudev. 'Nityananda is in my head; he is in my forehead. My beloved Nityananda is in both my ears. Nityananda is in the light of my eyes; he is in my throat. Nityananda is in my arms. He is in my hands. Baba Nityananda is in my fingers. He is the soul dwelling in my heart. Sri Nityananda is in my abdomen. He is in my back. Sri Guru Nityananda is in my thighs. He is in my knees, Nityananda is in my legs. He is in my feet.'

"Thus I installed him in my body. While touching all these parts, I continually repeated *Guru Om, Guru Om,* and felt him in each. What a joy! There was lightness in my heart, and its anguish vanished. Fresh, cooling impulses flowed through my being. I plunged into ecstasy."

Introjection of the object of contemplation in this way may facilitate the surrender of personal patterns of malfunction, and may thus radically affect the disease process—or make it irrelevant.

Faith

Letting go in the mind can also permit the release of the paranoia which forms our self-image as an isolated individual struggling to manipulate a hostile or indifferent environment. In Sufism, for example, the dissolution of the sense of "I," called *fana*, is complemented by *baqa*, the consciousness of survival in God (Arberry, 1950, p. 14). At the end of Attar's *Conference of the Birds* (1954, p. 131), the thirty bird-pilgrims come to the end of their arduous journey, and find the king they were searching for, the Simurgh. (*Si-murgh* means "thirty birds.")

"The sun of majesty sent forth his rays, and in the reflection of each other's faces, these thirty birds (*si-murgh*) of the outer world contemplated the face of the Simurgh of the inner world. This so astonished them that they did not know if they were still themselves or if they had become the Simurgh. At last, in a state of contemplation, they realized that they were the Simurgh and that the Simurgh was the thirty birds. When they gazed at the Simurgh, they saw that it was truly the Simurgh who was there, and when they turned their eyes toward themselves they saw that they themselves were the Simurgh. And perceiving both at once, themselves and Him, they realized that they and the Simurgh were one and the same being. No one in the world has ever heard of anything equal to it."

Fana and *baqa* have nothing to do with visions, physical sensations, or altered perceptions. They are related to something subtle and inward: a radical reorientation toward life and death, toward individuality and humanity. Those who are greedy for psychic fireworks or oceanic regressions must look elsewhere (Becker, 1974). The inner revolution of Sufism is the ultimate medicine for human suffering: by comparison, the other benefits of meditation look more like symptomatic relief.

Diagnosis, Prescription, and Contraindications

Each aspect of meditation has its powers of healing; many have specific uses and, unquestionably, particular dangers and drawbacks for certain individuals. The diagnosis and prescription of meditative practices for the many varieties of suffering is an art that has received far less attention than it deserves.

In general, concentrative practices should be avoided by individuals whose reality-testing function is poor, who are strongly paranoid, or who are likely to develop delusions of grandeur from the altered states of consciousness that these practices tend to produce. Carrington (1978) describes several clinical examples of this syndrome. People with overwhelming anxiety should probably avoid insight meditations, in which the anxiety level can reach intoler-

able proportions. Long periods of meditative practice (as in contemplative meditation) may precipitate psychotic episodes in susceptible individuals (French *et al.*, 1975). Like any other interest or activity, a person's meditation practice can be misused in a way that maintains psychopathology or family pathology—as, for example, when a meditator maintains a defensive feeling of specialness and tyrannizes the rest of the family into silence by the remote control of his or her daily meditation sessions.

Probably the safest course for those in the healing professions is to experiment with meditation practices for themselves, and then to share with clients and friends *only* those which they thoroughly understand. Also, in monitoring the meditation practices given above, the professional should bring to bear all the available tools of Western psychological analysis in evaluating the gain or the danger, regardless of the exotic or "sacred" origin of the techniques being studied. In the Bhagavad Gita, Krishna gives Arjuna some timeless advice that is relevant here: "Fear not, Arjuna, for what is Real always was and always will be, and what is not Real never was and never will be."

Suggestions for Further Reading

Bennett, John G., *Understanding Subud*. University Books, 1959.

Bentov, I., *Stalking the Wild Pendulum*, Dutton, 1977.

Carrington, P., "Using Modern Forms of Meditation in Psychotherapy," in S. Boorstein and K. Speeth, eds., *Explorations in Transpersonal Therapy*. Aronson, 1978.

Davidson, Roy W., *Documents on Contemporary Dervish Communities*. London: Hoopoe, 1966.

Dreissens, Georges, ed., *The Preliminary Practices of Tibetan Buddhism*. Burton, Wash.: Tusum Ling Publications, 1974.

Johari, Harish, *Dhanwantari*. San Francisco, Calif.: Rams Head, 1974.

Ouspensky, P., *In Search of the Miraculous*. Harcourt, Brace, and World, 1949.

Patanjali, *The Yoga Aphorisms of Patanjali: How to Know God*. Translated by Swami Parbhavananda and Christopher Isherwood. Signet Books, 1969.

Rajneesh, Bhavagau, *Meditation: The Art of Ecstasy*. Harper Colophon, 1976.

Sannella, Lee, *Kundalini: Psychosis or Transcendence?* San Francisco, Calif.: Sannella, 1976.

Sayadaw, M., *Practical Insight Meditation*. Santa Cruz, Calif.: Unity Press, 1972.

Shah, I., *Islamic Sufism*. Weiser, 1971.

Speeth, K., *The Gurdjieff Work*. And/Or Press, 1976.

Spiegelberg, F., *Spiritual Practices of India*. Citadel Press, 1962.

Suzuki, Roshi, *Zen Mind, Beginner's Mind*. Weatherhill, 1970.

Tuktu, Tarthang, *Gesture of Balance*. Dharma Press, 1976.

KATHLEEN RIORDAN SPEETH, *Ph.D., is a practicing psychotherapist in the San Francisco Bay Area. She has taught at the California Institute of Transpersonal Psychology, SAT institute, Nyengnia Institute, and JFK University, and is the author of* The Gurdjieff Work *and* The Essential Psychotherapies *(edited with Dan Goleman).*

Self-Hypnosis: Making It Work for You

Francis Dreher and Patrick Woods

SELF-HYPNOSIS can help you meditate, relax, or accomplish certain specific goals—changing habit patterns, increasing performance, improving health, and much more. In this article we present a simple, effective, step-by-step procedure for doing self-hypnosis. It should meet your needs, whatever they may be. If your goal is meditation or relaxation, ignore the *Preinduction* and *Utilization* phases. If you want to accomplish specific goals, use the entire process.

The design of this procedure lets you follow along, step by step, in as much detail as you need. For the first few times, read the entire text, including the *Explanations*. Later, once you are familiar with the process, you can simply read the *Steps* and *Instructions* to refresh your memory. With practice, of course, the whole process will become automatic.

An outline of the four phases of self-hypnosis appears at the end of this article so that you can follow each step clearly, referring to the body of the text only as needed.

Self-Hypnosis Procedure

I. *Preinduction Phase* (Creating a hypnotic affirmation)

Step one: Set a goal.

Instructions: Choose *one goal* at a time.

Explanation: Obviously, there are many different goals you might choose. The important thing is to choose *one goal at a time*. Once you have chosen a goal, it is best to use self-hypnosis at least once a day, and to work toward that goal for a period of time (generally four weeks) before moving on to another goal. Although you will be able to accomplish some of your goals much quicker than in four weeks—perhaps even instantly—four weeks is a reasonable period to allow for when using self-hypnosis. When

This article is an excerpt from the upcoming book, *Self-Hypnosis: Making Your Unconscious Mind Work For You*, by Patrick Woods and Francis Dreher.

you are communicating your conscious desires to your unconscious mind, *repetition* and *consistency* are extremely important. The unconscious maintains learned behavior patterns; therefore you will be repeating the new desired pattern (your goal) over and over so that your unconscious will adopt and maintain this pattern.

Be careful not to start off with a "shopping list" of problems or goals. Often, people choose one topic one day and another topic the next day. But this is a mistake—it does not give the unconscious ample time to redirect itself in a consistent direction. Remember: *one goal at a time*.

When you first start to use self-hypnosis, choose a goal that is important to you but that is not in the category of "a major life-change." Be patient; there is plenty of time. First get used to the process of using self-hypnosis, then gradually build up to bigger and bigger goals. If you address the "smaller" issues first, later on the "bigger" issues may not seem so big. Small changes tend to generalize—to go beyond their immediate effect—and to have a positive impact on your entire life.

Once you have a goal, the next step is to state it in a specially designed way.

Step two: State the goal in the positive, present tense.

Instructions:

1. State your goal clearly and concisely.
2. State your goal in the present tense (as if it has already been achieved).
3. State your goal with "positive phrasing" (no negative "I am not" or "I do not" statements).

Explanation:

You are now ready to create a hypnotic affirmation for the goal you have selected. As an example, let's say that you are afraid to speak in front of groups. To reprogram your unconscious, you would *not* say, "I am *not* afraid to speak in front of groups"—you would not state what you *don't* want. Instead, you must figure out what you *do* want. This positive instruction will give the unconscious a clear message about the direction in which you wish to go. So you may say something like, "I am calm and confident when I speak in front of groups." Now, check the phrase and make sure it is what you really want. If not, adjust your wording accordingly.

Note that in this example, we are speaking as if the change has *already* occurred. If you set the statement in the future—as in, "I *will be* calm and confident when I speak in front of groups"—then the unconscious may take the statement literally. It may think of the goal as something that is going to happen in the future; and since the future never comes, the goal may never be accomplished.

Now that your goal is properly worded, you need to know how to use this wording.

Step three: Use auditory, visual, and kinesthetic senses.

Instructions:

1. Repeat your properly phrased goal mentally to yourself. (Auditory)
2. Imagine yourself doing what you are saying to yourself. (Visual)
3. Add the phrase, "and I feel good" to the end of your "properly phrased" sentence. Imagine what it feels like to be doing what you are saying and visualizing. (Kinesthetic)

Explanation:

The more senses you are able to use, the stronger your affirmation will be. For hypnotic purposes, the three most easily usable senses are: auditory, visual, and kinesthetic. It is easy to activate the *auditory* mode—you are using it simply by saying your hypnotic affirmation.

As you say your hypnotic affirmation, try to form a *visual* image of yourself doing what you are saying. If the images come to you easily, fine. If you have difficulty picturing the scene, then do your best with simply imagining the situation.

To complete the hypnotic affirmation, tag the phrase "and I feel good" onto the end of your properly phrased sentence. When you repeat this phrase to yourself, imagine feeling good in the scene you have created. This activates the *kinesthetic* sense. You may find one or two of the senses difficult to experience at first. This is normal, and with practice you can improve.

Using the public-speaking example, your hypnotic affirmation would be, "I am calm and confident when I speak in front of groups, and I feel good."

You now have a completed affirmation. Store it in the back of your mind—you will use it later.

Next, you will learn how to go into trance.

II. *Induction Phase* (Going into trance)

Step one: Assume a comfortable position

Instructions: Choose a position that you can maintain comfortably. Sitting, lying, or any variation is fine.

Explanation:

You may prefer to sit, since this makes you less likely to fall asleep. Or, conversely, a reclining position may be best, since you can maintain it more easily without experiencing distracting body tension and pains. The important thing is to find a position that is comfortable. If you find yourself falling asleep, adjust toward a sitting position. However, sometimes you may want to go to sleep and will naturally choose a reclining position.

Step two: Maintain a comfortable breathing pattern.

Instructions: Pay attention to your breath. Adjust it so that it is relatively slow and deep.

Explanation:

You are going to be slowing down your body processes, and your breath is what guides those processes. So start by taking several deep, slow breaths to relax yourself. Next, begin to regulate the inhalation so it is comfortably deep but not forced. The exhalation should last at least as long as the inhalation. Regulate your breath in this way so that it becomes slow, even, and comfortable. You are going to maintain this breathing pattern throughout the induction phase. Upon entering the *Utilization* phase, you may continue with this pattern, or you may adjust to a different pattern; do whichever feels right for you.

Step three: Give waking instructions.

Instructions: Decide on a signal to awaken. The signal may be internal or external.

Explanation:

Before beginning the actual induction, you will need to give yourself suggestions on when to awaken. You may use either an *external* or an *internal* signal. If you want to use an external signal, you can use an alarm clock, a timer, or anything in your environment that is predictable. For instance, if you were sitting at a bus stop, the waking signal might be "when the bus comes."

If you want to use an internal signal, you must rely on your internal sense of time—you must suggest that you will awaken "X" minutes from when you close your eyes. The unconscious body-sense of time is quite accurate; it may surprise you after a little practice. The only drawback to the internal-clock method is if you happen to fall asleep. If you have a habit of falling asleep or are especially tired when doing self-hypnosis, use an external signal to awaken.

There is no danger about falling asleep while doing self-hypnosis. In fact, many people use self-hypnosis expressly to relax and help them sleep. If you do fall asleep and have no specific signal to awaken, you will simply sleep in a safe and normal way, and will awaken when ready (as you would any other sleep state).

Step four: Give general suggestions.

Instructions: Repeat the following suggestions to yourself:

I am relaxing into a state of self-hypnosis.
It is a safe and comfortable state.
I may wake whenever I choose.
I may go into a light or deep trance; either is fine.
I can adjust my body as I need, and this will help me go deeper.

ERICKSONIAN HYPNOSIS AND NEURO-LINGUISTIC PROGRAMMING: HOLISTIC APPROACHES FOR CHANGE

Francis Dreher and Patrick Woods

What Is Hypnosis?

HYPNOSIS is a state of consciousness in which our habitual patterns of thinking and behaving are temporarily suspended, thus allowing us to explore beyond our "normal" limits. Because our conscious experience defines reality within certain learned and fixed limits, suspending our familiar conscious patterns creates an altered state, often causing us to experience "reality" differently. Hypnosis lets us journey into the unconscious realm, where reality may be subjective and flexible. In the hypnotic state, different parts of the mind function: the subjective rather than the objective, the abstract rather than the linear, the creative rather than the fixed. Old realities may become irrelevant; new realities may be explored. Hypnosis lets us step out of the world of limits and into the world of potential. The conscious mind may get caught in the idea of failure, but the unconscious mind—the mind reached by hypnosis—operates, unimpeded, in the realm of solutions.

The hypnotic state is not a contrived one. Rather, it simply recreates naturally occurring phenomena, which the body and mind already know how to produce. Naturally occurring abilities often elicited through hypnosis include amnesia, age regression, pain control, time distortion, and control of the involuntary nervous system functions. The hypnotist does not *create* these hypnotic phenomena, but rather *elicits* them from the client's pre-existing abilities.

These "pre-existing abilities" are crucial to the hypnotic process: Inducing the hypnotic state simply means connecting the client with these abilities. It is natural to drift in and out of hypnotic states—we do it all the time. What driver has never experienced highway hypnosis? The conscious mind loses a portion of time, while somehow the unconscious mind navigates our car along the highway. And who has never "blanked out" while watching TV or a movie? So the hypnotic state is not foreign to us.

Ericksonian Hypnosis

Hypnosis has been used for many different purposes over the years, including therapeutic and ability-enhancing uses. The late Milton H. Erickson, M.D., whose clinical career spanned six decades (1920s–1980s), had a tremendous impact on the field of hypnosis and is considered the world's leading therapeutic hypnotist. His assumptions about the nature of the unconscious mind and of human behavior deviated radically from previous viewpoints, yet closely parallel the holistic health principles of today. He believed that people have the necessary resources within themselves to achieve the changes they desire, and that—on the unconscious level—people are always working with positive intentions, and will always select the best choice that is available at any given time. Single-handedly, Erickson created a new direction in the field of hypnosis, and attracted a new interest in, and acceptance of, hypnosis as a therapeutic tool.

The key to the difference between Ericksonian hypnosis and traditional hypnosis is the hypnotist's attitude. In traditional hypnosis, the hypnotist assumes that he/she knows what is best for the client; induces a hypnotic trance; and then, while the client is in a suggestible state, suggests (or demands) that the client follow his/her directions. In Ericksonian hypnosis, the hypnotist takes care not to impose any outside ideas of change on the client, but instead to carefully reinforce the client's abilities to generate change from within.

Because the Ericksonian hypnotist follows Erickson's beliefs about human nature and behavior, he/she needs simply to elicit, and sometimes to help magnify, the client's pre-existing resources and abilities. Thus, the hypnotist treats each client as an individual, with individual needs and abilities, rather than imposing the same general solutions on everyone. Further, the Ericksonian assumption that people's intentions are positive, reliable guides to making good choices, opens enormous possibilities of helping people help themselves. With this confidence in the unconscious mind the hypnotist may suggest that the client use the unconscious realm to explore many different possibilities and select the best ones.

Erickson often made suggestions of this nature. In the case of one overweight woman, he hypnotically suggested that she would "go home, look in the mirror and learn what she needed to learn in order to reach her desired weight." The woman did just that. In all of Erickson's work and teachings, what stands out is a trust in the unconscious mind and faith in human abilities.

Erickson often told the story of when he was a boy and a lost horse wandered onto the Erickson's farm. No one knew who the horse belonged to, so Erickson hopped on his back and rode him out to the main road. Upon reaching the road, the horse turned and continued walking. When the horse occasionally wandered off the side to graze, Erickson would nudge him back onto the path. Eventually the horse turned up a driveway and walked to a small farmhouse. The excited farmer ran out of the house exclaiming: "You found my lost horse. How did you know he belonged here?" Erickson replied: "I didn't know where he belonged, but the horse did. All I did was get him on the path and keep him moving."

Neuro-Linguistic Programming

Throughout the years, many people have studied Erickson's work. Two of the most notable are Richard Bandler and John Grinder, who organized many of Erickson's principles into a coherent, learnable system: Neuro-Linguistic Programming (N.L.P.) N.L.P.'s basic assumptions are rooted in Erickson's philosophy.

Since its beginnings in the early 1970s, N.L.P. has developed into a model of how people process sensory information and interact in the world. This model of human communication and behavior is a learnable one, enabling practitioners to promote rapid change. N.L.P. recognizes the wide diversities of human experience, and systematically looks at how people communicate and make sense of the world. The N.L.P. practitioner uses this information to help people achieve what they want. Much like Erickson, N.L.P. practitioners always look for the unique resources present in any situation, and use these resources to achieve the desired results.

A woman sought help from the authors of this article concerning her debilitating fear of heights. She would get dizzy and freeze at any height above six feet. Interestingly she wanted to overcome this problem so that she could go rock climbing with friends.

Thinking in terms of resources, we asked her what she would need in order to accomplish her goal. She replied that she would need to know that she could move. We then investigated some of the times in her life that she had known she could move in the way she needed. She remembered at time when she had had a particularly strong experience of that sort while running. She recalled, in response to our questions, that she had felt strong and confident, and in control of her body.

Of course when a person remembers something they also re-experience it. And with our assistance she remembered quite strongly what that resource experience was like.

Through a series of hypnotic and Neuro-Linguistic techniques we connected those abilities to the problem area. She went out and accomplished her goal of rock climbing, and no longer had an abnormal fear of heights. This was accomplished in one session without digging into the reasons (real or imagined) for the problem. She had what she needed all the time. All we did was connect her to her abilities. As simple as that.

Relation to Holistic Health

Looking at Ericksonian hypnosis and N.L.P. against the backdrop of holistic health, it is easy to see how these two modalities typify the idea that each individual can gain control of his/her health/life situation. In both modalities, the practitioner helps the client to set aside distractions and limitations, to find and use his/her resources and abilities, and to make the appropriate choices.

Both Ericksonian hypnosis and N.L.P. are true holistic modalities. Their fundamental philosophies involve trust in the individual, and confidence in each person's inner ability to generate and maintain healthful change.

The safe normal sounds around me help me go into self-hypnosis to the depth that is right for me.

Explanation:

These phrases are carefully worded to give you the hypnotic experience that is right for you each time you do self-hypnosis. You may need to read them a few times during this phase of the induction until they become committed to memory.

Step five: Do the induction.

Instructions: Count backwards from twenty to one.

Explanation:

You are now ready to go into trance (you may close your eyes at this point or focus your gaze on a spot in front of you and wait until they close naturally). Give yourself these two suggestions:

"As I count backwards from twenty to one, I relax more and more with each number I count."
"As I reach the number one, I will be in a safe, comfortable hypnotic state."

While counting backwards, coordinate each number you say with the exhalation of your breath (remember, you are breathing regularly).

In conjunction with saying each number as you exhale, to insure that you go into trance use one or both of the following hypnotic-induction methods:

Method one: As you say each number, visualize (or imagine) the number in front of you. What color is it? What size is it? What is it made of?
Method two: Imagine yourself walking down a safe, secure stairway. As you say each number, imagine yourself taking one step down on that stairway. What does the stairway look like? What is it made of? How much more relaxed do you get with each step down?

When you reach the number one (the last step), you will be in a safe, secure place of your choosing. It could be the beach, or the country, or anyplace in your imagination that is safe and secure. Here is where you will use what you have learned in this article to get the changes you want in your life.

Now it is time to remember your hypnotic affirmation and to use it in the *Utilization* phase.

III. *Utilization Phase* (Communicating desired changes to the unconscious mind)

Step one: Use the hypnotic affirmation you have created.

Instructions: Say, see, and feel your affirmation.

Explanation:

When you have reached this phase, you are in trance. It can be a light trance or a deep trance, or somewhere in between. Whatever depth of trance you are in, you will now use your hypnotic affirmation (as described in the *Preinduction* phase) to let your unconscious mind know the changes that you desire. Say, see, and feel your hypnotic affirmation over and over. Remember that trance is a relaxed state and that you can utilize your affirmation from time to time. When you notice that your mind has wandered, simply go back to your affirmation and pick up where you left off. This becomes easier with practice. Remember: for achieving your goals, you should use self-hypnosis *at least* once a day.

After repeating your hypnotic affirmation as often as your time allows, you are ready for the last step: the *Reorientation* phase.

IV. *Reorientation Phase* (Coming out of trance)

Step one: Wake up.

Instructions: Allow yourself, using whatever signal you have as a cue, to reorient into your surroundings.

Explanation:

If you wish to awaken at a specified time, then you have already decided upon a waking signal. When you become aware of that signal, you will know that it is time to reorient into your surroundings. Allow your eyes to open and your body to begin moving (as if you were awakening from any sleep or relaxed state). If you are slow to reorient from a deeply relaxed state, remember that you can go back to that comfortable state whenever you choose, and that you may indeed bring some of those good feelings into the waking state. Give yourself a moment to stretch and reorient before going back to your activities.

You have now completed an entire cycle of self-hypnosis. You may use the process whenever you want and for however long you want. The process will naturally get easier and quicker as you practice. Good luck. Enjoy yourselves.

I. Preinduction Phase (Creating a hypnotic affirmation)
   Step one: Set a goal.
   Step two: State the goal in the positive, present tense.
   Step three: Use auditory, visual, and kinesthetic senses.
II. Induction Phase (Going into trance)
   Step one: Assume a comfortable position.
   Step two: Maintain a comfortable breathing pattern.
   Step three: Give waking instructions.
   Step four: Give general suggestions.
   Step five: Do the induction.
III. Utilization Phase (Communicating desired changes to the unconscious mind)
   Step one: Use the hypnotic affirmation you have created.
IV. Reorientation Phase (Coming out of trance)
   Step one: Wake up.

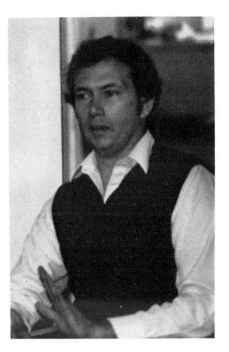

FRANCIS DREHER, *M.A. has been exploring the uses of hypnosis and self hypnosis since 1973. His integration of his master's work in Clinical Psychology with Eriksonian Hypnosis brought him to the Berkeley Holistic Health Center as a practitioner in 1980.*

He has lectured and taught throughout California, Colorado, and Oregon for various schools and organizations. Along with his private practice at BHHC, he is a trainer and co-director of the Hypnosis Training program at the Institute for Educational Therapy.

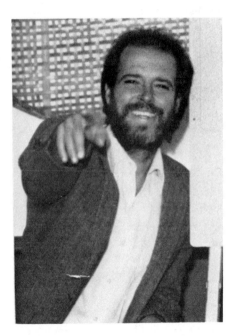

PATRICK WOODS *has been a practitioner in the holistic health field since 1976 and a core member of the Berkeley Holistic Health Center since 1977. His early practice as a deep tissue bodywork therapist lead him to an exploration of the mental and emotional correlates to body disease. He is now also an Ericksonian hypnotist and a "Master Programmer" of Neuro-Linguistic Programming.*

He has lectured and taught throughout California for various schools and organizations, and is a trainer and co-director of the hypnosis training program at the Institute for Educational Therapy in Berkeley. He is also a staff teacher at the National Holistic Institute (Oakland) and Heartwood College (Garberville).

Creative Visualization

Shakti Gawain

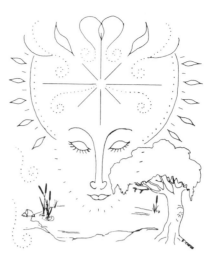

Visualizations are a creative means for developing imagination to positively transform any situations in our lives. Their power becomes real when the idea of "creating our own realities" becomes experience rather than theory. If we believe and act on the assumption that life is positive and that the universe is a safe, supportive place to be, this assumption will become a genuine reality.

CREATIVE VISUALIZATION is one of our most important tools for achieving and maintaining good health. It is the process of forming images and thoughts in our mind, consciously or unconsciously, and then transmitting them to the body as signals or commands.

Creative visualization is thus not really new or unusual; it is a process we already use continuously, every moment. The important thing is to learn to use it *consciously*, to create what we truly want, rather than unconsciously to create things we may not want at all. In a negative sense, we have used creative visualization to produce disease in the first place, and we can learn to use it positively to foster and maintain radiant health and vitality.

Conscious creative visualization is the practice of creating positive thoughts and images to be communicated to our bodies, instead of negative, constricting, literally "sickening" ones.

The key to *using* creative visualization is imagination. Imagination is usually associated with fantasy, daydreaming, "spacing out," with the impractical and ineffectual. In fact, though, our imagination is a powerful tool, closely linked with our natural creativity.

Imagination is the ability to create an idea or a mental picture in your mind. In creative visualization, you use your imagination to create a clear idea of what you want. Then you focus regularly on the idea, or mental picture, giving it positive energy, until you achieve the desired effect.

For example, suppose that certain situations make you tense and nervous. Your image of yourself as a tense, nervous person will tend to perpetuate the problem.

When you learn to use creative visualization constructively, you will spend short, regular periods of meditation, imagining yourself as calm and relaxed in formerly threatening situations. You will start to see yourself as a more easygoing, self-confident person. In this way you will gradually replace the negative image with a positive one. Eventually (sometimes even immediately), you will find yourself more relaxed and confident than ever before.

The same basic process can be used to treat physical problems. Often it is adequate therapy just to get in touch with the ways we created illness, and, using creative visualization, to replace negative concepts with healthier ones. Sometimes other forms of treatment are needed as well. But whatever type of treatment is used, from conventional medicine or surgery to more holistic therapies, creative visualization is always a helpful supplement, one that the patient can use himself in conjunction with what his doctor or practitioner advises.

Using Creative Visualization

There are an infinity of ways to use creative visualization as a meaningful part of our lives. Here are a few ideas.

Physical Health

As we've already discussed, almost any physical problem can be improved by means of creative visualization.

Self-image

Many people have at least some images of themselves that are negative; we see ourselves as in some sense ugly, stupid, selfish, or whatever. When we begin to visualize ourselves as beautiful, intelligent, wise, and so forth, we begin to become that way.

Food

Many people feel negative about food. We may be afraid that the food we eat is going to make us fat or unhealthy. But we can positively program ourselves that we will stay healthy and slim, regardless of what we eat. (Believe it or not, this works.)

One good practice is to make positive affirmations mentally while you eat. Here's another beautifully simple technique: at some point each day, sit down, relax, and drink a glass of water slowly, telling yourself as you drink it that this water is the elixir of life, purifying your body and bringing you perfect health.

Relationships

You can significantly improve almost any relationship—family, friends, lovers, co-workers—by visualizing increased harmony, better communication, more closeness, affection, or appreciation.

Forgiveness and Release

Many emotional and physical illnesses are related to old hurts and resentments from the recent or distant past that are still being held in the body or the psyche. One powerful technique is to picture anyone toward whom you feel hurt or resentful, forgive them, and send them a blessing. When felt deeply, this can totally dissolve and release blocked energy and stored negativity.

Goals

Just visualize and affirm having, achieving, or creating whatever you want. At the end of each visualization period, say the "cosmic affirmation": "This, or something better, now manifests for me in totally satisfying and harmonious ways, for the highest good of all concerned."

Conclusion: Making Creative Visualization Work

The basic technique, as we have seen, is quite simple. Yet creative visualization does not work superficially; it is not mere "positive thinking." It involves our deepest attitudes toward life and toward ourselves. That is why learning the techniques can become a process of deep and meaningful change and growth. In the process, we may discover many ways in which we are holding ourselves back, blocking ourselves from achieving satisfaction and fulfillment, because of our fears and limiting concepts. Once seen clearly, these feelings can be dissolved by means of the creative visualization process, leaving space for us to find our *natural* state of health, happiness, fulfillment, and love.

At first you may use creative visualization only at specific times and for specific goals. As your ability grows, and you begin to trust the results it can bring, you will find that it becomes an integral part of your thinking process.

This is the ultimate point of the practice: to make every moment of our lives a moment of wondrous creation, in which we just naturally choose the best, the most beautiful, the most fulfilling lives we can imagine.

Suggestions for Further Reading

Shakti Gawain, *Creative Visualization*. Whatever Publishing, 1978. Available from Reunion Center, 722 Alcatraz Avenue, No. 205, Oakland, CA 94609.

Marcus, Shakti, and Noj, *Reunion: Tools for Transformation*. Whatever Publishing, 1978. Also available from Reunion Center. Contains many good visualizations and meditations.

Catherine Ponder, *Pray and Grow Rich* (1968); *The Dynamic Laws of Healing* (1963); *The Dynamic Laws of Prosperity* (1962). Parker Publishing. The sensationalistic covers and Christian orientation of Ms. Ponder's works may turn some people off, but I have found them to contain some of the deepest understanding and greatest variety of techniques of affirmation and creative visualization anywhere.

Jean Porter, *Psychic Development*. Random House/Bookworks, 1974. A good guide to visualization with lots of practices.

Israel Regardie, *The Art of True Healing*, Weiser, n.d. A tiny book, containing a beautiful system of creative visualization derived from the teachings of the Kabbala.

Jane Roberts. *The Nature of Personal Reality*. Prentice-Hall, 1975. A clear and powerful explanation of how we create everything that happens to us, and how we can learn to do so more consciously.

José Silva, *The Silva Mind-Control Method*. Simon and Schuster, 1977. The same clear and simple approach used in the Silva Mind-Control Course (this week-long course is taught in most major U.S. cities).

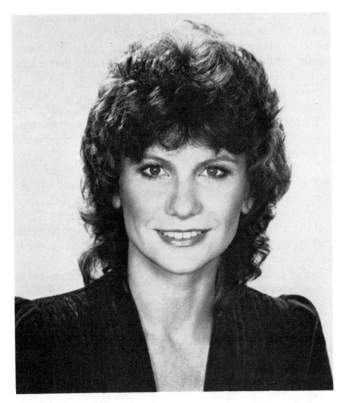

SHAKTI GAWAIN, *author of the best-selling* Creative Visualization *and* The Creative Visualization Workbook, *teaches people how to expand and focus their creativity in order to bring more satisfaction into every area of their lives. She has studied extensively both eastern metaphysical philosophy and western humanistic psychology and sees her work as a blend of these two disciplines.*

Shakti gives lectures and seminars on creative visualization and related topics all over the United States. She makes her home in Tiburon, California, where she maintains a private consulting practice. An articulate and entertaining speaker, she has appeared on many radio and television programs. Shakti is currently at work on her third book, Living in the Light.

Visualization: Producing a Good Harvest

Betsy Blakeslee Teegarden

ARILYN KING, three-time Olympian pentathlete, says she was not a natural athlete—and yet she ranked among the best. She attributes her success to hard training and visualization.

Visualization—the making of mental images—requires only an imagination. We can image any outcome we want, and by so doing feel better.

Psychophysiology of Visualization

How does visualization work in our bodies?

We are not sure. The brain may work better when different kinds of stimuli reach it at one time. During visualization, visual images, words, rhythm, and proprioception all stimulate the brain at once. The brain responds to images as if they were real. It may initiate endocrine and nerve responses that improve mood or health.

Since we visualize while in deep relaxation, we quiet the fight-or-flight response to stress. This alone helps many health problems.

When visualization helps infection or cancer, the following may happen: Neurotransmitters are biochemicals in the brain that carry messages from nerve to nerve—that is, they carry thoughts among cells in the nervous system. Lymphocytes are cells in the immune system that help us to fight infection and cancer. They are a category of white blood cell.

What do these two kinds of cells have to do with each other? The lymphocytes have receptors—places where other substances can attach to them—for neurotransmitters. Neurotransmitters can influence lymphocytes, or else lymphocytes would not need to have a place for them.

According to one hypothesis, during visualization, neurotransmitters travel from the brain—where we make images—to the lymphocytes. The information brought by the neurotransmitters then increases either the activity or the maturation of lymphocytes, or both. This hypothesis explains why there are more lymphocytes in the blood after visualization.

A greater number of neurotransmitters and mature lymphocytes not only helps us to fight infection and cancer, but may stir creative thinking and thus help us to achieve our goals.

How to Visualize

First, decide on your goal or outcome.

Second, follow a relaxation exercise such as the one shown toward the end of this article. We are more suggestible in the relaxation state.

Third, either allow mental pictures to emerge that symbolize your goal, or summon feelings or words instead of pictures to symbolize your goal. People use their senses in different ways.[1] (For those who are highly developed kinesthetically and less so visually, it is easier to feel or sense images to see them. Others whose auditory sense is most acute find it easier to state their desired goal in rhythmic words, sounds, or music. Use the sensory mode that works best for you.)

Now add detail to your image. Refine your picture, feelings, or words until they vividly symbolize your goal.

End with a firm vision of yourself reaching your goal. Step inside this image. Become one with it; feel yourself in a new state.

Finally, tell yourself that as you go through the day, you continue to get closer to your goal. Count from one to three, feeling refreshed and alert at three. Open your eyes.

For a few days, repeat and refine this first imagery. Then include a new sense in it—words, sensations, or pictures that symbolize your goal. Overlap this new sensory symbol with the earlier one.

If you do deep relaxation followed by visualization twice a day, you will usually get results. To improve health conditions, use visualization three times a day. Deep relaxation and visualization each take two to eight minutes.

Vignettes—one- to three-minute visualizations—are a good short cut. After getting calm via a short relaxation,[2] add a crisp, condensed image of your goal. Once or twice a day, vignettes can replace a longer visualization.

Whether you use the long or the short form, keep your visualization specific and simple. Tackle only one goal per visualization.

Use Visualization for:

1. Coping par extraordinaire with a stressful time of the day.
2. Coping par excellence with a stressful event, physical symptom, person, or work task.
3. Finding solutions to a problem.
4. Stirring yourself to action: Visualize yourself taking active steps toward a goal, then—some time from now—reaching the goal.
5. Healing an illness: First, understand how the body heals the symptoms you have.[3] Then visualize and feel the healing process speed up. For example, visualize and feel warmth at the site of an infection or tumor, then picture lymphocytes eating bacteria or tumor cells. For muscle spasms, picture and feel the muscle get warm and creamy. For arthritis or inflammation, visualize and feel coolness at the site of the symptom.

Suggested Imagery

Prevent interruptions. Remove glasses. Close your eyes. Sit or lie down comfortably in a quiet setting.

Draw your thoughts of the day to a close.

Count very slowly from 10 to 1. On each lower number, you go more deeply relaxed. Starting at 10, feel free to drop your tongue and jaw. As you do, loosen your lips, letting them part slightly. At 9, you can let your shoulders begin to go loose and limp. As you go down to each lower number, you become more and more calm. And as you feel the support of what's under you, sink into it. When you're ready, go down to 8, letting tension leave your chest and upper back. Feel your breath soften the muscles there. Each exhalation takes you deeper and deeper into a pleasant, relaxed state. And when you're ready, go down to 7, breathing into your abdomen and lower back. Little by little, let them soften completely. Let yourself sink even more comfortably, 6, deeply relaxed. The pelvis and buttocks—let any tension there soften, 5, deeper and deeper. And when you reach 1, you'll feel loose and calm. Four, your thighs become heavy and warm. Three, deeper and deeper relaxed. Two, The lower legs and feet become heavy and relaxed. And when you're ready, go all the way down to your toes, to 1. Good.

Take a moment to understand an important part of your life that you can influence. Choose an area that now is unsatisfying, but can improve. View it as a film clip—as it is now.

What part could you begin to influence now? Choose a part that, as it changes, will benefit you and those around you. Make it specific.

Let an image emerge that will help you to learn how to influence this part of your life.

See, hear, or feel yourself taking that first step—that step that can make a difference. That's it. What might you say? How would you feel? See yourself taking that step now.

Now, as if you had a time machine, project yourself into the future. Some time from now, many steps later, you look back, taking pride in that positive change you made. You *made* it, and it not only helps you, but also those around you.

Congratulations! Feel the self-confidence that this new change brings. It's good to know that at any time, simply by closing your eyes, you can picture this again and again, helping to make it happen.

When you're ready, count from 1 to 3. As you count, get ready to bring that new positive image back with you to this time and place. When you say "3," you'll feel refreshed and alert. One, two, three.

Problems and Solutions

1. There are two ways to create images—allowing them to emerge and directing them. If you have trouble allowing images to emerge, direct them. If you don't easily direct images, let them emerge. Read Lennart Nilsson's *Behold Man*[3] or Cooper Eden's *Remember the Night Rainbow*[4] to help you make images.
2. If you don't get results within four to ten weeks, examine the obstacles inside and outside yourself blocking your progress. Visualize yourself replacing the obstacle with something stronger than it. Try on your own, talk to friends, or see a therapist for help.
3. Are you trying to change too much too fast? Discuss your goals with someone you respect. Do your goals include changing someone else? Unless it's your own young child, forget it.
4. Do you need more information, insight, or inspiration before your path clears? We live in the age of information. Try books, magazine articles, selected television shows, conferences, classes, the newspaper.
5. You may not be able to influence some things using only your powers. As a seminary student said, "I pray as if everything depended on God. I act as if everything depended on me." Do your best, strengthen yourself until you're capable of more, then try a new tack. Don't try so hard that you become tense. If you don't notice change after awhile, forget this goal for now, and aim for something simpler.

Produce the harvest many times and it becomes good.

Notes

[1] Richard Bandler and John Grinder, *Frogs into Princes* (Moab, Utah: Real People Press, 1979)

[2] Charles Stroebel, *The Quieting Reflex* (New York: Putnam, 1982)

[3] Lennart Nilsson, *Behold Man* (Boston, Mass.: Little, Brown and Co., 1974)

[4] *The Merck Manual*, Ed. Robert Berkow (Rahway, N.J.: Merck, Sharp, and Dohme, 1977)

[5] Cooper Edens, *If You're Afraid of the Dark, Remember the Night Rainbow* (La Jolla, Ca.: Green Tiger Press, 1979)

Suggestions for Further Reading

Dennis Jaffe, "Healing from Within," New York: Bantam, 1982.

Shakti Gawain, "Creative Visualization," Mill Valley, California: Whatever Publishers, 1979.

Norman Vincent Peale, "Positive Imaging," New York: Ballantine Books, 1982.

Norman Shealy, "Ninety Days to Self-Health," New York: Bantam, 1977.

O. Carl Simonton and Stephanie Matthews Simonton, "Getting Well Again," New York: Bantam, 1980.

BETSY BLAKESLEE TEEGARDEN *has an M.S. in Health Psychology. In her private practice in Berkeley, California, she counsels and teaches imagery, self-hypnosis, and stress management. She trains professionals in these methods and is writing a book on how to use illness as a learning experience.*

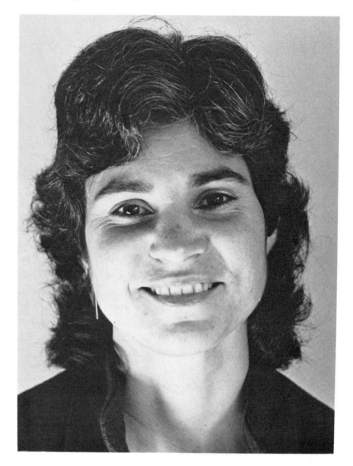

B. NOURISHING THE BODY

Dieting with the Seasons

Elson M. Haas, M.D.

I SEE SO many people in my office who have dietary questions like, "What diet should I eat?" "What is a balanced diet?" "Should I eat meat or be a vegetarian?" "Is this particular food right for me?"

Of course, there are no simple answers. It seems that dietary awareness is growing rapidly, and more and more people are asking themselves and their practitioners these questions.

The answer that I have found most reliable after working with myself and others the last 11 years is—your diet is an *individual* experience based on *personal needs*, your *climate*, i.e., where you live, and your daily *activity*. Food is the body's fuel; how you digest, assimilate, and use the nutrients in your diet create the energy on which you run your body—that magnificent machine.

Obviously, most people eat differently in the peak of winter than in the summer heat. It seems that heating and cooling the body through diet is a good balancing tool. When it is cold, you are naturally attracted to warm drinks and food; more cooked meals and concentrated foods that provide more *fuel*. During hot weather, it is the opposite: cool drinks, fruits and vegetables, and in general, lighter eating.

When you do physical work or exercise, your body needs more fuel. During inactive times the dietary intake needs to be diminished or the body can gain weight. Mental activity requires less total calories; however, the vitamins and minerals are used more readily. The business person who sits a lot, doesn't exercise, and eats three large meals a day may get into trouble around the waist and could more easily develop health problems.

The simplest weight loss program obviously requires eating less food and calories and being *more active physically*. Exercise is very helpful to good digestion, assimilation, and circulation.

Dietary Habits—The Five Truthful -lys
(words that end in lys)

There are very few broad generalizations you can make about diets and proper eating. Here are a few that seem to be most universally helpful.

1. *Moderately*—Eating too much at a meal or in your total diet is stressful on the body, may lead to poor digestion, and can slow you down. Eating the proper amount for you is the key to your diet.

2. *Simply*—Mixing too many different foods at one meal can also be stressful for the body, especially the digestive system. In my experience, food-combining is an important principle to follow to prevent intestinal gas and fermentation of simple foods like fruits.

3. *Early*—It is best to eat the majority of your dietary intake before dark if possible. Eating too close to sleep can lead to both poor use of the food and poor sleep.

4. *Naturally*—Eating as close to the garden and nature as possible is ideal. The more steps and processing a food goes through, the less vitality it has. The essence you get from foods comes from the sunshine, water, air, and earthly nutrients that go into them.

5. *Seasonally*—Eat according to the seasons; those foods that are naturally available in your locale. Growing some of your own foods if possible, and eating the current seasonal diet is the easiest way to be in harmony with nature.

Of course, listening to your body (being aware of how foods affect your energy), eating in a relaxed and inwardly calm atmosphere, eating a chemical-free diet, drinking good clean water, and chewing well, are other dietary habits to develop.

The Seasonal Diet

The premise of eating seasonally is to re-attune yourself to nature, as your ancestors lived in harmony with what nature provided. Their basic diet was fresh fruits and vegetables, grains, beans, nuts, and seeds. Also added were fish in the coastal and freshwater areas, and occasional beef in the range areas. Growing your own food and buying from local farmers is a beginning step for eating seasonally.

Two other factors affect what is available to you and what your diet will be. The first is the climate in which you live. Most of the United States has definitive seasons: cold and snow in the winter, and heat in the summer. The bounties of fresh foods come from later spring into autumn. The west coast and southern states have longer growing seasons, less dramatic seasonal changes, and thus, more available fresh foods.

The second aspect of the seasons affecting your dietary habits is the light and dark cycle of nature, i.e., the amount of sunlight and darkness. Summer is the longest daytime period and winter has the longest nights. This cycle of light and dark is common across the country. The equinoxes (spring and autumn) and solstices (summer and winter) are the demarcation points for changing seasons. This cycle influences your activity levels more than any other, and in this way influences your dietary needs. By affecting the actual temperatures, it also modifies your intake.

Spring

Spring is the cleansing and healing season. Everything is being renewed in springtime. Nature is returning from its inner season and beginning to green. The fresh greens are the revitalizing foods. High in chlorophyll, they tend to strengthen the blood and purify the body. The lettuces and spinach are available, plus a variety of local greens like dandelion, miner's lettuce, dock, sorrel, etc., may be available in your area. Other spring vegetables are also harvested, like asparagus, artichokes, chard, and celery.

Citrus fruits may also be available, especially in the west and south, and these foods tend to be cleansing to the body systems. In my book, *Staying Healthy With the Seasons*, I discuss fasting on a specific lemonade formula. It is often a powerful and healing experience.

Herb teas as spring purifiers may be beneficial. Sassafras bark, dandelion root, comfrey, nettles, mints, and more may be helpful to you.

Again, spring is the time for clearing the past, healing the present, and planning for the future.

Summer

The summer is usually the warmest of seasons and often a time of increased physical activity, so you may need additional nourishment as well as a lighter diet than usual. It is important to not overheat your system. Drinking plenty of good water, juices, and cool teas can prevent this.

Summer is the main fruit season of the year and nature is certainly wise to provide us with these most cooling foods during this season. With plums, peaches, apricots, and most of the berries and the melons, it is definitely a juicy time. Lots of vegetables for salads or sliced up for dips are also a good idea. In summer your heavier, cooked, or protein meal can be eaten later in the day as the temperature cools down.

Autumn

The light cycle changes as we move into autumn, and nights now become longer than days. This often means a cooling of the weather and a decrease in your activity.

Autumn is the *harvest* season, and everything is available—fruits like apples, pears, persimmons, and grapes; melons, too; bushels of vegetables like corn, carrots, beets, all the squashes; lots of beans, seeds, grains and nuts are being gathered.

So you will be adding more concentrated protein and complex carbohydrates to your diet, such as cooked grains, beans, squashes, and potatoes, that burn richer and hotter in your system. It is a good time to move more into work and school and re-focusing on your health and toning your body. A new exercise program is an ideal autumn venture as you begin to build your strength in preparation for the deep, upcoming winter.

Winter

Life seems to become more internal as you may spend more time inside during the winter. It is a powerful time for inner development, often reducing outer activities, and a strong family and friend time.

There is often more focus on food with lavish holiday preparations and parties. Winter can be the most food-oriented season and you'll have to find that balance between keeping your body well-heated and watching your waistline.

Again, the richer foods from autumn harvest are available, and cooked grains and root vegetables like carrots, onions, garlic, and potatoes can be eaten more plentifully. Also, the ocean foods, like fresh fish and seaweeds, and the high mineral foods, are very balanced together.

Eating a heavier diet often leads to reduced activity, and more rest and sleep as you can spend a bit more time in the dreamland of winter.

Conclusion

It seems that more and more people are turning back to nature and eating more simply. The upsurge in health awareness is creating new demands on the food industry to make more wholesome and chemical-free nutrition. This is concurrent with the general lifestyle changes that promote optimum health, such as more exercise, relaxation and stress reduction, healthier work environments—all which make current new demands on the health industry to address the issues of preventive medicine and health education.

The more subtle issues in regards to how you live your life on a day-to-day basis seem to most greatly influence your long-term health. Good air, good water, and good food are the beginning building blocks for the healthy body. As the wise ones know, "Good food, good thoughts, good actions."

Following the secrets of the centenarians, who live close to the land, often in the fresh air of the hills and mountains, and work and eat close to nature, is a direction you can all follow. Even living in a more stress-filled city, with the knowledge and practice of what you can best do for yourself and family to attain your current optimums in health is likely to add years to your life and life to your years.

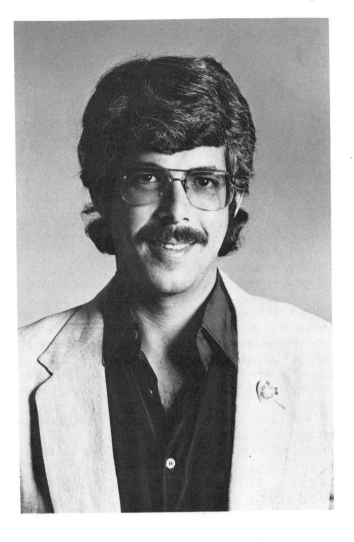

ELSON M. HAAS, *M.D., author of* Staying Healthy With the Seasons, *received his degree in medicine from the University of Michigan in 1972. Since then, he has undertaken independent studies in Chinese medicine, acupuncture, nutrition, herbology, and metaphysics which has led him to practice what he calls Integrated Medicine in his San Francisco Bay area offices. This article on Seasonal Diet is an outgrowth of his book which is in its fourth printing and has been translated into both German and Spanish. Dr. Haas is a lecturer and health educator in addition to his private practice.*

Eating Poorly, Eating Well

Peter Ways, M.D.

If doctors of today will not become the nutritionists of tomorrow, the nutritionists of today will become the doctors of tomorrow.

—Thomas A. Edison

E ARE experiencing a renaissance of nutritional awareness. More and more professionals and lay people are acknowledging that how and what we eat is vital to health. Medical schools are beginning to teach nutrition, and the legitimate purview of the subject is no longer just "obesity" and vitamin deficiency. Many other relationships between nutrition and health have attained widespread acceptance: high-fat diets increase risk for heart disease, fiber lowers risk of bowel cancer. Many others are subtle and still poorly worked out or not even generally recognized: the effects of food processing on the nutritional value of most foods; is refined sugar only "empty calories," or is it harmful in other ways as well? However, the most compelling reason for attending to the qualitative issues of nutrition is that people who do so feel better. It isn't a matter of "taking your medicine" to avoid disease, it's really an issue of enjoyment and energy.

Personal Health Competence includes attention to both these qualitative issues and the quantitative aspects of eating.

Current Nutritional Behavior of Most Americans and Its Consequences

For the last 50 years Americans have eaten a diet high in fat (average 42% of total calories), particularly saturated fats (the harder fats like lard, butter, and meat fat, in contrast to oils which are unsaturated) and cholesterol.

Our diet has also been high in refined sugar—18% of calories on the average. In 1976 each American consumed 126 pounds of refined and processed sugar in contrast with less than 40 pounds in 1825. We consume more salt than we need as well. An adult requires less than 1/10 of a teaspoon per day, but Americans average 1–4 teaspoons per day. Typical food also contains too little fiber, the indigestable part of many vegetables and grains that help food residues move through the bowel more rapidly. Finally, a significant number of people get more than 10 percent of their total calories from alcohol—which, in addition to its addicting properties, is, like sugar, "empty calories."

Table 1 summarizes the better-known consequences of such poor nutrition, not including vitamin deficiencies. Starred items are discussed in the paragraphs that follow.

TABLE 1: THE MEDICAL CONSEQUENCES OF UNHEALTHY NUTRITION

Poor Nutritional Behavior	Medical Consequence
too much salt	increased blood pressure★ in susceptible people
too much refined sugar	increases weight, empty calories, displaces nutritional food, dental caries, addiction
too much total and saturated fat, too much cholesterol	increases risk for heart disease★
too many calories (overweight)	increases risk for diabetes, arthritis, high blood pressure, gall bladder disease
too much alcohol	empty calories, liver disease, alcohol addiction, alcoholism, increases risk for some cancers★
too much fat	increases risks for cancer: breast,★ colon,★ rectum★
low fiber	diverticulitis, bowel cancer, higher blood cholesterol, constipation

From *Take Control of Your Health*, The Stephen Greene Press, 1985.

Hypertension—High Blood Pressure

There is an important relationship between the intake of salt (sodium chloride) and blood pressure. It is the sodium in salt, as well as other compounds, that is responsible for this relationship. While individuals react differently to high salt intake, the frequency of high blood pressure is related to the level of salt intake in most societies. In the United States, almost every processed food label reveals salt in the enclosed product. Salt is added to baby food to make it taste okay to mothers. Babies don't need it, but it's there, so another salt addict is born. Many people who develop high blood pressure add large amounts of salt to their food, though there are also people who ingest a lot of salt and never get high blood presure. Some individuals with mild hypertension (blood pressure levels of 140–160/90–105) show significant lowering of blood pressure on restricted sodium intake, although by no means all do. All people who have high blood pressure or who are at some added risk for developing high blood pressure, such as a family history of the condition, are wise to limit their sodium intake. Effectively this means no use of salt at the table, no cooking with salt, and giving up salty processed foods such as potato chips, tortilla chips, pretzels, and pickles.

Recent investigations indicate that a high calcium intake is beneficial for high blood pressure. When calcium supplements are used, rigid salt restriction is not desirable though excessive use of salt is still harmful.

Coronary Artery Disease

Heart attack and related problems are the leading cause of death in the United States. Volumes of evidence from population studies, laboratory experiments, and clinical observations tell us that there is a definite relationship between the blood (serum) cholesterol level and the chance of developing heart attack. An attack is usually caused by closure of an artery that supplies blood to the heart itself and is due to arteriosclerosis. Some of the same studies, as well as careful experiments on humans involving manipulation of dietary components, show that, for most people, lowering the total fat in the diet lowers the serum cholesterol. In addition, there are high correlations between total dietary fat intake in populations (particularly hard fats) and the incidence of coronary disease. People who have high cholesterol and/or blood sugar need to worry more about their fat intake. The intake of vitamins E and B_6 and lecithin may also be crucial to preventing arteriosclerosis, though research is still in progress.

Cancer of the Large Bowel and Rectum

A relationship between the amount of fiber in the diet and the incidence of bowel cancer (the more food, the less cancer) is increasingly apparent. The time required for food residues to travel from stomach to rectum is the crucial factor. Fiber provides bulk, and speeds this process. Because of refined foods and high-fat, high refined sugar intake, the fiber content of the average American diet is very low. Milling flour, for example, removes most of the covering of the wheat kernel, which is the part containing the bran. Bran is largely fiber. Natural foods, particularly oatmeal and granola, and bread made from whole-grain flours, are rich in bran. Pure wheat bran sold in natural food stores is inexpensive, and, unlike Kellogg's All-Bran and similar products, is whole bran. It tastes like sawdust, but is tolerable when mixed with salads or cereals. Corn bran is said to be more effective but is not so readily available.

The frequency of large bowel and rectal cancer is also increased by high alcohol and dietary fat intake over a number of years. High alcohol intake also increases the incidence of cancers of the lip, mouth, pharynx, esophagus, and stomach. Consumption of more than 8–10 alcoholic beverages a week may be the critical amount.

Cancer of the Breast

While many factors formerly thought to increase risk for cancer of the breast have been excluded (e.g., being Jewish, never having married, menstruation beginning before 12, daily consumption of alcohol) it now appears that a high-fat diet is the most critical risk factor yet identified. Some say the evidence is as compelling as that linking smoking with lung cancer.

Health Competence in Nutrition

To be health competent nutritionally means applying certain basic principles to your eating, and gradually changing to an alternative food pattern—of health competence.

The Principles of Healthy Eating

The following principles of healthy eating are a synthesis of the current thinking of nutritionists, medical people working in nutrition, and health maintenance enthusiasts. They also incorporate the dietary goals of the Senate Select Subcommittee on Nutrition (1979).

1. *Strive for variety* because, a) no single food or group contains all the nutrients you need, b) eating different foods will decrease likelihood of exposure to harmful contaminants that might be found in any one food. Select foods from each of the following groups: a) fresh fruits and vegetables, b) whole-grain breads, cereals, other grain products (corn, wheat, rye, rice), c) dry peas, beans (legumes), and nuts, d) animal products—red meat, poultry, fish and also milk, yogurt, cheeses. The amounts eaten from group d) must be limited. An eight-ounce steak contains 33 gm, or 300 calories, of saturated fat. This is half the fat intake an average person should have in a day. Meats are more likely to contain drugs and toxins because the animals are sometimes fed grains "doctored" with hormones to increase meat production.

2. *Use unprocessed foods* and (in general) non-fat foods—they have more vitamins and minerals per ounce or cupful. Processing can remove, reduce, alter, or destroy these nutrients. It may also add undesirable contaminants. In addition, most processed foods contain a lot of the salt, saturated fat, and sugar so prevalent in our diet.

TABLE 2:—COMPARING PREVALENT AND ALTERNATIVE FOOD PATTERNS

Caloric Density and Salt, Sugar, and Saturated-Fat Content of Common Foods

KEY: SF = SATURATED FAT; C = CHOLESTEROL; Sa = SALT; Su = SUGAR

	High Caloric Density (HCD)	Medium Caloric Density (MCD)	Low Caloric Density (LCD)
Alternative Food Pattern	Commercial baked goods and cakes made from mixes (SF, C, Sa, Su) Frankfurter (SF, C, Sa) Bacon (SF, C, Sa) Luncheon meat (SF, C, Sa) Ham, sausage (SF, C, Sa) Most regular cheeses (SF, C, Sa) Ice cream, ice milk (SF, C, Su) Creamy peanut butter (SF, Sa) Red meat (SF, C) Organ meat (SF, C) Butter (SF, C) Snack crackers (SF, Sa) Palm oil, coconut oil (SF) Hardened margarines (SF) Candy (Su) Fruit in heavy syrup (Su) Sherbet and frozen yogurt (Su) Salted nuts (Sa) Potato chips and other chips (Sa)	Buttermilk (SF, C, Sa) Egg yolk (SF, C) Whole milk (SF, C) Granolas with added salt and sugar (Sa, Su) Shellfish (C) Turkey franks (Sa) Roasting turkey injected with salt (Sa) Canned soups (Sa) Canned corn, beans, or peas (Sa) Frozen fish (Sa) Canned tuna (Sa) Biscuits, muffins, pancakes (Sa) Instant cereals (Sa) Dehydrated potatoes (Sa) All-Bran, Bran flakes, cornflakes (Sa) Soda crackers (Sa) Soft drinks (Su) *Low in fiber, but otherwise "heart healthy"* White bread, English muffins White rice Spaghetti and other pasta made from white flour Fruit juice without pulp	Bouillon (Sa) Consommé (Sa) Canned vegetable juice (Sa) Most canned garden vegetables (Sa) A few frozen vegetables (peas, succotash, lima beans) (Sa) Pickles (Sa) Sauerkraut (Sa) Melba toast (Sa) Salted popcorn (Sa)
Usual U.S. Food Pattern	All vegetable oils (*including* olive oil) except palm and coconut Avocado Honey Mayonnaise or salad dressing Natural peanut butter (no salt) Sesame butter Sesame seeds Soft margarine Sunflower seeds Unsalted nuts	Breads, lightly milled or whole-grain Brown rice Canned fruit (no syrup) Chicken without skin Common potato and corn Egg whites Fresh fish Fresh or dried fruit Fruit juice with pulp Granolas without salt or sugar Legumes (beans, lentils, peas, soy beans, garbanzo beans) Low-fat cottage cheese Nonfat milk Puffed rice Shredded wheat Spaghetti and other pasta (from partial whole-wheat varieties) Turkey Yams and sweet potatoes	Alfalfa sprouts and bean sprouts Artichokes Beets Broccoli Brussels sprouts Cabbage Carrots Cauliflower Celery Chard Cucumbers Fresh vegetable juice Green beans Lettuce Mushrooms Radishes Spinach and other greens Squash Tomatoes and most other garden vegetables Most frozen vegetables

From Farquhar, John W. *The American Way of Life Need Not be Hazardous to Your Health*, The Portable Stanford (Palo Alto, CA: Norton, 1978)

3. *Practice moderation*; it is OK to eat almost anything once in a while but moderation in total calories, salt, fat, cholesterol, sugar, alcohol, and caffeine are healthy.

4. *In certain physiological, stressful, and illness states "compensation" is necessary.* Women in the childbearing years may need iron supplements to replace iron lost with menstrual bleeding; pregnant or breastfeeding women need more iron, folic acid, vitamin A, calcium, and calories but most of these can be obtained by properly adjusting the diet. Infants and young children need more vitamins and minerals because they are growing. Elderly or very inactive people usually eat less, and should particularly avoid foods high in calories and low in vitamins and minerals. Persons under inordinant stress or with physical or mental ailments need more protein and calories.

The Alternative Food Pattern

The food pattern of health competence is much more compatible with health and well-being than the typical contemporary American diet. It depends heavily on the first three principles of good nutrition just outlined, and will help people avoid the disorders that are significantly related to our prevalent diet. In addition, people who have made the change consistently *feel better*, have more energy, and enjoy their food more.

The alternative pattern means more variety (principle 1), fewer processed foods (principle 2) as well as everything in moderation (principle 3). As a result of these changes total intake of fat, cholesterol, salt and refined sugar decrease, and the overall caloric density of the food gradually declines. In Table 2 one shifts from foods predominately above the line to ones mainly below the line. This involves eating less red meat, fewer high-fat dairy products (butter, cheese), less high cholesterol food and fewer processed foods. These are replaced by more whole grains, legumes (mainly beans and peas), fresh fruits, vegetables, and low-fat dairy products. It also means replacing foods high in caloric density with foods of lower caloric density.

It is not necessary or even desirable to eat all foods that show below the line or entirely to the right in Table 2, and it is definitely not necessary to make these changes all at once. It is far better to move into the alternative pattern in several phases, each 3–6 months long. Each phase can involve relatively easy changes but the *cumulative* effect over two years is a striking alteration in dieting pattern. John Farquhar's book, *The American Way of Life Need Not be Hazardous to Your Health* describes how to accomplish this phased change process.

About Vitamins

In the years I've been working on this book, no single question has confused me more than "should I take vitamin pills"? There are professional nutritionists who say we should use supplements and there are also those who say a balanced diet will provide enough vitamins. I am not going to summarize the evidence to both views; I favor supplementation. Here are my reasons.

1. The Recommended Daily Allowances (RDAs) for vitamins are felt by many experts to be too low. Dr. Pauling (a Nobel Prize winner in biochemisty, and more recently the most influential and persistent advocate of the use of

Vitamin C to prevent and minimize colds) believes we should call the RDA values the Minimum Daily Allowance (MDA) and then propose a Recommended Daily Intake for each vitamin presented as a range instead of just one figure (see Table 3).

2. The requirements for a given vitamin vary from individual to individual. This is true in the "normal" state of health. Greater variations occur during psychological stress, illness, surgery, physical inactivity, and with aging.

3. Many people do not, or cannot for economic and social reasons, eat nutritionally sound diets.

4. Many medicines antagonize, block, or neutralize the effects of vitamins. Our knowledge about this is very sketchy.

5. Various environmental hazards may increase our need for certain vitamins: pollution, chemicals in food, herbicides, pesticides.

6. Not enough is known about the effects of additives, heat and cold during the growing, preserving, transporting, and cooking of food, particularly large-scale cooking, on vitamin activities in the food.

7. Our knowledge about all of these things is only beginning to accumulate and be organized in useful ways.

There are a number of multivitamin preparations available which are inexpensive and provide adequate supplementation for average circumstances.

"Reading What You Need"

The uncertainties of good nutrition are apparent. To some extent we must rely on our own judgment to decide what is good for us and what is bad, what we should eat today and what tomorrow. Although I am not aware of scientific evidence to support this contention, I believe we are capable of developing and sharpening a *felt sense* about food— an ability to read our needs. Simply, this means that our bodies will tell us what and how much we need. Yearnings for a particular food are highly significant. If I want dried apricots and nothing else will do, my body is telling me there is something in dried apricots that it is important for me to have. No longer a regular meat eater, I have widely spaced yearnings for red meat. I accede to them. This also happens with certain nuts, a particular fresh vegetable, or fruit. If I keep my diet varied and fresh, I notice these specific yearnings occurring less frequently. I think a tuned mind-body is necessary to activate this sense in a highly refined way. People who are actively exercising and participating in activities which regularly enrich their emotional/spiritual health are more likely to have this sense. In this time of nutritional uncertainty it is a helpful, perhaps even a highly protective, mechanism.

The Depletion and Alternation of Food

In the next decade, depletion and alteration of food will be a major controversy in the health field. The following will provide some appreciation of the magnitude of the problem:

- Most food is grown in depleted soil artificially enriched by chemicals. Changes can occur in the levels of vitamins and protein in grains and other foods as

TABLE 3: THE COMMON VITAMINS

Vitamin	Main Sources	Properties	Function	Recommended Daily Allowance[f]
FAT-SOLUBLE VITAMINS				
A	Cheese, green and yellow vegetables, butter, eggs, milk, fish-liver oils	Lost by long cooking in open kettle. Toxic in large doses.	Growth, normal bone development, tooth structure, night vision, healthy skin.	4000-5000 IU[b], adults. 2000-3300 IU, child.
D	Fatty fish, eggs, liver, made by skin on exposure to sunlight.	Very stable. Toxic in large doses.	Intestinal absorption of calcium, metabolism of calcium and phosphorus, bone and tooth development.	400 IU
E	Widely distributed in foods, particularly vegetable oils, wheat germ.	Lost by long cooking in open kettle. Toxic in large doses.	Not definitely known for humans.	30 IU, adult. 20 IU, child.
K	Eggs, liver, cabbage, spinach, tomatoes. Made by intestinal bacteria.	Destroyed by light and alkali. Absorption depends on normal fat absorption.	Blood clotting.	Not established. Given to pregnant women and newborn infants.
WATER-SOLUBLE VITAMINS[a]				
Thiamin (B$_1$)	Meat, whole grain, liver, yeast, nuts, eggs, bran, soybeans, potatoes.	Stable in cooking but may dissolve in cooking water. Needed daily.	Carbohydrate metabolism. Promotes growth.	1.0-1.5 mg,[d] adult. 0.7-1.2 mg, child.
Riboflavin (B$_2$)	Milk, cheese, liver, beef, eggs, fish.	Stable in cooking of acid foods. Unstable to light and alkali.	Metabolism in all cells.	1.1-1.8 mg, adult. 0.8-1.2 mg, child.
Niacin (nicotinic acid)	Bran, eggs, yeast, liver, kidney, fish, whole wheat, potatoes, tomatoes.	Stable in cooking, may dissolve in cooking water.	Growth, metabolism, normal skin.	12-20 mg, adult. 9-16 mg, child.
B$_6$ (pyridoxine)	Meat, liver, yeast, whole grains, fish, vegetables.	Stable except to light.	Amino acid metabolism.	1.6-2.0 mg, adult. 0.6-1.2 mg, child.
Folic Acid	Liver, Green vegetables.	Not stored; need daily; water soluble.	Division of cells DNA & RNA metabolism.	.4 mg
B$_{12}$	Meat, liver, eggs, milk, yeast.	Unstable to acid, alkali, light.	Red blood cells production and growth.	1.0-2.0 μg,[e] adult. 3.0 μg, child.
Ascorbic acid (C)	Citrus fruits, cabbage, tomatoes, potatoes, leafy vegetables.	Very unstable to heat, alkali, air. Dissolves in cooking water.	Cellular metabolism; necessary for teeth, gums, bones, blood vessels.	45 mg, adult. 40 mg, child.

Footnotes: a. Other water-soluble vitamins seem essential to nutrition but are not as well understood, and deficiency is less common. b. International Units. c. Retinol Equivalents. d. Milligrams. e. Micrograms. f. Pregnancy and Lactation require 1.5-2.0 times the RDA.

the result of growth assisted by artificial fertilizers.

- Meat and poultry are produced with the aid of hormones and antibiotics. These medicines are used in high enough concentration so that some of the native material and/or its metabolic product persist in the meat throughout butchering and processing. They are consumed by the meat eater.
- There is widespread use of insecticides, pesticides, and herbicides in agribusiness. Less well known is the fact that small amounts of these materials are often found in consumer-ready food products. Some are poisons, but their effects on man have not always been adequately studied.
- There are thousands of different (estimates vary from 3000 to 12,000) chemical compounds and additives that may be used to alter or maintain the color, taste, and texture of food, to fortify food that has been depleted during processing, and to prevent premature spoilage. Some single artificial flavorings contain 100 or more untested chemicals. Relatively few of them have been tested for safety by the food industry or the FDA. Most people presume food additives are monitored *before they are used*. To emphasize the fallacy of this assumption, Dr. Herbert L. Ley, Jr., former FDA commissioner, said:

The thing that bugs me is that the people think the FDA is protecting them—it isn't. What the FDA is doing and what the public think it is doing are as different as night and day.*

- High-volume cooking, freezing, and thawing are commonplace in the preparation of processed foods. Potentially these procedures can deplete food of vitamins and minerals and/or cause other chemical alterations. There is definite evidence that this is so for some foods, but in the vast majority of instances *we do not know the consequences*.
- Americans' love of salt and sugar begins with baby food, to which needless salt and sugar are added.
- Although 35 percent of asthmatics are allergic to tartrazine (Yellow #5) it is found as a coloring agent in many anti-asthma medications.
- The red dye in one cherry soda can cause cancer in chick embryos.

Recently, the Environmental Protection Agency (EPA) has put severe restrictions on the use of Ethylene Di Bromide (EDB) as a pesticide in agriculture. It has been used

---

*N.Y. Times, December 31, 1969

particularly for corn, wheat, and other grains. Before its use, muffin mixes and flour grew weevils after being stored in the home for a while. For a decade, EDB has been identified as a potent cancer-causing agent in animals. As yet no definite links with human cancer have been shown. But the EPA in its statement says, "It is not acute effects we are concerned about—it is the long-term repeated exposure that may be dangerous." This is 1983. EDB has been used since 1948!

Thus it is obvious that with respect to the qualitiative aspects of food the number of variables is increasing at an enormous rate. Current knowledge is imperfect. We are in an age of nutritional approximation. Most foods are processed. Even fresh fruits and vegetables may be dyed, and most have been grown with pesticides. The situation is complicated by the politics and economics of the food industry. As often occurs under such circumstances, experts and personal experience enthusiasts offer guidance and solutions. Even those programs which are sound can involve principles counter to established eating habits and, often, economic capability.

There are no easy answers for consumers about how to deal with these problems. Packaging laws do not require that all additives be mentioned on the label, so it behooves all of us to keep informed as well as possible, to express concern when we feel it, and to boycott any products for which there is good evidence of harmful effects. Eating a variety of unprocessed foods as often as possible will minimize the unknown dangers, but unfortunately, under present controls, not make us immune to serious harm.

Suggested Further Reading

Ballentine, R., *Diet and Nutrition.*, Himalayan International Institute, Honesdale, PA, 1978. A comprehensive and authoritative analysis of many of the most crucial aspects of nutrition.

Hall, R.H., *Food for Nought, The Decline in Nutrition.* Harper and Row, New York, 1974. A critical analysis of the current qualitative issues in nutrition. Comprehensive and provocative. The author is a prestigious biochemist.

PETER WAYS, *M.D., developed an innovation in medical education, a problem-based learning segment designed to help students integrate basic science with clinical problems. He was Professor of Health Professions Education at University of Illinois where he helped develop strategies and materials for helping emerging countries learn effective health management practices. He is the author of* Take Control of Your Health: The Guide for Personal Health Competence. (*The Stephen Greene Press, 1985*).

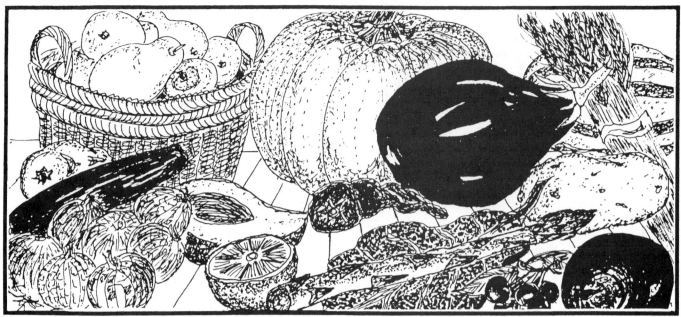

Illustrations by Maija Meijers

Organic Foods: How Can You Be Sure?

Michael Rozyne

I F YOU'VE ever eaten an organically grown carrot, you must have wondered "How do I know it's really organic? I paid 20 cents more per pound for this carrot than I'd pay for an ordinary one. It looks the same. It feels the same. Hmmm.... It does taste really *sweet*. But is that because it's organic...or is it just fresher? or better variety of carrot? Could this carrot be an impostor?

In your moment of doubt, you have acknowledged the possibility of consumer fraud. This may lead you to wonder what "organic" really *means*, and whether there is any way for the consumer to tell the difference between organic and "commercial" produce.

What is Organic?

"Organic" is not a product. It's a process, a method of production. There's no federal definition, and only three states (California, Oregon, and Maine) have legislated definitions. Farmers generally adhere to the standards set by

Whole Life Times (July-August 1983), 18 Shepard Street, Brighton, MA 02135. Reprinted by permission.

their local or regional organic growers' association. Although there are dozens of such organizations all over the world, virtually all of them would agree that organic foods must be grown, transported, stored, packaged, and distributed without the use of chemical fertilizers, insecticides, or herbicides (weed killers). In addition, the land where the crop is grown has to have been chemical-free for at least a year before organics were planted. Some certifying organizations require up to five years chemical-free before the crop can be labeled "organic"; this is one of the most hotly debated issues in the field.

What Price Purity?

At the Cambridge (Massachusetts) Food Co-op, organic sunflower seeds sell for $1.02 per pound, while commercial sunnies sell for 88 cents. Organic long-grain brown rice is priced at 72 cents per pound, its commercial counterpart at 40 cents. Organic Thompson raisins are ofered at $1.83 per pound alongside the commercial variety, currently from Mexico, selling for $1.23. Most consumers pay the hefty hikes for organic produce in order to avoid eating chemical residues which accumulate on food; some are also consciously supporting an alternative agriculture that is ecologically based and does not dump toxins into the environment.

The shopper who chooses organic raisins will avoid not only pesticide and herbicide residues, but also traces of methyl bromide, a fumigant applied to raisins in storage to kill insects. (Organic raisins are frozen instead—the only legal alternative to fumigation.) Scientific literature tells us little about what effect chemical residues have on our bodies. So buying organic is an indirect form of life insurance.

Organic foods may also be more nutritious, containing more nitrate and protein than chemically grown foods, according to recent experiments reported by Hardy Vogtman, director of the Swiss-based International Federation of Organic Agricultural Movements (IFOAM).

Proof Is in the Produce

Most of us examine food for a uniform, unblemished appearance, a measure of quality learned from food-industry hype. The wisest organic food shoppers look for different signs. Odd shapes and spots aren't uncommon, nor necessarily unhealthy. The concerned organics consumer should ask what written documentation the seller has to assure that the product was grown without pesticides or synthetic fertilizers. One cannot, of course, stride into the buyer's office and examine the files before making every organic purchase, but one should choose a co-op or retailer who has documentation on hand and is as interested in it as you are.

The simplest and least informative document is a grower affadavit—the farmer's notarized statement that s/he has complied with a particular organic code. The best documentation is that which develops from intimate contact between grower and first handler or between grower and certifier. Farm visits and lengthy questionnaires give the investigator substantial background about a farmer and his cultural (i.e., growing) practices.

For example, Little Bear Trading Company of Cochrane, Wisconsin, a miller and distributor of organic-grain products, requires an annual seven-page questionnaire of every farmer they buy from. A farmer must map out the location of every field and a four-year rotation plan for that field. The questionnaire also asks that a farmer distinguish self-owned land from rented land, specifying the owner for rented land. This enables Little Bear to trace the history of land a farmer may not know about. The last three pages require detailed information about fertilization, weed control, pest control, drying, and storing methods. Both the farmer and a Little Bear field person must sign a verification that the information is true.

A final on-paper check is an independent laboratory test for pesticide residues (techniques for discerning the use of chemical fertilizers have not been perfected). Testing one sample from a batch of grain can cost $70 to $300; such tests may be commissioned by a certifying organization, food-processing company, packer, or distributor.

Among those in the industry who swear by testing is Frank Ford, chairman of the board of Arrowhead Mills, who calls it "scientifically sound, subject to being proven without controversy.... It puts the rubber to the road."

Indeed, even if farm inspections are conducted annually, residue analysis can be a useful check, since an herbicide applied improperly or at the wrong time could leave behind an organic-looking, weed-choked field.

On the other hand, residue analysis is as subject to error or abuse as any other method. A farmer may be clean, but chemical sprays may drift onto the crop from nonorganic neighbors. The person ordering tests must be familiar with the entire spectrum of pesticides that are customarily used on a particular crop, in order to know which chemical families to test for. And there's no government certification program to help determine which laboratories do reliable work of this kind.

Ultimately your assurance that the carrot you're munching is truly organic depends on a chain of trust. From farmer to packer or processor, to distributor, to co-op or retailer, each person in the chain must depend on the integrity, motivation, and *knowledge* of the previous person who handled the food. I like to buy organic products from millers or packers who know farming well and who have a personal relationship with the farmers they buy from. Production questionnaires and residue analyses have greater depth when the certifier has firsthand, subjective experience with the farm, fields, and farmer.

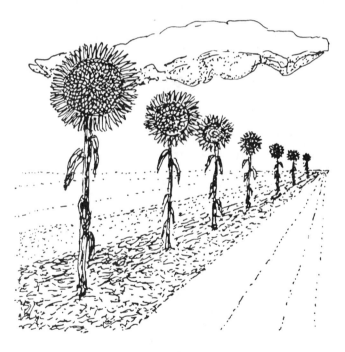

Sunflowers Under a Cloud

Last year I flew into Fargo, North Dakota on a bitter, overcast November morning. Boston had been deceivingly pleasant when I left, and as I stepped into the numbing subzero temperature outside Fargo's windswept airport, I thought fondly of my brown wool scarf and mittens, suspended on a hook in my bedroom closet. Even my ballpoint pen was frozen.

As a natural-foods buyer for the New England Food Cooperative Organization (NEFCO), my mission in Fargo was to investigate organic sunflower seeds. I had been purchasing from Red River Commodities for several months through New England Grain Buyers, a regional trade association of wholesale cooperatives based in western Massachusetts. One of the half-dozen largest sunflower-seed suppliers in the country, Red River started offering organic sunnies, which now account for 6 percent of its business, about a decade ago. Its price was excellent, significantly below the competition.

Frank Gunkleman, vice president of the confectionary (edible-seeds) division, had extended a warm invitation to me to visit their operation anytime I happened to be in the area. On Friday, November 12, 1982, spurred by rumors from reliable sources that something was amiss, I was there. Feeling anxious and numb, I met Gunkleman at his office in the early morning. He greeted me with a firm handshake, standing tall and lean, conservatively dressed, ready for business.

Gunkleman is both extremely self-assured and reassuring, creating a feeling of confidence in his listeners. He speaks emphatically. He presented a tough but realistic image of a cruel world laden with indiscriminate use of toxic chemicals, severe soil erosion, armies of hungry insects developing resistance to once-potent insecticides, and tired farmers facing foreclosures and bankruptcy. Next he presented a spotless certification and packing program that enabled Red River Commodities to jockey around these obstacles and emerge with a top-quality organic product at the best price.

"Our verification program for natural acreage is conducted in three parts," he told me. "First is a grower affidavit relating to [the farmer's] land history and cultural practices. . . . If someone is pulling our leg it tends to show up here. The second step is a field inspection by our field personnel. They look for super weed-free or pest-free fields. Every farm is visited at least once per year. The third and probably most significant step is the residue testing. . . . Every lot is tested except for a few small batches. . . . We do it even with the established growers."

A Dissatisfied Seller

But Wayne Anderson, an organic farmer who grew one hundred acres of organic sunflower seeds for Red River in 1980 and 1981, says he was never visited by a Red River field inspector, nor does he recall ever having his crop tested for chemical residues. "I thought, well heck, they don't care if I'm organic or not." Anderson, who has been on tractors since he was in the first grade, was 15 when his farming family planted its first crop of sunnies. In 1976, two years after starting his own farm, he became an organic farmer. "I'm a strong conservationist. Soil conservation and wildlife are really important to me. My desire for chemically pure, high-quality food came a little later."

When I questioned Gunkleman about Anderson's story, he responded that Anderson "may not have been aware that our field man was there. We know where the fields are. It's all legally laid out when the grower affidavit is signed."

The blank Red River affidavit Gunkleman gave me has no mapping provision; it's one sheet of paper that asks what, if any, insecticides, fertilizers, herbicides, and fumigants have been used on the crop.

Anderson later told me that he never filled out a grower affidavit, nor did he ever lay out the boundaries of his farmland to a Red River field person. I phoned Frank Gunkleman: How could Red River have conducted inspections? He explained that he knew where Anderson's fields were because he did business with a neighboring farm," adding, "I'm virtually 100 percent sure that I've got it [the grower affidavit] in his [Anderson's] file." He promised to retrieve it from the "archives" and send me a copy; at press time, two weeks later, this had not arrived.

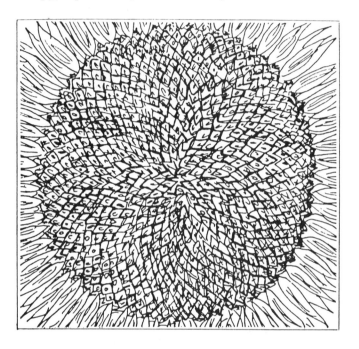

Unanswered Questions

I'd asked Gunkleman about another allegation: One afternoon, Anderson claims, he delivered a load of organic sunnies to a grain elevator in Anselm, North Dakota, where Red River was renting storage space. He noticed that his seeds were being mixed into a bin with other sunnies. Were these, too, organic? The grain-elevator employee on duty didn't know, Anderson says. When he asked whether the facility had provisions or instructions to keep organic seeds separate from commercial ones, he was told that they did not. Anderson brought this matter to the attention of Gunkleman, "who said he'd look into it," the farmer asserts.

"Impossible," was Gunkleman's comment. "If there was commingling it should have shown up in the residue testing and it did not."

Twice in the past I'd requested copies of Red River's residue analysis; each time Gunkleman had sent test results for red durum wheat, assuring me that exactly the same analyses were done on sunflower seeds.

My curiosity growing, I phoned the North Dakota Department of Agriculture to find out more about chemicals commonly applied there to confectionary sunflower seeds, one of the state's major crops. I learned that Treflan, a dinitro-aniline herbicide, is the No. 1 weed killer applied to sunflowers, methyl parathion the most commonly applied insecticide.

Gunkleman's sample residue analysis did not include

testing for Treflan. "I don't have to test for that," he responded. "We would know immediately, just by looking at the field."

We had come full circle. To this day I cannot say with absolute assurance whether Red River Commodities sells legitimate organic sunflower seeds. In its new, ultramodern, multimillion-dollar plant, Red River certainly has the storage space to receive all shipments directly from farmers, and to control every step in the sunnies' handling. The evidence suggests that prior to the opening of this plant last October, the company did not maintain adequate control over outsiders' handling of its organic products.

A Matter of Trust

The rest of Anderson's experience, however, points to something even more crucial: Gunkleman's relationship with his growers. Anderson's story may be an isolated mistake, a blotch on an otherwise clean portfolio. Even if this is so, one wonders why Gunkleman would claim to have his field people sleuthing about the plains of North Dakota in so covert a manner as to seldom meet the farmer face to face. It is impossible to understand a farmer's production strategy, let alone gain confidence in that farmer's dependability and trustworthiness, without lengthy personal conversation.

In any case, NEFCO plans to buy its organic sunflower seeds elsewhere this year.

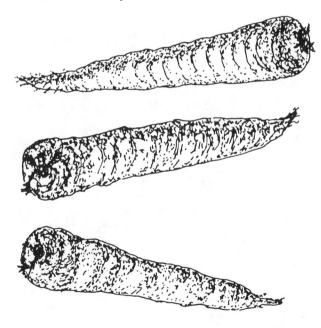

The Carrot Chronicles

From my perspective as a former worker in commercial farming, and buyer for NEFCO (one of eight consumer-owned food wholesalers serving 1,500 food co-ops in the northeastern United States and Quebec), I'd say that 90 to 95 percent of growers and packers of organic food are legitimate. They are handling products that were grown to be more healthful than the average crop, and therefore exhibit unusual concern for high quality and care. It's the other 5 to 10 percent I worry about. Somewhere mixed in

with the good stuff are some less-than-organic products, and this confusion I call the organic-food haze.

At times in this young industry's history, the fog has gotten pretty thick. "I would guess that, in the past, 90 percent of the carrots coming out of the state of California as organic were just conventional carrots placed in an organic bag," says Stuart Fishman, a produce buyer for San Francisco's Rainbow Grocery and one of the original organizers behind California's Organic Foods Act of 1979. "There are a number of large carrot-packing companies centered around Bakersfield. Half of them, before the law existed, were packing conventionally grown carrots and putting them into their private label bags with the word 'organic' on them. They were able to get an extra dollar per bag. I called a couple of these places and was *told* the carrots were not organically grown. Most of these companies have since admitted they weren't packing organic."

Fishman believes the deception has stopped except in one or two cases. His prime suspect is the L.A. Produce Company's Nature-Pak brand. "Several packers in Bakersfield have told me they've packed non-organic carrots into Nature-Pak bags," Fishman says, "last season, and recently. But the president of L.A. Produce denies it; he says their organic carrots come from small farmers, not those packers."

The legislation Fishman backed "really hasn't helped keep the industry clean," he believes, though is did largely clean up the carrot frauds. "That was a special case," Fishman explains. "These were several large packers from *outside* the organics industry. They didn't understand what organic was; they didn't know the process or the law." After the bill passed, the state health department—acting on complaints from Fishman and others—wrote to all of the offending companies. "Most of them decided the whole thing wasn't worth the trouble."

A Lack of Enforcement

Letter writing is about all the support the law is likely to get from the state, Fishman believes. "We knew before the legislation passed that there would be no money for enforcement," he notes. He would, in fact, rather see a strong, active trade association setting and enforcing standards; "but people point to the law and say that's taking care of it." Yet he doesn't regret the effort he put into passing the legislation. The campaign helped to organize the industry nationwide, spurring it to establish a benchmark definition of "organic," he explains, and began educating the rest of the natural-foods trade about organics, a crucial unfinished task.

"Most retailers don't know much about organic agriculture or about how the produce they sell is grown," he says. "I've had a packer tell me, '*All* my onions are organic. Organic means it was *grown in the ground*.' A farmer told me that organic means 'you can use any pesticides you want as long as you raise the humus content in the soil each year.' And a retailer said, 'It's organic as long as it doesn't have any DDT residue on it.'"

To assure the quality and validity of organic products, everyone involved in handling and marketing them must understand what "organic" means and how the process works, at least well enough to investigate and make judgments.

It would be madness if every consumer were to request written documentation for every organic product purchased; but it would be good for everyone in the industry if a consumer made an occasional spot-check.

The wholesaler who buys in 1,000-pound lots should have written documentation for every organic product in the warehouse. The retailer—the buyer for your neighborhood co-op or natural-food store—should have confidence in the organic labels she chooses to offer. And she should, at least, know how to obtain and evaluate organic verification, if she has none on file.

Until uniform organic standards are accepted and enforced throughout the natural-food industry, good information about a product will remain as precious as the commodity itself. The consumer who wants to be absolutely sure should not wait to catch the worm in his food. He should request written proof that the product is organic, and make certain that somewhere in the line of distribution, a trusted seller or manufacturer has left a footprint among the weeds that grow beside those carrots.

Epilogue:

In late July, 1983 the Northedge office received a phone call from Larry Leitner. Mr. Leitner had recently assumed the position of National Sales Director at Red River Commodities and expressed a wish to re-establish our confidence in his company. A conversation with him rapidly confirmed all suspicions regarding Red River's "organic program." Although all the sunflower seed lots we had been purchasing from them had been lab-tested and "certified residue-free," they had not necessarily been grown by accepted organic methods. No field visits were made, no standards were established. In short, said Leitner, Red River has never sold sunflower seeds that could be considered organic in the sense of that word widely accepted in the natural food industry. Frank Gunkelman had "misled" Northedge buyers.

By not insisting on written, verifiable documentation, Northedge and the Northeast co-op food distribution network had unwittingly taken part in the serious misrepresentation of a product. Purchasing organics can be a treacherous business. Let's hope that this lesson will serve us in our effort to build a reliable, believable structure for marketing organically-grown foods.

MICHAEL ROZYNE *is a Buyer for the Northeast Cooperative consumer-owned warehouse in Cambridge, Massachusetts which serves 400 food co-ops in greater New England. He first became involved in food and agriculture when living in Bombay, India as an AFS foreign exchange student in 1974. Before joining Northeast Cooperatives, Michael worked as Marketing Manager for Estabrook Farm, a commercial vegetable farm-greenhouse operation in Yarmouth, Maine.*

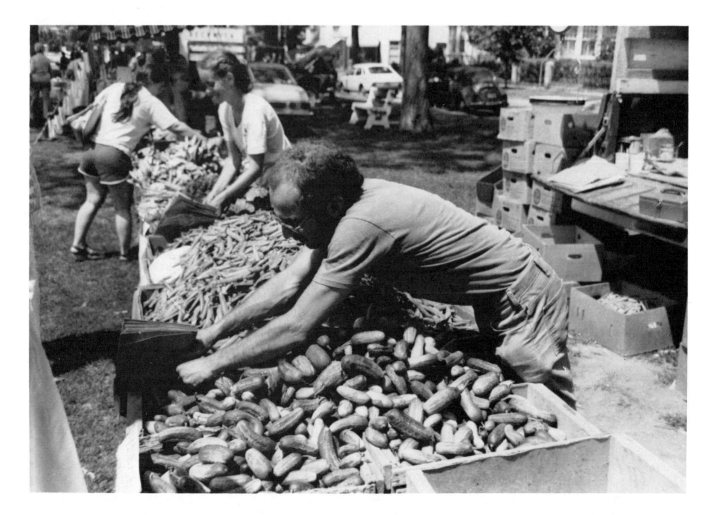

I Fasted—And Lived

TRUE CONFESSIONS OF A CULINARY ADDICT
WHO SURVIVED FOR SIX DAYS WITHOUT FOOD

Jerry Howard

A S A young boy in my grandmother's kitchen, I learned critical skills of self-survival: the preparation of chicken livers sauteed in Amontillado sherry, of eggs scrambled with gruyere cheese and sweet cream. Her kitchen, with its porcelain jars of fudge brownies and butter almond cookies, was my temple, and its icebox was my altar. I don't believe I ever passed it without pausing for meditation and communion. It inevitably groaned with cold chickens and deviled shrimp, crocks of pâté and rich butterscotch puddings.

It was to this haven that I escaped from my parents' apartment, where food, I had convinced myself, was a controlled substance, meted out in meager portions and monitored by unseen guards. I made predawn forays past my parents' open bedroom door to plunge my chubby digits deep into peanut butter, and retreated hastily in fattened guilt.

One bleak morning my father caught me on a stool with my paws clutching a fistful of Nabisco butter cookies. He sentenced me then, in a flash of grim humor, to a diet of butter cookies until the entire box was gone. I think there were 35 in all, and I have never eaten another one since. I retaliated swiftly and often, raiding his bureau for small change which I converted into Hershey bars and Hostess cupcakes. So persistent was my obsession that at the wizened age of 12, I dared to vandalize a pumpkin pie that was cooling for Thanksgiving dinner.

Over the years, I have come to harness my indulgences, if not my desires, and have acquired what others of healthy countenance might deem a reasonable diet—of mostly vegetables, grains and fruits, with eggs and cheese in moderation, all of which I have learned to prepare in the sumptuous manner to which life in Granny's kitchen accustomed me. Occasionally I have chicken or fish, and I suffer chronic lapses into ice cream, chocolate or coffee,

which I largely avoid by keeping them out of the house. To this day, if cookies appear, so do the fat little hands of the child. Sufficient is never enough.

As years passed, I came to observe a pattern: my binges increased in direct proportion to my stress, with predictable toll on my body. My remedy was always swift and severe discipline for the naughty child: extreme exercise and stringent diet until the symptoms receded.

After one virulent siege of sugar and caffeine two years ago, I confessed to a friend my dread of the inevitable medicine. She listened with tolerance while I intoned my litany of bodily woes, which I concluded with the mournful declaration that I was quite ready for Geritol.

"*Nonsense,*" she snapped brightly. "*All you need is a good fast.*"

It had never occurred to me. Imposing a *diet* was bad enough. I always dieted about as willingly as a cat takes castor oil; the noun itself I found tainted with innuendos of deprivation and distress. But *fasting* was a word I had succeeded in keeping out of my working vocabulary for 34 years. "Fasting" made diet sound like "picnic." The only fast I'd ever suffered was in Navy Survival School, when I was forced to go a week without food except for a midweek snack of rabbit and dove, which I was required to kill and dress with my bare hands. Fasting was for flagellants and faddists, withered people with walnut skin you'd find somewhere south of Los Angeles.

"*No,*" I finally replied to my friend with a wan smile. "*I think not, thank you.*"

The conversation ended there, but the idea came up again, as appropriate notions are wont to do with persistence once you decide to resist them. Friends appeared, beatific on the fifth or ninth day of a fast, announcing that they felt simply *wonderful*. So I became curious. It was the sort of curiosity one reserves for water moccasins and rabid bats, but I allowed myself to listen.

I liked much of what they told me: I would give my organs a needed rest, and scour my innards of accumulated toxins. My body, cut off from food, would begin to nourish

From *Whole Life Times*, 18 Shepard Street, Brighton, MA 02135. Reprinted by permission.

143

GUIDELINES FOR A CLEANSING FAST

Dori Smith

DEFINITION: A fast is abstinence from food and drink for a period of time. A *cleansing fast*—for the purpose of physical detoxification and rejuvenation—is what we refer to here. Abundant water and/or fruit and vegetable juices are used to facilitate elimination of such toxins as uric acid and heavy metals. We focus on the one- to seven-day fast; longer fasts require more experience and supervision.

Some general fasting guidelines are given below, compiled from a variety of medical sources. There is general agreement on many points, and specific differences of opinion on some. Radical fasting practices can be dangerous; be moderate and gentle, especially if you are not experienced.

Fasts should be tailored to the individual. Length of fast, frequency, and choice of cleansing aids may be determined from the following:

1. *The type of accustomed diet.* Heavy meat/starch eaters need to be more cautious, beginning with one-day fasts and increasing gradually. People on whole-foods diets can undergo more strenuous fasts.
2. *Individual strength or weakness.* Some practitioners recommend building up the strength of a weak or chronically ill person through diet before attempting fasting. Others recommend fasting under well-supervised conditions, to assist the ill to regain health.
3. *Initial reactions to the fast.* (See "Side effects," below.)

There is common agreement that fasting is useless if not accompanied by an improved diet. Some stress a raw food/sprout diet; others suggest a balanced vegetable-fruit-grain-bean diet with some animal products. The "bad guys" are refined sugars, excess protein and salt, and processed and fried foods.

Several practitioners emphasize the importance of cleansing the body's organs of elimination—especially liver, kidneys, and intestines—for a more comfortable fast *and* for better health after the fast. (See "Aids to Cleansing," below.)

Benefits claimed:

1. Rest for the body's internal organs.
2. Improved organ and system functions (digestion, circulation, etc.) by elimination of interfering toxins. On a distilled-water fast, heavy metals may be drawn out of the tissues.
3. Rebalancing of blood chemistry.
4. Heightened mental and spiritual clarity.
5. Mastery through self-restraint.
6. Elimination of drug cravings.
7. Restful sleep.
8. Reduction of overweight, if fast is paired with an improved diet.

How often and when to fast:

Let the body tell you—for instance, by general sluggishness. You may fast one day per week, or several days a month. In addition, if you are strong, you may wish to undergo a fast of longer duration (four to ten days) once or twice a year in the fall and spring.

How to prepare for the fast:

1. An *attitude* of joyful expectation is vital; look ahead to a period of rejuvenation. You need will power

itself on my own fat and unhealthy cells. I would feel lighter and more spirited. I like that. But I did *not* like the idea of going without food; my stomach convulsed at the very thought.

Soon enough, the bloated Monday arrived when I knew I could resist the fast no longer. It was as much vanity as poor health which drove me to it: my favorite pants felt like tourniquets on my thighs, and my waist had begun to seep over my belt. I sat at my desk much of that first day locked in a rigid posture of self-denial, having periodic discussions with my stomach that went something like this:

"Get some ice cream down here quickly."

"We're not eating today."

"What is this, some kind of puritanical fascism? You better shovel something down here in a big hurry."

"We're giving you organs a vacation. Why don't you go visit the liver or colon or something?"

"I'm a workaholic; I need food. NOW."

"Look, we're trying to improve our physical vehicle for the betterment of body, mind and spirit."

"You sound like a holistic parrot."

That first attempt got as far as nine p.m., when I succumbed to a mad craving for peanut butter and thoroughly clogged my works. But a week later, I actually *wanted* to fast; there would be no struggle now.

Day One

This would be at least a three-day fast, and I would sip diluted apple or lemon juice, and perhaps some fresh vegetable juices toward the end. This first day I spend doing

to carry out the fast, but a forceful approach can be harmful. Heed bodily or environmental messages that may intervene to say "not yet" or "no more."

2. It is good to fast when workload and stress are minimal; however, shorter fasts can be undertaken while working, with adequate time for rest.

3. Fasting is a wonderful time for increased inner exploration—meditation, dreamwork, and journal writing. Plan to visualize and affirm positive changes in body and mind throughout the fast. One suggestion is to list separately the negative qualities ("mental toxins") you would like to eliminate, and the positive qualities ("mental nutrients") you'd like to increase. Then read the list over each time you take in water or juice.

4. It helps to lighten your diet for a few days before fasting.

5. Plan for the materials you will need; have them assembled and ready.

Aids to cleansing:

Abundant water (preferably distilled or spring water) is the foundation for the cleanse. To help your body eliminate toxins thoroughly and quickly, and thus feel better while on the fast, consider the following aids:

1. To keep solid wastes moving, use an enema or herbal laxative for three nights, beginning the night before the fast. Some people prefer taking a colonic irrigation before and after the fast. Additionally, use a good intestinal cleanser made with a ground psillium-seed base (this invaluable item may be obtained through health-product distributors or stores). Shake a heaping teaspoonful in four ounces of water or juice, then follow with an additional twelve ounces of liquid; take this five times daily for three to six days.

2. Fresh fruit juices in moderation, especially diluted lemon juice, are rapid cleansers. Cranberry juice, fresh watermelon juice, and diuretic herb teas, such as fresh parsley, specifically help kidneys eliminate toxin-laden fluids.

3. Yoga postures and massage are very helpful to hasten elimination by way of the lymph glands.

4. If you're feeling especially sluggish, take this opportunity to give your liver a "flush." For three mornings, blend well and drink: juice of an orange, a grapefruit, and one-half lemon; 2 large garlic cloves; and 2 to 3 tablespoons good olive oil.

5. Fresh vegetable juices, such as carrot, celery, spinach, and beet, taken toward the end of the fast, reportedly will begin nourishing the cells in preparation for your return to solid foods.

Side effects to expect:

People often experience headaches, dizziness, sluggishness, nausea, body odors, or other effects, especially in the first three days. This usually is a sign that the organs are overloaded by toxins being drawn out of the tissues. Some choices of action:

1. Step up the use of eliminative aids.

2. Temporarily reduce the rate of detoxification by ingesting raw vegetables or veggie broth.

3. If you are physically strong, wait it out—it's worth it. After this difficult period, you should begin feeling light and clear.

4. End the fast; then return to it after improving diet or reducing stress.

Coming off the fast:

Fatigue may be a clue, telling you your body wants nutrition again. Re-introduce solid foods slowly, eating lightly and chewing carefully for a period almost as long as the fast itself. You will be amazed at how delicious the simplest food is now! Here are some suggested foods: steamed greens; raw salads; vegetable broth; fruits and juices. Lastly, add small amounts of proteins and grains.

---

odds and ends about the house. About mid-afternoon I pick up on a gravitational pull toward the kitchen. I find myself at my desk starting for the peanut butter, and check myself. I find myself with hand on the refrigerator door, and stop. I begin to record each time I have one of these urges; by dinner time I record 23 habitual starts for food in four hours. How much, I wonder with alarm, do I actually eat without any awareness?

This day, I discover a new cache of time; I am liberated from the tyranny of preparing and cleaning up after meals. I go to bed hungry, and satisfied.

Day Two

The second day, as I pedal about town doing errands on my bicycle, I find myself tantalized again by every fast-food den that had snared me in the past. I revisit each small crime, and am shocked to find how many I've erased from memory promptly after commission. Ambient smells in the air provoke sensuous recollections of feasts I have long forgotten: my first shrimp curry at the age of 10... the first Julia Child Bourgoignonne I prepared all for myself one lonely summer when I was 18... the duck roasted in cognac and cherries, my last supper before surrender to the Navy at 22...

As the day wears on my body begins to complain, joining the chorus my mind began the day before: dizziness, hunger pangs, itchiness... I become thoroughly irritable, and my body feels plugged.

Then I remember something else I'd promptly forgotten: an enema. Enemas, I was told, were essential to a fast and felt wonderful. My last enema I'd had about 25 years ago; my one experience with a colonic irrigation had been 45 minutes of torture.

Grimly, I try—lying on the bathroom floor, hoping the warm water will go in to do its thing. It won't. I recall the joke about the shipwrecked parrot and the dowager, adrift together on a log. "So how's yer ass?" the bird remarked. "Oh SHUT UP!" retorted the indignant lady. "So's mine," said the parrot, "must be the salt air."

I recall that coffee enemas are supposed to be especially effective. The aroma of coffee brewing reassures and relaxes me, and it works at last. They were right about enemas after all. I sleep like a child.

Day Three

The third day, I feel a new lightness: my hunger is completely gone, and my mind is beyond temptation or culinary fantasy. I spend much of the day at work in a delicate cloud, like the mist of a spring morning. I am weak and move slowly, but I can think clearly and write, if I let my body set my pace for me. When I speed up or think hard, I get a headache. When I relax, it instantly disappears.

In a conference that afternoon, I sit less than an arm's reach from a bag of roasted almonds, unmoved. My fellow workers seem unusually forceful and urgent, humorless as stones. They say I smell. I smile, and move away. All those chemicals are oozing out of my system at last.

I have vegetable broth this evening to fortify myself, and go to sleep very early, resolving to end the fast by morning if I don't feel stronger.

Days Four and Five

By the next morning my body has made the awkward transition from eating food, to eating nothing, to eating *itself*—a long-awaited feast on fatty tissues. I awake with a new burst of stamina, a tremendous vitality and excitement that remain soft and gossamer as the day before, but no longer misty. This day and the next, I bike the 10 miles to work and home again, and swim half a mile or more in the evening. And as I pump along in the cool sun of these crystal June days, I have minor revelations.

I see myself as if I am watching a cinema verite film. I am in my kitchen, cramming raw peanuts and coleslaw into my mouth with the same emotional hunger and mindless compulsion that must goad the 400-pound man I see eating M&Ms on the subway. I judge this man for his weakness; I make myself virtuous because I gorge myself in private with healthy foods.

I see that fully half of what I eat goes in because an alarm goes off in my brain or stomach, or because I don't know when to put down my fork. I see the complex machine of habit that I allow to drive me: habit, legacy of a childhood where I learned to eat to fill some hole in my heart. Habit, abetted by the restrictive ministries of a caring and loving father who wished only to spare me the pain he had endured as an obese schoolboy.

Habit, nourished by a society where doctors reward the courage of small children with lollipops; where dripping steaks loom in megasize about our thoroughfares; where

chocolate in heart-shaped boxes means love. Chocolate, the substitute for love anyone can buy at the corner drugstore. Chocolate, I love you.

And I multiply myself by many millions late that afternoon, as my arms slice through the mirrored surface of the lake where I swim. I am one with the industries that thrive on our collective indulgence; I embrace the countless families whose livelihood depends on the making and marketing of foods no one needs. I am an entire culture mesmerized by food, and I am another culture deadened by scarcity.

I see that I have spent as much time thinking about food, pursuing it, preparing it, consuming it, digesting it, resisting it, suffering from too much of it, as a Cambodian woman my age has spent with hunger dull or raging in her stomach. As I try to tempt my daughter into eating this or to dissuade her from eating that, the woman prays for her child with the swollen belly.

For the first time, this business of world hunger is real for me. It is not because I have paid my token obeisance to want, but because I have cleaned out the glut which has clogged my vision. My empathy goes beyond intellect, beyond sense of duty; it goes beyond my guilt and dissolves it. On this fast I have become a brother, a fellow traveller on the planet. It is not a feeling that words can describe very well, and it is very powerful.

I am not for an instant angry or disheartened by what I see, because in this vision that unfolds as I pedal and swim, I see only *possibility*.

I feel the ecstasy of my own enlightened body, sleek and soft and 10 pounds lighter than it was just days before, a body far happier for having had far less. I see myself beyond compulsions, beyond slavery to needs that are not real. And in this bright mirror, I see a world, perhaps in our lifetimes, *where we will eat to live*: where more of the world's people will eat less, enjoying it more and without guilt; where more of us will come to know our daily bread as a birthright and not a rare blessing.

I am not sure just how this will happen. I think it will not be my mailing doggie bags to Biafra, by screaming at corporate exploiters of the Third World, or by whipping ourselves after each excessive feeding. As our consciousness awakens, it will simply be something we will all need to see done.

It is now midnight on the fifth day of my fast; I am working in my darkroom, euphoric with the freshness of morning. I recall with fascination the countless people I have watched eating today—so many people so obsessed with something so utterly irrelevant to me, people goaded by screaming neon and billboards to cram even more down their gullets. People like me, a week ago. It is at once riotously and poignantly absurd, humans and food. I no longer understand the need to eat anything at all.

The Sixth Day

And I know, in the next sober moment, that it is time to come back. I decide to end my fast on the next day, my sixth, before I lose all touch with the fact that physical bodies need nourishment.

I work most of this day in the garden; the touch and

smell of the earth grounds me. Dinner that evening is a potluck feast with friends in celebration of the summer solstice. I am supposed to eat only a little fruit or vegetable, I know, but I sample everything, infinitesimal nibbles of carrot and onion, chickpea and lettuce . . . of nut bread, or peach, even of barbequed chicken. The flavors and textures of these new substances are beyond description, and I revel in delight.

I know even as I taste that the time will come soon enough when I will forget what my hand stuffs into my mouth, when food will again become a routine obsession. And that my body will announce that the time has come to fast once more. But tonight I am eating God's food. I am part of God now with a new body, in summer pants that billow loose in the soft breeze of the midsummer evening, sparkling with the glow of fireflies.

Several References:

Viktoras Kulvinskas, *How to Survive into the 21st Century.*
Paavo Airola, *How to Stay Slim and Healthy with Juice Fasting.*
Alan Cott, *A Way of Life.*
Dr. John Christopher, *Dr. Christopher's 3-day Cleansing Program and Mucousless Diet.*

JERRY HOWARD AND DORI SMITH *are both Boston-based writers, photographers and former editors of* The Whole Life Times. *Jerry's principle concern is improving relations between humans and their landscapes; Dori is developing a dimensional multi-media portrait of Russia and the Soviet Union. Jerry is a partner with Margarite Bradley in* Positive Images, *a stock and assignment photo agency. They break their fasts on peanut butter and pizza, respectively.*

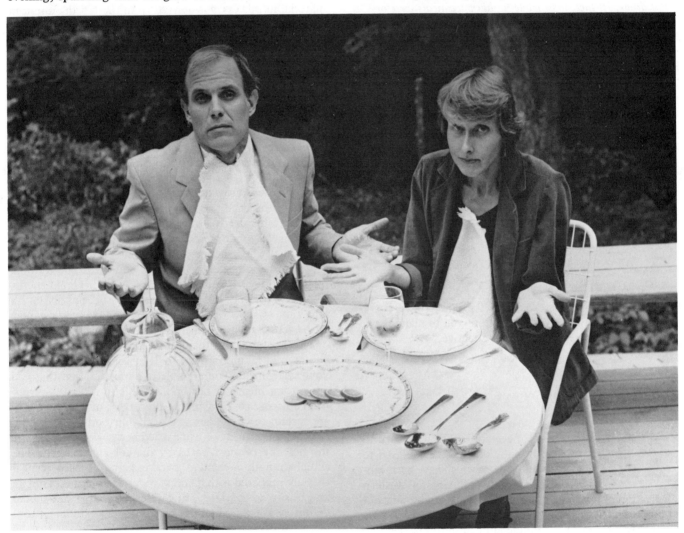

Positive Images

The Way of Herbs

Michael Tierra

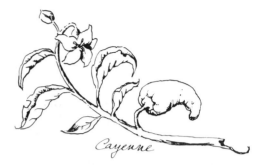

Cayenne

The use of herbs as healing agents is universal. Herbs can catalyze potent healing without the harmful side effects of drugs. In fact, most modern pharmaceuticals were originally derived from botanical sources. Once again, we are returning to the whole plant as food and "medicine" for the planet. We are, so to speak, rediscovering our roots.

Herbs are found everywhere; they are so common and tenacious that they are often labeled weeds. Yet these so-called weeds carry life-giving properties which millions overlook in their search for a wonder drug. The abundance of herbs is a statement of the Earth's beneficence, a source of health freely available to all.

In this article, Michael Tierra shares his reverence for and practical knowledge of the healing virtues of herbs.

"God of his infinite goodnesse and bounty hath by the medium of Plants, bestowed almost all food, clothing and medicine upon man."

> Thomas Johnson
> Gerard's Herbal, 1636

"O plants and herbs! You have the power to rescue this sufferer! I call upon and adjure you to make the remedy I prepare powerful and effective."

> Atharva Veda

HERBS HAVE been and still can be used to save lives. In addition they can be used to help regenerate bodies which have been subjected to the various pollutants of Western civilization. More and more we see both young and old seeking their way back to the ways of nature as lived by the Native Americans, Chinese, and Eastern peoples.

There are probably as many systems for using herbs as there are herbalists, because herbalism is more an art and a tool of divine nature than a science. You will probably discover the "magic" of herbs after you get involved in the gathering, growing, and use of them.

Herbal traditions vary from one culture to the next, both in the specific herbs used and in their application. The material in this essay is derived from the North American tradition, which includes both the American Indian and certain white herb doctors, such as Samuel Thompson, Dr. Shook, Dr. Nowell, Jethro Kloss, and Dr. Christopher.

Preparation of the Tea

Bitter herb teas should be taken unsweetened, especially if they are for digestive and related disorders. You may add a little licorice to cut the harsh effect if you wish. For other kinds of teas, you may want to add a little honey, mint, or other aromatic herbs for flavoring. The healing effects of the herb teas will permeate more quickly when they are taken warm, as is always necessary for sweating teas. On the other hand, the diuretic properties of herbs are helped when the tea is taken cold.

When using herbs, you should stay with one formula for several days in order to experience any healing benefits from it. This does not mean that herbs necessarily take a long time to show results; rather, you must recognize how herbs actually work, which is to nourish a particular part or system of the body that is in need. *Have faith.* Providing you are not taking in more toxic or acid-forming foods in your system than you are able to eliminate, and that you are getting plenty of rest and are able to remove yourself from all causes of tension, the proper use of herbs and diet are certain to strengthen and heal your body.

When purchasing or using dried herbs, you can evaluate the potency of most herbs by the color and smell. The actual strength of the teas is increased up to 30 percent if they are prepared with distilled water. If you cannot obtain any, be sure to use pure spring water. Of course, one should definitely not use alumium or any other toxic metal containers for preparing teas.

The standard method is to bring the water to a full boil; add the herbs, and continue to *simmer* coarse roots, barks, stems, and hard leaves for one hour. The pot should be tightly covered to prevent the escape of essential volatile oils. More delicate leaves should simmer or steep for 20 or 30 minutes.

The proportion is one ounce of dried herb to one pint of water. If you are fortunate enough to have fresh herbs, you should increase the amount of herb by half. For convenience you may prepare three or four days' worth all at once, and keep refrigerated in a tightly capped jar.

The standard dosage is one-half to one cup of the tea, three or four times a day. It may be taken in a little fruit juice. Frequent small doses are more effective than a few large doses. If herbs are to be taken over a period of several weeks, it may be more convenient to grind them into a powder and put them in gelatin capsules; or a small amount of the powder could be taken wrapped in a small wad of rice paper.

For quickest results and especially in severe acute ailments, you will find it best to take the herbs while fasting or doing a special cleansing diet. However, the healing power of the herbs will be working, though more slowly, without fasting. This has to do largely with the body's ability to eliminate more toxins than it is taking in, as mentioned above.

In acute symptoms you can generally expect to notice the effect within three days. Longstanding chronic ailments may take longer. In fact, a good measure is one month for every year of disease to complete healing.

"An acute knowledge and application of a few critical herbs is better than a smattering of many."

Dr. Christopher

Nine Useful Healing Herbs

Cayenne is the most powerful natural stimulant and is completely safe and nonirritating. At the first sign of sickness, you should begin taking one-fourth to one teaspoon of good quality cayenne in a little cold water.

Comfrey is the most powerful healer known, and is also useful as an astringent capable of drawing out infection from the body. It can be applied internally or externally.

Elder flowers are a good blood purifier and sweating herb when taken in the most famous formula of all, ½ oz. elder flowers and ½ oz. peppermint to a pint of water. Taken cold, it serves as a good diuretic.

Yarrow blossoms, like elder flowers, are a good diaphoretic and blood purifier, but also first-rate as a nervine and tonic. They are a specific for all glandular complaints, menstrual troubles, and nervousness.

Raspberry leaves should be used for all flus and fevers. They can be given with good effect for any sickness, even when you're not sure of the cause. In addition they are a specific for digestive disturbances and any problems relating to the female generative organs.

Lobelia is the best muscle-relaxant herb there is. It has the unique virtue of not only relaxing the muscles and removing all spasm from any part of the body with which it comes in contact but also, because of its stimulant properties, speeding up the circulation while relaxing the affected area, thus setting the stage for effective healing to occur. It is frequently combined with cayenne, both in small doses, to act as a catalyst and thus intensify the effect of other herbs in the formula. It is an herbal first-aid remedy for pain when applied locally to the affected part. One of the best poultices I have ever used is made of three parts comfrey, one part lobelia, and one part cayenne.

Plantain is a valuable herb because it is usually found anywhere. There are two varieties: broadleaf and lanceleaf. Both are equally good as a poultice for drawing, as a mild blood purifier, diuretic, and external pain reliever, and for bringing down inflammations.

Garlic is useful externally for neuralgic complaints and skin disorders; internally to avoid bacterial complications that might occur in conjunction with since it is more palatable than the cloves. It can also be used externally for ringworm, scabies, lice, etc.; a strong garlic tea should be prepared and used three times a day as a wash, followed by an application of garlic oil. (This should be kept up for two weeks.)

The syrup of garlic can be used for catarrh, asthma, tuberculosis, difficult breathing, regulating blood pressure, heart weakness, internal ulceration, etc.

Aromatics: A few drops of oil of anise, oil of caraway, oil of fennel, oil of cinnamon, or peppermint oil will effectively cover the odor and taste of garlic.

Golden Seal: If there ever were such a thing as a cure-all, Golden Seal would be it.

Some of the properties of this remarkable plant are: tonic (will return tone and strength to body tissue), astingent, emmenagogue, oxytonic. Too much Golden Seal is not good, however. No more than one-fourth teaspoon per day should be taken by an adult, since excessive amounts can dissipate B vitamins.

It is best to combine a small amount of Golden Seal with herbs for specific organs of the body to direct its healing effects to that part of the body: squaw vine and Golden Seal for uterus; cascara and Golden Seal for lower bowel; turkey rhubarb and Golden Seal for small intestine; centaury and Gold Seal for stomach and liver; eyebright and Golden Seal for eyewash.

Golden Seal as well as ginseng will grow in this part of the hemisphere, and since the popular supply is being threatened by impending F.D.A. restrictions, people should pursue this possibility.

Golden Seal has antibiotic properties; but this is not its best use. Its strongest use is as a tonic-stimulant.

Herbs for Specific Areas of the Body

In natural medicine it is unnecessary to have a precise diagnosis of the exact nature of a disease, such as an analysis of the particular virus or bacteria that would be associated. All diseases have to do with the inability of a particular organ or system to receive proper nourishment because of improper diet or because toxicity is causing faulty assimilation of nutrients. That is why natural systems of diagnosis as Chinese pulse diagnosis or iridology (iris diagnosis), base their treatment on a malfunction of a particular organ or organ system within the body.

Every herb has properties which tend to have a special effect on a particular organ or system within the body, nourishing it and eventually restoring it to normal function.

Hair: rosemary, sage, henna.

Brain: lily of the valley, ginseng, gotu kola.

Ears: eyebright, Golden Seal.

Nose: for the sinuses, make a snuff of one part powdered bayberry bark and three parts Gold Seal root powder.

Mouth and Gums: tincture of cayenne rubbed directly on the gums for any gum infection; the more you do it, the quicker the relief. Bayberry bark, oak bark, or rhatany root make a good mouth wash.

Throat: mullein, sage, Golden Seal, slippery elm.

Bronchioles: For steaming, use benzoin, eucalyptus, bay, or poppy seeds; to expel mucus, yerba santa, bloodroot, hyssop, or elecampine.

Lungs: comfrey, mullein, lobelia, oat straw (for TB), pleurisy root (for pleurisy), lungwort, and garlic.

Heart: three tbsp. wheat germ oil a day, hawthorne berry tea; tansy should be used for pounding of the heart.

Blood pressure: European mistletoe, apple bark to lower, and asafoetida to increase.

Stomach: raspberry leaf, dandelion root, angelica, centaury, agrimony, calamus, wormwood, and Oregon grape root.

Small intestines: turkey rhubarb root, slippery elm.

Large intestines: cascara sagrada bark, squaw vine for the transverse colon.

Liver: Oregon grape root, dandelion, agrimony, maple bark, mandrake.

Gall bladder: olive oil, bayberry bark, comfrey, and the above-mentioned liver herbs.

Spleen: maple leaves and bark, hyssop tea taken with steamed figs, bayberry bark, angelica.

Pancreas: cedar berries, yarrow, periwinkle, dandelion.

Kidneys: dandelion root, uva ursi, white poplar bark, sandlewood, parsley.

Bladder: same as above, including juniper berries, buchu, wild carrot seed, gravel root, and hydrangea for stones anywhere in the kidneys or bladder.

Prostate: pumpkin seeds, a combination of echinacea and saw palmetto berries, uva ursi, gravel root.

Fertility: sarsparilla, false unicorn, damiana, licorice.

Uterus and Vagina: dong kwai, squaw vine, Golden Seal root, oak bark, white pond lily, trillium or beth root, uva ursi, angelica, myrrh, yarrow.

Muscles: comfrey, alfalfa, saw palmetto berries to increase weight.

Bones: comfrey, horsetail grass gathered in late summer.

Arteries: remove salt from diet, kelp, hawthorne berries, wheat germ oil.

Skin: chickweed, walnut husk tincture (see formulas).

Circulation system: cayenne (most powerful, fast-acting, nonirritating if uncooked, anti-inflammatory), ginger, bayberry bark, prickly ash (for the joints and extremities), myrrh.

Digestive system: hops, papaya, mustard seeds (one-half tsp. of whole seeds in a cup of warm water 20 minutes before eating), apple cider vinegar and honey (a tsp. of each in a glass of warm water 20 min. before eating), tonic bitters (should be taken unsweetened) including centaury, gentian, agrimony, Oregon grape root, wormwood.

Endocrine gland system: ginseng, sarsparilla, yarrow, licorice, false unicorn root, true unicorn root, pumpkin seeds, kelp.

Respiratory system: cayenne, lobelia, hyssop, elecampine, oat straw, garlic (best carrier of oxygen in the body).

Urinary system: dandelion root, parsley root and herb, wild carrot seed, juniper berries, uva ursi.

Nervous system: skullcap, valerian, hops, lobelia, lady's-slipper root, passion flowers, linden flowers.

To develop chi *energy in the body*: Fo ti-tieng, gingseng, dong kwai (for women).

The Preparation of an Herbal Formula

Since most herbs have more than one property, it is possible to increase the effect of a formula by thoughtfully combining a number of herbs with similiar and/or complementary properties. For instance, *cleavers* is a diuretic herb with blood-purifying properties, whereas *uva ursi* is a diuretic herb with astringent properties. In combining these two essentially diuretic herbs, one may also have the benefit of astringency and blood purifying in a formula that is essentially a diuretic.

To this formula, of course, you would want to add a small amount of *licorice root*, which will serve both for flavoring and as a necessary demulcent for the kidneys, and perhaps an even smaller amount of gingerroot, as a stimulant to intensify the action. Thus, you would have a perfectly wonderful diuretic formula made up of 4 parts each of uva ursi and cleavers, 2 parts licorice root, 1 part gingerroot. This is a good formula for most conditions in which a healing diuretic is required, such as bladder and kidney infections.

To take another example, what is needed for rheumatism or arthritis is something that will increase elimination, relieve pain, break up inorganic calcium deposits in the joints, clean the blood, and correct the toxicity in the bowel which precipitated the trouble in the first place. This is a lot to ask of an herbal formula, but it can be done effectively by studying the properties of the herbs. Blue flag root is a strong blood purifier that combines laxative and diuretic properties; sassafras is another blood purifier, good for the joints with both stimulant and diuretic properties.

It is very difficult for an herbalist to tell specifically why he would use this or that herb in a formula. From a deep understanding of the properties of the herbs, he is able to use the very same herbs that a layman would use, but in a combination that would be far more immediately successful. Though there are standard formulas, such as lower-bowel tonics, nerve tonics, etc., there are also particular combinations of herbs that would apply to a person's individual needs. The ability to use herbs in this way can be developed only by experience. By the study of their properties, you will come to understand the signature of the various herbs, and after a time find yourself putting special formulas together for yourself and your friends.

Formulas

I think you will find the following formulas most helpful. However, you must understand that although herbs in themselves sometimes display fast curative powers, they have the quickest and surest effects in conjunction with other therapeutic measures, such as rest, fasting, and the cleansing diet. Furthermore, some of the formulas—the lower-bowel tonic, nerve tonic, Red Clover combination, eyewash, and female corrective, for instance—should be taken regularly for enough time, say, two to three months, to attain complete healing with no recurrence of symptoms. Best results occur when they are taken six days a week for six weeks, then one week off (or six months and one month off, etc.). By going through each formula and asking yourself why this or that herb is included, you can learn a lot about the conceptual basis of healing with herbs. To help you in this train of thought, I will attempt to reason through each of the ingredients included in one of Dr. Christopher's best formulas, his lower-bowel tonic, as follows:

1 part *barberry bark*: tonic, purgative, and antiseptic.

2 pts. *Cascara sagrada bark*: laxative, tonic; good for the liver; regulates digestion; for habitual constipation; strengthens the muscles of the lower bowel, restoring it to normal function.

1 pt. *turkey rhubarb*: astringent, laxative, tonic, stomachic, aperient; a simple and safe laxative with special effects on the small intestine; very good for digestion.

1 pt. *Golden Seal*: tonic, stimulant; especially good tonic for mucous membranes, such as the lining of the stomach and bowels.

1 pt. *red raspberry leaves*: muscle relaxant, astringent, stimulant; to aid digestion, relax abdominal muscles, and pave the way for the herbs to have best effect.

(The next herbs are included mainly to serve as carriers or as a catalyst for the other herbs to take effect.)

1 pt. *lobelia*: stimulant, antispasmodic; a very useful herb because it relaxes muscle spasm while stimulating the flow of energy and blood.

1 pt. *ginger*: stimulant, carminative, expectorant. A longer-lasting, more diffusive stimulant than cayenne; also very good for digestion.

Thus you may understand how this lower-bowel tonic is not a mere laxative, although it certainly can be just that, but also helps the entire system of absorption and elimination. Taken daily as a powder in two gelatin capsules three times a day between meals for a few weeks or months, it can restore the lower bowel to normal function completely.

Antispasmodic Tincture

One oz. each of powdered lobelia seed, skullcap, skunk cabbage root, granulated gum myrrh, black cohosh, ½ oz. cayenne.

To prepare, take one pint boiling water, steep the powdered herbs in it for ½ hour, strain, and add one pint apple cider vinegar; bottle for use.

Dose: 8 to 15 drops in half a glass of hot water every hour or so, or as needed. This is an excellent all-purpose first-aid remedy for a variety of emergencies, including shock, cramps, epilepsy, hysteria, lockjaw, poisonous bites, and stings. It is also good as a gargle to clear the voice, to

cut mucus, for pyorrhea, and sores in the mouth, or applied externally for strains, pains, and muscular spasm.

Composition Powder

    1 oz. bayberry bark
    2 oz. ginger
    1 oz. white pine
    1 dram of cloves
    1 dram of cayenne

The composition powder is a basic item to be used hourly during the acute stage of disease.

Steep one tsp. in a cup of boiling water for 15 minutes, covered. Drink the liquid poured off from the sediment.

Jethro Kloss' All-Purpose Liniment

Two oz. powdered myrrh, 1 oz. powdered Golden Seal, ½ oz. cayenne, 1 quart of apple cider vinegar. Mix together, shake every day for seven days, strain, and bottle.

Red Clover Combination

Following is the famous Hoxsey Formula which has been used in the treatment of cancer. This herb formula has great curative powers when used along with other therapies. As an all-purpose blood purifier, it is one of the best.

    4 parts licorice root
    4 pts. red clover
    2 pts. burdock root
    2 pts. stillingia
    2 pts. berberis root
    2 pts. poke root
    1 pt. cascara amarga
    1 pt. prickly ash bark
    1 pt. buckthorne bark

Directions: along with organic iodine (kelp), begin by taking one gelatin capsule on the first day, two on the second, etc., until you can work up to a tolerance level of 36 a day, which should be sustained for two years.

Take no vinegar, pork, or tomatoes.

Stay away from meat and dairy products as much as you can, substituting almonds in the middle of the day for protein.

Nerve Tonic

One part each black cohosh root, cayenne, hops, lady's-slipper root, skullcap, valerian, wood betony HB, mistletoe. Powder and mix these ingredients thoroughly and place in gelatin capsules; take two capsules three times a day.

Dr. Christopher's Comfrey Paste

This can be used topically to heal burns, fractures, sprains, and cuts. For third-degree burns, wash the affected area thoroughly and apply with a bandage; do not disturb for three days, thus allowing granulation of new skin tissue to take place. The honey will keep the burn free from danger of infection.

½ part wheat germ oil, ½ part honey; 3 parts ground

comfrey (either herb or root) and 1 part powdered lobelia. This will keep indefinitely if stored in a wide-mouthed jar.

Poultice

This formula is good for drawing infections out of painful and swollen joints.

Three parts each mullein, comfrey, marshmallow root; one part lobelia and a pinch of cayenne.

Take equal parts wheat germ oil and honey, and blend with the above mixed herbs until a paste is formed. Spread on gauze and apply over the painful area; cover with plastic, and leave on all day and night if possible.

An Herbal First-Aid Kit

Charcoal, used externally for drawing
Oil of garlic
Composition powder
Cayenne (African birdpepper)
Antispasmotic tincture, or tincture of lobelia
Herb salve, or eucalyptus oil, or tiger balm
Jethro Koss' liniment
Cascara extract for constipation
Peppermint oil for nausea
Sweating herbs: ½ elder flowers, ½ peppermint

Conclusion

Historically, people have used herbs daily for self-healing. Herbs can supply all the vitamins and minerals the body needs without the danger of toxic side effects. Herbs are a natural balance of many substances which can affect the bodymind, whereas synthetic vitamins and minerals, although equally potent, can cause damage and imbalance, because these substances are not easily eliminated from the system.

We must keep open to the fact that there are many different healing approaches. The measure of their effectiveness should not be some abstract or theoretical idea, but whether or not they work. Spiritual healing, herbs, diet, acupuncture, and the many other methods of natural healing not only are very powerful alternative healing methods, but may be the only way some persons can regain their health, since orthodox Western healing methods are often not able to cure certain kinds of sickness.

Likewise, we must also remain open to the fact that the highest methods of healing with herb and food may not be convenient, or the individual may not be psychologically disposed to deal with sickness in that way. In such a case, the patient should take whatever the allopathic physician prescribes and be encouraged to take the herbs along with it, and continue for at least two months after all the acute symptoms have subsided.

Herbs are a reminder of nature's cycles. According to the Chinese, one of the major causes of disease is our inability to respond to the changes within our environment. Inflexibility leads to sickness; flexibility is a sign of health. Thus, we become sick in the fall if we don't let go of summer, and we get sick in the spring if we're too anxious for winter to be over. Anything that will impair the smooth flow of the life force in nature will lead to disease, and disease itself has the positive aspect of forcefully separating us from the tension of our desires.

Suggestions for Further Reading

John R. Christopher, N.D., *School of Natural Healing*. Provo, Utah: Bi-World Publishers, 1976.

John Lust, *The Herb Book*. Sun Valley, California: Lust Publications, 1974.

Naboru Muramoto, *Healing Ourselves*. Swan House and Avon Books, 1973.

Edward E. Shook, N.D., D.C., *Advanced Treatise on Herbology*. Mokelumne Hill, California: Health Research, 1976.

MICHAEL TIERRA, *N.D., C.A., C.H., has been a prominent lecturer, teacher and leader of the herbal renaissance. He is author of* The Way of Herbs *(published by Pocket Books) and formulator of the Planetary Line of Herbal products combining distinctive herbal formulas using Eastern and Western herbs together; he is also author and director of the East-West Course in Herbology, a comprehensive correspondence course of the study of both western, ayurvedic, and Chinese clinical herbology. For further information write: Box 712, Santa Cruz, California 95065.*

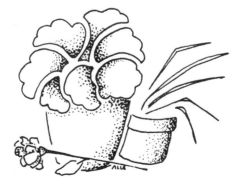

Roots of the New Herbalism

Ethan Nebelkopf

THE ROOTS of the New Herbalism go back to the beginning of humanity. Archaeological analysis of pollen grains at neolithic burial sites in Iraq indicate that Neanderthal tribes used such herbs as yarrow, thistle, and ephedra over 60,000. Healing plants mentioned in the Bible include garlic, onions, mandrake, hyssop, aloes, mint, nettles, coriander, cassia, frankincense, and myrrh. The ancient Egyptians used licorice, fennel, juniper berries, thyme, and senna for medicinal purposes. Pieces of licorice were even found in King Tut's tomb.

The old herbalism was largely a trial-and-error affair. Different cultures used locally available herbs to deal with a multiplicity of physical and spiritual ills. These therapeutic "secrets" were passed on from generation to generation, interwoven with religious practices and ritual mores. Bodies of herbal medicinal knowledge developed in pockets around the planet, exhibiting a remarkable cross-cultural validity—many of the same plants were used for similar purposes in a wide variety of cultures.

The Chinese developed an herbalism based on the relationships of the elements earth, fire, water, wood, and metal. In North America, the Native Americans practiced a unique brand of herbalism. When intermingled with western European herbal lore, this gave birth to a home-grown, eclectic naturopathy in the nineteenth century, only to be superceded by modern medicine with its reliance on chemical drugs and sophisticated surgical methods.

Fortunately, the self-help and holistic health movements of the past few years have rekindled interest in the gentler, more natural healing methods. Herbs as alternative medicine are once again becoming popular in America. The New Herbalism represents a renaissance in natural healing—a breath of fresh air amidst the chaos of modern civilization.

Chinese Medicinal Herbs

Today in China, herbal preparations and acupuncture are well integrated into the mainstream of established medical practice. Such integration doesn't happen overnight, so it's no wonder that the earliest treatise on medicinal herbs was written in China 5,000 years ago.

The most famous of Chinese herbs are ginseng, ma huang, and ginger. Ginseng, *panax ginseng*, is the fabled herb of immortality, used by the Chinese as a panacea for many different ailments. Modern research has demonstrated that ginseng helps the body adapt to stress. Ginseng is a tonic for the endocrine glands and is soothing to the digestive system.

The Chinese used ma huang, *ephedra sinica*, as an herbal stimulant to improve circulation and open up bronchial passages. It wasn't until the late nineteenth century that scientists isolated the alkaloid ephedrine from this plant. This drug is commonly used today for hay fever, asthma, and the common cold.

Ginger is the most popular Chinese herb used in cooking. It stimulates the circulatory system and aids digestion. Chinese herbal medicine relies on complex herbal formulas that are designed to balance the body's energy flow.

The Golden Age of Herbalism in England

In western Europe, herbalism was practiced in ancient Greece and Rome. Hippocrates, who is regarded as the father of Western medicine, used herbs in conjunction with diet, fresh air, and exercise.

English herbalism was grounded in the elf magic of the Saxon culture, whose mystical beliefs were steeped in a deep involvement with plants. The sacred herbs in the Saxon tradition were mugwort, plantain, chamomile, nettles, chervil, and fennel.

In 1551 William Turner published his *Newe Herball*, inaugurating a more formal, scientifically rigorous interest in herbs as medicine, and ushering in the Golden Age of Herbalism in England. In 1597 John Gerard, a Tudor surgeon who was apothecary to James I and superintendent of the Royal Gardens of Queen Elizabeth, published his herbal text. In it he listed over 200 plants, including their common and scientific names, descriptions, and therapeutic uses.

The most controversial of the English herbalists during the Golden Age was Nicholas Culpeper, a physician who incurred the wrath of the Royal College of Physicians by publishing an unauthorized translation of the Latin *Pharmacopeia* in an attempt to demystify the medicine of that era.

Culpeper popularized the *doctrine of signatures*, which put forth the belief that certain parts of a plant might resemble some part of the human body in form or color. The healing properties of each herb were indicated by its shape, texture, or manner of growing in relation to the part of the body it resembled. Thus a person needed to develop the sensitivity for perceiving the plant's *signature* in order to understand the plant's medicinal use.

According to Culpeper, "Modern writers may laugh about it, but I wonder in my heart how the virtues of herbs first came to be known, if not by the signature. The moderns have them from the writings of the ancients—the ancients had no writings to have them from."

Native American Folk Medicine

The herbalism of the Native Americans was rooted in a deep feeling of unity among people, plants, and animals. Native American tribes used golden seal, slippery elm, chapparal, sarsaparilla, witch hazel, cascara sagrada, and echinacea, among many other herbs, for healing purposes.

Chapparal was used by the Dieguenos as a potent blood purifier. This tribe also used yerba santa for respiratory ailments. The Cherokees used golden seal root to heal sores and arrow wounds.

Slippery elm bark was called *oohooska* (meaning "it slips") by the Iroquois, and was used to soothe sore throats. The Kwakiutls made sarsaparilla as a spring tonic, and the Sioux used echinacea as an antidote for snake bites and bee stings. Cascara sagrada served as a laxative for West Coast tribes. The Menominees of Wisconsin boiled the leaves of the witch hazel plant to alleviate muscular aches and pains.

Thomsonian Naturopathy

As orthodox medicine in Europe and America moved away from the Hippocratic model of natural healing and began using blood-letting, leeches, and powerful chemicals such as mercury, a distinctly American folk medicine emerged in the eighteenth and nineteenth centuries, cross-fertilized by European and Native American herbal traditions.

American folk medicine paved the way for Thomsonian naturopathy. Samuel Thomson, a poor uneducated New Hampshire farmer, studied with the local herbalists and developed a variety of gentle, naturopathic home remedies as alternatives to the harsh chemicals popular with the physicians of the time. Thomson used such herbs as cayenne, lobelia, and red clover to cleanse and remove toxins from the bloodstream in an attempt to restore metabolic balance to the body.

The Shaker community was the first group to produce and distribute herbs on a national basis. The Shakers, a large communal group on the East Coast, were dedicated to building a society free of crime, poverty, and misery.

They grew acres of cultivated herbs and also gathered herbs in the wild. These they processed into a variety of herbal products, including extracts, powders, oils, elixirs, and syrups.

Naturopathy caught on in the nineteenth century—it was accepted by the public, but not by the burgeoning pharmaceutical industry and organized medicine, which posed considerable opposition. The big issue at this time was the licensing of physicians: The first state licensure laws allowed herbalists to practice, but forbade them from collecting fees for their services. Needless to say, this did not please the Thomsonian naturopaths and they began a campaign to repeal medical licensure—a campaign that succeeded. By the time of the Civil War, the practicing of medicine was open to anyone—a policy that brought in the snake oil era of patent medicine. Coca-Cola, for example, started out as a patent medicine and headache cure containing extracts from the cola nut (caffeine) and coca leaf (cocaine). Other popular snake oil medicines contained opium, a powerful painkilling herb, but it wasn't until the invention of the hypodermic needle and the laboratory synthesis of morphine that modern medicine began to emerge as a powerful force.

The Ascendence of Modern Medicine

With improvements in laboratory methodology, the opium poppy was transformed into morphine, and morphine could be injected into the human body with the hypodermic needle. Thus, modern medicine lost touch with its herbal roots, depending more on advanced technology than on plants. The discovery of quinine—made from red Peruvian cinchona bark, which natives had used for centuries by natives to treat fevers—was the next breakthrough in the pharmaceutical laboratory. The foxglove plant was the source of another significant breakthrough: From this herb, the glycoside digitalis was isolated. Digitalis is still the treatment of choice in cases of congestive heart failure. From the belladonna plant, the alkaloids atropine and scopolamine were synthesized. Today these alkaloids are used in cold remedies sold over the counter, even though they are highly toxic in larger doses. Atropine opens the bronchial passages, and scopolamine produces a "twilight state" of consciousness.

Even aspirin had its herbal beginnings. White willow bark, *salix alba*, was used externally by Native Americans as a painkiller for rheumatism, arthritis, gout, and headaches. White willow bark contains salicin, which is transformed in the laboratory to acetylsalicylic acid—aspirin—today's most widely used medicine for headaches and pains of the muscles and joints.

The New Herbalism: Seeds for the Future

By prescribing drugs to treat most ailments, the medical establishment perpetuated drug dependence as a way of life. By the middle of the twentieth century a new age of snake oil permeated the fabric of American society. Amphetamines, heroin, cocaine, methadone, LSD, marijuana, alcohol, tranquilizers, barbituates, coffee, tobacco, and sugar were readily available. The self-help movement originated on a grassroots level to improve a health-care system that was concerned more with profit than with people.

Holistic health arose as a specific alternative to established medical practices. It emphasized prevention over treatment, and strove to integrate the physical, emotional, spiritual, and mental aspects of health for the *whole* person. As an alternative to drugs, chemotherapy, and surgery, the new healing technologies included natural methods such as herbs, exercise, organic foods, massage, and fresh air. As we come back full cycle to the original Hippocratic notions of medicine, a renaissance of healing arts begins to emerge—and flourish. By the year 2000, every household is likely to have an herbal first aid kit to deal with such simple disorders as colds, anxiety, stomachache, diarrhea, and constipation.

The New Herbalism is a return to the roots of medicine. Our lives are interwoven with the plant kingdom far more than we realize. The seeds planted by the New Herbalism today will produce abundant fruit tomorrow for our children.

Suggestions for Further Reading

Nebelkopf, Ethan, *The Herbal Connection*, Orem, Utah: BiWorld Press, 1981.

Nebelkopf, Ethan, *The New Herbalism*, Orem, Utah: BiWorld Press, 1980.

Nebelkopf, Ethan, *White Bird Flies to Phoenix: Confessions of a Free Clinic Burn-out*, Eugene, Oregon: Jackrabbit Press, 1974.

Nebelkopf, Ethan, "Holistic Programs for the Drug Addict & Alcoholic," *Journal of Psychoactive Drugs*, Volume 13 (4), 1981.

Nebelkopf, Ethan, "Herbs and Drug Addiction," *Well-Being*, #28, 1978.

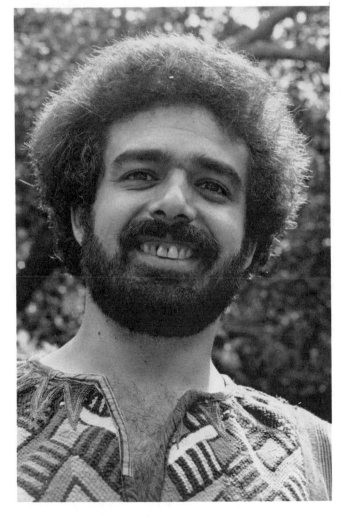

ETHAN NEBELKOPF *is a family therapist who has helped many addicts get off drugs by using herbs. During the 'sixties he received a Master's degree in Clinical Psychology at the University of Michigan. In the 'seventies he studied herbs, developed a program of alternative medicine at White Bird Free Clinic in Eugene, Oregon, and served as herbalist at the Berkeley Holistic Health Center.*

Currently, Ethan is Aftercare Coordinator at Walden House, a drug program in San Francisco. He is the author of several books, including The Herbal Connection *(BiWorld Press, 1981) and* The New Herbalism *(BiWorld Press, 1980).*

Natural Cosmetics

Rosemary Gladstar

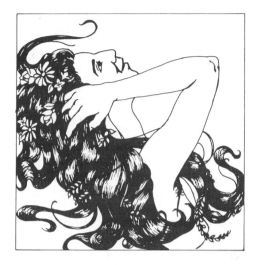

As we approach a more holistic way of living, we seek to be aware of what we take in, what we put on. We look for natural, unadulterated foods, non-synthetic clothing, a pleasing environment, soaps that don't pollute our water. We look for cosmetics that heal and enhance us instead of acting as a facade between us and the world.

Women's magazines often describe skin and hair as "dry, oily, combination, or normal," as if these were inevitable, chronic conditions. They suggest use of preparations whose ingredients are either undisclosed or comprehensible only with the aid of a pharmaceutical dictionary. No wonder men and women alike often come to say, "I hate my hair," or "My skin is a mess," and to feel that nothing can be done about it.

Rosemary Gladstar has another approach, gentle and more positive. She says, "Take tender care of your face and hair—the care of a gardener who loves all the seasons of the garden." Here she shares rituals and recipes, inspiring us to bring some much-needed love and nurturing to our hair and our skin, the meeting ground of the inner self and the outer world.

MORE THAN 2,000 years ago the Greeks spoke of hair as a "natural crown" and of skin as the "royal robe of the body." It was they who gave to us the word cosmetic. Stemming from the word "cosmeo," it meant restoration of balance and harmony. (Ironically, today its meaning has been twisted to mean an artificial or covered-up appearance.)

Contained within this royal robe are many secrets of the universe. Our skin, which contains our body senses, is the meeting ground where the inner self meets the outer world. When there is a balance within, harmonious beauty manifests itself on the borderline. Imbalances can often be corrected by the gentle tuning of nature's cosmetics.

Cosmetics, then, are among our tools for restoring harmony of the body. Gifts of nature, they flow from the rivers, spring from the mountains, are found in the forest. The art of preparing them is part of the magic of their effectiveness.

Just as in cooking, there are basic formulas, or recipes to follow, but the great chef is the one who has an innovative spirit. Use my recipes only as guides to express your own immense creativity. The following suggestions will prove useful in this creative process:

1. Learn what each ingredient *does* in the basic formula (i.e., is it a solvent, emulsifier, liquifier?).

2. Develop a thorough understanding of the properties of each ingredient. When using herbs, treat them as your best friend. Know their properties and uses. Know where the beeswax comes from and what it does. Understand each ingredient for a purer knowledge of the finished product.

3. Make only small amounts when creating the first mixture of anything, and write your recipes down.

Blessed with an Armenian wizard for a grandmother, I've been making my own cosmetics since childhood. Although I gleaned many recipes from early herbals, most of my creations were whims of imagination. What I share with you will be the simplicity of nature: her waters, her minerals, her flowers. When you use these simple creations, embrace the harmony as your own. Then look for your reflection on the mountaintop.

Bathing

Botticelli's beautiful image of Venus being born from the sea embraces the renewing effects of bathing. Warm, clear water, the fragrant essences of flowers, and the healing virtues of herbs are among nature's great tools for restoring harmony.

Water is deeply relaxing or powerfully invigorating, depending on its temperature. Addition of herbs heightens the effects of water. It takes very little time and brings great pleasure to prepare an herbal bath. Any of the following methods work well:

1. Simmer 1 cup of herb mixture in 2 quarts of water for 15 to 20 minutes. Strain and add liquid to your bath.

2. Place a large handful of herb mixture in a muslin (cotton) bag. Tie to faucet of bathtub and let hot water pour through. Adjust water temperature for bathing. Use the bath bag as your aromatic washcloth. These bags are good for 3 or 4 baths before they should be emptied and replaced with fresh herbs.

3. Herbs may be placed directly in the tub. This is best done with blossoms and best done outdoors. There is a certain calm experienced in bathing outdoors, the incense from trees wafting over you, while rose and lavender blossoms float about your thighs and open your heart.

Rejuvenation and Stimulation Baths

I. Equal amounts of
    lavender
    peppermint
    comfrey leaf
    comfrey root
    lemon verbena

II. Equal amounts of
    sage
    patchouli leaf
    sandalwood chips
    lemon thyme (or any thyme)
    eucalyptus or bay

III. Equal amounts of
    peppermint or spearmint
    chamomile
    roses
    rosemary
    comfrey root
    bay leaves

Calming, Relaxing Bath Formulas

I. Use a mix of
    2 parts chamomile
    1 part linden flowers
    1 part mistletoe
    1 part violet leaves

II. Use a mix of
    1 part comfrey
    1 part hops
    1 part chamomile
    ½ part valerian root (do not simmer this mixture; steep in warm water 20 to 30 min.)

Blossom Blends

Any number of aromatic blossoms can be used: acacia, rose, honeysuckle, jasmine, lavender, marigold, pansy, carnation, fuchsia, and so on into the flower garden.

For oily skin.

I. Equal amounts of
    witch hazel bark
    lemon peel
    white oak bark
    peppermint
    orange flowers or peel

II. Equal amounts of
    raspberry leaf
    strawberry leaf
    lemon grass
    lemon peel
    chamomile flowers

For dry skin.

I. Equal amounts of
    comfrey leaf
    comfrey root
    chamomile
    roses
    rosemary

II. Equal amounts of
    acacia
    chamomile
    violets (leaves and flowers)
    roses

As you can see, there are many herbs that lend themselves beautifully to bathing. Listen to your intuition; it will guide you to your favorite recipes.

Store your bath mixtures in a procession in the bathroom. Glass jars with tight-fitting lids, bath bags ready to be filled, and a large seashell for a scoop will make it easy for you and your friends to enjoy these herbal baths.

Bath Salts for Scents and Softness

Here's one recipe; don't hesitate to change it.

    1 cup Borax
    ⅛ cup kelp powder (valuable minerals from the sea)
    ⅛ cup oatmeal ground fine (soothing, smoothing)
    ⅛ cup sea salt (draws any impurities)

Place in a glass jar and sprinkle your favorite essential oil(s) over the mixture. Allow to dry for a few hours. Mix well with your hands, powdering any lumps that may have formed. Store in a glass jar with tight-fitting lid. To use, place about 4 tablespoons in bath.

Dusting Powder

I love talcs, love the scents they come in, the silky cloud they dust over my body. Too bad there's not one good one on the market: the asbestos used has sometimes proven carcinogenic; the scents are synthetic; and many are composed of harsh ingredients. So I make my own.

    1 cup finely powdered white clay
    ¼ cup finely powdered orris root
    ¼ cup finely powdered oatmeal

For variety, add finely powdered roses, lavender, or chamomile. For a woodsy scent, add yellow sandalwood, cedar, patchouli leaves, or spices such as allspice, lemon peel, or cinnamon, all finely powdered.

Mix ingredients thoroughly and place in a bowl. Sprinkle with your favorite essential oil to augment the fragrance. Allow to dry, and powder any lumps that have formed. Store your fine dust in a fancy jar, and use the soft magic of feathers to powder it on.

For babies with diaper rash I prepare the following formula.

    1 part white clay
    1 part volcanic mineral ash
    1 part slippery elm powder
    ½ part powdered myrrh

To prepare, follow the instructions for dusting powder, leaving out the essential oil if you desire.

Herbal Oils for Bath, Body, Massage

Richly organic, fruit and vegetable oils blend readily with the fragrant essence of flowers and herbs. You can feel, smell, and taste the difference in the oil as the properties of the various plants are absorbed. Make several different kinds for you and your friends. The basic recipe is easy.

Place herb mixture in a jar with tight-fitting lid. For each cup of oil, add 10,000 I.U. of Vitamin E. With lid on, let oil jar sit in a warm place in direct sunlight for two weeks. Strain. This procedure may be repeated for stronger oil.

Oils may also be ever so gently warmed in the oven. Place herbs and oil in a pan with a tight-fitting lid. Turn oven on to lowest temperature (about 100°). Let oil infuse for 2 or 3 hours.

The herbs and flowers you choose determine the essence of your oil. Don't hesitate to use your own favorite mixture, but understand each plant you use. Know its properties, its strengths, a little of its personal history, so that your oil will be richly alive for you, a product of your imaginative skill.

Basic oil blend

1 part apricot
1 part almond
½ part olive
          or
1 part almond
1 part soy
1 part peanut

You may blend fruit and vegetable oils in any number of combinations or use a single oil. To each cup of oil, add ¼ cup of herb mixture. In the summer months, gather fresh lilac, honeysuckle flowers, roses, lavender, marigold, and acacia to make fragrant blossom oils. Bay, eucalyptus, basil, and pennyroyal make effective insect-repellent oils, and are easily available since they grow wild. Many of your garden herbs make wonderful oils as well for body, bath, and massage. Here are a few recipes from my files.

Rosepourri

2 parts roses
2 parts lavender
1 part chamomile
1 or 2 drops rose oil and lavender oil

Insect repellent

2 parts pennyroyal
2 parts eucalyptus leaves
2 parts bay leaves.

A couple of drops of eucalyptus or pennyroyal oil may be added if scent is not strong enough.

Relaxeze

2 parts chamomile
2 parts hops
2 parts comfrey
¼ part bay
add a drop or two of cedar oil

Stimulant oil

2 parts peppermint
1 part bay leaf
1 part yellow sandalwood powder
1 part rosemary leaf
1 or 2 drops sandalwood oil

Faces

Far better than names, faces are remembered. Reflecting inner states of being, the contours of our faces flow to form the mountains and valleys of our thoughts. Distant twinkling of the stars, the touch of dew, an early morning sunrise linger on the face of one who lives close to the laws of nature. Take tender care of your face, even more care than a gardener takes who loves all the seasons of her garden.

Facial Steams

For deep pore cleansing, softening, and tonings, there is nothing better than an herbal steam.

Herbs to use. Chamomile, roses, lavender, acacia flowers, elder blossoms, mint, rosemary, sage, chickweed, slippery elm bark, comfrey leaf and root, raspberry leaf, strawberry leaf.

How to prepare. Add a couple of large handfuls of herb(s) to 2 quarts of water. Bring to a simmer, and simmer for 5 to 10 minutes. Remove pan from heat. Cover your entire head and pan with a towel, forming a tent. Dream while you steam away for 5 to 10 minutes. Finish treatment with a splash of cool water or the Queen of Hungary's water.

Queen of Hungary's Water

Bestowed with the honor of being the first herbal product peddled throughout Europe, the Queen's water was used as an astringent wash, aftershave, deodorant, hair and skin tonic, and a bracing headache remedy. This same formula sells in exclusive department stores for $7 an ounce. You can make it for about $2 a quart. Those gypsies knew a good thing when they saw it.

Basic formula

1 part each of roses, lavender, rosemary, sage, orange peel, and lemon peel
2 parts mint

To each pint of apple cider vinegar, add 2 oz. of herbal formula. Place in a glass jar with a tight-fitting lid. Let sit in a warm place for two weeks. Strain. To each pint of Queen's water, add 1 to 1½ cups pure distilled rosewater. Rebottle, label, and date. Enjoy daily this bracing skin tonic that reputedly saved the life of the Queen.

Facials

As colorful as the palette of nature, facials are adaptable to every skin type. Like a great organic feast for the face, they feed, nourish, and tone the skin, while they draw forth impurities. One of these evenings when the moon is shining just right, invite your friends over for a facial party. Have bowls of clay, yogurt, Brewer's yeast, and honey ready. Also have clean towels, astringent washes, and apricot or olive oil for massaging in afterward.

To give a facial, wash the face. Then mix ingredient(s) into a paste. The thicker the paste, the more drying and drawing it is. Delicate or dry skins respond best to a thinly applied light paste. Apply facial over entire face area except on the delicate skin surrounding the eyes. Let dry completely, about 15 to 20 minutes. Rinse off with warm water. If skin is oily, finish with a light splash of astringent toner, Queen of Hungary's water, or a pure rosewater. For dry skin, complete your facial with a protective layer of apricot kernel or olive oil.

Dry skin

white clay	honey
blue clay	watermelon
avocado	honeydew
peaches	pears
cream	

Normal skin

red clay	honey
Jordan clay	egg
yogurt	bananas
brewer's yeast	cucumbers

Oily skin

green clay	egg
red clay	tomatoes
yogurt	cucumbers
brewer's yeast	strawberries
honey	

Here are a few of my favorite facials.

Brewer's yeast. Its high protein and B-vitamin content make it an excellent skin food, both inside and out. Mix with warm water, chamomile tea, or rosewater to form a paste. For dry skin, mix in cream or mashed avocados and water. For normal to oily skin, enrich with yogurt and/or an egg.

Yogurt. Like Brewer's yeast, yogurt is an excellent skin food. Prepare in any of the ways listed for Brewer's yeast.

Honey. I wake up every morning with a quick honey facial. Pull hair securely back from face. Spread a thin layer of room-temperature honey over entire face. Massage in thoroughly; then begin to pat vigorously until the skin, like elastic, pulls and stretches readily. Washes off easily with warm water.

Oatmeal. Oatmeal is a delicious facial nourishment on a cold winter's morn. When you are preparing oatmeal for breakfast, skim off a tablespoon of the thick cream that forms just before the cereal is done. Let cool. While it is still warm, spread over your freshly washed face. Let dry. Rinse off.

Clay. Powerfully absorbant, stimulating, and cleansing, clay is a recognized facial around the world. Use as a weekly facial, either by itself or mixed with other facial ingredients.

Lotions and Creams

A long time ago, when cosmetics truly were "cosmeos," tools for restoring harmony to the body, creams and lotions were created as skin foods. Made with fruits, vegetables, aromatic herbs, and fruit oils, they provided the skin with external nourishment.

The following recipes are recreations of those early formulas. I have provided several basic formulas for you to play with, and a list of variations. When making a lotion/cream for the first time, make only a small amount.

Skin Food

1 part lanolin
1 part coconut oil
1 part aloe vera gel
Vitamin E oil (10,000 I.U. per cup of lotion)

To prepare, melt lanolin and coconut oil together. Remove from heat and beat in aloe vera and Vitamin E.

Facial Cream

2 tablespoons lanolin
2 tablespoons coconut oil
2 tablespoons apricot kernel oil
2 or 3 tablespoons distilled rosewater or orange-flower water

To prepare, melt oils together. Remove from heat. Beat in flower water, and beat until creamy.

Orange Mint Face Cream

5 oz. lanolin
3 oz. almond oil
3 oz. distilled orange-flower water
1 or 2 oz. strong mint tea

To prepare, melt oils together. Remove from heat. Beat in orange water and mint tea until creamy.

Milk Moisturizer

Not the traditional lotion, but worth making. Boil 1 cup steel-cut oats in 1 pint water for about 30 to 45 minutes. Strain. Beat in distilled rosewater or orange-flower water to create a milky consistency. Keep refrigerated. Use cotton balls to apply after showering or washing.

Hand and Body Basic Lotion

3 oz. almond oil or apricot kernel oil
1 oz. lanolin
1 oz. aloe vera gel
2 oz. rosewater or herb tea

To prepare, melt oils together. Remove from heat, and beat in aloe vera gel and rosewater or tea.

Variations

You can add any one or more of the following ingredients to each cup of the above recipes: 5,000 to 10,000 units of Vitamin E oil; 50,000 units of Vitamin A oil; 1 or 2 tablespoons of aloe vera gel; 1 teaspoon of honey; ½ teaspoon of tincture of benzoin; or 1 teaspoon glycerin. You can also substitute cocoa butter or avocado, sesame, soy, olive, or any combination of vegetable oils for oils in recipe, and you can greatly improve the quality of the oils by adding herbs to them as discussed above under "Herbal Oils."

Hair Care

I'm a lover of hair! Reaching down to my waist since I was a child, my hair at times has been so long that I have been able to sit on it, wrap it up in exotic styles, braid it, feel it flow in the wind and hang dripping with the smells of rain. More deeply, I've been willing to appreciate my hair as the "natural crown" of my physical body. A gauge of inner states of well-being, our hair registers tension, emotional stress, and diet as surely as any personal indicator that we have been given. Treat your hair with care, and it will flourish.

Brushing

A simple ritual enjoyed by thousands of people daily, brushing distributes natural oils, promotes circulation, and stimulates hair growth. It also is a good way to release tension and raise the energy level.

Having your hair brushed or brushing another's is a real treasure. Here's a ritual to enjoy! Gather a group of friends together. Be sure everyone brings natural bristle brushes (*no* others will do) and rosemary oil or hair oil (recipe given). Form a close circle, sitting back to front. Massage, brush, and stroke the hair in front of you. Serve mellow tea, listen to favorite melodies, light the candles! It's a beautiful way to come closer to friends and to share energy. It is also a good way to get your hair brushed!

Conditioners

Pure rosemary or lavender oil (either alone or together) have been cherished for centuries for their conditioning qualities. Brush or massage a few drops daily into hair. (Some people find rosemary oil drying; naturally, don't use it if this is true for you.)

Hair Oil

A favorite daily conditioner for dry, lifeless hair.
>   1 cup olive oil
>   25,000 I.U. Vitamin E oil
>   ¼ cup mixture of horsetail, rosemary, sage, and
>   comfrey

To prepare, simmer herbs and olive oil in double boiler for 20 minutes. Strain. Add Vitamin E oil, and a drop or two of pure lavender oil. Brush or massage a few drops daily into hair.

Herbal Hair Rinse

As far back as my memories carry me, my mother made her rinses of vinegar and herbs. She'd step from the bath, her black hair shining with blue lights, skin soothed with the oil of her homeland. Now in her sixties, she is still admired for her hair, which naturally flows in black waves.

Here is her simple recipe:
>   1 quart apple cider vinegar
>   ¼ to ½ cup herb mixture (use herbs listed under
>   "Shampoos")
>   1 quart water

Simmer gently 15 to 20 minutes. Strain. Shampoo and rinse hair. The herbal rinse should be cool enough to use by then. Place a basin under hair to catch excess flow. Rinse and repeat several times. This is your final rinse; no need to rinse it out with water.

Shampoos

Here's a basic shampoo that is easy to make and effective. Don't hesitate to experiment with the list that follows.

Basic recipe
>   1 oz. pure liquid castile soap (available at most
>   natural food stores)
>   1 oz. herb(s) from the following list
>   8 oz. water

To prepare, simmer herbs in water 15 to 20 minutes. Strain. Stir in liquid castile soap. Add a drop or two of your favorite essential oil.

Herbs

For oily hair: peppermint, spearmint, quassia chips, lemon grass, witch hazel bark, white oak bark, nettle, willow bark, sage, orange peel, raspberry leaf, strawberry leaf.

For dry hair: acacia flowers, elder flowers, comfrey leaf and root, rosemary, orange flowers, chamomile.

For dark hair: sage, cloves, rosemary, nettle, raspberry, yarrow.

For light hair: marigold, chamomile, American saffron.

For problem scalp (i.e. dandruff, itchy scalp): witch hazel bark, white oak bark, yarrow, artichoke leaves, nettle, willow bark.

Variations
>   Add these only to the amount used at each shampooing.
>   1 teaspoon honey, beat in well;
>   1 teaspoon liquid collagen protein;
>   beat in an egg;
>   dissolve 1 tablespoon clay in a little water, and
>   add;
>   a little cream for a milky rich shampoo;
>   a little mashed avocado, peach, or apricot for a
>   tasty treat.

After shampooing, rinse with a homemade rinse, dry hair thoroughly, and brush until the shine and the glow create a fitting crown for the temple of your thoughts.

Henna

An ancient herb, henna was valued by early civilizations for both its conditioning and its coloring properties. Men especially valued the deep earth tones of henna and used it to color their nails, nipples, and navels. It was believed to concentrate energy and heighten one's awareness, and was often painted on the chakra centers of the body.

Today, henna is most valued for its hair-conditioning and coloring effects. Available in a variety of shades, henna deepens and heightens the natural tones of one's hair.

Color chart.

Red: brings out red highlights in dark and auburn hair. For blonde and brown hair, red henna will flamboyantly color the hair anywhere from carrot color to bronze red.

Burgundy: a deep, rich red. Beautiful in dark brown, auburn, or black hair.

Brown: tones and highlights shades of brown and blonde.

Black: deep blue-black coloring.

Neutral: no color; conditions and tones.

For best results, mix various shades to match your own hair. Henna should highlight, not disguise, your natural coloring. Powdered cloves, quassia chips tea, walnut hulls, chamomile, marigold, etc., are often added to augment its effects.

To condition and color, 2 oz. of henna are usually sufficient for shoulder-length hair. Place henna in a glass or ceramic bowl, and mix with hot water to form a thin paste. Dampen hair. Apply henna to hair (pack it on!). Cover with a plastic bag, then wrap a warm towel over all. Leave on for 1 or 2 hours. Do not let it dry in your hair! Shampoo thoroughly, and rinse with an herbal rinse. When it is completely dry, walk into the sunlight and brush! brush! brush! Sunlight and shiny hair do wonders for the spirits.

Conclusion

Creating inner harmony is the true essence of natural cosmetics. It is that gentle bit of caressing that people so often neglect for themselves. A bath richly enhanced with herbs, skin that's been stroked with the oils of nature, hair that shines and glows, all do much to maintain balance and joy in our daily lives. Learn to experience as a family or with others the joys of these simple cosmetics. Walk together in nature gathering the flowers and herbs that you will need. Make your bath time a renewing ritual, your daily brushing a family meditation. With the sensuous oils you've made, massage one another. Let your natural cosmetics be to you what they were meant to be in ancient days, pleasures used to elevate the mind and body to a harmonious relationship with the world at large.

Suggestions for Further Reading

The Calendar Book of Natural Beauty by Virginia Castelton. Harper & Row, 1973. Beauty editor for *Prevention* magazine, Virginia Castleton provides simple, easy to prepare cosmetic recipes for all seasons. I enjoy her nutritional approach to beauty, diet, exercise, herbs, and balanced living.

The Herbal Body Book, 1976, and *Herbs and Things*, 1974, by Jeanne Rose. Grosset & Dunlap. Both highly recommended. Jeanne Rose is a practicing herbalist, creator of a line of purely organic cosmetics, and author of several books.

ROSEMARY GLADSTAR *has maintained a deep relationship with nature since childhood, when her grandmother taught her the lore of herbs and wild plants. Years of backpacking, camping, and riding her horses into the wilderness of the northlands further increased her friendship with all of nature. Choosing herbs as her vocation through visions she had as a child, Rosemary dedicated herself to the healing arts. Kept busy with her garden, teaching, and writing, she finds time for facilitating seasonal holistic health retreats, seminars, and celebrations of well-being. Her latest project is the founding of the California School of Herbal Studies, dedicated to the furthering of the herbal arts.*

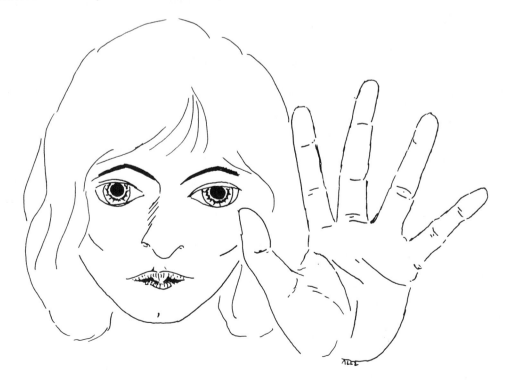

Dick Gregory

CRUSADING FOR HEALTH
AND A BETTER WORLD

Peter Barry Chowka

STRIDING TO center stage of the imposing John F. Kennedy Center in Washington, D.C., Dick Gregory projected an image of natural poise and dignity. At the podium—perfectly attired in stylish evening clothes—Gregory addressed the large crowd that had gathered for the gala celebration of Martin Luther King's birthday. The nationally televised event, featuring entertainment by the country's leading black artists and performers, was a benefit for the Martin Luther King Jr. Center for Non-Violent Social Change in Atlanta.

Solemnly, without a trace of his typical satiric humor, Gregory managed in one minute and 20 seconds to articulately review King's educational background, his decision early on to dedicate his life to the ministry, and his unique contributions. "Martin," he concluded, "was able to take a formal education and add that spiritual upbringing and that spiritual force together to talk about love and peace and the horrors of war and to talk about the downtrodden and the oppressed and world hunger . . . to talk about why hatred was not only bad but went against God. And because of that the world will never be the same." Dick left the stage to sustained applause.

It was simply another of the roles—there seem to be as many as days in the year—that Dick Gregory plays with aplomb. His public career began in 1960 when, as a comedian, he broke the color barrier and became the first black comic to work in first-line white nightclubs and supper clubs. A self-described "social satirist," he was performing at black clubs in Chicago when someone suggested to Hugh Hefner that Dick stand in one night at the Playboy Club for a comic who had canceled. Dick was so popular that he appeared at Playboy for three weeks, during which a critic from *Time* spotted—and loved—him. Soon, by the force of his enormous talent, he was a regular guest

on national television shows, indelibly embedding himself in the public mind with trenchant one-liners: "I spent six months once sitting at an Atlanta lunch counter, and when they finally served me, they didn't have what I wanted." "When I left St. Louis, I was making $5 a night. Now I'm getting $5,000 a week for saying the same things out loud I used to say under my breath." Robert Ruark called him "The Will Rogers of the Atomic Age."

Throughout the turbulent '60s Dick's roles expanded: He joined the budding civil-rights movement, spent many days in jail, and, inspired by Gandhi, began in 1967 to experiment with prolonged fasting in protest of the Vietnam War. Physicians who studied him during a 100-mile walk following a 70-day fast were stunned at the feat, the *New York Times* reported (September 28, 1981). In the process, he became one of the nation's leading advocates for meatless eating and better health.

Today it's almost impossible to list the myriad activities of Dick Gregory. Although still often referred to as a comedian, he seldom appears in purely entertainment settings. "I walked out of nightclubs in 1973," he relates. "How could I say alcohol and drugs are bad and then say, 'Come to my nightclub and have a taste and catch my act'?" Instead he travels non-stop around the world, speaking at more than 200 campuses and political and health events each year, demonstrating, researching and networking—as his biography notes, "making people laugh, making people listen, and ultimately helping them understand one another."

My first extensive contact with Dick came several years ago when I spent the day with him as he addressed and met individually with students at a racially troubled suburban Boston high school. I was impressed with his complete sincerity and talent for reaching people, winning over the audience with humorous anecdotes and one-liners, while not neglecting problems of the world and conditions at the school. He received a standing ovation from the street-wise adolescent audience.

Later, he gave his full attention to each person who

Whole Life Times, March 1984. 18 Shepard Street, Brighton, MA 02135. Reprinted by permission.

approached him, often reaching into his bulging briefcase for a document or clipping to prove a point.

During the drive back to Boston, Dick's other worlds and other selves seemed to be manifesting. He became alternately gibing and sarcastic, self-questioning and reflective. I envisioned the once-poor kid, a "good talker" as he admitted, who had made it to the top on the strength of his considerable intelligence and wit, but who had not forsaken his roots. Often straining to hear Dick's quiet voice amid the highway's roar, I recalled, too, Boston television interviewer John Willis's description of Dick as "one of the gentlest people alive."

Lately, with the problems facing the planet seemingly on the increase, Dick Gregory is focusing even more on individual diet and health as a common ground, a practical starting point, for healing and change. He feels, for example, that scientific information generated by his supervised fasting may be relevant to contemporary world problems: excessive food consumption, degenerative disease, and dulling of the senses of people in the West, undernutrition and starvation in Third World nations.

Constantly on the road and in demand, Dick is never in one place very long. When I finally caught up with him this time, he was in Atlanta, late on the night of Martin Luther King's birthday, several hours after the taped broadcast of the Kennedy Center celebration gala and at the end of the weekend of national celebrations honoring King. It was a special moment, the spirit of King that weekend having touched the nation.

PBC: Your name is a household word. Millions of people know of you: as an activist, comedian, runner, health expert.... Do you have a definition in your own mind of the role you're playing on the planet?

DG: I've been fortunate in that I've never had to designate one role for myself. Oh, I'm a father, a husband, a comedian—whatever you want to call me. Civil rights, peace, sexism, poverty—I've been able to be involved with all these. But you have special obligations being a celebrity. I started smoking and drinking because my heroes smoked and drank. I never saw John Wayne say violence was *not* the answer. I never saw John Wayne pray. We came up in a society where it was cool to drink and smoke. But thanks to a whole lot of people now we're beginning to see a turnaround—in the not too distant future it's going to be cool to be healthy.

PBC: You've described how in the early '60s you were an alcoholic, grossly overweight—generally in bad shape. Is there one event or person you can recall that helped to turn it around for you?

DG: The event was the civil-rights movement, and the person was Martin Luther King. Because the movement embraced non-violence I decided I wanted to change my lifestyle—change my eating habits to include nothing that had to be killed. I met Dr. Alvenia Futon in Chicago, who exposed me to knowledge on nutrition.

And Dr. King—everything that people see in him today I was able to see back then. The power, the effect he's had on people—not just for black folks in America but around the world. He's stronger now in death than he was in life. If you went around the world today with pictures of Reagan—of many current celebrities—and Dr. King—the one person who would be guaranteed to be known is Dr. King. He was more than just a leader, he had a moral, honest, ethical force that can never be duplicated.

PBC: How did you get into fasting?

DG: I decided to go on a 40-day fast to protest the war in Vietnam. And I knew as little about fasting as I'd known about vegetarianism; all I knew was you just stopped eating.

Then Dr. Fulton came to me—she's black, owns a health-food store [Fultania] on the south side of Chicago, and is a foremost authority on fasting. She taught me everything about fasting. I went to something like 63 cities, made 70-some speeches in 40 days. I went from 280 pounds to 95 pounds. And on about the 21st day I started feeling this *energy*.

That first fast I wasn't into prayers. The second one, I was praying. And what a difference! That's when I realized there's something to prayers, because the second fast was almost like not fasting at all. And all I had added was prayers.

PBC: In your experience, what was the most difficult part of making the transition to a healthier lifestyle?

DG: The belief I had that eating animal products was right. I became a vegetarian for moral reasons, not health reasons. So I had this fear. You see, I'd never *believed* that segregation was right, or racism was right; I always heard my grandmother and grandfather say it was wrong. But I thought you *needed* a ham sandwich to survive—if you didn't eat it you would die.

Then 18 months into not eating animal products, my sinus trouble left; it used to hurt so bad that I could understand people committing suicide. One day it just left! About six months later, my ulcers went away. I was still drinking a fifth of scotch a day and smoking, so the only thing I had altered was what I was eating. I realized then that there's something about food that we hadn't been told about.

My mother, my father, my school, my church, my government had never told me that eating meat was wrong—that sugar was the No. 3 killer on the planet, that cholesterol will mess up your heart. Hey, man, my mother gave me candy as a *reward*. Now are you going to tell me she was killing me?

I have never, ever underestimated the power of misknowledge, misinformation, particularly on poor folks, oppressed folks. People start drinking cow's milk and sugar water the first day they're born. So when you talk about changing your diet, to me it's like the problem of drugs and alcohol multiplied by a trillion. Remember that our fathers felt that a meal wasn't complete without meat, and that the more you ate, the more of a status symbol it was. You have to have compassion for folks and know how scary it is for them. There's Grandma saying, "God, son, you got to *eat*"; your kinfolk slipping cookies to your children, and looking at *you* as a bad, evil man. They're not doing that because they want to hurt your kids.

People are into an eating thing, and to go against that takes a long time.

PBC: Why do you think there's so much misinformation around about food and health?

DG: Disrespect for human life on the part of a handful of people who run and manipulate this country.

PBC: Your comment suggests that you believe in a conspiracy...

DG: I've always believed that. Look at the record: 6 percent of the American population controls 97 percent of the wealth and pays less than 14 percent of the income tax. When you look at all the scientific knowledge we have: Can our scientists send us all the way to outer space and not know that red dye no. 2 was poison? And not know that asbestos in the homes and schools would cause cancer? And not know that all the chemical waste that we're dumping is hazardous to Americans' health? Is it really conceivable that Harvard and MIT, Mayo and John Hopkins, these schools that pride themselves on some of the finest research on the planet, do not know what the body is about? Somethin's wrong.

PBC: So what you're describing is, at root, an economic conspiracy.

DG: No. They've *got* all the money already. It's got to do with control. We live in a country that's hooked on nicotine, caffeine, cocoa, whiskey—on drugs. The wino has always been looked down on by the whiskey drinker, the reefer smoker thinks he's hipper than the whiskey drinker, the cocaine snorter thinks he's more sophisticated than all the rest. Big Brother is drugs, Big Brother is alcohol, Big Brother is caffeine, nicotine, cocoa, chocolate. Big Brother is the passionate disrespect we have for ourselves.

PBC: What can individual Americans do to help solve these problems?

DG: It's difficult to say.... It goes all the way back to our lifestyle—to the disrespect we have for our neighbors, poor folks, women, minority folks, and for other nations—to valuing trinkets and money over human values.

But things are changing fast, interesting to see *how* fast. Newspapers are finally coming out and saying cholesterol will kill you, that "die" comes basically from diet. People are begging me for literature: "What can I do to change?"

Basically, I tell people to change their diets, to look into themselves. That's where the difference begins.

PBC: A lot of people see a spiritual resurgence in American and note that originally the United States was founded on a religious ideal—people seeking religious freedom.

DG: I don't know that—how can we profess to have founded this country on religious ideals, religious freedoms, when we stole Africans, made them slaves, and came over here and beat up the Indians? That's a hell of a bloody start for religious freedom.

God needs no leaders, if we're willing to serve God and willing to go out and plant the seeds that will make the change. Crops growin', harvest time's comin'—that's left in the hands of God.

PBC: Could you describe your own principal spiritual interest, practice, or focus?

DG: I get up in the morning and watch the sunrise, and it smacks the nighttime and cleans out the sky and never makes a sound. And I know that's the God force. There's no Russian or American military might, or nothing Hitler and the Nazis ever put together, that could make the nighttime disappear.

Once you get clear spiritually it's gonna clear up everything you do. You shoot dice better. You see color better. Your reasoning gets better. And then a lot of old petty things that you normally get hung up with, you don't anymore.

PBC: 1984 is being viewed by many people as a turning point. Are you optimistic?

DG: It *is* a turning point—negative as well as positive. If we don't do something to deal with stress this country's going to be in trouble. But if we can understand physical fitness and see how it relates to the health of the nation, we'll be in good shape.

If 1984 is going to be business as usual like 1983, then this country's in trouble, on the brink. The problems that are confronting America, though, are *not* problems where we've gone beyond the point of no return!

PETER BARRY CHOWKA *is a contributing editor of* Whole Life Times.

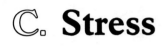 C. Stress

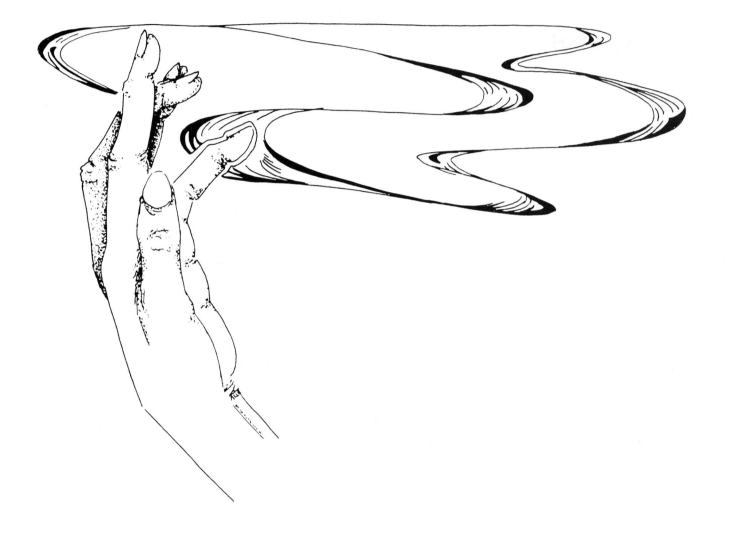

Coping with Burnout

Rick Ingrasci, M.D.

"**I** CAN'T TAKE another day of this," you may find yourself thinking at the end of a particularly hard day at work. You feel exhausted, drained, irritable, but after a pleasant evening and a relaxing sleep, you're ready to go again the next morning, good as new.

But what do you do if you *don't* feel so hot the next morning—and the next, and the next? What if, every morning, you wake up wishing you could just sleep the day away? You find yourself overreacting to the slightest setbacks; tears flow easily; your resilience seems to have just disappeared, along with your zest for life. "What did I ever see in this job in the first place?" you may begin to wonder. Physical symptoms start to plague you: your back aches, or you're tired even when you've scarcely lifted a finger. If this seems like an accurate desription of your life—not sometimes, but day in and day out—it may mean you're burned out, or well on your way there.

Burnout, a combination of mental and physical fatigue, was first identified in the early '70s by psychiatrists studying volunteers who worked long hours with difficult cases at free clinics. It's now known that burnout can occur in *any* profession (and even among the unemployed). At highest risk, writes Dr. Kenneth Pelletier in his new book *Healthy People in Unhealthy Places*, are idealists who approach their work with "unrealistically high expectations of making the world a better place"—a profile that no doubt fits many *New Age Journal* readers.

Burnout is essentially a maladaptive response to stress in the workplace, reflecting an inability to cope with the inner and outer pressures of one's job. Researchers have identified three stages:

People suffering from first-degree burnout feel chronically fatigued, emotionally exhausted, drained and depleted. The most obvious solutions seem elusive, as reason loses ground to aggravation. Paranoia blooms; people often feel under attack, or else trapped by their work. They dream of getting away or escaping, but somehow can't see their way clear.

In second-degree burnout, chronic frustration and dissatisfaction lead to cynicism and callous, insensitive disregard for people. Alienated statements such as "I'm only in it for the money," "I'm not going to knock myself out," or "Whatever I do won't make any difference anyway" are characteristic of this phase.

By the time they've reached third-degree burnout, people tend to feel like total failures, as if all job efforts have been utterly futile. They can become almost completely dysfunctional, staring off into space, unable to focus. Since depression affects the body's immune system (its capacity to fend off disease), disillusionment this deep places individuals in serious danger of developing physical illness.

It's important to remember, however far along you may be, that burnout is not a disease you can catch; rather, it's a process in which you actively participate. Though there may be many external factors contributing to your burnout (e.g., long hours, inadequate vacation time, excessive workload, or lack of social support), it is the internal factors—principally, your attitude, your self-esteem, or your sense of personal power—that determine your *response* to the stresses at work. The tendency to burn out is rooted in negative self-images and self-defeating attitudes which come in all shapes and sizes. The following are a few of the more prevalent attitudes; don't be surprised if you find a little bit of yourself in more than one.

• *Worriers* tend to be in constant state of performance anxiety. They'll say things like "I'm not going to get this right," "I should have...," or "I'm going to get myself in trouble." A certain type of worrier can go to work, feel too frazzled to function properly, accomplish next to nothing, yet end up totally exhausted by the end of the day. Other worriers actually accomplish a lot but burn out because they think that they have to try even harder, or could have done more. Everybody has a bit of the worrier in them, but when this attitude predominates, the fear and insecurity can be very draining and, in the long run, incapacitating. Worrying takes a lot of energy!

• *Overachievers* are easy to spot. They're the ones whose calendars are crammed with nonstop commitments for the next six months—enough activities to keep six people busy.

Rick Ingrasci, M.D., "Coping with Burnout." *New Age*, 342 Western Avenue, Brighton, MA 02135 January 1984, pp. 11–13.

Overachievers have very high expectations of themselves and want to do anything and everything remotely interesting that comes their way. This is because their self-worth is tied to their accomplishments; unless they're busy achieving, they tend to feel as if they have no value. The idea of relaxing or resting is dismissed as a waste of time and, if attempted, can actually make overachievers quite uncomfortable.

• *Pleasers* are people who can't say no, because they are always trying to please everybody. Many of us have been brought up to believe that it is wrong to pay attention to our own needs and wants. Yet taking good care of ourselves—through self-assertion and by setting limits—is essential. Otherwise, it's easy to get overextended or overwhelmed, and end up unable to please *anyone*.

• *Self-criticizers* feel guilty or nervous when their nose isn't to the grindstone. Because of their poor self-image, they feel as if they should be working all the time, no matter how much they've already accomplished. Self-critics lack a sense of rhythm—they pour their energy out but never stop to take an in-breath. They drive themselves mercilessly, rarely stopping to enjoy the fruits of their labor, because it's never quite good enough.

• *I'd-rather-do-it-myselfers* have a fine-sounding but self-defeating motto: "To do the job right, you've got to do it yourself." Maybe, but these insecure—if self-sufficient— people have a hard time delegating even the most mundane of tasks. They tend to be distrustful of others' competency, and ironically, their negative expectations tend to attract co-workers who do in fact let them down. By projecting their own lack of self-trust and self-confidence onto others, do-it-myselfers set the stage for their own burnout.

• *Rescuers* abound in the helping professions, where service and some degree of self-sacrifice are built into the job. Many rescuers learned to be "little helpers" as children and continue to overidentify with the role as adults. They tend to become immersed in their work, doing things that they don't really want or need to do. True altruism is a great and wonderful thing, but rescuers need to consider whether their "doing for others" is an attempt to circumvent a secret fear: that unless they're taking care of someone, they have no value in and of themselves.

Burnout comes in infinite guises, but the good news is that it's totally preventable—and it can also be healed at any juncture. Says Pelletier: "Treatment or prevention can be as simple as one executive's decision to 'make sure that every day I sat down with a real person and talked about a real problem, instead of pushing paper around.'" Dennis Jaffe, a California-based psychologist who is writing a book on the subject, suggests a three-tiered approach to self-care:

1. Self-awareness may seen like an obvious first step, but it's surprising how easy it is to lose perspective once burnout starts to creep up on you. "I'm not anxious," you may tell yourself as you pace around your office, wringing your hands. "What do you mean? I'm not irritable!" you may snap at an associate. The best thing to do is sit down, and quietly assess your situation; from there change can begin. Self-awareness will involve becoming aware of the many patterns in your life as they relate to your work. Are you drinking more, watching lots of TV, overeating? These and other compensatory behaviors may tell you something about the degree of stress you're encountering on the job; with awareness you can come up with better ways to cope. Are you suffering from headaches, insomnia, stomach pains, or other bodily complaints? If detected early, these stress-related symptoms are less likely to develop into serious physical ailments.

2. Self-management is the key to changing the personal patterns that lead to burnout. Though you may not be able to change certain aspects of your work environment, you *can* change your own response. Developing new, more flexible attitudes toward yourself and your work is a good place to start. You may need to go through a period of self-exploration and/or counseling. Creating a support group with friends or co-workers to discuss new goals and vent frustrations and feelings can be a lifesaver. Some people also find books or courses on assertiveness training and other "office survival skills" helpful. Mastering time management is an absolute must: Jaffe estimates that at least 25 percent of the "I have to" work that we each do is unnecessary. Managing your time will help you to learn to set priorities, delegate work, and ask for help when you need it.

3. Self-renewal—alternating work with rest and relaxation—involves treating yourself like any other valuable resource (we all know what happens to overgrazed land). Take time off—the more, the better. You'll need more than a weekend to stand back and take stock, so set up a real vacation. During your time off, don't work too hard at playing. Hang out with your friends or family, explore new ways of interacting. You might take up a new hobby, or look into some stress reduction techniques, such as meditation. While you're regaining your strength, plenty of sleep and good nutrition are essential. Who knows? The new habits you're forming may help offset the stress once you're back on the job.

All of these self-care suggestions share an underlying premise: that basically you like your work, even though it's often trying. But what if you don't? What if, for example, you find your work totally meaningless and boring, or you're only doing it for the money, or you're caught in a miasma of office politics that shows no signs of ever improving? Then perhaps you should consider changing or restructuring your job. Think twice, though, if your misery stems from a *particular* interpersonal difficulty: chances are, even if you leave, you're going to run into someone at your next job that you can't get along with either. This is a good opportunity to do some inner work. Hang in there: if you can confront this person in a positive way, and negotiate a resolution to the conflict, you'll have learned something valuable that you can take with you wherever you go. And while you're at it, you may discover some inner strengths that will help you break the bonds of burnout.

Suggestions for Further Reading

Healthy People in Unhealthy Places by Kenneth Pelletier (Delacorte Press/Seymour Lawrence, $16.95).

Burnout: The High Cost of Achievement by H. J. Freudenberger (Anchor/Doubleday, $3.95).

Burnout: Stages of Disillusionment in the Helping Professions by Jerry Edelwich (Human Sciences Press, $26.95/12.95).

Managing Professional Stress and Burnout: A Workbook by Leroy Spaniol (Human Services Assoc., 49 Leslie Rd., Belmont, MA 02178; $14.95).

RICK INGRASCI, M.D., M.P.H., *is a physician/healer whose practice includes both individual and group psychotherapy. He uses a psychospiritual approach to the healing of people with cancer and other psychosomatic illnesses. He received his medical training at Cornell University, a Masters of Public Health at Harvard, and psychiatric training at Boston State Hospital. He is Co-President of the Association for Humanistic Psychology, President of the Interface Foundation, and Health Editor of the New Age Journal.*

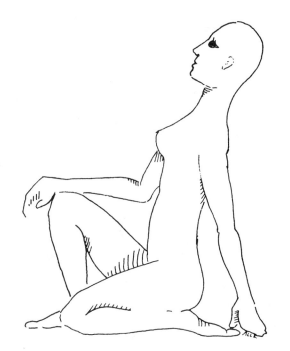

Eliminating Anxiety
and Dis-ease
in the Classroom

Gordon Edlin, Ph.D.

HOW MANY of you experience serious anxiety before taking an exam?" I once asked my class of about 30 freshman students. By "serious," I meant more than just a feeling of heightened anticipation, or even the common "butterflies in the stomach," but actual physical symptoms. To my surprise, more than half the students raised their arms emphatically. "What do you mean by 'serious anxiety'?" I asked them further. "What are the physical consequences of your mental anxiety?" "Headaches," they responded. "Vomiting, diarrhea, feeling awfully sick." I'd known for many years that persistent anxiety can produce emotional stress and physiological changes that might eventually develop into physical illness. But what I had not known was how many students suffer moderate to severe physical symptoms before exams.

In this country, most of us spend from 12 to 25 years in some sort of educational environment, completing at least grammar school and high school. Success within the educational system inevitably depends on performance on quizzes, midterms, aptitude tests, and entrance and placement exams. Students justifiably feel that their grades and exam scores will determine their ultimate success in life, both personally and in terms of their place in society. By now it is almost axiomatic to equate educational success, academic degrees, and professional licenses with attainment of important life goals, particularly financial ones. Consequently competition in the classroom has increased and intensified. Students compete for entrance to prestigious schools and for particular courses; they compete for points on exams and for grades in courses; they compete with one another because they feel that there is less and less room at the top of the social ladder.

Reducing Exam Pressure

What *is* exam anxiety, how can we understand its workings in our lives, and how can we deal with it? Since the holistic approach to health focuses on personal responsibility—on the nutritional, physical, emotional, and environmental situations that we choose for ourselves—the solution to exam anxiety and its associated physical symptoms lies in personal change in not forcing the educational system to change (desirable as that might be). Each of us can *choose* how our personal environment will affect us.

Over the past several years I have worked with students, both individually and in groups, on ways to reduce exam anxiety and feelings of competitiveness and, as a result, to increase their general health and well-being. I will briefly discuss the origin and reasons for exam anxiety, and then suggest a specific mental technique that can help students cope with exam anxiety and can also help eliminate or reduce the undesirable symptoms it produces.

Why We Experience Exam Anxiety

Automatic as it may feel, the fact is that exam anxiety is learned behavior. It probably began quite early in life. (Can you recall the first time you experienced it?) Like any learned behavior that is undesirable or harmful, it can be unlearned or changed—if you are motivated to do so. In attempting to change the undesirable behavior of exam anxiety and its concommitant physical symptoms, you need to realize that exams themselves contain absolutely nothing frightening or dangerous; the danger is in how we *think* about them. For example, if you had no stake in the outcome, you could take any exam for *fun*. The anxiety that you experience relates directly to the importance you attach to your performance on the exam and to how well you do relative to all the other people taking the exam. Obviously, if you feel that your whole life and future hinge on how well you score on the exam, then you are constructing a situation in which severe anxiety and physical symptoms such as headaches or diarrhea may result.

Taking Responsibility

It's not that exams are unimportant or that they should not be taken seriously; exams *are* important, and high grades serve students better than low grades. But the real issue is often the choice between health and an overzealous desire to succeed. You must ask yourself whether all A's are worth getting an ulcer. Or whether a migraine headache is the price for being the best. Or whether going through college on daily tranquilizers is a necessary sacrifice for getting into medical school. So one way to start taking responsibility for how you experience exam situations is to sort out your deeply felt academic plans and goals.

Another technique can be used to obtain relief from exam anxiety. It is more immediate, and it frequently improves class performance as well. The technique? Visualization. Visualization can be used to deal with the onset of anxiety. We all know from painful experience that when panic (anxiety that's out of control) begins, intellectual ability invariably erodes—indeed, logical thought all but vanishes. Panic blocks thought processes and memory so effectively that your mind may "go blank" during the exam and recover only when you have left the exam and regained your calm. Who among us has never experienced that post-exam teeth-gritting moment of realizing, "I *knew* all those answers; I just couldn't think of them during the exam!"

Image Visualization

For reducing stress and eliminating the physical symptoms of exam anxiety, image visualization is a powerful and useful technique. It also helps change other undesirable behaviors or symptoms caused by anxiety or stress. There is nothing bizarre or mystical about image visualization—it is basically what people do when they "space out" during the day and remember some experience from the past that is stored in their memory.

Here's how it works: The first step is to teach your mind and body how to relax. Choose a comfortable place (an environment where you feel secure) and a quiet time (when there will be no disturbing distractions). Sit in a comfortable chair or lie down on a couch, bed, or floor. The main thing is to get physically comfortable. If music helps you relax, play some of your favorite instrumental music. But keep it low—it should not become intrusive.

Next, close your eyes and ask your mind to recall a place from your memory where you felt content and happy. Let it be a place where you have the kind of positive feeling you would like to have all the time. Use your imagination to reconstruct this place where you felt so good. It might be a vacation spot, a beach, or mountains where you went hiking. It might be a place where you live now or where you lived a long time ago. The main thing is to let your mind freely choose what place or memory feels most comfortable, and to let yourself become totally immersed in that scene. It's just like having a daydream, except that you are directing the dream yourself. While your mind is engaged in this pleasurable activity your body automatically becomes relaxed and free of tension.

Once your mind and body have become comfortable and relaxed, turn your attention to a more specific scene—such as an upcoming exam. Using the same image-visualization technique as before, in your mind see yourself taking the exam in a relaxed and confident way. Since your mind and body are already relaxed, and since you are secure and comfortable, your mind will extend these positive feelings onto the image of exam-taking. Using your imagination, see yourself taking the exam; see yourself being calm and confident as you write down the answers to the questions or essay topic. Put in as many details of a real exam situation as your mind can provide: Visualize the exam room and where you are sitting. Notice that you can read and understand the questions without any effort. Pay attention to how you feel as you take the exam, and note the absence of anxiety or any uncomfortable physical symptoms.

Continue doing this visualization until you feel comfortable with it—and with the experience of taking the exam. Repeat this exercise for several days prior to the real exam. When you actually take the exam, you probably will be surprised at how nervous and anxious you *don't* feel—and you will be even more surprised and pleased at how much your grades improve.

This is how one student used image visualization to reduce exam anxiety.

When I closed my eyes, I immediately saw myself on my favorite beach. I had a golden tan and was wearing a white summer smock. I could feel the sand crunching beneath my feet and the sea breeze cooling me off from the hot sun. Soon I could see the sun starting to set, and as I turned around I saw my boyfriend walking towards me. I reached out and we hugged each other. It was wonderful!

I was feeling so relaxed I had no problem picturing myself walking into my English class, sitting in my seat, reading the essay topic, and writing a good essay without feeling pressured for time. I had a feeling of success. An hour later, when it was time for me to really go to English class and write my essay, I still had that same successful feeling. The pinched nerve in my back was gone, and I wrote a terrific essay.

The following week I used the same exercise before my calculus and German tests. I pictured myself biking to class, locking my bike, walking into the classroom, sitting at my desk, looking over the tests, and taking them with ease. When it came time for me to actually take my tests, I was very calm because I had the feeling that I had done this before. I scored 40 points higher on this calculus test than the previous one, and 20 points higher than the previous German test.

Anyone can use image visualization to increase relaxation and concentration. It effectively reduces exam anxiety as well as other kinds of anxiety. It requires no expertise other than a willingness to try and a little practice.

Good luck and good health.

Suggestions for Further Reading

Samuels, Mike and Nancy Samuels. *Seeing with the Mind's Eye.* New York: Random House, 1975.

Pelletier, Kenneth R. *Mind As Healer—Mind As Slayer.* New York: Dell Publishing Co., 1977.

GORDON EDLIN *is Professor of Genetics at the University of California Davis. He is the author, along with Eric Golanty, of a holistically oriented college text,* Health and Wellness, *Boston: Jones and Bartlett (1982). He also has written a genetics text for college students majoring in the humanities,* Genetic Principles—Human and Social Consequences, *Boston: Jones and Bartlett (1984). This text shows how applications of genetics in our society affect our lives. In addition to teaching and doing research in genetics, Dr. Edlin has presented numerous workshops on relaxation techniques and ways to heal with the mind. He is basically a lazy person and enjoys lying down.*

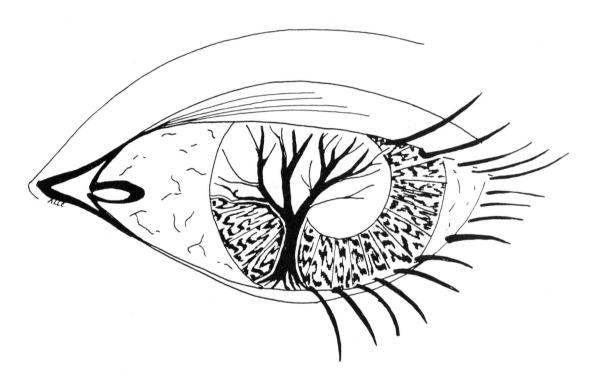

Preventing "Terminal Illness"

Craig Brod, Ph.D.

FROM THE mental-health point of view, encouraging people to get more and more involved with a computer turns out not to be such a wise move. Even some of the most vigorous champions of teaching computer skills to young children have suddenly developed misgivings. Recently MIT's Seymour Papert, who invented the LOGO programming language for children, warned that the computer whiz kids whom we now praise so handsomely may grow up to be a generation of psychotics.

The computer can wreak havoc with the brain. For example, a word processor encourages twice as much productivity as a typewriter. In typing, we experience traditional interruptions to the flow of mental processes: we pull out the paper when we are finished, or we apply white-out to correct our mistakes. But this human-paced rhythm is conspicuously absent in word processing. And when we consider the fact that stimulating feedback can engage the brain in two-dimensional interaction, the stage is set for overly high levels of mental activity.

The engagement with the computer can be so seductive that people can lose themselves in operating it. Managers complain that employees often won't take breaks from computer work, even when asked to; wives complain that their husbands have abandoned them for a relationship to a terminal, leaving them computer widows.

Technostress, the inability to adapt to computers, is the result of overinvolvement with the computer. It is most likely to strike people who have a high need for achievement, are somewhat overly responsible, enjoy mental excitement, and are slightly shy in social situations. In other words, most people who use computers are at risk.

The catch is that most people will not experience technostress until they attempt to switch from computer work to relating to people and find that they cannot.

The symptoms of overuse of the terminal are:

- Edginess and shortness—the result of mental fatigue;
- On-and-off communication patterns with others: yes ...no...yes;
- Impatience—because people take too long to get to the point; or the book has too many descriptive words, or the situation is too ambiguous;
- Fewer contacts with people, less time spent outdoors, less physical activity;
- Heightened longing for quiet time, extending well into the evening after work.

Technostress differs from all other forms of stress in that it is caused not only by mental fatigue, but also by the inner psyche's being shaped by the logic of the machine: yes-no statements, deductive reasoning, and demands for instant feedback. This is what makes the technostress victim different from the workaholic and the Monday-night football fan.

Technostress victims are trapped in a vicious circle: Stressed by people, they return to the terminal to seek solace from a source more predictable than other humans. Then, because they are unable to unhook from their fascination with the machine, they become more exhausted mentally, thus requiring isolation and increased recuperation time. People who experience technostress are essentially lonely, a feeling they attempt to overcome by working more at the terminal.

So should you throw your computer out the window? No. Instead:

- Put limits on computer use, just like the limits you would put on watching T.V. or drinking alcohol. It's natural to lose a sense of time when working on the computer, so put a clock beside the terminal—and set an alarm to help you leave the terminal when it's time.
- Train yourself to recognize the signs of mental fatigue, such as taking deeper breaths or making more mistakes. Realize that when you feel these symptoms, it is time to stop work. You can relinquish the problem you are working on either by logging it on the computer or writing it in a notebook which you keep near the computer. This will free up short-term memory, so that you don't have to worry about the problem.
- Allow for (at least) a 20-minute transition time be-

tween computer work and dinner or time spent on other family or personal relationships. If you don't, you will spend half the time at the dinner table thinking about what you just left on the computer instead of conversing with those around you.

• Make a conscious effort to spend non-technological time with others every day. This means not watching T.V., not working on the computer terminal, not working on the car, and not talking about new gadgets. Take time to value simple playfulness and discussions that include feelings and emotions.

Technostress is a new and widespread addiction, but it can be eliminated. With conscious effort, it will most likely become manageable as we learn to live with computers in an intelligent fashion.

Change is upon us, and we must all take collective responsibility in choosing constructive steps that we as a society must take. We must learn what computers can and cannot do, study how they are used and can be used in the future, question their impact, and develop appropriate strategies that allow high performance and personal well-being to coexist. Only through broad-based interest and participation can technostress be eliminated. Above all, we must get into the habit of trusting our perceptions. If people are complaining, we should pay attention. If people are anxious, we should investigate the source of their anx-

iety. We must resist the temptation to buy into the myths of the computer; instead, we need to make unhurried, critical, and imaginative evaluations of the computer environment.

Suggestions for Further Reading

1. Cooley, M. *Architect or Bee*. Boston: South End Press, 1980.
2. Cooper, C., Current Concerns in Occupational Stress. New York: John Wiley & Sons, 1980.
3. Dreyfus, H. *What Computers Can't Do*. New York: Harper & Row, 1972.
4. Fromm, E. *The Revolution of Hope: Toward a Humanized Technology*, New York: Harper & Row, 1968.
5. Gardner, H. *Art, Mind, and Brain: A Cognitive Approach to Creativity*. New York: Basic Books, 1982.

CRAIG BROD, *Ph.D., is a psychologist and psychotherapist who has been in private practice for ten years. A consultant to government and industry on how to integrate new technologies into the workplace, he has also lectured at the University of California at Berkeley, Extension/Continuing Education for Business and Management, and is the author of several articles on computers and adaptation. His experience with computers includes creating programs designed to build a more sensitive match between the individual and the machine. Dr. Brod lives in Oakland, California.*

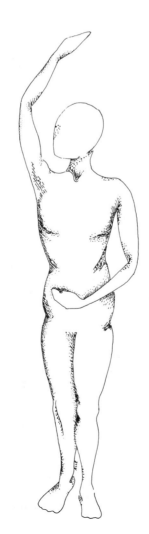

D. Self-Care

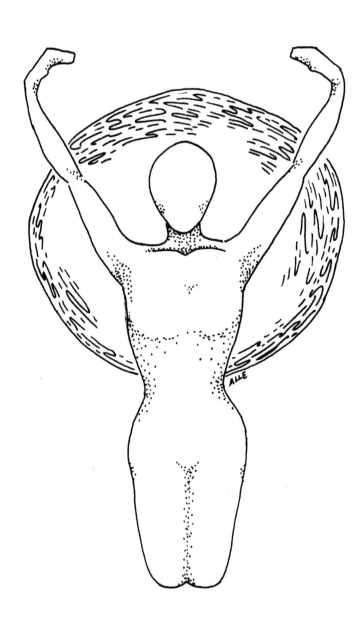

The Anatomy of Breath

Andrew Leeds

Breath is the only body function that can be either controlled or automatic. As such, it can act as a bridge between our conscious and unconscious functions. We can observe our breath to find out where it is and how we're feeling, and we can also change our breath to change our energy or our mood. Breath, as an integral part of the ancient system of yoga, has been developed and perfected over the centuries. More recently, its importance as a tool for physical and psychological well-being has been recognized in the West. In this article Andrew Leeds gives us a physical perspective on breath, offering an explanation of the diaphragm's workings, as well as some practical breathing exercises.

OR THOSE interested in developing well-being, the breath is one of our most valuable tools for increasing vitality and awareness. The breath can be looked at in many ways: as a physical system, as a biochemical system, as an energy system, and as an expression of our emotional state. Of course, all these perspectives overlap, and the different systems are interacting with each other all the time.

There are two crucial features of the breath as a physical system that are important in developing an understanding of how the breath is connected with our whole being. The first fact is that the organs of breathing, the lungs, are passive. Unlike the heart, the organ of blood circulation, which is a powerful muscle, the lungs depend for their function on the diaphragm and the external muscles of respiration in the rib cage and shoulder girdle.

The role of the diaphragm as a passage or connection between the chest and the abdomen is significant not just for physical health, but also emotionally and spiritually. Alexander Lowen in his *Bioenergetics* discusses the crucial importance of the diaphragm in allowing a feeling connection to the heart, where our emotional impulses influence our sexual feeling and functioning (as well as our sense of our personal connection and our interactions with others). Many spiritual teachers emphasize the importance of diaphragmatic breathing and breath exercises for "opening the heart."

Chronic restriction in the diaphragm and the muscles most closely associated with it interferes with our well-being. Birth trauma, physical accident, poor posture, stress, and repressed feelings can lead to inhibited functioning and tightness in the diaphragm.

The effects of inhibited functioning of the diaphragm and poor breathing are more common than you might think at first. For instance, problems among sedentary workers often result from lack of adequate exercise and failure to fully use the breath system. Also, people who feel a lack of connectedness within themselves frequently suffer from restricted breathing patterns. These patterns may be very deeply rooted in the body as well as in the mind, and often do not respond to verbal expression, verbal therapy, or conventional medical treatment alone.

For sufferers from poor breathing there are positive steps to be taken. And this brings up the second feature of the breath as a physical system—the unique connection of the breath with both the autonomic nervous system (involuntary) and the central nervous system (voluntary).

The breath is continuously and automatically adjusted to eliminate carbon dioxide (and other wastes) and to bring in oxygen at the rate that will meet the changing needs of our metabolism in every conceivable kind of physical situation, from quiet sitting to high-altitude climbing. We don't have to remember or think to breathe, unlike dolphins and whales, who must remain actively breathing and who cannot sleep for more than a moment without drowning. The muscles that do the work of breathing for us run on autopilot; consequently, most of us develop a habitual breath pattern that fits our activity range, our ability to transform and use energy, our beliefs about how we should feel, and the type of character structure we have created for ourselves.[1]

Yet in contrast to most other autonomic functions, at the same time that we have this marvelously automatic, self-regulating breath, we also have the capacity to become aware of the breath, to feel the movements of air, of rib cage, diaphragm, and the other muscles of respiration. And not only can we feel the breath, but we can choose to alter our breathing, to take a deep sigh or to allow the breath to become quieter and more shallow.

The breath is thus a kind of natural biofeedback apparatus. And it is this joint energizing of our breathing system by both involuntary and voluntary nerves that allows us to use the breath to learn about and to alter our habitual breathing patterns and other neuromuscular habits, including chronic tension and nervousness. This knowledge may be used to improve body awareness and coordination, and to develop "effortless effort" or efficient body use.

The significance of breath, and its potential as a vehicle for personal change and evolution, has long been recognized in the East. *Pranayama* and other forms of breath exercises, including chanting and meditating with the breath as the object of concentration, have been developed and perfected over the centuries. More recently, in the West, the breath has been recognized as a tool for personal growth and developing awareness as well as for its critical importance in cardiovascular fitness.

Wilhelm Reich pioneered in using the breath to increase the energy level or "change" in the body mind. Reich's work has influenced many other health educators and therapists. These include Alexander Lowen, developer of Bioenergetics; Ida Rolf, developer of Structural Integration; and Magda Proskaur, creator of Breathing Awareness, among others. These approaches to well-being recognize the central role of the breath for our whole being. Although philosophy and specific techniques vary considerably among these different methods, they are all based on the same physical and energetic principles. By reading, observation, and direct experience you can best decide which of these different systems might be most effective and valuable for you.

There are many different ways of working with the breath. The following will give you an idea of some methods and their intentions.

Probably the most basic and important way of maintaining good breathing is by regular exercise. Basically, anything which alters your activity pattern will affect your breathing. If you sit or stand without moving for long periods, walking, running, or swimming will promote adequate breathing. This type of activity also develops and

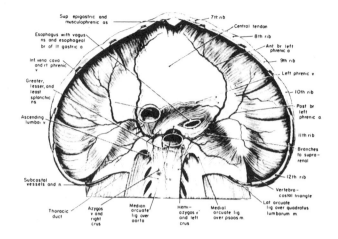

Figure 2. Inferior surface of the diaphragm. Important nerves pass through the diaphragm—vagus, phrenic, and splanchic—which help control the functioning of the organs in the abdominal and pelvic cavities.

maintains balance and coordination, by means of rhythmic activity on both sides of the body (cross-pattern movement). Many activity patterns, such as gardening, carpentry, and some games and sports, use the body asymmetrically, although they *do* involve at least moderate exercise. But running, walking, and swimming help balance the body at the same time that they promote adequate breathing and cardiovascular fitness.

One of the most widely available forms of breath work today is *pranayama*. *Pranayama* is a Sanskrit term that literally means "restriction or control of breath/spirit." *Pranayama* is the fourth stage of yoga, and emphasizes measured and controlled breath exercises. These exercises often involve precise timing of inhalation and exhalation. The aim of this method is to control, develop, and master the breath, and by means of the breath, to do the same with other body functions and ultimately the mind as well. *Pranayama* is often done in conjunction with Hatha Yoga. It is important in both these disciplines to find an accomplished master for instruction, particularly in the early stages, so that poor habits and initial difficulties may be overcome.

Reichian and Neo-Reichian breath work share a foundation in Reich's theory of energy, excitation, and discharge. This work requires long-term commitment in order to achieve lasting results. This very powerful way of working with deep chest and belly breathing patterns and some body movements often includes the letting go or decontrolling of habitual limits in the emotional body, often by means of catharsis or release, using yelling, crying, laughing, pounding, or kicking. The aim of this work is to develop the capacity for soft pulsations of energy, feeling, and movement throughout the whole body. Because of the use of hyperventilation and deep emotional release, it is crucial to work with a skilled therapist for Neo-Reichian and Bioenergetic work: a therapist who has both the years of training and the experience necessary to do this work properly and safely. Originally Reichian practitioners were all medical doctors whose training included long-term personal therapy.

Breathing Awareness is an approach to the breath that

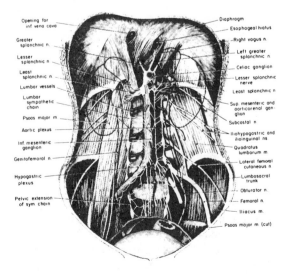

Figure 1. The posterior abdominal wall. The important muscles that permit running, walking, and bending (the psoas and quadratus lumborum) pass through small openings between the diaphragm and the lumbar spine.

was developed by Magda Proskaur. This work is part of the training at the Lomi school. Some Lomi practitioners also have training in Neo-Reichian breath work and *Pranayama*. Breathing Awareness emphasizes our ability to direct awareness and energy to different parts of the body, and is based on the close relationship between concentration and relaxation. This work encourages individuals to allow their own natural and unique breathing to develop rather than to impose a measured breath pattern. Slow, relaxed breathing in lying or other comfortable postures is used with imagery and small and often subtle movements, to develop deep relaxation combined with clear attentiveness. This combination of breathing relaxation and awareness provides a dynamic method for releasing chronic tensions, developing greater body awareness, and improving body use.

In order to release tensions, one must first become aware of them. Contracting areas of tension, acknowledging the tension, and then allowing a release, helps develop an evolutionary attitude toward growth and change.

Change cannot be forced; yet at the same time, change is inevitable. Efforts to change can lead to the opposite of the desired outcome. Truly effective and lasting change comes from the direct experience of what is. This experience can be cultivated with good will by means of relaxation, concentration, and the breath.

Exercises

In doing the following experiments with the breath, it is important to set aside enough time to work at your own pace. Find a room or a very quiet space outdoors where you will not be disturbed. Have a friend read the instructions for you or tape-record them first, so that you won't have to search for the directions in the middle of your experience.

Three-Dimensional Breathing

The first experiment is a breathing-awareness sequence that was developed by Renée Royak-Schaler, a Lomi practitioner in Washington, D.C. This sequence is designed to give you an experience of what Renée calls the "first principle," that we are three-dimensional, that we breathe, move, and exist in three dimensions.

1. Lie on your back. Place your hands on your upper chest and send your breath there. Focus your attention on the exhale; expel all the stale air and then allow the inhale to enter. Inhale into the upper chest and exhale, sending the breath down the arms and out the hands. As you breathe, feel yourself expand in all three dimensions: top to bottom (from head to mid-chest) side to side (between the shoulders), and front to back (from sternum to upper thoracic vertebrae).

2. Place your hands on the lower rib cage, in the area of the diaphragm. Visualize the diaphragm moving beneath your hands: as you inhale, see and feel it moving into the abdomen; as you exhale, see and feel it relaxing upward into the chest. Feel the expansion and contraction of this part of your body in all three dimensions. Feel your ribs lift up away from your spine. Feel how your rib cage expands and contracts at your sides. And feel how your body lengthens and contracts here at your middle with each breath.

3. Place your hands on the lower abdomen, just below your navel. As you inhale, feel your breath move into your pelvis. Then exhale, sending the breath down and out through the legs. Feel your pelvis expanding from front to back (from the abdominals to the sacrum), from side to side (feel the movement at the sides of your pelvis), and top to bottom (feel your lower back release and lengthen with each breath).

4. Place your hands where they are most comfortable. Allow a complete exhalation, and let your inhalation be natural and full. Focus in turn on all three areas. As you breathe, track your breath from top to bottom, feeling how you lengthen from head to toes. Track your breath from side to side in your pelvis, belly, rib cage, and shoulders. Track your breath from front to back, noticing the changing space between your back and the front of your chest, at your diaphragm, and in your pelvis.

5. When you are ready to move, first make some small movements and then roll over on your side. When you are ready, use your arms to help you to a seated position. Take your time; enjoy whatever new spaces you have created.

Deep Abdominal Exercise

Here is a Bioenergetic exercise that works with the deep abdominal muscles, which are seldom mentioned (except in dance), but are very important for supporting the lower back. It is especially important in this exercise to do what feels "right" without straining, although some effort will be involved, especially after many repetitions. These are the same muscles (the psoas and quadratus lumborum) that are closely involved with the diaphragm. You may be surprised at how this exercise affects your breathing.

1. Lie on your back. Then sit up and place the soles of your feet together, hands behind you on the floor. Tilt your pelvis forward so that your belly hangs over your pubis. Release your pelvis back. Repeat this several times. Lie down and rest.

2. Sit up again. Place the soles of your feet together and your hands behind you. This time tilt your pelvis forward and let your head fall forward. Notice how you breathe in relationship to your movements. Repeat this movement several times, noticing your breath. Rest.

3. Repeat instructions for (2), but reverse the head movements.

4. Use the same position and pelvic movement as in (1). This time roll your eyes upward as your pelvis moves forward and roll them downward when you release your pelvis back. Do this without much head movement. Then rest.

5. Repeat sequences (1)–(4), placing your elbows behind you for support instead of your hands. Rest as long as you need to between sets of repetitions.

6. Now, with the soles of your feet together, sitting with your hands supporting you again, push your belly to your right side, allowing your right knee to move toward the floor. Repeat this movement to the right several times. Rest. Repeat this on your left side. Rest.

7. Repeat movements in (6), but also move your head

THE FUNCTION OF THE DIAPHRAGM

Andrew Leeds

The diaphragm is the large and powerful dome-shaped muscle that is responsible for most of the action of respiration in "normal" breathing. The diaphragm forms the floating boundary between the thoracic cavity above and the abdominal cavity above and the abdominal cavity below. On the right side it rests on the liver, and on the left on the stomach, spleen, and left kidney.

When you inhale, the diaphragm contracts and descends, creating a partial vacuum in the (pleural) chest cavity. If the upper respiratory passages are open, air will rush into the many small sacks—alveoli—of the lungs. The lungs will then expand outward and down into the chest as they fill with fresh air.

During exhalation, the diaphragm relaxes and returns upward to its resting place, supporting the lungs and the heart. The upward movement of the diaphragm creates a pressure around the lungs greater than normal atmospheric pressure, which forces the air from the alveoli and out through the upper respiratory tract. The diaphragm is not attached to the lungs. It is the partial vacuum created during the downward contraction of the diaphragm and the pressure created during its return upward that breathes the lungs.

However, in deep or labored breathing, the action of the diaphragm is aided by the so-called "external" muscles of respiration between the ribs (internal and external intercostals) and in the shoulder girdle (trapeius, pectoralis, and serratus posterior). Together these serve to raise the ribs at the front and sides, expanding the rib cage from without. The upward and outward movement of the ribs augments the partial vacuum in the lungs during inhalation, and the contraction of the rib cage during exhalation adds to the pressure around the lungs to aid in the complete expulsion of air. The greatest movement in the rib cage occurs in the lower ribs.

When the diaphragm descends, it moves the contents of the abdominal cavity, providing direct stimulation to the liver, stomach, spleen, kidneys, pancreas, colon, and other viscera. This rhythmic stimulation of the vital organs with each breath is crucial to their normal functioning. Bile is moved from the liver to the gall bladder; the contents of the stomach shift; the movement of lymph in the thoracic duct is aided; the contents of the colon move on their journey up, across, and down; the kidneys and the adrenals receive their periodic massage.

The diaphragm contains openings for the aorta, the thoracic lympatic duct, and the esophagus. Important nerves pass through the diaphragm, including the tenth cranial or vagus nerve, the phrenic, and the splanchic nerves. These nerve fibers, along with the twin simalganglion chains which pass between the spine and diaphragm, supply nerve endings and control the functioning of the organs in the abdominal and pelvic cavities.

The important muscles that support the trunk and permit running, walking, and bending (the psoas and the quadratus lumborum) pass through small openings between the diaphragm and the lumbar spine. Thus any chronic restriction in the breath function which impairs the normal movement or flexibility of the diaphragm can affect the lower back by inhibiting the antigravity job of the psoas and quadratus.

One way to visualize the function of the diaphragm is as an inverted funnel connecting the chest with the abdomen and pelvis. Smooth and relaxed functioning of the diaphragm is important not just for easy breathing, to avoid overworking the external muscles of respiration, but also for normal functioning of the digestive, eliminative, and sexual systems.

---

in the same direction as your knee and belly. Do both sides.

8. Repeat these movements again to one side and then the other, moving the head toward the other knee (the one moving up slightly).

9. This time, with the soles of your feet together and hands behind you, with your head remaining in line with your spine, allow your eyes to move in the same direction as your belly and knee. Repeat this several times and then rest. Do these movements to the other side. Rest.

10. Repeat the movements of (7), (8), and (9) using your elbows for support.

Allow enough time to rest in between each set of repetitions. When you have finished the sequence, lie down and bring your knees up. Feel how your breath has changed. Feel where your breath is moving. Allow this movement to be full. Allow yourself to visualize an image in your pelvis; imagine that you can move into your pelvis to see it; now let yourself go there to see it. Rest.

Roll on one side and then stand up. Notice how you feel

as you begin to walk around. If you want to, talk about what you saw and experienced with your partner.

One-Breath Meditation

Here is the last exercise. It is short and easy to do anywhere and any time; yet it is as effective as any other exercise I know with the breath. This is the "one-breath meditation" which I learned from Dr. Michael Ash when he was in Santa Cruz in 1977. His work in radiesthesia and the energy fields of the body have some interesting consequences for the role of the breath.

Sit comfortably on a chair or the floor. Sit up straight and relaxed. The one breath begins with a complete and relaxed exhalation. Exhaling all the stale air from your lungs rids you of the low-energy-potential, carbon-rich air that accumulates in your lungs, and allows room for high-energy-potential oxygen to enter. As you exhale, allow your spine to curl slightly forward and allow your head to move forward toward your chest. Empty yourself. Let out your ego. (Dr. Ash pronounces this *aygoo*.) Then let yourself really fill up with fresh air, fill up with inspiration, with the spirit. Let your breath lift up your heart!

Notes

[1] Character structure is a term developed by Wilhelm Reich to describe the neuromuscular pattern of strengths, weaknesses, areas of flexibility or rigidity which are the physical foundation and expression of our personality, how we express ourselves energetically in the physical body. See the article by Richard Hoff.

ANDREW LEEDS *received a Master's Degree in Clinical Psychology from Goddard College. He is an Associate of the Lomi School of Mill Valley, a Lomi Body-Work practitioner, and Program Coordinator for the Institute for Life Development in Aptos, California. He has also written for Well-Being Magazine.*

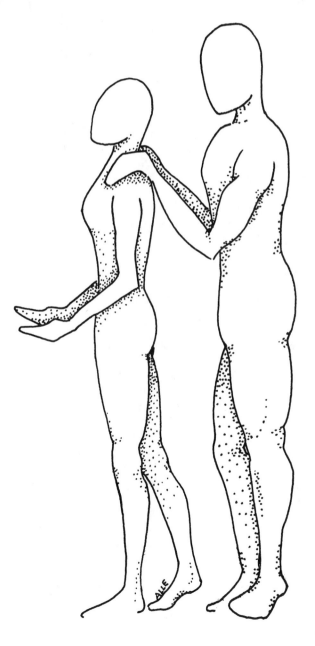

Preventive Dentistry

Frederick A. Aaron, D.D.S.

In very obvious ways we are responsible for our dental health. When we are negligent, problems will crop up to remind us to pay attention. Dental health is directly related to diet, digestion, physical energy, attitude, and the five minutes a day it takes to clean our teeth. Our rewards for diligence here are a minimum of dis-ease and of time and money spent at the dentist's office, and a maximum of happy smiling teeth to last a lifetime.

Here Dr. Aaron introduces us to the simple practices that control decay, gum problems, and plaque.

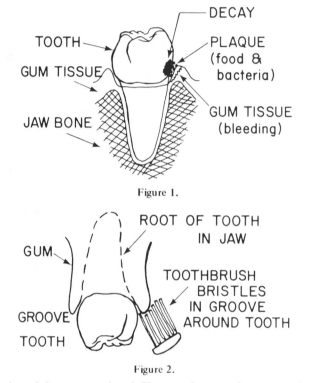

Figure 1.

Figure 2.

"Teeth hadst thou in thy head when thou wast born to signify thou cam'st to bite the world."

Shakespeare

TODAY ANYONE can have good dental health. We know the causes of dental disease, and we also know how to control it. All that is necessary is to commit oneself to good oral health and then invest some time and effort toward that goal.

The material that causes dental disease (bleeding and cavities) is a whitish-yellow material that sticks to the teeth. It is called "plaque," and is composed primarily of bacteria and food. These bacteria love sugar especially, since it is easily digested by them. As the bacteria that live in the plaque use this food, they give off a waste product that is an acid. It is this caustic acid that can burn a hole in the side of a tooth, and this hole is what we call decay or a cavity. The acid can also cause the gum tissue to bleed; we call this gum disease, gingivitis, or pyorrhea. The entire process can be written as a formula:

$$\text{Tooth} + \text{Food} + \text{Bacteria} \rightarrow \text{Plaque} \rightarrow \text{Acid} \rightarrow \begin{array}{l} \text{Tooth decay} \\ \text{Bleeding gums} \end{array}$$
(sugar)

The process is illustrated in Figure 1.

There are several ways to know whether plaque exists in your mouth. One particularly effective way is by the use of disclosing tablets. These tablets are easily obtainable at pharmacies or grocery stores. They contain a staining dye that, when released by chewing, stains any plaque that is present in your mouth and allows you to see exactly

where it has accumulated. You can then set about removing these very visible stains. The disclosing tablets are especially effective with children, who respond well to the bright colors of the tablets and the raspberry-cherry flavoring. Adults can also use the tablets after they have cleaned their mouths to check themselves. The results are sometimes a complete surprise.

Once you know that plaque is present in your mouth and have decided to remove it, the question becomes, "How do I do it?" There are many answers to this question. The important point to remember is to remove the plaque. If you use your fingernail and you get the results you want (i.e., no bleeding and no cavities), by all means keep using your fingernail. It is the result that counts, not the ritual.

There are more customary ways, however than your fingernail that will get the proper results. One, of course, is to use a toothbrush. The toothbrush is ideal for the surfaces it reaches, mainly the biting, cheek, and tongue surfaces of the teeth. There is a small groove of gum tissue that encircles each tooth, and it is important to get the bristles of the brush into this groove, since plaque accumulates quite easily in this space (see Figure 2).

Illustrated by Marlyn Amann

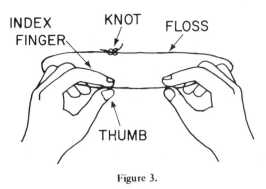

Figure 3.

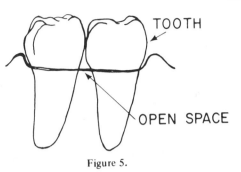

Figure 5.

The motion of the brush depends on each individual, but most people seem to like to use small rotary movements, followed by a brisk, whisking motion on the side of the tooth. For the biting surfaces, make sure that the bristles are aimed down into the small grooves around the tooth. To repeat, use any method that is comfortable, but make sure the plaque is removed from the tooth.

The toothbrush has its limitations. It can't get in between the teeth, where, in fact, most cavities and bleeding gums begin. The use of dental floss can effectively clean these areas. Floss is a commercially made string that can fit easily between the contacts of the teeth where a toothbrush can't go.

By using a six-to-eight-inch piece of floss, one can get into all the areas that the toothbrush misses. Tie the two ends of the floss together, making a loop. Then hold the loop in each hand, using the index fingers and thumbs for support (see Figure 3).

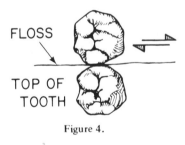

Figure 4.

When you see-saw the floss back and forth between two teeth, it will pass into an open space (Figure 4). Once the floss is into this space, wrapping the floss around the tooth allows it to pass into the small groove of gum tissue that surrounds the tooth (Figure 5). Several up-and-down strokes will be enough to loosen or remove any plaque material present. This technique should be used between all contact points at least once every 24 hours. Plaque takes approximately 12 to 24 hours to form; therefore, if it is removed during this time period, not enough can ever collect to do any damage to the teeth or gum tissue.

There are several different kinds of floss: waxed, unwaxed, and dental tape. If you have many fillings that are rough, it may be easier to use the thicker tape or waxed floss. If you are having fluoride applied to your teeth (a good idea especially in children below 18 years of age), unwaxed floss is preferable, since it will not leave a film of wax on the teeth that retards the tooth's fluoride pickup.

Whichever floss you use, use it with moderation. Don't press it so hard that you injure the gum tissue. At the same time, make sure you get deep enough to remove all the plaque that is present. A good rule of thumb is to go just deep enough to be able to feel the floss meet the junction between the tooth and the gum tissue.

With prudent use of the toothbrush and dental floss, most people can keep free of dental disease indefinitely. For some, however, it is difficult to use them adequately. Your teeth may be overlapped or tilted. Your tongue may be large, and may inhibit a toothbrush from effectively cleaning the insides of the lower teeth. For these situations, another dental aid can be employed that is simple to master and easy to obtain—the toothpick!

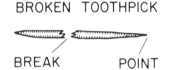

Any round toothpick is acceptable. World's Fair and Fairmount Dome are two very good toothpicks for this function. To use the toothpick effectively, first break it in half (Figure 6). Place the point of one end in the groove of gum around the tooth you are going to clean, at about a 45-degree angle (Figure 7). Gently move the pick around the circumference of the tooth until it hits the next tooth. Continue this until all the teeth are done. As the toothpick is used, the saliva will soften the point until it is acting like a miniature toothbrush. If it gets too soft, switch to the second half.

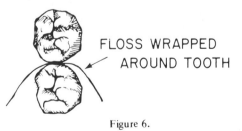

Figure 6.

This technique is particularly useful on the insides of the lower teeth and the outsides of the upper back teeth. Many people use this method on all of their teeth, since it provides an invigorating massage as well as an effective cleaning.

The toothpick can also provide an excellent means for removing stains from the teeth. If the end that has been

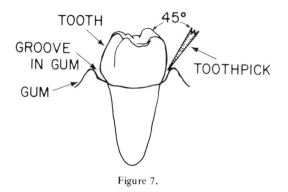

TOOTH   45°
GROOVE
IN GUM
GUM
TOOTHPICK

Figure 7.

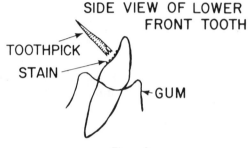

SIDE VIEW OF LOWER
FRONT TOOTH

TOOTHPICK
STAIN
GUM

Figure 8.

broken is placed against the tooth (Figure 8), it will act like a stiff brush and remove most stains. This technique is best applied on the inside surfaces of the lower front teeth.

Of course, there are many variables in maintaining good oral health. Diet, fluoride therapy, exercise, and heredity can all play important roles in a person's state of oral health. The most important factor, however, is the energy that the individual puts into it. By investing a small amount of time (usually less than five minutes per day), one can maintain good dental health for a lifetime.

Suggestions for Further Reading

Charles A. Amanta, Jr., D.D.S., and Robert C. Brachett, D.D.S., M.S., *Dialogue on Preventive Dentistry*. March Publishing, 1971.

Thomas McGuire, D.D.S., *The Tooth Trip: An Oral Experience*. Random House/Bookworks, 1972.

Joe McKeown, D.D.S., *Everybody's Tooth Book*. Happy Valley Apple Press (Box 456, Santa Cruz, California 95061), 1973.

DR. FREDERICK AARON *maintains a private dental practice in Berkeley, California, geared toward disease prevention. He obtained his D.D.S. from the University of Detroit in 1970, and also an English Degree from the University of Michigan. He is a member of the dental staff at Alta Bates Hospital and a dental consultant to several convalescent hospitals in the area. He has conducted prevention workshops for dayschools and kindergartens in the Berkeley School System, and is a member of the Berkeley Dental Society, California Dental Association, American Dental Association, and the American Society for Preventive Dentistry.*

Iridology

Armand Ian Brint

Iridology is a 100-year-old system of health analysis that interprets the neural-optic reflexes in the sensitive tissue of the iris (the colored part of the eye). Simply stated, each part of the iris reflects the dynamic changes occurring in distinct areas of the body.

We know that dis-ease in one part of the body is often reflected in another. For example, faulty elimination will show up as a yellowish coat on the tongue. As Doctor Bernard Jensen says, the body is a marriage of its individual parts.

Iridology is a sophisticated system of reflex associations, and although there is a great deal of research yet to be done, it offers an exciting approach to preventive health care.

L ET US begin with a short definition of iridology, by Dr. James T. Carter, O.D.: "Iridology, or iris diagnosis, is the art and science practiced through the observation of the texture, pigmentation, and density of the iris whereby the physical condition and activity of all special organs and/or systems of the body are directly and most profoundly observed. Structural defects, chemical imbalances, toxemias, inherent weaknesses and predispositions, tensions, endocrine disorders, *et al.*, are observed through direct iris examination. The location, and often the etiology or cause, can likewise be determined. Reflex responses to diseases in other areas are most readily detected. The basic premise from which this definition is derived is that each organ or tissue area of the body has a corresponding locus within the iris, which undergoes 'microinflammatory' change simultaneous with the change at the organ level during its imbalance or disease states."

Metaphor, Myth and Mandala

"Eyes without speaking confess the secrets of the heart."

St. Jerome.

Eyes are perhaps the most important link we have between our outer and inner worlds; they bridge the gap between the physical universe and the eternal unseen realities within us. "These lovely lamps, these windows of the soul" lie at the threshold of two worlds; they mediate the outer light of the sun and the inner light of the soul.

Greek mythology also suggests this esoteric function of the eyes. Iris was the goddess of the rainbow. Her role, along with Hermes, god of medicine, was to transfer information about reality from Olympus to Earth. We can read in this myth the very similar function of our physical iris, the rainbow bridge which connects two realms of consciousness, the soul (like Olympus) and the body (like the Earth).

From an Eastern point of view, the eye may be viewed as a *mandala*. This Sanskrit word means, literally, *circle* or *center*. For ages, in many cultures, the circle has symbolized the entire cosmos, and, with a dot placed within it, the essence and source of all things. The mandala links the microcosm and the macrocosm.

Jose and Miriam Arguelles, in their book *Mandala*, say, "A mandala consists of a series of concentric forms, suggestive of a passage between different dimensions. Through the mandala man may be projected into the universe and the universe into man."

The mandala expresses the notion that all parts of the whole are interrelated, and that each part contains a seed picture of the whole. Recent scientific evidence supports the application of these ideas to study of physical health. The discovery that each cell of our bodies contains a tiny DNA blueprint for the complete life-form is an example.[1]

In iridology, the macrocosm and the microcosm are linked in our eyes. The eye is the single most obvious mandala in our physical body. We may easily view it as a small world reflecting the entire person behind it.

Development

The eye was highly revered in ancient cultures, as a symbol of omniscience. It naturally followed that examination of the eyes was a part of the healer's attempt to ascertain the nature of one's illness.

The civilizations of Mesopotamia and the Indus Valley acknowledged the appearance of signs in the eyes as being often the first indication of disease. It is well-documented that, for centuries and to the present time, Chinese medicine has included an examination of the eyes as part of any diagnostic procedure. The Native American peoples of the southwestern United States developed long ago the sister science/art of sclerology, reading one's health by means of the tiny blood vessels in the whites of the eyes.

Western medicine was slower to discover and accept the

reflex correlations within the eye. In the later years of the seventeenth century, several European doctors discovered a relationship between changes in the iris and certain disease states. Yet it was not until the end of the nineteenth century that two independent Western researchers brought out books outlining the specifics of iridology. Ignatz von Peczeley, a Hungarian doctor, is credited with the discovery of modern iridology. He published his text in Germany in 1881, complete with charts correlating sections of the iris with organs and systems of the body.

From long observations of his patients, he arrived at a system of visible density changes in the fibers of the iris that corresponded to acute and chronic conditions. Shortly after von Peczeley's work appeared, Nils Lilequist, a Swedish minister and homeopath, published his *Diagnosis From the Eye*, which recorded his observations of changes in iris pigmentation that resulted from toxic accumulations in the body of chemicals, drugs, and minerals popularly used at the time, such as quinine and iodine.

Iridology was introduced to the United States in 1904, with the publication of *Iridology, the Diagnosis From the Eye*, by Henry Lahn, M.D. More recent American texts include *Irisdiagnosis*, by Henry Lindlahr, M.D., a student of Dr. Lahn, and the internationally acclaimed work, *The Science and Practice of Iridology*, by Bernard Jensen, D.C., N.D., first published in 1952. Today there are an estimated ten thousand practitioners of iridology in Europe and one thousand in the Unites States, according to Iridologists, International, an organization based in Escondido, California.

Theoretical Background

Dr. James ("Josh") Carter, who helped develop the "contour" soft contact lenses, has been using iridology in his Marin County, California, optometry practice for many years.

Why does iridology work? Dr. Carter believes it is because the irises are intimately connected with the brain and the nervous system as well as the circulatory system. Iris pigment, which is unusual because it has nerve endings, is constantly replaced as the eye color is maintained. Any abnormality in the body chemistry can disturb this process. According to Carter, researchers have observed iris color spotting caused by injections of certain chemicals into the blood. The irises, he says, actually absorb and retain toxic drugs.

The iris, because of its connection with the sympathetic nervous system, can respond to stress and inflammation. A serious injury, for example, can release fatty acids in the iris, causing its fibers to spread apart. Such alterations in the normal pigment or iris-fiber uniformity are observed and interpreted by the iridologist.[2]

Chart Orientation

Figure 1 is a chart of the iris as it is viewed by the iridologist. A miniature human body is represented in the iris. The left iris is a picture of the left side of the body, the right iris of the right side. The head is at the top of the iris and the feet at the bottom; other areas of the body are arranged in proper relation to each other. Symmetrically placed organs and paired organs, such as the kidneys, are found in both irises.

The topography of the iris has two main characteristics. These are the specific organ and gland locations and a series of "radial zones," extending from the pupil to the iris margin, indicating specific bodily systems (the nervous, circulatory, lymphatic, etc.).

According to Theodore Kriege, a well-known German iridologist, if we divide the iris into three concentric circles, the first one (closest to the pupil) corresponds to the organs of food preparation and absorption. The second one corresponds to the organs of transport and utilization. The third (outermost) circle corresponds to the organs of structure, support, and "ultimate utilization, including detoxification and elimination."

These concentric divisions of the iris reveal the relationship between the inner and outer portions of the body. In addition, the internal parts of any one organ will be found pupilward, whereas the outer layers of that organ will always be found toward the iris margin.

If you study the iris chart, you will see that it looks like a wheel, with the pupillary zone as the hub and the ciliary zones as the spokes radiating from it. Most iridologists agree that the integrity of the body's energy is reflected by the quality of energy in this hub, or core. The vitality of the gastrointestinal system greatly affects the systemic equilibrium. The small intestines and the colon, through links in the autonomic nervous system, have a tremendous influence on the other organs of the body. We know that the small intestine and the colon are the only major organs with links to three plexuses of the sympathetic nervous system. In addition, they may be connected with other cranial nerves as well as the vagus nerve.[3]

On the chart, the intestinal zone is actually delineated by the autonomic nerve wreath. It is this intimate relationship and integral connection of the autonomic nervous system with the rest of the body that brings much of the iridologist's attention to bear on the "hub" area.

One of the advantages of iridology is that it is a system whereby the interdependence of the body's constituent parts may be ascertained.

Iris Signs

If you look closely at an iris, you will see many fibers radiating out from the pupil to the iris periphery, almost like a tiny sun sending contiguous rays of light into the atmosphere. An iris whose fibers are straight and lie close to one another is said to have fine density. One whose fibers are wavy or unevenly arranged, with openings between them, reveals a looser density. Dr. Jensen uses the analogy of fine silk and the coarser texture of burlap to describe density. This "weave" of the iris reflects one's inherent constitutional strength and recuperative powers, information which can be vitally important in deciding on individualized treatment.

It is important, however, not to estimate strength or weakness from the iris alone, but to take into account the unique qualities of each individual. Iris density indicates a general constitutional dispostion; yet a delicate consti-

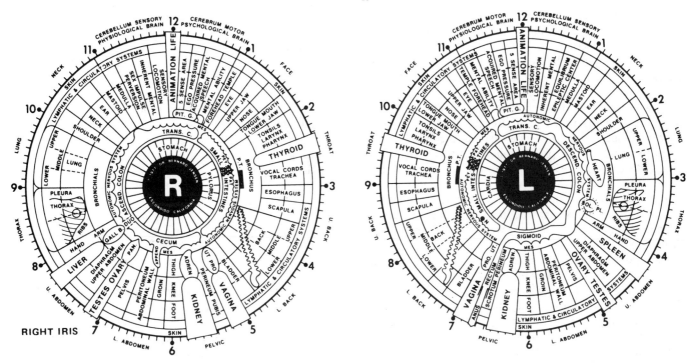

Figure 1. Iris Chart. © Dr. Bernard Jensen.

tution may enjoy the same degree of health as a stronger one, given the proper attention to health maintenance.

The markings in the iris range from light to dark, that is, from acute (hyperactive) to chronic (hypoactive) conditions.

Iris signs may generally be divided into two major categories. The first comprises changes in density, which reflect inherent or acquired organic weaknesses. The second category, pigmentation or coloration change, reflects the accumulation of drugs, chemicals, and other toxic substances in the circulatory systems.

Most iris signs can be viewed as stages of inflammation, according to Dr. Jensen. The *acute inflammatory signs* show as white or a lightening of color in the brown eye. The surface fibers swell and appear elevated. These signs may represent acute inflammation, congestion, pain, etc., and show up more readily than the chronic signs. According to Theodore Kriege, acute signs typically appear as *lines* (straight or zig-zag), *flakes*, or *clouds*, which are larger than flakes and indicate a broader area of involvement. The organs corresponding to the places where these marks are found are said to be undergoing changes of an acute nature.

Darker signs are viewed as indications of a deeper imbalance, which requires more time and energy to heal. They occur in the following ways:

(1) *a thinning of density*; that is, the uppermost-surface iris fibers separate enough that the underlying, darker layer of iris tissue is exposed;

(2) *a crypt*, whereby the iris fibers diverge in small or large arcs, thus exposing the second darker iris layer (crypts may be entirely or partially closed);

(3) *radii solaris*, which are small or large spokes, usually beginning in the intestinal-tract area, that indicate channels of toxic absorption and nerve weakness in the areas they run through;

(4) *contraction furrows*, or nerve rings, which are concentric interruptions of iris fibers resembling rings and which indicate peripheral nerve tension and/or cramping;

(5) *a shurf ring*, which is restricted to the skin area and appears as a darkening, indicating poor elimination and tone. This last mark may be confined to one area of the skin, or may make a complete circle around the perimeter of the iris.

Inflammation passes through graduated stages as health declines. A typical pattern for a blue eye would begin with a white sign (acute) and move into yellowish (subacute), grey (subchronic), and black (chronic). The reverse of this process can be observed as health is recovered. This is referred to as the *healing crisis*, and is explained in Dr. Jensen's book *The Science and Practice of Iridology*.

Pigmentation change appears as large bands of color that differ from the normal iris color; as localized spots of color, called *toxin flecks*; as a *lymphatic rosary*, which looks like a string of smallish white balls arranged in a uniform pattern in the lymphatic and circulatory zone (this indicates congestion of the lymph nodes); or as an opaque white ring at the outer margin of the iris, known as a *sodium ring*, which indicates inorganic deposits of sodium, other minerals, cholesterol, or other agents which contribute to ossification of tissue.

Anemia is described as a hazy quality or lack of definition in the iris margin. This sign may encircle the iris, but is usually found in the upper rim, because the brain proportionately demands the greatest supply of blood, and therefore circulatory problems first show up. Anemia may indicate sluggish circulation and/or a deficiency in the blood.

The most gratifying signs to read are known as *healing lines* or *calcium luteum lines*. These tiny white lines begin filling in areas of darkness, typically crisscrossing one another in a honeycomblike pattern. They indicate that the body has generated enough vitality to slough off old tissue and to replace it with new, bringing, as Dr. Jensen says, "light to dark places."

Iris signs appear to be dynamic, changing with time in relation to the cumulative change in corresponding bodily tissue. There is one exception, when an organ has been surgically removed. It is reported in these cases that the corresponding iris reflex point freezes in its presurgery condition, and never registers a tissue change again.

Iris markings often represent inherent rather than purely acquired weaknesses. Usually one or both parents will display similar signs in their own eyes. It is not uncommon to observe a baby with nerve rings, crypts, toxic accumulations, etc. This startling realization impels us to strengthen our bodies for our own sake and for that of future generations.

One iridologist says our genetics are as dynamic as our bodies. He has several cases on file in which patients who exhibited numerous weaknesses cleaned and strengthened themselves before conceiving a child. They bore children with beautifully clear eyes, even when their older children inherited defects.

I do not intend to provide here a definitive guide to iris markings, but merely to outline some common signs likely to be encountered. For greater detail, see Dr. Jensen's work and Theodore Kriege's *Fundamental Basis of Iris Diagnosis*. It is proficiency at locating and interpreting the signs that determines the skill of the iridologist.

Eye Color

According to Kriege, there are three primary eye colors: blue, grey, and brown. Each color has its own set of inherent characteristics. For example, he refers to the blue eye as the rheumatic, lymphatic, tubercular type, meaning that there is a predisposition to weakness in these areas.

Admixtures of colors may represent simple variations from the inherent inclinations designated by the basic color "types," or may result from an organic or chemical imbalance of the types described in the preceding section.

Eye color often becomes lighter as the body eliminates old toxic deposits and weak tissues. It is not uncommon to see an ostensibly brown eye change to green, and even to blue, during a period of recovery. In Dr. Jensen's words, "In a state of good health, the colors are bright and clear; in ill health or a toxic condition, the colors are defiled and dull."

Evaluating Well-Being

Paul Lynn, M.D., defines a toxic condition as "an evolving but reversible condition, where the normal eliminative and building patterns of the tissues have been disrupted by

(1) accumulation of wastes,
(2) poor blood supply,
(3) poor lymph drainage,
(4) excessive contraction or atrophy,
(5) malnourishment of the nervous tissue."

Dr. Jensen lists several facets of iridology which help one discover the relative balance between toxicity and health and thus the degree of well-being, within the body. His list of indications that can be assessed from the iris includes:

(1) the general constitution of the body, including inherent strengths and weaknesses,
(2) the presence and stages of inflammation,
(3) drug accumulations,
(4) degree of acidity,
(5) the unity of symptoms of the whole body, and
(6) the process of healing.

By examining the iris, using various techniques (which range from a simple, direct examination in natural light to the use of a biomicroscope, or slit lamp), the iridologist can pinpoint key areas of treatment. The standard equipment involves nothing more than a 4X magnifying lens and a penlight, which is held at an angle in order to illuminate the depth of markings. This simple method contrasts markedly with the use of allopathic tests, almost all of which can be physically and psychologically traumatic for the patient.

Iridology can be easily learned, according to Dr. Carter. Some of the skills involved are mechanical, but others are definitely intuitive.

What kinds of cases lend themselves to iris diagnosis? Carter says, "the technique ... has very good predictive value.... The primary value is that it is an early warning system." For example, it is possible to detect signs of an impending heart attack or a cerebral stroke by examining the areas of the iris that correspond to the organs responsible for fat metabolism, and by looking at the whole circulatory system's sufficiency: the distribution, quality, and quantity of blood circulated. One can evaluate how efficiently the organs responsible for absorption and utilization of nutrients in the body are performing by examining the section of the iris which records the changes in the intestinal tract. If certain toxins are being ingested or internally formed, they will also be shown by changes in iris pigmentation.

Dr. Carter suggests that iris diagnosis is best used as an adjunct to other diagnostic skills. "Any good diagnostician doesn't pin everything on one technique." When it is indicated, Carter will suggest nutritional or herbal treatment, but if there are indications that other medical procedures are required, he refers patients to appropriate medical practitioners.

About diagnosis of specific diseases by means of the eyes, Dr. Carter states: "The iris doesn't lend itself to microcellular, biochemical distinction in disease. We can find [the] location and intensity of a condition, but we can't tell the type of cancer cell present, for example, unless there is actual tissue destruction involved. The iris shows inflammation at the energetic tissue level." The same principle applies to the presence of gallstones. "Gallstones aren't a condition *of* the gall bladder; there are stones *inside* the bladder. There has to be some weakness of the gall bladder to create the stones, but you can't look today and tell if

IRIS ANALYSIS

Armand Ian Brint

Here is a brief analysis of an iris photograph. This is not a thorough examination, but merely a description of the outstanding features of this iris. It is always a good idea to conduct additional evaluations in order to corroborate iris findings.

The density of this left iris is above average, indicating a sound constitution with fine recuperative powers. The hub of the iris displays underactivity (deficient energy) in the digestive tract. This condition suggests a general impairment in the functions of digestion, assimilation, and elimination. The overall constriction of the autonomic nerve wreath indicates a tendency toward tightness in the bowels (possible constipation), and a general nervous hypersensitivity and tension (excess or blocked energy), especially since it is accompanied by several sets of nerve rings (ciliary body) and wavy radial fibers. Although it does not show up clearly in this black and white photograph, a discoloration around the wreath indicates a potential accumulation of waste in the circulation of blood and lymph (deficient energy). Radii solaris, found throughout the body of the iris along with a slight lymphatic rosary (periphery) confirm the above observation. The lymphatic rosary specifically points to a tendency toward

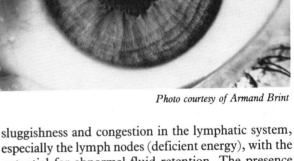

Photo courtesy of Armand Brint

sluggishness and congestion in the lymphatic system, especially the lymph nodes (deficient energy), with the potential for abnormal fluid retention. The presence of a skurf rim represents weak peripheral circulation and an atonic condition of the skin (deficient energy), suggesting poor elimination of waste through the pores.

there are no stones and then look tomorrow and find stones."

A possible diagnosis might be "gall-bladder blockage," which is not precise, but does indicate that the bladder is not functioning normally. Further study would be needed to discover whether the malfunction were caused by hormones, some mechanical effect, a circulatory imbalance, or even a postural situation. As more areas of the iris are studied, more insight may be gained into the causes of such imbalances.

Pregnancy, because it is a normal condition of the female body, does not create inflammation; so it is not revealed by an iris examination. Inflammation, trauma, and toxemia are readily observed. Should a person fall and receive a cut from a rock, the trauma of both the fall and the wound would be recorded in the iris and would leave a permanent mark related to the severity of the injury. If certain toxins were ingested, their accumulation would be revealed; the change that the resultant toxemia causes in the iris tissue is different from that caused by tissue inflammation.

Nervous disorders that arise from the cellular level can be observed in the iris, because the iris records changes in the cellular structure. Even some behavioral conditions have a predictable and characteristic effect on the body; anger is one. By incorporating the principles of Oriental medical philosophy with iridology and by integrating bio-

chemical and nutritional concepts, Dr. Carter has found an interesting and dynamic place for iridology in the area of mental health.

Diagnostic Advantages

There are at least six primary advantages to iris diagnosis:

(1) the whole body is simultaneously visible in the iris;
(2) the technique is noninvasive;
(3) the skills are transferable, since it can be easily learned;
(4) it can be used as an early warning system before a medical crisis occurs;
(5) it can be accurate adjunctive technique when used with other processes of health evaluation;
(6) it has significant value for public health when used in the screening of large populations.[4]

Conclusion

Much could be written concerning the appropriate use of iridology, but a few simple reminders will suffice:

(1) Complete a comprehensive course of study in iridology. Investigate a broad range of literature, as there are numerous theories, charts, and applications.

(2) *Do not use an iris analysis to diagnose medical conditions.* As in the practice of acupuncture, the benefit of iridology is derived from assessing deficiencies or excesses of *energy* in the system.

(3) Iridologists should have a working knowledge of natural remedial agents for the conditions identified in the iris, or be able to refer clients to the appropriate health-care practitioner.

(4) Remember that many of the markings in the iris are inherent or constitutional; they can be strengthened, but are not likely to demonstrate dramatic change. Concentrate on differentiating acquired from inherent signs, and make recommendations accordingly.

(5) In any given set of eyes, you are likely to see several systems that are out of balance. The iridologist's job is to concentrate on the system(s) that will prove most pivotal in balancing the entire body energy, or to work with the system most immediately in need of care.

(6) You should obtain as much information as possible in order to corroborate and hone the iris analysis, including a health history, dietary survey, and analysis of lifestyle factors.

In closing, I would like to underscore the point that iridology is truly an holistic or integral study. It may be summed up as the interpretation of the picture that arises from the interplay of body, mind, and spirit. It is a microcosm of your entire being. According to Matthew 6:22–23, Jesus said, "The light of the body is the eye: if therefore thine eye be single, thy whole body shall be full of light."[5]

Notes

[1] David Keil, "A Look At Iridology" *The Berkeley Monthly*, vol. 7, no. 8, p. 7.

[2] See Keil.

[3] See Wolf, *Well Being*, no. 24, p. 3.

[4] E. M. Oakley, "Iridology: Your Eyes Reflect Your Health" *New Realities*, vol. 1, no. 3, pp. 51–63.

[5] In addition to my own experience, I have depended heavily in this essay on the articles by David Keil, E. M. Oakley, and Harri Wolf, and wish to acknowledge my gratitude to them.

Suggestions For Further Reading

M. Hogan, *Histology of the Human Eye.* Sanders, 1971.

Bernard Jensen, D. C., *The Science and Practice of Iridology.* Escondido, Calif.: Jensen, 1952.

Theodore Kriege, *Fundamental Basis of Irisdiagnosis.* London: Fowler, 1969.

Henry Lindlahr, M. D., *Iridiagnosis and Other Diagnostic Methods.* Chicago: Lindlahr, 1922.

Harri Wolf, *Applied Iridology.* San Diego, Calif.: Wolf, 1979.

ARMAND IAN BRINT *is the founder of the Berkeley Holistic Health Center, and co-editor of the* Holistic Health Handbook *and its companion volume, the* Holistic Health Lifebook. *Armand is a charter member of Iridologists International and has taught iridology and related health practices throughout California. He currently is the administrator of a mental health clinic in Oakland, California.*

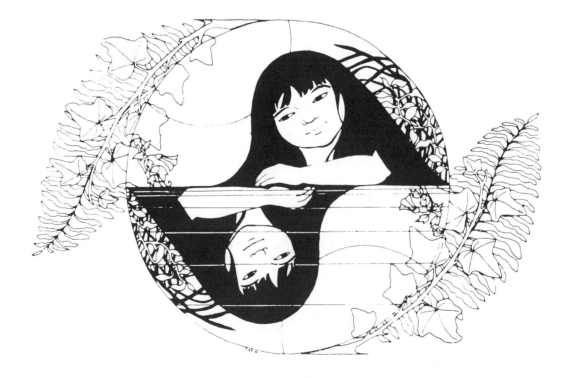

Improving Eyesight: The Bates Method

Gerald Grow, Ph.D.

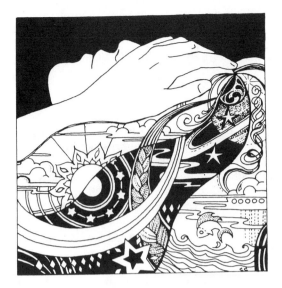

Dr. William Bates was educated as an ophthalmologist to believe that most common eye disorders were permanent and could not be effectively alleviated. But after years of practice, he came to believe that vision is at least 50 percent a mental process, and that when the mental states of his patients improved, often their vision improved also, as did their eyes. Dr. Bates realized that organs function best when properly used, and that proper use can often cause organic defects (such as eye problems) to improve or disappear completely.

Dr. Bates developed a system of mental and physical exercises to teach his patients to use whatever vision they had as well as possible. He almost always recommended either giving up glasses completely or using the least amount of correction and going without the glasses whenever possible.

At a time when it was considered quackery to heal the body by means of the mind, Bates worked on the eyes by encouraging the systematic use of the memory and the imagination. He emphasized the bad effects of staring, and invented special methods of relaxation, pointing out that relaxed minds and organs function better than tense ones. His methods for relaxing the eyes were so powerful that they often cured other conditions as well. His techniques resembled meditation, and anticipated certain principles of biofeedback and stress-reduction training.

In 1939 Aldous Huxley used the Bates method to recover from near blindness caused by severe illness. He recounts the story of his recovery in his book The Art of Seeing.

In this article on the Bates method, Gerald Grow discusses his approach to the Bates work and offers us instructions for beginning to use this holistic method of visual re-education.

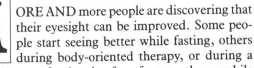

MORE AND more people are discovering that their eyesight can be improved. Some people start seeing better while fasting, others during body-oriented therapy, or during a new health diet, or after jogging for a few months, or while on a meditation retreat. A very nearsighted woman re-

ported to me that, after a deep back massage, she could see perfectly for four hours.

Although such changes are usually temporary, since bad habits will reassert themselves, they have awakened a tremendous interest in the possibility that eyesight may be permanently improved, and have led to a sweeping revival of the Bates method of visual re-education. Invented by ophthalmologist W. H. Bates in 1920, this system of "eye and mind exercises" almost faded from sight in the '60s, but has returned in rejuvenated form.

I will try to give you a feeling for the Bates work, and for how it is now increasingly practiced, in the context of personal growth and holistic thinking.

The Tune-In

At the heart of every vision problem lies *stress*: subtle, long-term, usually undetected tension. Stress builds upon a disharmony between the body's rhythms and the rhythms of the mind or environment. You can start reducing stress, therefore, by focusing first on body rhythms, and gradually restructuring your lifestyle around them, instead of against them. Here's a way to start.

Whatever posture you happen to be in, relax into it. Give yourself all the room you can in your chest and belly, to allow space for *breathing*. Begin to remember *rhythms*: breathing, heartbeat, walking; waves on the beach. Imagine you are on a boat being rocked by the waves, rocked in a hammock or a cradle, breathing. Wherever one of the following exercises calls for movement, tune into these rhythms, and allow one of them to rise up out of you and to move you. Then you will know how fast to move: by not moving, but by being moved from inside.

Blink, Breathe, and Relax

With rare exceptions, vision problems are accompanied by immobilization of the eyes: *staring*. Most people are unaware of this; it is hard to tell when you are staring. Staring, though, is part of a larger pattern that includes holding (or dampening) of the breath, and a general tensing-up.

To start remobilizing your eyes, then, learn to identify when you are *holding your breath* (which is easier than discovering when you are staring). Then *blink, breathe, and relax.*

Glasses

Although glasses help you see clearly, they do nothing to change the underlying causes of vision problems, and may aggravate them. Go without glasses whenever you can do so safely and *without strain.* As an intermediate measure, you can use less-powerful lenses, which will allow you to see enough to get around, but will give your eyes room to improve.

Do the following exercises without glasses or contacts.

Palming

If you go out and do "eye exercises"—visual calisthenics—you may do more harm than good. Start instead by learning to relax your eyes deeply. Palming teaches this.

To palm, sit with your elbows propped (on a cushion, table, back of a chair, etc.). Shake out your hands to relax them, then place—snuggle—your palms over the orbits of your eyes, but without touching the eyelids at all. Gently, softly, close out the light. Let your eyelids close. Breathe.

Once you have settled into position, do the Tune-In, then do one of the following.

(a) Relax each part of your body in turn, toes to scalp.

(b) Pay soft attention to every facet of every breath, altering it as little as possible. After each breath, count it. Relax, watch, let go. If you find yourself thinking, go back to counting breaths.

(c) Go on a fantasy trip to the beach, mountains, woods, desert, down a river in a canoe, to an art gallery, the zoo. Invite yourself to see everything in vivid color and depth. Frequently shift focus from near to far. Imagine movement and follow it with your eyes. Choose scenes that are peaceful and expansive.

(d) The most important palming meditation is this: when you are palming, begin to remember times in your life when you felt really whole, expansive, at one with yourself, when you were vibrant, relaxed, alive, and fully yourself. Invite visual memories to come to you. Cultivate this inner place of healing wholeness.

If you are *nearsighted,* do the following while palming. Imagine seeing something clearly up close, then imagine it moving slowly into the distance, but *staying clear.* Let your imagination have perfect sight.

If you are *farsighted,* do the opposite. Imagine something clearly visible that moves slowly closer. You might imagine walking toward a tree, seeing limbs at first, then leaves, then veins, and finally the little luminous hairs on the stems, with tiny insects crawling in the hairs and their tiny legs with even tinier feet. In imagination, allow your sight to be perfect at all distances.

If you can *imagine* seeing clearly at a distance that is normally blurred for you, this imagination helps remobilize the eyes and the attention, so that they work together to provide better sight at that distance. Whenever you imagine something, your eyes focus as if you were looking at it.

Exercise your imagination, and let your imagination exercise your eyes.

When you come out of palming, open your eyes slowly, blinking softly. Let yourself receive the world for a few moments with all the wide-eyed, open-eyed wonder you can find. Cultivate a large mind, an open heart, and an innocent eye. Better sight needs such a habitat to grow in.

Sunning

Along with palming, sunning is the best way to rejuvenate your eyes.

With eyes closed (that's *CLOSED*), sit or stand facing the sun. Do the Tune-In, then allow your head to begin to turn gently from left to right, through an easy angle of about 90°.

Under your closed lids, keep your eyes facing the direction your nose is pointing, so that your eyes cross and recross the full light of the sun.

DAILY DRILLS FOR EYES

Gerald Grow

1. *Morning warmup:* deep breathing, stretches, face massage and wrangling, swinging, tapping head, *neck-loosening exercises.*
2. *Sun:* five minutes, four times a day, or equivalent.
3. *Palm:* five minutes, four times a day, with mental imagery, or counting breaths. Once a week, palm for 30 minutes to music. In your mind's eye, allow yourself to have perfect vision. Visualize in color, depth, movement.
4. *Swing:* three times a day for three minutes each. Relax. See apparent movement.
5. *Count:* objects, colors, shoes, patterns, anything: in quick, easy glances.
6. *Edge:* slowly trace the outlines of objects, especially at the distance you cannot see clearly. Allow illusion of apparent motion in the direction opposite to that in which your eyes are moving.
7. Play *games of movement* without glasses: ping-pong, catch, frisbee, etc. Follow movement with your eyes and head.

ON THE ART OF SEEING

Aldous Huxley

Ever since ophthalmology became a science, its practitioners have been obsessively preoccupied with only one aspect of the total, complex process of seeing—the physiological. They have paid attention exclusively to my eyes, not at all to the mind, which makes use of the eyes to see with. I have been treated by men of the highest eminence in their profession; but never once did they so much as faintly hint that there might be a mental side to vision, or that there might be wrong ways of using the eyes and mind as well as right ways, unnatural and abnormal modes of visual functioning as well as natural and normal ones. After checking the acute infection in my eyes, which they did with the greatest skill, they gave me some artificial lenses and let me go. Whether I used my mind and bespectacled eyes well or badly, and what might be the effect upon my vision of improper use, were to them, as to practically all other orthodox ophthalmologists, matters of perfect indifference. To Dr. Bates, on the contrary, these things were not matters of indifference; and because they were not, he worked out, through long years of experiment and clinical practice, his peculiar method of visual education. That this method was essentially sound is proved by its efficacy. My own case is in no way unique; thousands of other sufferers from defects of vision have benefited by following the simple rules of that Art of Seeing, which we owe to Bates and his followers.

From *The Art of Seeing*, by Aldous Huxley. Copyright ©1975 Montana Books.

(a) Sunning is first of all a breathing exercise. Breathe.

(b) Sunning is next a *relaxation* exercise. It is *essential* to relax into the light. Please do not squint, strain, frown, or otherwise fight the light. If necessary, start with partial shade or a weak lamp. Use the amount of light you can relax into. (If you sun regularly, you will have little need for sunglasses.) Sunlight is best, but when there is no sun, you can use an ordinary 150-watt "reflector spotlight" found in most hardware stores.

(c) Sunning is an *awareness* exercise. Feel. Feel the warmth of the sun gently penetrating all the tissues of your face in turn: brow, cheeks, temples, mouth, jaw, chin, nose, eyebrows, eyelids. Then feel the warmth penetrating your eyeballs themselves, and deep into your eye-sockets, warming and relaxing the muscles that surround your eye and extend far back behind the eye, muscles that cradle the eye as your hand might cradle an orange. Relax these muscles all the way back, almost to the center of your skull.

(d) People often tense against the light in order to keep the world at a distance, to shut out what they do not want to see. Some people even remember how, as children, they made a conscious choice to stop seeing: "This is too painful; I'm shutting it out." I suspect that any eye problems arise from the choice not to see.

If this is true for you, you can reopen your eyes and learn again to let the world in, and see. You can learn to change defenses, tension, and overexertion. You have the strength and power to deal with anything the visual world presents to you through your eyes. You do not need to close it out with squinting, frowning, furrowing, or blurring—or the mental equivalent.

Learn gradually to open your eyes, to open yourself, and to expand your capacity to assimilate what you see—by means of more generous, compassionate understanding. Expand your "vision" of life, and you will be capable of seeing more.

Sunning can be your time to *practice nonresistance* by allowing light to come into you. Be naked to the light, soft, vulnerable as a newborn baby. Receive the gift of light. Relax. Feel glad. Trust yourself. Forgive. Give thanks. These attitudes open your sight better than any exercise can.

When sunning, allow the light to seem to penetrate all the way into your brain—softening and expanding, relaxing and making it more spacious, more easy, all the way to, and through, the back of your head. Let the warmth go all the way through you, till you can imagine it warming and relaxing the back of your head and neck. Let any resistance melt away.

After a few minutes of sunning, turn away from the light and open your eyes, blinking softly. Allow yourself to see whatever you see. Don't work to see better. Look softly into the blur. Make room for better sight to find its way to you. It will.

Swinging

Swinging helps you relearn how the eyes feel when they move rapidly in a spontaneous, relaxed, effortless manner.

Stand with your feet comfortably apart. Do the Tune-In, and, with your eyes open, begin to turn your head and shoulders from right to left, increasing till you are shifting your weight first to the ball of one foot, then onto the other, in a gentle turning, twisting, swinging rhythm. Breathe and blink normally. Move with a lazy precision.

GUIDELINES

Gerald Grow

Keep These in Mind as Much as Possible

1. *Blink, breathe, and relax.*
   (a) Learn to identify when you hold your breath, then blink, breathe, and relax.
   (b) Whenever you are going into a difficult situation, monitor yourself to consciously blink, breathe, and relax.
   (c) Set up arbitrary times to consciously blink, breathe, and relax: until the light changes; to the next freeway sign; until *X* stops talking; until the interruption is over; until the pain stops; until the craving goes away; etc.
2. Keep your eyes *moving*: shift focus from near to far, and scan the world from side to side. Look in quick glances. Pick out outlines, details. Shift your eyes around the face of persons you are talking to.
3. Check your *posture* often. Expand into width, height, spaciousness, balance, ease—an easy strength.
4. Turn your head to face the direction you are looking in.
5. *Relax*: Once a day, relax from head to foot, deeply. Practice relaxed action—just the right amount of effort for the task. Relax your mind by palming visualizations, fantasy, meditation, prayer, forgiveness, positive attitudes, innocence, problem solving, delight. Allow yourself to be imperfect, improvisational, learning, in process. Laugh at yourself. Allow mistakes and learn joyfully.
6. Practice *effortless seeing*: no straining, squinting, frowning, etc. Invite, nourish, *allow* seeing—don't force it. Accept the present state of your vision: see what you can see. Practice looking into the blur while you accept it, relax, blink and breathe, scan, encourage the best vision you have. Learn good seeing habits, and allow vision to come to you.

Keep your eyes open, facing the direction your nose is pointing in. And do the following.

(a) Imagine a thin black line drawn at eye level across the most distant things you can see. In this thin black line, imagine a small, blacker dot moving easily, smoothly, swiftly just where your eyes are pointing. Imagine this black dot to be like a magnet, pulling the point of your focus along smoothly down the line, across all the objects the line is drawn on. Make no effort to see anything. Just focus on the black line and blacker dot moving in it, and let the world slide by. Breathe, blink, relax.

(b) While following the black line and swinging, now begin to notice how objects nearby seem to be in *apparent motion* in relation to you. As you move one way, they seem to move in the opposite direction. Let go of the illusory stability of the world; cultivate this sense of movement; relax into it. Let your body move; breathe, blink, relax; swing; focus on the black line; and let your attention settle down into that alert, quiet, wondering part of your mind that allows the world to *move by* as you move.

Breathe and relax through a hundred swings. Vary from an easy pace to a very slow, continuous swinging.

Relaxed Seeing

You will need to make an eye chart of different-sized letters. You can cut them out of magazines and paste them on white cardboard. If you have trouble seeing in the distance, make the chart from large and medium type sizes. If you have trouble seeing up close make the chart from small type sizes. Place this chart at a distance where you can see the lines of large letters, but not the smaller ones.

In this manner, locate your *borderline of blur*. By working with this borderline of blur, you will be able to tell immediately when you are doing something right, because your vision will clear up noticeably. The chart acts as a biofeedback device, letting you know at once when you are seeing in a more relaxed manner.

Please note: you can temporarily clear your vision by squinting, straining, frowning, tensing, narrowing your eyelids, tilting your head, or other "tricks." These are strictly for emergencies, however, and if you use such tricks very much, they will strain your eyes and worsen your sight.

Instead, locate your borderline of blur on the chart and practice relaxation. First of all, practice looking at the blur and doing nothing about it. Stop *trying* to see better. Give up the *effort* of seeing. Rather, just see what you see. *Allow* your sight, encourage it, invite it. Any *effort* you *make* to see *better* will use the conscious, voluntary nerves of focus, and these are relatively clumsy emergency mechanisms. But if you scan the line of blur gently and continuously, and alternate using the chart with sunning, palming, swinging, and relaxing, you can begin to allow the unconscious, involuntary nerves of focus to perform their delicate "fine tuning" of vision. This fine tuning does not appear until you relax out of strain and conscious effort. But when it comes, your mind and eye will—by a process of trial and error—discover how to focus better.

Work first with one eye for a while (with the other covered lightly by a patch or handkerchief or your palm). Then work with the other, then with both together.

And remember: relax, give up effort, be patient, invite vision, and wait for it to come to you from a place inside you that you can cultivate, but not command.

Flashes

As you relax through these exercises, the subtle, involuntary "tuning" of mind and eye can begin to reassert itself, and you may begin to experience sudden clearings of sight: "flashes" of clear vision. If you have such a flash, close your eyes before it goes away, tune into yourself, and feel what you are doing inside yourself that makes this possible. When you begin to learn how to live from that feeling, you have solved half your eye problem. You solve the other half when you learn new, healthy habits for the moment-to-moment use of your eyes. For more help with both, consult a vision teacher or one of the recommended books.

The Gift of Seeing

Improving your vision is not a selfish act. You can learn to see someone else in such a way that both are healed by that seeing. On a larger scale, the universe gives us light, and we give back perception. It is by means of our sight that the universe sees itself. We bear witness. Our sight can celebrate, center, and confirm what is most real. Seeing is your gift. Give it generously.

Suggestions for Further Reading

Margaret Corbett, *Help Yourself to Better Sight.* Wilshire Books, 1949.

Aldous Huxley, *The Art of Seeing.* Montana Books, 1975.

"Improve your Eyesight Without Glasses," an LP record of Bates exercises, available from Wolf Records, 615 E. Pike, Seattle, WA 98122.

Note: Dr. Bates' original book was heavily edited after his death and reissued under the title *Better Sight Without Glasses.* It is somewhat difficult to read and use, and I recommend you read one of the above books before trying it.

GERALD GROW *attended Harvard and Cambridge Universities, and received a Ph.D. from Yale in literature and drama. After teaching at San Francisco State and St. Mary's Colleges for five years, he became trained in the body-oriented therapy of Wilhelm Reich. He then studied Bates Method vision training under Anna Kaye—a vision instructor—and Ray Gottlieb, O.D. He has been concentrating on vision work since 1975. He has a private practice in Berkeley, gives workshops across the country, and is a published author and cartoonist.*

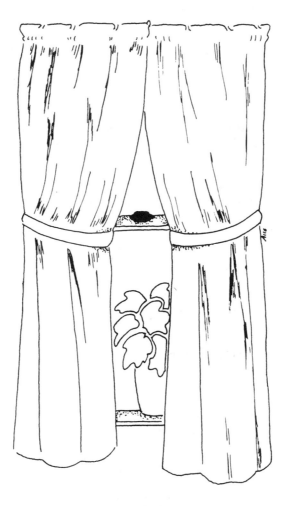

Meet Your Colon

William LeSassier, N.D.

THE COLON is not easy to clean, rebuild, or even strengthen. The colon responds to many inputs of energy: vertebrae position, the condition of the internal flora and the mucous membrane, the acid/alkaline balance, parasites, emotions, etc. One must create optimum conditions in and for this organ in order to regain and maintain physiological balance.

There has been controversy about how many bowel movements a person is supposed to have daily. It has been stated that a bowel movement after every meal is best, and this frequency would indicate highly active peristalsis. However, I think it is normal for elimination to vary greatly from person to person, depending on the proportion of bulk in the diet, on how much is eaten each day, and on what types of food are eaten. Most people agree that the morning is the time of greatest elimination. The time of greatest bowel activity is between 5 and 7 A.M. Certainly sleeping too late in the morning will throw the colonic activity off schedule. However, given the diversity of colons and opinions, it is difficult to establish a standard. It is a matter of individual balance. A healthy colon responds to nerve stimuli, and normally eliminates by means of both peristalsis and gas (not the fermented "methane"-type gas, which everyone dislikes, but normal, occasional, healthy "wind").

Constipation

Many think that constipation is a cause in itself of disease, but this viewpoint is incomplete. Colon imbalances are symptomatic of imbalances in other systems within the body, and, of course, affect other parts of the body as well. Because it is an organ of elimination as well as nutrition, the colon reflects what other organs are doing or not doing. For example, if the liver is sluggish, the colon will not function properly. A very common cause of constipation, and one that many overlook, is excessive urination when there are not enough fluids in the body to compensate for

the loss. Anyone who takes diuretics (agents which promote water elimination) without taking in enough fluids will have dry stools. Improper food combinations can also produce this dryness, by causing so much fermentation that the colon becomes hot. The body then sends fluids to the surface of the body, to cool the body by evaporation. When one has this kind of dryness in the system, one must use herbs that will expel gas, cool the system, and moisten the stool. A combination of fenugreek, cascara sagrada, and slippery elm will surely relieve the symptoms of dry stools.

The best laxatives to use are actually foods. Carob pods, pecans, agar-agar, tapioca, and ripe fruits are all good. Prunes and figs are laxative, and can also regulate the acid/alkaline balance in the colon. Always soak dried fruit overnight before using it as a laxative. Prunes soaked overnight increase the acidity of the colon, expel excess mucous, and eliminate many bacteria, but in excess they can kill the flora and can irritate hemorrhoids or sensitive spots in the mucous lining. Figs are alkaline, emollient, soothing, and cooling to the large intestine. They are bulky, give tone to the colon, increase flora, and are excellent for hemorrhoids.

It is very important to have the proper proportions of fiber in the diet, which should therefore include wheat bran, carob, and coarse foods. Fenugreek and wheat sprouts will help keep anyone's colon healthy. The sprouts, eaten when they are seven days old, will help digest leftover waste, which sometimes cakes onto the walls of the colon. These sprouts are cleansers as well as builders.

Pregnancy

Many herbal laxatives are definitely suspect as toxic to fetal activity. Such herbs as mandrake (American), senna, and aloe are to be avoided. Even cascara sagrada, buckthorn, or other rhamnus species are to be avoided, for although they are not directly toxic, they can be irritating.

The safest laxative for pregnancy are manna, butternut bark or root, flax seed, slippery elm, and lemon verbena (very mild). These may be combined with an aromatic, such as fennel or anise seed. Take about one tablespoon of the herb to each cup of water. Drink up to three cups daily. However, it is not wise to use much of any kind of laxative except under the care of a competent herbalist. The herbs I have mentioned here are the least toxic.

Hemorrhoids

Hemorrhoids are an engorgement of the blood vessels around the rectal lining. They can become irritated, ulcerated, and quite painful. They are caused by blocked flow of blood in the veins of the colon. In pregnancy they are common, because of the pressure on the pelvic floor, which reduces circulation (and thus also causes varicose veins). Cayenne taken internally will stimulate the circulation in the body. The dosage varies greatly from person to person. If you wish to take it, start with small amounts in food or tea, increasing the amount if it does not bother you. Agents like nettles and Irish moss increase blood circulation, which is helpful. Any constipation should be treated also, and excess amounts of salt should be avoided, since salt creates thick, heavy blood. Heavy uses of curry, black pepper, ginger, and cinnamon can also be irritating to the rectum.

If there is ulceration, irritation, or ineffective elimination, a potato suppository may be useful. Whittle out a piece of raw potatoe about the size and shape of your little finger. This is inserted overnight and really aids in the healing of hemorrhoids. Slippery elm or flax seed can also be used to soothe this condition. Take them in either tea or suppository form.

Diarrhea

Diarrhea is sometimes caused by a weak spleen. If the spleen is functioning properly, it will neutralize toxins which enter the system; they then pass out of the body unnoticed. Also, if the intestinal flora are weak, they will be unable to destroy unfriendly flora, such as are often found in spring or winter runoff water. Diarrhea attacks can also result from weakness of liver functions.

Whatever its cause, diarrhea can cause loss of the precious electrolytic fluids (digestive waters) that enable the digestive tract to absorb nutrients. Debilitation can follow, because the body loses its ability to obtain nourishment. To prevent this, drink barley or rice water (boil one cup of rice or barley in eight cups of water for one hour). Celery juice, coconut milk, or lime juice can be added to this to cool the colon.

Herbal astringents which help check excessive discharge may also be useful. Blackberry root, bush monkey flower, white oak, bistort root, and cranesbill have been found effective. Also antiseptic herbs may be useful if the condition has been brought on by amoebic or toxic floral invasions or by parasites.

Intestinal Flora

Healthy intestinal flora are essential, since they manufacture B vitamins. These friendly flora are also guardians against unfriendly flora, consuming and digesting them as they pass through the system. Some things that help create healthy flora are kefir, yogurt, miso, nuts, and seeds (peanuts, almonds, and sesame seeds in particular). Of course, a good diet will help maintain healthy flora.

Some things which weaken flora are: excessive use of garlic (this varies from individual to individual); Golden Seal in excess of three double-0 capsules a day (except under a physician's specific care), enemas in excess, colonics, antibiotics, and, of course, diarrhea attacks. You must re-establish healthy flora by eating a proper diet, after heavy cleansing of the colon.

Please realize that your intuition is your guiding force. Sometimes one must recultivate intuition about how to eat and take care of the body properly. But do not mistake "cravings" of all sorts for true intuition.

Happy floral digestion!

WILLIAM LeSASSIER, N.D. *is the founder and director of the Christos School of Natural Healing, Taos, New Mexico.*

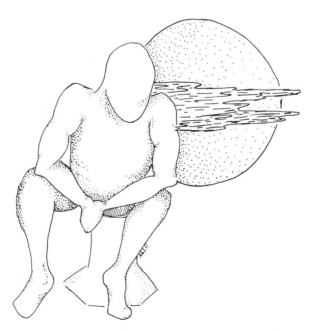

Reflexology

Lew Connor and Linda McKim

Our feet connect us with the Earth. They are our foundation; yet an awareness of them is often literally the farthest thing from our minds. This article approaches the feet with appreciation and understanding of their integral relationship to the whole being.

Learn to give a complete reflexology treatment for its therapeutic value as well as the pure relaxation. And if you have never paid attention to your feet, you can look forward to developing a new relationship with yourself.

"Early man roved over plains, through forests, and stepped on sharp objects which pressed into his feet, reaching the tiny electrical reflexes, furnishing a natural massage. . . . The electrical shock stimulated the portion of the body for which that part of the foot was responsible, and the body as a whole was in rhythm with the universe"

Mildred Carter,
Helping Yourself with Foot Reflexology

ROUND 1913 Dr. William Fitzgerald introduced Zone Therapy to the United States. He found that pressure on certain reflex points brought about a more normal functioning of body organs and frequently a decrease or cessation of pain. Actually, he rediscovered a practice which has its roots in ancient Chinese acupressure. Since then, many people have adopted and modified his ideas. Each has his or her own approach to the subject, which has come to be known as Reflexology; it is up to you, as a student of the healing arts, to pick the approach that best suits you. We offer here an approach that our experiences have shown to be effective.

Why Does Reflexology Work?

Reflexology refers primarily to reflex points on the feet and hands, but there are many other usable reflex points throughout the body.

There are several theories on how reflexology works. Some say that each of the 72,000 nerve endings on each foot connects to a different body area; in massaging those nerve endings, we send a stimulation to a corresponding body area. Others say that we are activating energy points along meridian lines as in acupressure. Dr. Fitzgerald's zone theory divides the body into ten zones, five on each side (see Figure 1). Each zone has its own nerve-stimulation pattern, so that when a pressure is applied at a reflex point on that zone, a stimulation is sent to a corresponding organ or gland on that zone. A large gland or organ which overlaps zones will also have reflex points on all the zones it extends into. We feel that all these ideas have validity, but are only a part of the total healing process, which involves the body, mind, and spirit.

We are all affected by our environment, and for many of us that means stress, tension, and worry. A combination of any of these can cause imbalances, which we usually experience as some sort of symptom, such as colds, flu, or headaches. We continually find that specific reflex points during these times are congested and painful, and very often they feel as if there are grains of sand under the skin. These grains are composed mostly of uric acid or calcium

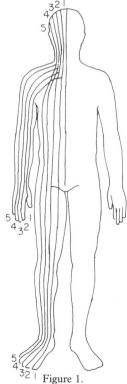

 Figure 1.

Illustrated by Marlynn Amann, Lew Connor

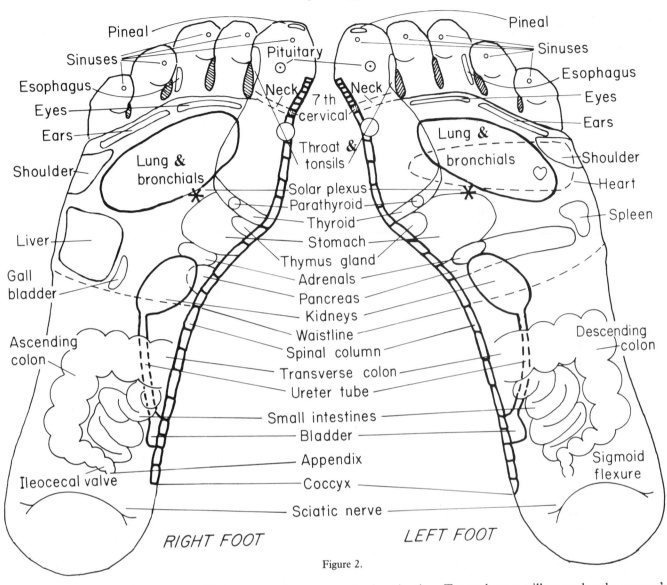

Pineal
Sinuses
Esophagus
Eyes
Ears
Shoulder
Liver
Gall bladder
Ascending colon
Ileocecal valve
Pituitary
Neck
7th cervical
Throat & tonsils
Solar plexus
Parathyroid
Thyroid
Stomach
Thymus gland
Adrenals
Pancreas
Kidneys
Waistline
Spinal column
Transverse colon
Ureter tube
Small intestines
Bladder
Appendix
Coccyx
Sciatic nerve
Neck
Pineal
Sinuses
Esophagus
Eyes
Ears
Lung & bronchials
Shoulder
Heart
Spleen
Descending colon
Sigmoid flexure
Lung & bronchials

RIGHT FOOT   LEFT FOOT

Figure 2.

crystals. When our bodies are out of balance, we do not metabolize our food correctly. By-products of incomplete metabolism include uric acid and excess calcium, which crystalize around nerve endings in the feet and other areas in the body. These crystals cause a blockage around the nerves and cut down on normal stimulation of glands and organs.

Reflexology can assist the body by relaxing it and stimulating the blocked nerve endings, thereby stimulating sluggish glands and organs to regain their normal functioning. The crystals around the nerve endings can be crushed, so that they are reabsorbed by the blood and lymph system and excreted out of the body. Used frequently, reflexology can give the body a general toning to enhance vitality and one's sense of well-being. It is also a wonderful gift to give to a friend.

Suggested Techniques for a Foot Reflexology Massage

First make your friend comfortable, in a position where the spine is straight. Reclining chairs or massage tables are best and easy to work with, but not always available; so

be imaginative. Try to have a pillow under the person's knees so the legs are not locked straight. Next, sit in a comfortable position yourself, facing the soles of the person's feet. Before massaging someone's feet, make sure that your thumbnails are clipped and filed so that you don't inflict discomfort. Also, check with the person to make sure there are no problem areas on the feet, such as rashes, cuts, warts or bruises. If so, avoid these areas, so that they are not further irritated.

Now introduce yourself to each foot, one at a time, by generally rubbing, stroking, kneading, and massaging it. Relax the person by doing this for about a minute on each foot, and by requesting that the person take a few deep breaths to relax his or her body. Each of us has our own techniques for relaxing someone, and you will soon develop your own style.

The first area to approach is the solar-plexus reflex. The solar plexus itself is a major nerve center located in front of the diaphragm and behind the stomach. It is often called the "abdominal brain," since it fires off many fine thread-like nerves to the entire abdominal area, including the diaphragm and adrenal glands.

The reflex to the solar plexus is therefore an excellent

area to massage for relief of tension, stress, fright, anger, or nervousness. Working this reflex area first provides overall relaxation, and increases the person's receptivity to your massage. The solar-plexus reflex is located just below the ball of the foot, about in the center (see Figure 2). There is a crevice-like area that your thumb will fit nicely into. Take hold of both feet, place the pads of your thumbs in these areas, and slowly begin to apply pressure. Ask the person to focus his or her breathing into the area where you are pressing. Use a medium-strong pressure, one that is not uncomfortable for either of you.

During this time, you can coordinate your breathing with your friend's by inhaling and exhaling simultaneously with him or her. This will help relax you both, and aid in establishing an energy connection. You can also visualize yourself as being a channel for healing energy that flows through your hands into his or her feet. A sigh or deep exhalation often signals that the person is beginning to relax.

The actual massage movements are mostly done with the thumb. By using the end of the thumb (Figure 3), you can maintain a steady pressure and crawl across the foot if you flex and extend the thumb by bending the joint closest to the thumb nail. The other fingers can be nesting on the top of the foot while the thumb crawls across the sole. Put the fingers of the other hand between the top of the foot being massaged and the fingers of the hand doing the massage. This prevents the fingers of the actively massaging hand from digging in to the top of the foot. It also helps to stabilize the foot.

By using this massage technique, you can have pin-point control in order to isolate the painful points of the foot, and to more easily break up the crystal deposits. You will find that by moving the thumb only in a forward direction, you will cover the foot more thoroughly than if you tried moving it backward across the sole as well (see Figure 4).

After the solar-plexus reflex, the next area to massage is the toe area (corresponding to the head). Next, work down the foot, going from the outside toward the inside. On the outside edge of the foot, halfway between the heel and the toes, you can find a bump caused by the fifth metatarsal bone. This is the indicator of where the waist can be found. Draw an imaginary line across the sole. Above the line will be the glands and organs located above the waist. This line also indicates where the transverse colon is located (figures 2 and 5). When working the colon reflex, start at the ileocecal-valve reflex on the right foot (the entrance to the large intestine) and work up to the waistline, then across the foot to the instep. Change feet

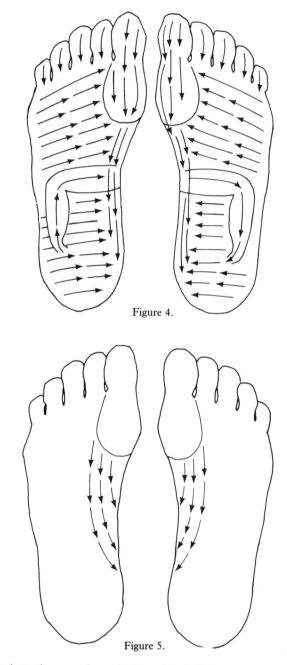

Figure 4.

Figure 5.

and continue on the waistline of the left foot, working from the instep out toward the side of the foot; then work down the side of the sole of the foot until about even with the ankle. Finish by working in toward the center of the foot. The colon reflex is worked in this way to follow the flow of elimination in the colon.

Massage a little on one foot, then switch to the same area on the other foot in order to keep a nice balance while doing the massage. After massaging both feet from outside to inside, covering the entire sole, work the adrenals, kidneys, urethra tube, and bladder by massaging from toe to heel (Figure 6). To work the spine, begin about halfway down the outside of the big toe and follow the bone that creates the arch. Don't massage directly on the bone itself, but on the underside, continuing down until about even with the ankle.

Massaging the top of the foot is easy. Start at the outside heel and massage around to the inside heel (Figure 7). The

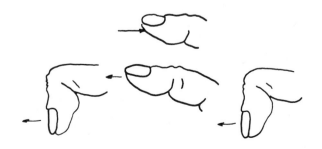

Figure 3.

reflexes located between the toes are especially important. This area corresponds to the thoracic lymphatic ducts, which are located under the clavicle between the shoulders and neck. The lymph system plays a major role in removing toxins from within the body, and working the lymph reflexes stimulates this action. In order to drain the lymph system via the reflexes, place the index finger on top of the foot, between the tendons and bones, about 1″ to 2″ away from the web of the toes. With the thumb on the bottom of the foot, squeeze the thumb and index finger together and with a squeeze/release/squeeze motion, mas-

sage toward the web. Repeat this motion with all the webs of the toes. Following this, gently stroke the feet to finish the massage.

During the massage, whenever we find a spot that is extremely tender, we massage it for about a minute, then return to it a couple of times during the massage. We massage tender areas with a pressure that just borders on pain. Excessive pain creates undue body tension, and one of the aims of this massage is to keep the person relaxed.

Usually we massage the feet for about an hour. However, if a person is very ill or toxic and in a stage of heavy elimination already, we do not want to release too much toxic waste at any one time, so we work on them lightly and only for a short period of time each session (five to ten minutes). We then try to work on them often, about every three to four hours if they are acutely ill, or daily with a more chronic condition.

Sometimes people feel tired or rundown the day after receiving a reflex massage. This indicates that the body is

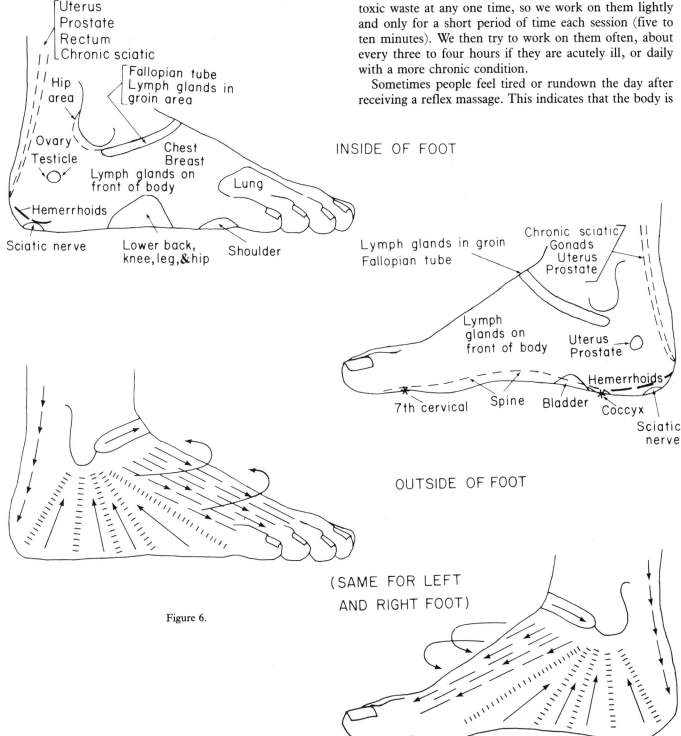

Figure 6.

eliminating blocked toxic material, which is released first into the bloodstream before being eliminated. We encourage people to eat lightly and to drink a lot of liquids to aid the body in the process of elimination. Eating pure natural food that has not been sprayed or injected with chemicals, additives, or hormones is essential for good nutrition, and is a strong complement to natural healing methods such as reflexology. A little processed food goes a long way in causing organ or glandular malfunctions.

Often during reflexology treatments, people will ask what areas of the body tender reflexes are related to. There are three things we suggest you *not* do in response.

1. *Don't diagnose*. Even if you know from your experience that a tender area that you are massaging is related to a specific organ, don't tell the person what it is. Just say that your massage is intended to relax the body so that it may heal itself. Thoughts and words have a force that is manifestable. If you tell someone they have "thyroid trouble," that might just be negative enough to start them imagining, and guess what? They may develop "thyroid trouble."

2. *Don't prescribe*; that means anything. Even telling someone to take a glass of water every day is prescribing. So be careful.

3. *Never treat for a specific ailment.* If someone comes to you and says they have a colon problem, don't go to the colon area and say that working on this area will cure it. Reflexology aids the body in healing itself.

And remember that in most states only M.D.s have the license, according to law, to prescribe, diagnose, and treat.

Energy and Spiritual Awareness

Whenever you do bodywork, you are in essence acting as a healing channel from the Creator (or whatever you might call the higher universal healing power). Before you start your massage, you can affirm that the healing is from the Creator, that you wish only that the Creator's will be done, and that the person about to be massaged may be open to accepting whatever healing they are ready for at that time.

Some of you may have experienced massaging someone with a headache and found that, when the massage was over, the patient's headache was gone, but you had acquired it. This sometimes happens when the person doing the massage is too open to accepting that energy. One technique to avoid this is to envision a bright protective white light around your elbows, and affirm that this light shield will prevent your body from accepting any negative energy. A good time for an affirmation like this is at the beginning of the massage, when you are holding onto the person's solar-plexus reflex.

If during the massage your hand gets heavy, cramped, or uncomfortable, it may be an indication that you are absorbing negative energy. Stop and shake your hands; this rids them of any unwanted energy, and relaxes them as well. It is also helpful to wash your hands in cool water when you finish the massage.

Remember to always keep your shoulders and neck relaxed while massaging someone. The looser you are the more effective you will be and the more relaxed your client will become.

Massage with love and walk in balance.

Suggestions for Further Reading

Devaki Berkson, *The Foot Book: Healing with the Integrated Treatment of Foot Reflexology*. Funk and Wagnalls, 1977.

Mildred Carter, *Helping Yourself With Foot Reflexology*. Parker Publishing, 1969.

Eunice D. Ingham, *Stories the Feet Have Told*. Ingham Publishing (Box 8412, Rochester, NY 14618).

Eunice D. Ingham, *Stories the Feet Can Tell*. Ingham Publishing.

LEW CONNOR *and* LINDA MCKIM *are Co-Directors of the Reflexology Institute of California.*

E. HEALING

How to Choose a Holistic Practitioner

Don Ethan Miller and
Shelly Kellman

How Do You Decide...

where to go for medical or therapeutic help? If you wake up one morning feeling like a giant is pressing his 500-pound hobnailed boot into your lower back, what's your next move? Do you call your health-maintenance organization or clinic, a hospital, or your family doctor? Do you check out that chiropractor you've been meaning to call? Look up the nearest osteopathic doctor (D.O.) in the Yellow Pages? Send a friend to the bookstore for a copy of *Maggie's Back Book*? Seek out a healer, a massage therapist, a Rolfer, a Soma bodywork expert? Do you call a friend who always seems to know about these kinds of things? Check with your yoga or T'ai Chi teacher? Or simply treat yourself with aspirin or Valium and lay up until the pain subsides?

This article will outline the major steps involved in finding and choosing treatment systems and individual practitioners—whether for preventive health and personal improvement or a pressing problem.

What Are You Looking For?

When choosing a medical practitioner of any kind, you should be sure about your primary purpose for seeking help. Are you looking for **health maintenance** (disease prevention or health enhancement) or **treatment** (the attempt to cure or control an illness or injury)? Perhaps you are simply trying to become acquainted with a range of trusted experts—from an acupuncturist to an herbalist to a family doctor—to call on in times of need.

Mainstream Western medicine reigns supreme, and often succeeds magnificently, in certain areas of treatment and cure: traumatic injury, surgery, and antibiotic therapy for bacterial infections, for example. Health modalities known as "holistic," on the other hand, are the best for teaching one how to build a healthy, sound body-mind that resists

disease well, heals rapidly, and degenerates as little as possible with age. After an ambulance crew pulls one through a heart attack and a surgeon performs a miraculous coronary bypass operation, it may be a combination of a nutritionist, aerobic fitness specialist, and psychotherapist who can design the most well-informed, effective program for recovery and prevention of further trouble.

In between prevention and the acute crisis is the wide gray area where most health complaints occur, where conventional and alternative therapies debate each other and sometimes compete, and where sometimes neither has a definitive solution or track record with the problem. How do you treat a cold or other virus, a low-grade bacterial infection, muscle aches, digestive upsets, nervous tension, headaches, backaches, allergies, and the like?

If you want a variety of options at your disposal, you must look into the philosophies and methods of many different therapies. (See sidebar on "Educating Yourself.") If you have a specific problem or desired area of self-improvement, you might work with a variety of modalities at once, or try one at a time to see what works. There are no hard and fast rules. Your choice of a practitioner may ultimately depend more on your feelings of trust and confidence in the individual than on whether she is a chiropractor or physical therapist.

Defining Your Problem/Need

The first question to ask is whether your problem is an emergency or a serious, life-threatening condition. Unconsciousness, severe bleeding that can't be stopped, oppressive chest pain, internal hemorrhaging, accidents (which often cause shock even if there are no injuries), broken bones, etc., are all emergency problems and are probably best dealt with by orthodox medical care: EMTs, (emergency medical technicians), hospital emergency rooms and local doctors.

Early warning signs of cancer, heart disease, and diabetes also fall into the life-endangering category (you should

Whole Life Times, November 1983. 18 Shepard Street, Brighton, MA 02135. Reprinted by permission.

familiarize yourself with these signs, from any good medical guide for the layperson), and should spur at least a diagnostic visit to a clinic or hospital—even if you ultimately choose a different form of treatment (i.e., diet modification, stress reduction, and aerobic exercise instead of anti-hypertensive drugs for high blood pressure).

Assuming your problem is not obviously life-threatening, you should then define or "prediagnose" your condition by asking yourself the following questions:

1. What are the **symptoms?** Be sure to include both the overt symptoms (pain, swelling, difficulty with swallowing, etc.) and the more subtle ones—general loss of energy, change in eating or bowel habits, mood swings, etc.
2. What is the **history** of your condition? Is it chronic, recurrent, or appearing for the first time? What can you remember about the origination of your symptoms?
3. What other factors seem related to the condition: Do certain foods, exercise, stress, or certain environments aggravate it, precipitate it, or diminish your symptoms?
4. What **treatments** have you tried in the past and how successful were they?
5. What is your intuitive sense of the disorder? What are your feelings about it? What, if any, is the **psychological** or emotional component of the problem and your reaction to it?

Write down your answers to these questions if possible, being as complete and honest as you can. Include any other associations, memories, or information you have about the problem. From this information and your research into various health modalities, you can select the kinds of experts you want to consult.

Seeking Help

We asked several holistic practitioners *their* major criteria in choosing where to go for help.

Julian Miller, former program director for the Eustress Institute in Hanover, New Hampshire, and author of *Breaking Through: Freeing Yourself from Fear, Helplessness, and Depression*, responded: "You should become as knowledgeable as possible about your condition. Learn the credentials and track record of the practitioner in dealing with your kind of disorder. You might ask for the names of other patients you can speak to. Ultimately, you should choose someone you can trust, who will inform you intelligently and objectively about what's wrong—but will also give you the freedom to feel positive and in control. Get second, third, even fourth opinions if necessary. *Never relinquish your control to the professional*—whether a holistic person or a mainstream medical doctor."

Michael Janson, M.D., director of the Cambridge (Massachusetts) Center for Holistic Health, also emphasized self-responsibility. "You have to be your own guide first," he said. "I wouldn't care if my orthopedist knows about vitamins; when a car runs over my foot, I'd only care that he knows what he's doing... A big problem in holistic medicine is that so many systems claim to be able to cure everything."

Janson speaks about *triage*, the process of categorizing disorders and referring patients to the most appropriate form of help. "It's important to choose a practitioner who's good at triage, who's willing to refer you to someone else if they can't help you themselves." Traditionally the general practitioner or family doctor has played this role. "You want to find someone who's open to new things, but remains critical—constructively critical," Janson adds.

Unfortunately, the classic relationship of medical authority figure and obedient patients (See "Unwhole Healers", *Whole Life Times*, January/February 1983) seems to repeat itself far too often among holistic practitioners and their clients. Individuals sometimes accept the most far-fetched remedies uncritically, putting themselves unquestioningly in the hands of nutritionists, bodywork therapists, spiritual gurus, naturopaths, and chiropractors (to mention but a few)—wanting them to be all-knowing and magically effective. And some practitioners keep the patient coming back for treatment, rather than teaching the client everything possible about self-cure, self-care, and prevention.

This all-too-prevalent pattern leads not only to a personal loss of control over one's health and healing, but also to the perpetuation of inferior, ineffective, and even fraudulent practitioners (both conventional and alternative) who profit from unassertive, ill-informed patients.

A Consumerist Approach

To deal with the latter problem, Dana Ullman M.P.H., a San Francisco area health educator who specializes in homeopathic medicine and alternative health care, emphasizes consumerist principles: "It's very important to know who you are going to, what formal and informal training they've had, what on-the-job experience they have. Sometimes the experience is more important than the training." He mentions a new type of practitioner, who does not treat patients but is solely concerned with directing them to appropriate care: "There are some people going into practice whose role is basically to be an ombudsman... they're called holistic-health educators, or clinical-health educators, and their role is to help people decide what direction they should go for treatment." His recommendation for tightening up the standards of practice in both the allopathic (conventional) and holistic medical worlds: "It's time that consumers demand, and practitioners give, detailed professional disclosure statements." These would include the practitioner's formal and informal training, where it took place, accreditation status of the trainer, the practitioner's experience, etc. It could even include the practitioner's record in malpractice suits, if applicable. "The more that we can begin to become self-critical, and not just accept anything and everything that everyone does as wonderful holistic bliss, the better off the overall movement will be."

Here, then, are some guidelines in choosing the holistic practitioner that may be most effective for you:

1. Select one or more types of treatment appropriate for your problem or goal.
2. If possible, get a referral to a specific practitioner (or to several) from a source you can trust—a friend,

another medical-care professional, a practitioners association.

3. Check practitioner's background, training, credentials, experience, track record, etc., as appropriate. Don't hesitate to get the names of other clients to contact.

4. Don't hesitate to interview practitioners. Many alternative healers provide introductory lectures or free first visits, screenings, or evaluations. Its your chance to evaluate them as well.

5. Observe the practitioner's modus operandi as closely as possible. Is the office clinic, or workspace clean, organized, *healthful*? Don't make the mistake, however, of equating expensive furnishings and slick advertising with high-quality care; these things may only mean high overhead and high fees.

6. Are you treated in an honest, concerned, thorough manner? Do the practitioner and staff take *time* to really listen to you and genuinely attempt to understand your problem and your perspectives? Too many professionals are busy selling you their specialties—whether elective surgery or vitamin E—and pay little or no attention to what your real needs are.

7. Ask all the questions that are on your mind, even if they seem silly, picky, or naive to you. *You* are the person who needs to feel comfortable with the healer and treatment. Look for a professional who is patient (but not condescending) and thorough in answering your questions and discussing your fears—one who respects your need to know and discuss.

8. Is the practitioner honest about the possible outcomes, risks, and side effects of treatment? In the case of a procedure like surgery, what is the success rate?

9. Does the practitioner conduct a thorough diagnostic process (including a detailed history and appropriate tests) or too quickly decide on a course of treatment?

10. Does the practitioner *explain* at least some of his thinking and procedure, sharing the decision-making process with you; or does he simply announce, "This is what you need"? Does he respect your need to stay informed and in control, or does he insist that you simply do as he says, without input?

11. Does the practitioner appear to be someone of high intelligence and expertise, with a critical mind—rather than someone who merely repeats by rote what she learned in medical school or chiropractic college?

12. Is the alternative healer willing to consult with your medical doctor and other healers?

13. Don't be afraid of disappointing or insulting the caregiver with your questions or decisions. The practitioner should not act or be treated as someone who is superior to you, or has any special power. He is simply someone who has particular expertise and information that you may want. You are your own healer; the practitioner is your assistant. (Research is beginning to appear showing that cancer patients who argue with their doctors and sometimes defy them recover more frequently than patients who are quiet and obedient.)

14. Use your intuition about the practitioner, too. If your heart says no, there may be a good, though not obvious, reason.

15. Be skeptical of anyone who tells you a health problem is all in your mind, but don't rule out the psychological component of any illness.

16. Whenever possible, consult with several different practitioners before beginning any course of treatment. Second and third opinions will often produce markedly different diagnoses and therapeutic solutions, and you should be in a position to judge and choose, rather than accepting only one person's methodology.

Self-Healing Processes

While there is much that a professional can do for a patient that he cannot do alone, nonetheless to maximize the effectiveness of any treatment it is essential to incorporate *personal* practices that promote wellness and healing. A brief listing of these includes.

1. Maintain a positive attitude, including hopefulness, cheerfulness, inner calm. (This does not mean you should suppress feelings of anger, pain, or fear when they arise.)

2. Reduce environmental and emotional stressors as much as possible, particularly during the healing period.

3. Cultivate Eustress—Hans Selye's term for "positive stress"—positive, curative experiences such as exercise, nature and wilderness contact, aesthetic, sensual, and sexual experiences.

4. Maintain a sense of humor and *fun*.

5. Eat a nutritious, healthy, non-toxic diet (even if this is not part of your "treatment").

6. Maintain supportive and caring relationships.

7. Use meditation, visualization, and imagery techniques both for mental serenity and to optimize the healing process.

8. Get appropriate psychotherapy or counseling, if needed.

Monitoring and Re-evaluation

Once you have chosen a practitioner and embarked upon a course of treatment, you should continually monitor your progress and evaluate whether the treatment is effective. On one hand, it's important to be patient and give a therapeutic system time to work. "Sometimes people expect more from alternative therapies than they can offer," Ullman notes. "People are looking for instant gratification, immediate improvement, when sometimes nature moves in a slower way. Also, we have to measure treatments not only by their ability to get rid of symptoms, but also by their ability to improve the overall health of a person."

Ullman also points out that it's vital to give feedback to the practitioner, letting her know how you feel, if you're satisfied, and to what extent the treatment has been effective. However, if it is clearly not helping, this fact should be faced squarely and honestly. Sometimes even competent, well-meaning people cannot cure a particular condition.

Janson comments: "You have to be willing to change practitioners if their treatment isn't working—whether it's your ophthalmologist or your iridologist."

The Best Holistic Practitioner

Holistic medicine, by definition, takes into account all aspects of a person's life—diet, personal history, emotions, stress patterns, lifestyle, exercise and movement, posture, breathing, environments, relationships, spiritual values, humor, work, dreams, attitudes—as well as the functioning of the body's organs and systems. By this standard, there are few truly *holistic* practitioners, but rather many specialists in individual disciplines that focus on one aspect of the whole: nutrition or spinal alignment or emotional expression or stress management.

It is unreasonable to expect any single person to be able to understand and treat all dimensions of every client, or to know all the factors in your intricate, unique body-mind makeup. What we call "holistic" methods are really only "whole" when taken all *together*—as an array of options available to us. The only sane and reliable approach in getting effective help is to maintain a sense of responsibility for your own healing and well-being—using those elements of conventional American Medical Association medicine, unconventional and non-Western systems, and anything else that works and is appropriate at a given time. In the final analysis, there is only one practitioner who can have a truly holistic perspective on your health and your therapeutic needs—and that is yourself.

Educate Yourself on Health Alternatives

Although researching the medical literature on lordosis and scoliosis is inopportune at the moment you are aching with lumbar pain, self-education *is* an essential element in a successful healing process. Ideally, you should begin acquiring information before a problem becomes acute, and should continue even after symptoms have abated or treatment has been concluded. You *must* become knowledgeable both about your particular condition(s) and about the types of treatment available, inside and outside conventional medicine.

If you have a "problem" back, for example, that repeatedly causes you pain, you should learn about the back-care theories and methods of chiropractors, osteopaths, mainstream orthopedists, sports-medicine specialists, massage therapists, physical therapists, and probably a few others as well. With any disorder, it is extremely helpful to read the medical descriptions, diagnostic methods, analyses, and current treatments used by mainstream medicine. These can be found in a good layperson's medical guide (such as *Symptoms*, an Avon paperback), a general medical reference (such as *Merck's Manual*), or in more detail in a medical textbook or medical journals. To ignore or be unaware of such important information is as serious an error of judgment as to trust in the medical establishment completely.

To give yourself real options, either in a crisis or in a quest for self-improvement, you should be investigating the systems of healing and health-enhancement that are collectively termed "alternative" or "holistic." A brief listing of these follows:

Alternative Therapies and Healing Methods: A Partial List

acupuncture	macrobiotics
aerobic exercise	massage (various forms)
Arica	meditation (various forms)
autosuggestion (self-hypnosis)	
	naturopathy
	nutrition
Bach flower remedies	
bioenergetics	orthomolecular therapy
bioenergy healing	osteopathy
biofeedback	
bodywork (Feldenkrais, Rolfing, Soma, Trager, etc.)	polarity therapy
	psychic or "spiritual" healing
bowel cleansing	psychotherapies (co-counseling family therapy, Gestalt, primal, psychosynthesis, rebirthing, etc.)
chiropractic	
dance therapy	
Do-in	shiatsu
	Silva mind control
fasting	stress management
herbs	
homeopathy	T'ai Chi
imagery and visualization	yoga (various forms)

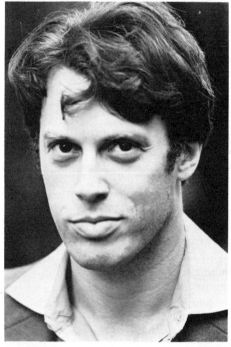

DON ETHAN MILLER *is a holistic martial arts instructor and has written extensively on body-mind disciplines. He has trained in Gestalt therapy, yoga and healing; as well as Tai Chi, aiki, karate, judo, and kickboxing. He is the author of* Bodymind *(Prentice-Hall, 1974),* The Conquest of Aging *(co-author; Macmillian, 1985), and articles for the* Atlantic, Village Voice, Runners World, *and* Whole Life Times.

SHELLY KELLMAN *is Senior Editor of* Whole Life Times.

Belief Systems and Management of the Emotional Aspects of Malignancy

O. Carl Simonton, M.D., and
Stephanie Matthews-Simonton

The following lecture is one example of pioneering efforts in the application of transpersonal techniques as an adjunct to standard medical treatment. According to Dr. Elmer Green of the Menninger Foundation, "Carl and Stephanie Simonton are pioneering in the domain of mind-body communication and are getting remarkable results in cancer control by coupling visualization for physiological self-regulation with traditional radiology."

The Simontons outline some basic personality traits that are typical of a vast majority of cancer patients. They also shed light on how family attitudes toward the patient directly affect that person's journey to recovery. They present a form of therapy used in their clinic in Texas that supplements traditional methods of treating cancer. These methods integrate the emotional and stress factors, and involve the patients themselves in creating the major lifestyle changes that are often necessary to complete their healing process.

THERE ARE over 200 articles in the medical literature covering different aspects of the relationship of emotions and stress to malignancy, as well as other very serious diseases. The interesting thing about the literature is that, in all these articles, the conclusion is that there is a relationship between the two. None (to my knowledge) conclude that there is no relationship. The question is one of degree of importance and how to influence it, not whether or not emotions are a factor. So I'd like to begin with a quotation that has had a profound effect on my own thinking by a cancer specialist who was president of the American Cancer Society in 1959, Dr. Eugene P. Pendergrass. I'm quoting from his presidential address, and these are his concluding remarks.

"Anyone who has had an extensive experience in the treatment of cancer is aware that there are great differences among patients.... I personally have observed cancer patients who have undergone successful treatment and were living and well for years. Then an emotional stress, such as the death of a son in World War II, the infidelity of a daughter-in-law, or the burden of long unemployment, seems to have been a precipitating factor in the reactivation of their disease, which resulted in death.... There is solid evidence that the course of disease in general is affected by emotional distress.... Thus, we as doctors may begin to emphasize *treatment of the patient as a whole* as well as the disease from which the patient is suffering. We may learn how to influence general body systems and through them modify the neoplasm which resides within the body.

"As we go forward... searching for new means of controlling growth both within the cell and through systemic influences, it is my sincere hope that we can widen the quest to include the distinct possibility that within one's mind is a power capable of exerting forces which can either enhance or inhibit the progress of this disease."

To summarize what I consider the salient points from the literature and my own experience in working in these areas for four years now, the biggest single factor that I can find as a predisposing factor to the actual development of the disease is the loss of a serious love object, occurring six to eighteen months prior to the diagnosis. This is well documented in several long-term studies. Now, the significant thing about this is that obviously not everyone who undergoes a serious loss, such as loss of a spouse or a child, develops a malignancy or any other serious disease. That's only one factor. The loss, whether real or imagined, has to be very significant; and even more important is the feeling that it engenders in the patient. *The loss has to be such, and the response to the loss such, that it engenders the feeling of helplessness and hopelessness. Therefore, it's more*

This article was first delivered as a lecture at a University of Florida symposium in June 1974, and was published in the *Journal of Transpersonal Psychology*, vol. 7, no. 1 (1975). It is reprinted here by permission.

than a loss—it's the culmination of the life-history pattern of the patient. And this also is well defined in the literature.

Personality of the Cancer Patient

I believe the work that has come out in *Type A Behavior and Your Heart* (Friedman and Rosenman, 1974) shows clearly that there is a life-history pattern in the development of heart diseases, and I believe that, if we continue to look, we will find predisposing psychological factors in the development of all disease. Those predisposing factors most agreed upon as (negative) personality characteristics of the cancer patient are:

1. a great tendency to hold resentment and a marked inability to forgive;
2. a tendency toward self-pity;
3. a poor ability to develop and maintain meaningful, long-term relationships;
4. a very poor self-image.

I believe one of the big underlying factors behind all the more superficial personality characteristics is *basic rejection*. The patient usually feels that he has been rejected by either one or both of his parents, and consequently develops the life-history pattern that we see so commonly in the cancer patient. All of us have a certain amount of this in our own personality. I probably have more than many. Of course, I developed cancer when I was 17; so I should have more than many. Just as Dr. Friedman, in *Type A Behavior and Your Heart*, points out the problems of personality in heart disease, he shows that they are very changeable. I strongly feel—and I certainly hope—that the cancer personality is changeable. Otherwise, I'm in a difficult spot. But if we don't bring it to the level of awareness, it is difficult to change. And just as Friedman and Rosenman point out in their book, the patient is very resistant to looking at the basic problem. That is, one very large factor contributing to heart disease is the person's response to stress. Supposing this same thing is true in cancer, which seems very strongly to be so, then as surely as the heart patient resists the fact that he has this type of personality, the cancer patient resists even more strongly. The heart-disease personality is basically a much more socially acceptable personality than the cancer personality.

Important Factors in the Patient's Progress

So how do we do anything about this? How do we go about changing the life-history pattern? As I have stated before, this is a very difficult business in my experience. You're questioning things that so many people never consciously question. But let's look at some of the more pertinent factors that influence how patients present themselves and how they progress throughout the course of treatment. *I believe there are three extremely important factors that need to be recognized and brought to light. One is the belief system of the patient. The second is the belief system of the family and those people who surround the patient and are meaningful to him. The third is the belief system of the physician. I'm going*

to elaborate on all of these and the role that I feel they play.

Belief System of the Patient

Let's begin with the belief system of the patient. I feel his beliefs about his disease, his treatment, and himself are very big factors, having a significant role in the course that his body takes during and after treatment. If we look at cancer as a disease, most patients see it as synonymous with death and something from without that there is almost no hope of controlling. Most patients have very negative feelings about treatment, whether it's radiation therapy, chemotherapy, or surgery. From the extensive psychological experimentation in expectancy, any thinking person must see that what a person believes will happen with his treatment and disease is related to the eventual outcome. The psychological experimentation concerning expectancy points strongly toward this.

The last part is the patient's set of beliefs about himself. Now, I previously outlined the basic negative personality characteristics of the cancer patient. I said he had a very poor self-image. You see, he's got three strikes against him already! His belief about himself influences the course of his disease and his response to treatment. Therefore, this is an area where it is mandatory to modify early if you're going to modify the course of this disease significantly. Most patients see themselves as victims of the disease and not as having participated in the development of it. They also can see almost nothing that they personally can do to help themselves get well. Or at least this is the belief system that most of my patients present to me.

Belief System of the Family

The belief system of the family is also vital, because we communicate what we believe to those around us. The patient is with the health-care personnel a small part of the time compared with how much of the time he is with his family. So, you see, education of the family and changing their beliefs about the parameters of the disease are also vitally important in influencing the course of the patient.

Belief System of the Physician

The last area is the belief system of the physician. Most physicians are not aware of the fact that their thoughts about the treatment and the patient's own ability influence the outcome, but they most definitely do. You see, where the real problem comes in is when the physician's belief system parallels that of the initial belief system of the patient, namely, that the disease comes from without, that it's synonymous with death, that the treatment is bad, and that the patient has little or nothing that he can do to fight the disease. This is all too common a belief among physicians. I know, because I have a large number of acquaintances who are cancer specialists, and I've heard them make statements like, "There is nothing that can be done." This, to me, indicates how they really feel about what a person can individually do to heal himself much more strongly than what they might intellectually tell me.

Spontaneous Remission and Visualization

When we look at spontaneous remission or at unexpectedly good responses and try to figure out what happens in common, we find the same spontaneous occurrence of visualizing oneself being well. You analyze these people; you sit down with them, and you find out what their thoughts are during that period of time, from the time they were given their diagnosis to the time that they were over their disease with no medical treatment: I have not found a patient that did not go through a similar visualizing process. It might be a spiritual process, God healing them, up and down the whole spectrum. But the important thing was what they pictured and the way they saw things. They were very positive, regardless of the source, and their picture was very positive.

I find that the converse is true of my patients. Whenever I have a person visualizing, and I ask him to go through his visualization with me, how he pictures things tells me a tremendous amount about how he pictures his disease, his treatment, and his own ability to fight it. If I had nothing but one tool to use in looking at my patient's attitude, it would be how regularly he is relaxing and what his imagery is. This tells me so much more than he could tell me consciously, because he isn't even aware of what he's telling me. Too often in his visualization he sees the cancer as some big powerful thing, and the treatment as some little weak something that doesn't do much. He sees his white blood cells, his own immune mechanism, as really nonexistent, and he's trying to coax it into working. These are to me very unhealthy signs. I say they are unhealthy signs because patients who verbalize these things are, in general, doing very poorly at the time they tell me this.

Then we begin to take a different approach, not just using behavior modifications, but looking at the reasons behind why the person has these images of the disease, the treatment, and himself. We begin to work with him in a conscious way, to modify these images to the point that they will be more meaningful in his body's ability to fight the disease. One of the things that I do early is to show the patient visually some of the best responses that I have ever seen, with some of the least side-effects to the treatment. I do this so that he can have a very powerful image of what is possible. I show him a series of slides, not typical responses, but among the best I've ever seen. This is so he might see what the potential of the body is, both in getting rid of the disease and in the minimal reaction to treatment.

Correlation of Attitude and Response to Treatment

When I arrived at Travis Air Force Base, I decided to duplicate two studies that had previously been done, correlating the patient's response with different personality characteristics and attitudes. I set up a study in which, at the completion of treatment, five staff members assessed each patient on their attitudes, from doubly positive to doubly negative, based on each one's clinical experience. I also had each staff member independently vote on what

the clinical response had been, again based on their own experience, grading these responses from excellent to poor. Then when we averaged these together, giving one score for each patient, we found essentially a one-to-one correlation, which was similar to what Dr. Stavraky had found in her work in Canada. Those patients with positive attitudes had good responses, those with negative attitudes had poor responses; and out of 152 patients over an 18-month period, only two did not fall into the predicted categories (see Table 1).

Table 1. CORRELATION BETWEEN CLINICAL RESPONSE AND ATTITUDE.

Clinical response	− −	−	+ −	+	+ +	Response totals
Excellent	0	0	0	11	9	20
Good	0	2	34	31	0	67
Fair	0	14	29	0	0	43
Poor	2	17	3	0	0	22
Attitude totals	2	33	66	42	9	152

These were 152 consecutive cases as they presented themselves in the department. Now, out of the 10 patients who had excellent responses, 11 of them positive and 9 of them doubly positive, 14 had less than a 50 percent chance of a five-year cure, and only 6 of them had better than a 50-percent chance for a five-year cure. We found that the correlation was with attitudes and not with severity of their illness.

Now, it should be strongly stressed that this was a very artificial environment, in a very protective atmosphere—that of a treatment center. These statistics did not last after they were out of that environment. Many patients who were very negative and had very poor responses changed after this study was over. In talking about it, they said they didn't like the positivity, trying to see themselves getting well. After they got through treatment, there was a turnaround. They gained some degree of perspective, were much more pleasant to be with, and their health changed. Many of the patients with severe diseases had been very positive in this protective environment, but, when they got back to their home situation, they changed attitudinally, and we saw that their diseases changed correspondingly. So to try to extrapolate from this or draw any far-ranging conclusions is foolish, because the study was designed to look at patients under very controlled conditions. I did this study to see how our responses would correspond with the work done in Canada and UCLA, and found a very comparable correlation. I also learned many other things as a result of doing this study.

I've asked my partner, Stephanie, who also happens to be my wife, to go into some of the specifics of what we do in beginning to allow the patient to see the role he's played in the development of his disease, and bring these things to his awareness so he can participate in the course of his disease. Stephanie will discuss the specific aspects of this portion of the therapy, since she coordinates this in our office.

Type of Practice and Type of Patients

Stephanie Simonton: In order to explain the specifics of what our psychotherapy consists of, I think it would be best if I give you an overview of the type of practice we have and the type of patients we deal with. The treatment varies from patient to patient. We have to assess the patients' belief structures when we first see them and try to fit our treatment to their needs. We find that, if we get into a conflict with their beliefs, they constantly fight us, and will almost get worse in spite of us, or *to* spite us.

We have a private practice with another radiation therapist in Fort Worth. The large majority of our patients come to us through normal referral channels from other physicians in our community, as most other cancer specialists receive their patients. These are about 80 to 90 percent of the patients we treat. We treat them with both medical treatment (radiation therapy or chemotherapy, or whatever is appropriate) and psychotherapy. Most of them come to us not knowing that they are going to receive psychotherapy with their regular radiation therapy. It should be pointed out that, of the patients that we receive through normal medical channels, who come to us with no preconceived ideas about what our treatment is, over half of them will not participate in any form of psychotherapy. They will not attend group therapy. They will not use the relaxation and visualization techniques we prescribe. Many of them not only will not talk about, or allow us to talk to their families about, the psychological aspects of their disease, but they might even go back to their physician and ask to be referred to another doctor. That was a shock to me; yet as I continue to work with the patients, I am beginning to understand more of this. So let's begin with an understanding of where the consciousness of most of our patients is.

One of the other types of patients we are beginning to receive from our local community do not have active disease currently. They may be patients who have been free of disease for a year or two or three, but are coming to us for help in dealing with what we now know is one of the real residuals of cancer, and that is fear . . . the fear of recurrence, fear of reactivation—are they going to die? It is interesting to note that, before a person has cancer, he may have a tennis elbow that aches occasionally. However, once he has had cancer, that aching tennis elbow suddenly represents the fear of metastases. Every time it hurts he thinks, "Is that a new cancer growing in there?" These patients need concrete techniques they can use to deal with aches and pains. Particularly after knowing that the mind participates in our becoming ill, it certainly doesn't help to worry and visualize cancer growing in new places.

The other type of patient that we have is generally referred from out of town and out of state. They are very few in number and we're extremely selective, but we are accepting some patients who come to us just for psychotherapy. They're usually receiving medical treatment from their local physician in their own community, or there may

be no appropriate medical treatment for their case. They come to us believing there is a psychological component to their disease, and asking for help in understanding how to participate more positively in their future prognosis. These are extremely rewarding patients. They're probably the ones that we learn the most from, because they already have grasped so many concepts concerning their own disease process. Basically I think the biggest thing we do for these patients is give them reassurance and a greater awareness of themselves.

Concepts Underlying Treatment

Now let me go over some of the concepts underlying our treatment, and then I'll get into the specifics of it. The first concept, and probably the hardest one for our patients to deal with, is our general concept of disease—the idea of personal responsibility. It's a difficult one. I think I can best refer to it as a double-edged sword. The idea that we have no participation in disease, that it's an outside agent acting on our body and we have nothing to do with its getting there, may be comforting in its denial. On the other hand, if you believe that concept, it doesn't make sense that you then can have any control in the progression of your disease. There's a double-edged sword there. In order to really grasp the concept that they can mentally influence their body's immune mechanism, they must eventually realize that their mind and emotions and body act as a unit and can't be separated. There is a mental and psychological participation, as well as a physical one, in the development of their disease. Once they can understand the psychological as well as physical reasons underlying their disease, they seem to get a better grasp on the future and how to deal with that. If you want to understand—and it took me a while to grasp it—how difficult psychotherapy is when you're ill, try an experiment. The next time you have the flu or a cold, ask yourself that very difficult question, "Why did I need this? What purpose does it serve?" It's a strange thing that happens to those of us, the staff, who work with the patients. If you're talking to a person who has cancer about his mentally participating in both the development and the progress of his disease, and suddenly you develop a cold, you have to get in touch with that. You can't continue to talk to them about influencing their cancer when you can't influence your own cold. So it causes all of us to do a great deal of self-discovery, which is not easy.

For some reason we have a conception of responsibility being the same as blame. This is one reason for our inability as a society to deal with the emotional aspects of our diseases. We feel that, if we accept responsibility, we are to blame, should feel guilty, or have done something wrong. We try to convey the idea to the patient that it's just as if you were to deny your body food for too long; we know that you would eventually die. The same thing is true emotionally. A human being doesn't survive just by food, clothing, and shelter. We have emotional needs that are very real and very concrete, and if these are denied, life loses its meaning. We will begin to seek the end of our life. *We stress not that they should feel guilty, but that they have emotional needs that are not being met.*

WHAT CONSTITUTES SCIENTIFIC PROOF?

O. Carl Simonton, M.D.

One topic I am frequently required to address is that of medical or scientific proof. Before I began this study and had only the ideas, most of my colleagues told me that I would never be able to prove anything because there were too many variables involved. As I have accumulated more and more results, I still find that the question of scientific proof is a very difficult one. About a week ago I came across an article which meant a great deal to me, and I would like to share it with you.

The article was about a psychiatrist who was doing some rather unorthodox work with schizophrenic patients approximately twenty years ago and was obtaining some very good results. Because of the nature of his techniques, however, his colleagues were reluctant to listen to him. He wrote approximately ten articles on the subject, but their standard response was, "Well, you haven't really proven anything." So he continued his work and wrote about ten more articles, and people continued to say the same thing. He began to wonder just what it is that constitutes scientific proof. He did still more work and published more papers, with the same result. He became determined to investigate thoroughly this question of scientific proof.

Being the editor of a psychiatric journal, he decided to hold a symposium on the subject. He wrote letters to several leading scientists, asking their participation in a study to determine what constitutes scientific proof. The first reply came from a man who sent a very short note: "The question," he wrote, "is much too difficult for me." He went on to say, briefly, that he doubted that he could make a significant contribution to so complex an issue.

This answer was more than the humility of a great man; it was more than the reflection of scientific honesty. It was at the root of a great man's whole philosophy of being. The letter was signed, "Albert Einstein."

From a talk by Dr. Simonton presented at the Dimensions of Healing Symposium at U.C.L.A.

The "Secondary Gains of Illness"

We do this in the beginning by trying to get patients to see what we call the "secondary gains of illness." One of the things we try to get them to do is to see how much different their life is now than before they developed the disease. This is the clue to what we call the secondary gains. Let me give you an example of a woman who has breast cancer. Typically, a couple of years prior to the development of her disease, her children were suddenly growing up, graduating from school, and beginning to enter their own lives. Her husband had become very preoccupied in his business, and she had suddenly felt unneeded. Since the development of her disease, her husband is now showing her attention that he has not shown her in years. Now that's fine. It's good that he's giving her affection because she needs that. But what we try to get her to see is that if the disease is the only way she can get that, then the disease must continue in order for her to get that secondary gain, this affection. We don't try to get her to cut off that affection, but rather, we help her develop healthier ways of getting the support she needs emotionally. In essence, the concept we use is not that one regains health first and then goes back to living a normal life, but that patients do better when they do both simultaneously.

I'm reminded of an unusual situation we had recently in one of our group-therapy sessions, where we had two patients who had almost identical diseases. They were within a few years of age of each other, and both men had lung cancer that had spread to their brain. One man had had the disease for over a year, but had not missed work other than a few hours each time he had a treatment. Early in the development of his disease he had gotten in touch with a lot of things that were causing life to lose meaning for him. He started to spend more time with his family, taking his family with him on business trips. I remember him saying one day, "You know, I'd forgotten that I didn't look at the trees. I hadn't been looking at the trees and the grass and the flowers for a long time. And now I do that." It was interesting to watch him; every week he improved, getting stronger, healthier.

The other man who had lung cancer which had spread to his brain stopped working practically the day he received his diagnosis. He had gone home to sit in front of the television set all day. His wife said that what he did every day was to watch the clock to make sure she had given him his pain medication on time. He was in constant pain. He could not even bring himself to go fishing, which is something he liked to do. He died in a short period of time. The other man is still getting healthier day after day. This is the kind of thing that we try to show our patients. The treatment for both patients was the same medically; the diagnosis was the same; the patients' ages and physical conditions were almost identical. The difference was in attitude, the way the patients reacted once they knew the diagnosis.

Significance of Choice in Reaction to Stress

When we begin our psychotherapy, based on Dr. LeShan's findings that cancer patients have an emotional trauma six to 18 months prior to the development of the disease, we found ourselves trying to get patients in touch with the event, and to change certain things about their lives so that life could gain more meaning. In essence, we were trying to accomplish in a period of four to five weeks, in once-a-week group therapy sessions, what it takes years of psychoanalysis to do—if it's ever accomplished. As you can imagine, that became very frustrating. We then began to realize that not every woman who goes through a divorce develops cancer, not every man who retires from work develops cancer, not every person who experiences an unhappy marriage develops cancer as a result. And these are some of the common stresses we see. The difference, then, was not the stress: that was not the problem. The problem was the person's *reaction* to that stress. We try to get them to see that here is something they do have control over. They may not be able to control their husband when he makes them angry or their children when they frustrate them, but they can control how they choose to react to that situation. And I stress the word *choose*.

Relaxation and Visualization Technique

Now, let me describe the actual tools we use. During the first week a patient comes to our office, he attends what we call an orientation session. He attends with as many family members and close friends as he would like to bring. We know that a person doesn't become sick in a vacuum, nor does he get well in a vacuum. We do best when we mobilize all the forces within the person's environment. So early on, we try to educate the entire family. Many times the patient never brings his family back again after the first session. But we do generally get him to bring some of his family with him, at least his spouse. During the orientation session, we explain our concept of disease, how the mind interacts with the body, and how attitude plays a major role. We teach our patients a technique which we call relaxation and visualization. You might call it biofeedback without a machine, meditation, autogenic training. There are lots of names for it, but it is a basic relaxation technique in which the patients are told to visualize their disease, their treatment, and their body's own immune mechanisms (we call them white blood cells to make it simple) acting on that disease. We tell them to do this three times a day, every day.

At that orientation, they are given a tape recording of the relaxation process that they can take home with them and listen to. All they have to do is put it on a cassette tape player and turn it on. We also give them the book *The Will to Live*, a short paperback by Dr. Arnold Hutschnecker that more fully elaborates the principles of the mind-body concept. They are told at that session that they may attend what we call group classes or group-therapy sessions once a week. Again, I estimate that over 50 percent of them will not come back at that point. Many of their families come to us and say they understand the psychological component in their relative's disease, but can't get him or her back to the group sessions.

In the group sessions, on a twice-a-week basis, we talk primarily about the relaxation and mental-imagery process and how many times they are doing it. Again, we find that the majority of the patients, if they ever use the technique, use it rarely, once a day instead of three times a day, or maybe three times a week. We talk about why they are not using the technique. And very often the things that are preventing them from quieting themselves, from listening to themselves and mentally picturing their own disease process, are the very things that are causing life to lose its meaning. In the group we tend to discover those things that are preventing them from getting well.

Let me give you an example of the kinds of things we talk about in groups. Remember the man I described to you who had lung cancer that had spread to the brain, the one who was doing poorly? He kept insisting that he was using the meditation or the relaxation technique three times a day. His wife said she did turn on the tape recorder and he was listening to it. So one day we asked him to describe to us what he visualized. We asked him what his cancer looked like to him and he said, "It looks like a black rat." When we asked what his treatment looked like (he was receiving chemotherapy in the form of little yellow pills), he replied, "They look like little yellow pills, and they go into my bloodstream and they look like tiny pills." We also asked what happened between the pills and the rat. He said, "Once in a while the rat eats one of the pills." We asked what happened when he did and he said, "Well, he's sick for a while, but he always gets better and he bites me all the harder." When we asked about his white blood cells, he replied, "They look like an incubator. You know how eggs sit under the warm light? Well, they're incubating in there and one day they're going to hatch." That was his visualization, three times a day, which gives you a good idea of the way he visualized his disease.

Current Studies

I'll conclude by describing some of the studies we presently are engaged in. We instigated a control study with another radiation therapist in Fort Worth five months ago. Between his office and ours, we treat approximately three-fourths of the patients given radiation therapy in the city. Both offices administer standard doses of radiation therapy, and our patients are treated on the same equipment, by the same technicians. The difference between the two is the psychotherapy administered to our patients. This study should show some interesting statistics, as to whether we can change both the quality and the quantity of the patient's survival time by influencing his attitude. In addition to this, we are cooperating in a study with the Carl Jung Institute of Los Angeles, using Jungian analytical techniques to study more fully the psychological aspects of our patients.

A good deal of research has been done on the personality of the cancer patient. One of the most intriguing aspects of this work is the suggestion that the behavior pattern of the patient can even be correlated to the exact location of the malignancy. For instance, the breast-cancer patient has a behavior pattern different from the lung-cancer patient, etc. We are currently quantitating this in our patients.

I recently finished reading the book *Type A Behavior*

and Your Heart, and was very excited by the possible implications it could have on medicine in the future. The similarities between their work and ours has led me to hope that we will begin to look at disease in a new way, that instead of being entirely concerned with the disease process itself, we will also take into account the patient and his environment as a whole, and see disease as a symptom of the general and total well-being of the patient.

Suggestions for Further Reading

H. Benson. *The Relaxation Response*. William Morrow, 1975.

B. Brown. *New Mind, New Body*. Harper and Row, 1975.

M. Friedman and R. H. Rosenman. *Type A Behavior and Your Heart*. Knopf, 1974.

R. Glasser. *The Body Is the Hero*. Random House, 1976.

Elmer and Alice Green. *Beyond Biofeedback*. Delacorte, 1977.

A. A. Hutschnecker. *The Will to Live*. Cornerstone Library, 1977.

Lawrence LeShan. *You Can Fight for Your Life*. Evans, 1977.

S. Peller. *Cancer in Man*. New York International University Press, 1952.

Kenneth R. Pelletier. *Mind as Healer, Mind as Slayer*. Delta, 1977.

E. Revici. *A New Concept of the Pathophysiology of Cancer with Implications for Therapy*. Yale University Press.

Michael and Nancy Samuels. *Seeing with the Mind's Eye*. Random House, 1975.

J. M. Schneck. *Hypnosis in Modern Medicine*. Charles Thomas, 1959.

M. E. P. Seligman. *Helplessness*. W. H. Freeman, 1975.

Hans Selye. *The Stress of Life*. McGraw-Hill, 1956.

A. M. Weitzenhoffer, *Hypnotism: An Objective Study in Suggestibility*. Wiley, 1953.

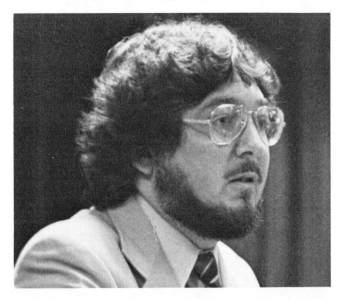

DR. CARL SIMONTON *is a cancer specialist who earned his M.D. degree from the University of Oregon Medical School where, after his internship, he also did a 3-year residency in Radiation Oncology. While at the University of Oregon, he developed a model of emotional support and emotional intervention in the treatment of cancer patients. This process was then implemented at Travis Air Force Base where Dr. Simonton was Chief of Radiation Therapy. The project was supported by the Psychiatry Department and approved by the Surgeon General's office in 1973. This was the first systematic emotional intervention program used in the treatment of cancer and, as such, has attracted much national and international attention. Dr. Simonton has co-authored* Getting Well Again, Stress, Psychological Factors and Cancer, *and numerous articles.*

STEPHANIE MATTHEWS-SIMONTON *is a psychotherapist who has specialized in counseling cancer patients. She pioneered the development of a model for emotional intervention in the treatment of cancer which considers a patient's emotional health a significant factor in combating the disease. That program, which has become known as the Simonton Approach, was approved by the Surgeon General's Office in 1973 and has gained both national and international attention. She designed a professional training program to teach medical and psychological professionals the treatment program.*

She founded the Cancer Counseling and Research Center of Dallas, Texas, a non-profit treatment, training and research facility.

In recent years, she designed corporate prevention programs, applying the principles used to treat cancer to healthy individuals who wish to improve and maintain their health. She is a frequent lecturer at medical, psychological, and various industry meetings on the subject of the psychological aspect of health.

A more recent development has been the conceptualization and refinement of new strategies which deal with the family system as the basic unit and focus of therapeutic intervention in the disease process. She has co-authored Getting Well Again, Stress, Psychological Factors and Cancer *along with numerous articles; and authored* The Healing Family *scheduled for publication by Bantam Books in February 1984.*

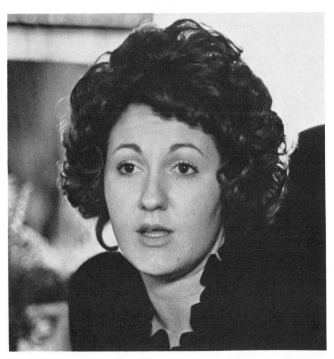

Hempel Photography

The Feminine Approach in Healing

Anne Langford, Ph.D.

A Knowledge of Textbook Bodies But No Experience of My Own Body

ECAUSE I was an allied health professional, I knew about the etiology and treatment of diseases. I learned to help cope and adapt their lifestyles to the effects of disease. I learned the medical language well and can confidently speak with any other medical, nursing, or allied health professionals. But over the years I learned nothing beyond symptoms and treatment, and nothing about myself as a multi-leveled, precious, deep person, guided by a principle of life: love.

From my years of experience beyond my professional beginnings, I learned of the interconnectedness of the many parts of myself—the spiritual aspects, feelings, emotions, mind, thoughts, desires, purpose, and so on. Yet despite my health background, I was barely conscious of my physical body. Although I knew how the nervous system worked, and although I knew about the origin and insertion of muscle groups, and although I knew about the enzyme reaction of a *textbook* body, I knew very little about the experience of my *own* body. And I trusted it even less. People would talk about "bodies as temples," and although I understood this conceptually, in actuality I saw my body as important only to hang beautiful clothes on.

My Illness, My Teacher

Cancer appeared when the time was right, and it taught me about my body very fast! With an advanced life-threatening disease (and with the pressure of the popular belief that cancer means impending death), my focus abruptly shifted. Every moment became precious. Cancer gave me the opportunity to scrutinize my own beliefs and habit patterns, as well as the medical profession, with its conventional surgery and medications.

I had the surgery, and once it was over I took some time to recover from it. At that point, I was satisfied with the

doctors' proclamation that there was a 99 percent chance for cure! Nine months later I realized that I was not cured—nothing had altered within my person, the one who had fostered the cancer. I sensed that the way I lived my life created the fertile soil for cancer to manifest. All aspects of my being worked together for it to occur. It did not just happen. And just because a part of my body was removed did not mean that I was cured. What would prevent my body from developing cancer again somewhere else? However, surgery had given me time to embrace my panic and fears of death so that I could begin to think about healing—its source and meaning in my life.

Something was wrong, but I could not put my finger on it. Who would listen to my hunch that my body was not healthy? I had no obvious symptoms. Silently I asked for guidance; gratefully I received the people with answers that life brought to me. The first thing I did was to shift my diet to macrobiotics. Within three days I dramatically felt emotionally stronger. Then, through the use of acupuncture and Chinese herbs, I began to feel even stronger. I thought I had the answer—but I was merely touching the tip of the iceberg. When, through electro-acupuncture, I received a diagnosis of severe pre-cancer, I was jolted into more committed action.

It became "the year of the body" for me, and I charged full steam ahead to learn what healing would really mean. I chose to take charge of my own program, but my doctors, my "healing assistants," provided valuable insights. A physician trained in psychosynthesis taught me about the unconscious concepts I had about my body. Another physician monitored me weekly with electro-acupuncture and homeopathy. Another administered Chinese acupuncture. I also received weekly lymphatic massages and spinal adjustments.

We Are Already Whole

However, the real key to my personal healing was that I was choosing life and surrendering to the innate natural wisdom of the healing process in my body. I did not depend on book learning anymore. Once again, I was on the battlefield with my body and cancer, but this time I knew that the old way of attack and retreat was not going to "cure" me. This time, healing meant that I had to remember that I am already whole, and that every cell in my body wants to function in its rightful way. Indeed, when I gave them the chance, all my cells responded, letting go of old habit patterns. This took a great deal of love, faith, and trust in myself, in my body, in my spiritual values, and in the universe's natural cycle of degeneration and regeneration. I had no guarantee that I would heal my disease, but this did not matter. What did matter was that I was fully engaged in a process of enhancing the quality of my life, regardless of the effect on my cancer.

Disease is a signpost that something far greater is emerging. It is a friend begging for attention, trying to let us know that we are out of balance, askew. It is like a volcano that has a great deal of unknown depth and strength to support us, but which may hold hidden dangers if we fail to understand it or ignore it.

The human organism is a miraculous instrument. It can take a great deal of abuse before it begins to break down. When a disease symptom finally manifests, long-activated patterns have already contributed to the breakdown. How we are and how we express or fail to express ourselves develops into patterns. These patterns occur as attitudes, behaviors, feelings, movement, and goals. Under certain stresses, these patterns can facilitate a disease. To be aware of and responsible for ourselves and the environment surrounding the disease is the interrelational feminine approach in healing. It recognizes our true nature—that we are already whole.

A Felt Sense of the Body

On the other side of the coin, today's medical and allied health professions have their concepts and approach to healing rooted in the masculine approach, which assumes we are not healthy or whole, but moving towards it. They focus on disease symptoms that are observable either to the naked eye or under a microscope, or that are audible or touchable. The symptom must show itself in a concrete way. It will not do for a patient to have a "sense" or a "feeling" that something is wrong with his or her body.

For the most part, healing in our culture has been delegated to the medical and allied health professions. Their frame of reference is to return us to the status quo. We live according to habit patterns, and when our body or mind becomes diseased or disturbed, we go to a professional to alleviate our problem so we can continue to live according to our familiar pattern. We focus on staying "normal," and when we fall short of this, we become alarmed. We go to someone who can realign us to "normal." Life seems to be a struggle to remain within certain fixed patterns.

Viewing ourselves this way has served us and continues to serve us. Many cures or remissions occur, but I question whether this approach facilitates the necessary awareness shifts that are needed to heal life patterns. There is some-

thing more beyond "normal." There is an opportunity to expand beyond our standard of "normalcy." There is an opportunity to join in the excitement of life and enjoy its continual movement, rather than maintaining the constricted focus on the status quo.

Masculine Healing, Feminine Healing

I would like to delineate the qualitative differences between the concepts of the feminine approach in healing and the masculine approach. Healing does not occur in such separated thinking: The essence of wholeness within the masculine archetype includes the feminine, and the masculine is included in the wholeness of the feminine archetype. However, if we are to work with this wholeness, we must explore and internalize the separated facets. Healing occurs when we can have *bifocal* vision and deal with the separateness while maintaining a vision of wholeness. It is like a dance—both sides need to be actively engaged with each other. Unfortunately, in our educational model of health we have gotten stuck in polarized thinking; we uphold one side, while disclaiming the validity of the other. The following breakdown between the feminine and masculine approaches to healing is a way to see the separation, yet to keep in mind that both polarities must have an impact on the other for healing to occur.

The Feminine Approach

- looks at the whole, the entire person beyond any part
- recognizes that the person is already whole
- creates a condition, or environment, or context for healing to occur
- surrenders, lets go
- embraces and includes the procedure
- has faith in the power of a higher order of things
- cooperates with: the natural healing process, aggressive procedures, a universal wisdom, family, friends, and professionals, the environment
- creates an opportunity to act, to participate in one's own healing process, to be self-responsible, to unfold and remember one's own perfection
- accepts the process as having no guarantees, accepts surprises and movement, is in a state of flux
- is in equal relationship with the disease process, sees disease a partner with the life force, has an interchange and interaction with the environment
- maintains a loving approach, is an open system, forgives, and has the attitude of compassion
- uses the creative unconscious as a healing tool, expresses self through imagination and images, creates a pattern for development of the psyche in our lives, holds complexities, looks at the unconscious and the irrational, looks to develop a different relationship to disease, considers disease as a symbol that creates an opportunity, wonderment, adventure, possibilities
- finds the piece that is missing, includes the unexplainable, asks the question, "What is happening?"

- allows personal vulnerability to be part of the healing process (the wounded healer)
- engages and focuses on life
- sees disease as a lens to create meaning in life and to find out and express our needs and wants, rather than focus on the symptom, includes the dark, mysterious, hidden
- a process that remembers it is already whole and understands this organically from the inside out

The Masculine Approach

- looks at the parts
- assumes the person is moving toward wholeness
- works on the person, works with the symptom, intrudes
- converges, does
- defends itself from the procedure, sees the procedures as other, an attack or a life-saver
- feels the responsibility of the professional, deals with cause and effect
- obeys authorities and internalizes their belief system
- lets professionals have the responsibility to tell us what we should do
- wants things to be a definite way, attached to an end result, works through form, structure
- has a topdog vs. underdog attitude: "You are either more powerful than the disease or the disease is more powerful than you," sees disease as the adversary that needs to be controlled, wants status quo, is cautious about going beyond the medical model
- has a strong will and separative approach, is a closed system
- uses the linear thought process to get to meaning, is single-pointed, looks at what is conscious and rational, defines disease as other than ourselves, can create guilt for having a disease, considers disease as something wrong or a problem
- deals with symptoms, asks, "Why me?" "What has gone wrong?"
- affirms personal invulnerability
- engages and focuses on death
- sees disease as a static, fixed entity that is intruding, focuses attention on the symptom, wants the light, clarity
- a process looking for wholeness outside itself, wants to learn in order to become something more.

Symptoms—A Game of Hide-and-Seek

In general, today's medical, nursing, and allied health professionals look at the disease—the part—rather than the environment surrounding it. Professionals are highly trained specialists, products of a specialized educational system. Their frame of reference is focused on curing disease or malfunction. This perspective can be necessary to alleviate pain, and can even be life-saving. There are many times when this is the best intervention.

The symptom presented in the doctor's office has the potential of being removed by our current sophisticated high technology. When confronted with medication, surgery, or radiation, the symptom quickly receives the mes-

sage that it is not wanted, nor appreciated, nor has anything to teach the patient. Unless it has been around for too long to be irreversible, it often retreats and the patient is pronounced cured, or at least in a temporary remission. But because the underlying contributing pattern provoking the disease is usually not addressed, another symptom may possibly emerge after some time. Thus, the game of hide-and-seek is perpetuated. The symptom hides for a while, but then gets caught by the medical profession. It is removed—or rather, suppressed—for a while longer until inner or outer environmental stresses provoke it to come out again.

Medical, nursing, and allied health professionals have a very specific language that alienates and mystifies most people. Usually by the time patients seek help, they have become vulnerable and helpless, experiencing an obvious or subtle form of panic. In this state, patients readily give their power over to anyone. Their life is on the line, and the internal working of their body is an area of pure mystification.

A patient who is diagnosed to have a severe illness is threatened with the loss of a body part, with a restructure, or with ultimate death. Impending death can be a powerful teacher of personal values and meaning. It is a threshold of transformation and enables a person to gather strength and consider one's priorities and purpose. It can also be a great motivator and helpmate. In an ultimate sense, whether we choose the masculine or the feminine approach, either one will be only a stepping-stone on our path toward eventual death. From this point of view, it does not matter which approach we choose. But what does matter is how we enhance the quality of our life for whatever time we have. The feminine approach in healing offers us this opportunity. It *includes* the masculine approach. Denying one approach and replacing it with another is not a characteristic of the feminine. I see the feminine approach as inclusive of the masculine approach, not an alternative.

Surrendering to the Life Force

The feminine approach in healing is an attitude, a way of being. It cooperates with systems, e.g., the medical and allied health professions. It is about relating gently to the condition or disease, not fighting it, for it is not looking for a cure. It is not about having formulas and procedures that will lead to certain results in a certain length of time. Rather, it focuses on enhancing and balancing the quality of life that surrounds the disease. It is about creating internal and external environmental conditions so that the natural process of wholeness resurfaces to take its rightful place in our lives.

The feminine approach in healing recognizes disease as an opportunity to learn and grow—for symptoms contain messages that, when listened to, can be enriching. Disease is like an entity in its own right. It first appears hostile, even life-threatening, but beyond this lies a wealth of information to guide us in remembering our *inherent* completeness and wholeness.

Within the entire healing cycle, there is a proper time to evoke our strengths and do battle against hostile disease forces. But there follows a time to be receptive and surrender to our life force. The point at which one shifts from the battle mode to the cooperative mode is not clear-cut or rational. It requires great courage to continue on this unknown path, and even greater faith to know that we are guided by the primary force in the universe, which I call love. Are we able to surrender to this inner stream of direction, and trust where it will take us—which may mean an immediate physical death? Allowing and participating in the flow of love, of life, is the joy in the healing process.

From the perspective of the feminine approach, the focus is not on a desired end—whether or not we are cured, or die. Cooperating and surrendering takes us into the unknown, the unexplained, the hidden, the dark. But the seeds of healing germinate in the dark, as seeds of spring flowers lie dormant in the darkness of bleak winter. Some of the seeds die, some of the seeds come right up, and some come up the following year. The feminine approach in healing recognizes that it does not matter when the seeds bloom into flowers. It is being with the rightness, the movement, and the joy of the process that counts. It takes a great deal of integrity to stay with this approach, especially in the face of immediate death.

While the masculine approach toward healing focuses on *doing*, going outside yourself to find the source, the feminine approach affirms *un-doing*. It is going within, accepting the reality and truth of the inner source. We need support (both inner and outer) to shift to the feminine frame of reference in the face of a life-threatening disease, where most of the people around us want us to *do* something—like have chemotherapy, radiation, or surgery. Our culture does not validate us for relying on our inner source of wisdom. And, in the face of a life-threatening disease, the intensity of impending death is increased. Sometimes it is our loved ones' fear of death we encounter, not our own. Panic and a great deal of confusion surround the diagnosis of a disease. Clarity eludes us. This is when it is crucial to have an impartial health professional to help *us* decide what is really most appropriate.

It is important to find a practitioner who understands and embodies the feminine approach in healing, not just the masculine approach. Unless the practitioner has personally experienced the feminine approach they, too, will possibly come from the cure or "doing" frame of reference, except their approach will be disguised in popular language. They will have only substituted alternative therapies, e.g., Shiatsu or biofeedback, for medical prescriptions—but they are still prescribing. A truly holistic practitioner creates a context for a client to explore their own attitudes about disease and facilitates the client's own choice-making process. Holistic health, as the name implies, incorporates and includes all the factors inherent in a client's life that contribute to disease. It acknowledges that the client inherently knows his or her own answers. Holistic health is a way of being, and a client can sense when a practitioner embodies this frame of reference.

Swimming Against the Current

In both the masculine and feminine approaches to healing, the issue of choice is crucial. The extremes are either to

choose to let people do things to you or to choose to be entirely independent. But healing is not an either/or issue. It is in the middle, where you are actively surrendering. To an outsider, it may look like you are simply engaged in the available medical or nonmedical procedures, but the impetus that motivates you is radically different. You choose these procedures from trust, surrendering to your life force, rather than having something happen to you. You are choosing to move toward a fuller life, rather than to move toward death.

Wholeness in healing includes and blends both the strictly masculine *and* strictly feminine approaches. It pays attention to the value of the medical and allied health professionals without giving away personal integrity. It takes a great deal of courage and faith to hold true to yourself and be steadfast in the face of proclamations of how you are, or how you should be, or how you will be. It goes far beyond just taking responsibility for yourself, for it also includes the relationship to others, who for the most part do not believe you know what is right for yourself. It requires inner strength to listen to your personal wisdom, surrendering to your own life's direction and flow, and at the same time include external help.

Few people realize how much struggle a person with a proclaimed diagnosis must go through to do what they know to be right. It is an exciting challenge—and it is work—but well worth the attention. Getting yourself into a healthy internal and external environment can be exhausting, but it can be done. It is like a salmon swimming against the current. The end result for both is transformation and an opportunity to fully participate in the cyclic nature of life.

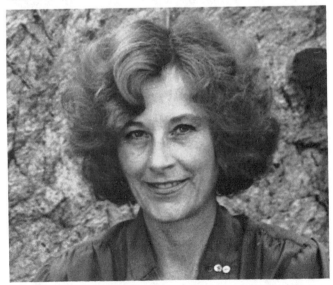

ANNE LANGFORD, *Ph.D., is the director of the Masters Program in Clinical Holistic Health Education at John F. Kennedy University Graduate School of Consciousness Studies, Orinda, California. She is a registered occupational therapist and a marriage, family, and child counselor engaged in a private practice that blends health issues with psychosynthesis. She is the author of* Meditation for Little People *(DeVorss and Co., 1975); is currently completing another book for children,* The Divorce Drawing Book; *and is coauthoring* The Healing Book *with Naomi Remen, M.D.*

The Sufi Way of Healing

Hazrat Inayat Khan

This article is excerpted from The Book of Health *by Inayat Khan,[1] a twentieth-century Sufi Master from India. In this work he discusses the basic laws of human nature and health, extending the notion that the mind and body reflect one another, with the mind having the deeper resonance. He emphasizes the need for greater awareness of the possibilities which spiritual healing can offer to suffering mankind in conjunction with medical science.*

ILLNESS IS an inharmony, either physical or mental, caused by a lack of tone and rhythm. *Prana*, which may be translated as life or energy, is the source of rhythm. In physical terms, the lack of circulation means congestion; and the lack of *Prana* means weakness. These two conditions attract illness and are the causes of dis-ease. In mental terms, rhythm and tone indicate the condition of the mind, whether it is strong, firm, and steady, or weak and scattered.

Susceptibility

The body which is already lacking in health is more susceptible to illness than the body which is perfectly healthy. Likewise, the mind which already has a disorder in it is more susceptible to every suggestion of disorder, and in this way goes from bad to worse.

Scientists of all ages have found that each element attracts the same element, and so it is natural that illness should attract illness. We see in everyday life that a person who has nothing the matter with him and is only weak physically, or whose life is not regular, is always susceptible to illness. Then we see that a person who ponders often upon inharmonious thoughts is very easily offended. A little disruption here and there makes him feel irritated; because irritation is already present, it wants just a little reinforcement to make it a deeper irritation.

Health is Harmony

The harmony of the body and the mind also depends upon one's external life, the food one eats, the way one lives, the people one meets, the work one does, the climate in which one lives. There is no doubt that under the same conditions one person may be ill and another may be well. A person who revolts against the conditions around him is likely to bring upon himself disorder and subsequent illness. Inoculation is a contemporary practice to put a person in harmony with the thing that is opposed to his nature. By accepting that to which there is no means of getting away, it becomes a healthy stimulus, and not a threat to one's well-being. Woodcutters do not as a rule get sunstroke; seamen do not catch cold easily.

Tone and Rhythm

There is a certain tone which the breath vibrates throughout the body, and this tone is a particular tone unique to each person, continually resonating. Now, if a person does not take care of himself and allows himself to be influenced by every wind that blows, he, like the water in the sea, goes up and down, disturbed by the air. Health is being able to stand firm through fear, joy, all the change inherent in life. When a person becomes sensitive to every little distraction that he comes across, it changes the note of his tone; it becomes a different note, to which the body is not accustomed, and that causes an illness. Likewise with rhythm. Once a rhythm is broken, pulsations change. Regaining rhythm must be a gradual process. It requires patience and strength. In every movement one makes, in every step one takes, there must be rhythm. Regularity in habits, in action, in repose, in eating, in drinking, in sitting, in walking, in everything, gives one that rhythm which is necessary and which completes the music of life. The wisdom is to understand oneself. If one can locate and sustain the proper tone and rhythm for oneself, that will be sufficient to keep one healthy.

Movement is Life and Stillness is Death

All different aspects of diseases are to be traced to congestion, caused by lack of movement. The mechanism of the body is maintained by a perpetual rhythmic movement, centered in the breath. Death is a change that comes through the inability of the body to maintain its life force or magnetism, and hold onto what we call the soul. We must learn to respect the human being and realize that a human soul is beyond birth and death, that a human soul has a divine spirit in it, and that all illnesses and pains and sufferings

[1]From *The Development of Spiritual Healing* by Sufi Inayat Khan, Sufi Publishing Company, Ltd., UK 1978. © International Headquarters of the Sufi Movement, Geneva. Reprinted by permission.

are only his tests and trials. The healer raises the consciousness of the patient to see that his illness is but a discordant vibration of his true, essential tone. The different remedies that man has found in all ages often bring cure to sufferers for a time, but will be incomplete until the true cause of the disease is brought to light and corrected at the level of its origin.

Belief

Everything that exists in the objective world has its living and more important part existing in the subjective world and is held by the belief of the patient. As long as the patient believes that he is ill, he is giving sustenance to that aspect of his disturbance. Even if the germs of the disease were destroyed, not once but a thousand times in his body, they would be created there again; because the source from which the germs spring is in his belief, and not in his body, as the source of the whole creation is within and not without.

The outer treatment of many such diseases is just like cutting the plant from its stem while the root remains in the ground. In order to drive away that illness, one must dig out the root by taking away the belief of illness even before the outer germ is destroyed. If the source of its sustenance is once destroyed, then the cure is certain. It has also been noted that the more a person is afraid of something, the more he is pursued by it, for unconsciously he concentrates on it.

When a person lives in a certain condition for a long, long time, that condition becomes his friend unconsciously. He does not know it, he may think that he wants to get out of it, yet there is some part of his being that is holding his illness just the same.

Exhaustion of the Nerves

Most cases of physical and mental illness come from exhaustion of the nerves. Not everybody knows to what extent to use nerve force in everyday life and to what extent to control it. Very often a good person, a kind, loving, affectionate person, gives out his energy at every call from every side, and so, continually giving energy, in the end he finds his nerves troubled and weakened. When the funds of energy have expired, then there is no control, there is no power of endurance, and there is no patience to take things easily. Then the person who once proved to be good and kind becomes irritable and troubled and tired and disgusted with things. Very often it may be called *abuse of goodness*. Constant giving out is not a balanced condition of body and mind. In the presence of that person, others will feel depleted, because he has no energy left. He is trying to give out what little he has, and the irritation and strain fall upon the others and make them nervous also.

The whole secret of magnetism is in the nerves. Strength gives one more power, weakness causes a greater weakness. The proper condition of the nerves enables one to impress. A person nervously depleted, even if he be in the right, cannot impress it upon another, because there is no strength behind it. He will be at a loss for what to do, lacking the power to go forward and stand up for his own right.

Nervous diseases are often treated by giving medicines. There is no medicine in the world which can do good to nerves; for nerves are the most natural part of one's being. Nervous energy is a kind of battery for the whole mechanism of the mind and body. There is no better remedy for nerves than nature, rest, repose, quiet, proper breathing, proper nourishment, and someone to treat the patient with love and understanding.

Thought Power

It is the attitude of mind, the willingness to be cured, the desire to get above one's illness, the inclination to fight against disorder, which help one to health. No doubt if a person is a hindrance to healing influences, then even a healer cannot do his work properly; but if a person's attitude is right, if one believes that spirit has all the power to cure, certainly one can be cured.

The Secret of Healing

The secret of healing is to rise by the power of belief above the limitations of this world of variety, that one may touch by the power of intelligence the oneness of the whole Being. It is there that one becomes charged with the almighty power, and it is by the power of that attainment that one is able to help oneself and others in their pain and suffering. Verily, spirit has all the power there is!

The Path of Intuition

No doubt the more a person evolves, the more he gains insight into the lives of things and beings. The first thing is to understand the condition of one's own body, mental and physical, and then to see the condition of other people. Then intuition is born and becomes active. As a man develops intuitively, he begins to see the pains and sufferings of people; and if this sympathy grows and becomes vaster, his sight becomes more keen, and he begins to observe the reasons behind the complaints; and if he goes still further in the path of intuition, he begins also to see what remedy would be the best one for the person who suffers.

The Best Remedy

The regular life, pure diet, good sleep, a balance between activity and repose, and right breathing, all these help one to health; but the best remedy for healing oneself of an illness and infirmities of mind is belief. If a person says, "I believe," that does not mean that he believes, for belief in its perfection becomes faith. When faith is attained to a certain degree, it will grow as a plant. Cure is brought about by faith in all cases. So great as the faith is, that quickly is the cure. Without faith even medicine cannot help. No treatment can give good results where faith is lacking. Faith is the first remedy; everything comes afterwards. All our failures, sorrows, disappointments, difficulties in life are caused by our lack of belief. Difficulty arises when illness becomes belief. The power with which one wishes to remove his illness is smaller than the power which is already established in him by illness. A shift in consciousness is the move out of the pit of self-pity and despair.

Faith

Faith is so sacred that it cannot be imparted, it must be discovered within oneself; but there is no one in the world who is without faith, it is only covered up. And what covers it? A kind of pessimistic outlook toward life. There are people who are pessimistic outwardly, there are others who are pessimistic unconsciously. They themselves do not know that they are pessimistic. Is faith attainable by perserverance in belief? Things of heaven cannot be attained by perseverance; they are the grace of God. To open to this and trust in it is how belief is crystallized into faith. We cannot pay for it in any form, in any way, by our goodness, by our piety, by our great qualities, merits, or virtues; nothing. It is a gift, and all we can do is receive it.

God is Love

The grace of God is the love of God, love manifested in innumerable blessings, known and unknown to us. Human beings live on Earth in their shells, mostly unaware of all the privileges of life, and therefore ungrateful to the Giver of them. In order to see the grace of God, one must open one's eyes, raising one's head from the little world that one makes around oneself, and thus see above and below, right and left, before and behind, the grace of God reaching one from everywhere in abundance.

Therefore it is not only for the sake of truth, but for life itself, that one must find belief in oneself, develop it, nurture it, allow it to grow every moment of one's life, that it may culminate in faith. It is that faith which is the mystery of life, the secret of salvation.

Suggestions for Further Reading

Hazrat Inayat Khan, *The Soul: Whence and Whither.* New Lebanon, N.Y.: Sufi Order Publications, 1977.

The Sufi Message, Vol. IV. published for the International Headquarters of the Sufi Movement, Geneva, London: Barrie Books, 1962.

Martin Lings, *What is Sufism?* University of California Press, paperback, 1977.

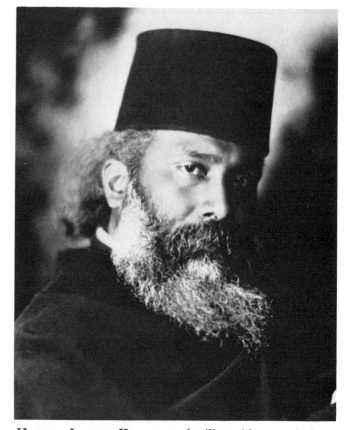

HAZRAT INAYAT KHAN *was familiar with every shade of human existence, and his teachings show his great reverence for life and the value he placed on integrating the best qualities found in humanity everywhere.*

Hazrat Inayat Khan was born in Baroda, India, on July 5, 1882, into a family of great musicians. After establishing himself at an early age as a master musician and then working for the revival of interest in the spiritual heritage of Indian music, he received initiation from his Sufi teacher and was trained in the four major Indian schools of Sufism: Chishti, Naqshebandi, Quadiri, and Suchrawardi.

In 1910, when his training was completed, he left India for the West. He lectured extensively in Europe and America. There are many volumes containing his teachings. Hazrat Inayat Khan died in February 1927.

Psychic Healing

Petey Stevens

What Is "Psychic"?

THE RECENT emergence of psychic awareness is an acknowledgement of a longstanding truth: All People Are Psychic! The origin of the word "psychic" comes from the Greek word *psychicos*, which means "of or pertaining to the soul." To be psychic is to recognize the existence of a reality beyond the physical world. In turn, this acceptance of another dimension of the self gives us the greatest opportunity to have a clearer perspective of our human condition. It allows us to see the connection between the body and the soul. This understanding of body and soul permits a level of responsibility that gives us the freedom to run our lives autonomously, with each soul responding to and influencing its own body. Only in this way, by taking full responsibility for our own well-being, can we make deliberate and real changes. The process by which this level of responsibility and influence is assumed is called *Opening Up*.

Opening up psychically can be viewed as a three-step process:

1. Self-discovery. You learn to recognize all that is you: your thoughts, considerations, ideas, opinions, feelings, dreams, wants, health, needs, style, loves, hurts, abilities, and potential; everything that is *You*.
2. This step follows when you know and accept who you are and can distinguish your own creations and personality patterns from all others. Your degree of "wellness" or "illness" directly relates to the constancy, flow, and integrity of your own essential "soul self" or "energy body."
3. This last step occurs when you take full control of your soul energy and take responsibility for the consequences of your personal choices on others and on our mutually co-created reality.

All things are energy. The floor that you walk on; the chair that you sit on; the clothes you wear; your thoughts, feelings and memories. Even your body and soul are made up of many millions of particles of energy vibrating at different frequencies and traveling at varying velocities. We see the particles of energy that are moving very slowly as dense masses; we understand them as physical matter. The particles that move most quickly appear less dense; we consider them to be massless. However, someone sensitive to such frequencies of energy can see them. We all have the ability, or possibility, of being sensitive to these higher frequencies of energy. We can develop this sensitivity through the discipline and study of energy during meditative states of consciousness.

Our whole universe is one large pool of energy. We each have our own individual energy systems, which are nestled in and swimming within a large "reality pool" shared by all. Our personal safety and freedom in the psychic pool depends upon how well we know ourselves (our personal energy) and on our ability to maintain our own psychic boundaries. We will understand energy better as we learn to translate and interpret the energy around us. Each person's energy unit or energy body is like a psychic computer that has its own internal communicative system programmed to translate that energy language into personal characteristics. The following color chart is an example of the types of metaphoric translations that could occur, given the respective color and shade of input.

The Energy Body

Each person has an energy body with specific patterns of energy that regulate and organize information and experiences. Certain functional parts of the energy body are the grounding cord, energy channels, the chakras, and the aura.

Grounding Cord

Your grounding cord is the psychic attachment to the planet on which you live. It serves as a commitment that binds you—the spirit or "soul"—to your body. This attachment helps you to be responsible for your actions and reactions toward the various situations and people in your everyday life. Your grounding cord serves as a release valve, or laundry chute, where you can let go of any excess energy. You may also let go of any energy that resides in your space that is not yours, through the process of grounding.

COLOR CHART

Color	Shade	Characteristic Attributes
Gold	pink gold	supreme love
	yellow gold	supreme intelligence
	white gold	supreme power
White	white	purity
Violet	ultraviolet	spirituality
	light violet	high aspirations
	violet	enthusiasm
	lavender	self-esteem
Purple	light purple	compassionate healing
	purple	compassion
	indigo	religious
	dark purple	dogmatic
Blue	silver blue	certainty
	sky blue	clarity
	royal blue	devotion, royalty
	dark blue	fanaticism, seriousness
Green	turquoise	humor, playfulness
	light green	calm, quiet, peaceful
	forest green	growth
	dark green	greed, jealousy
Yellow	light yellow	wisdom
	yellow	intelligence
	dark yellow	intellectualizing, rationalizing
	mustard yellow	manipulative, cowardice
Orange	peach	nurturing, love
	light orange	vitality, healing
	orange	creativity
	burnt orange	hysterical, mischievous emotions
Red	pink	love
	rose pink	hope, optimism, cheerfulness
	red	passion, stimulation
	wine red	negative emotions, hate, anger
Brown	copper	harmony with the planet
	light brown	earthy
	brown	groundedness
	dark brown	negativity, maliciousness
Black	silver	power
	grey	confusion
	dark grey	depression, apathy, loss
	black	extreme negativity, frozen energy

Grounding exercise. Sit in a straight-backed chair, with your hands and feet separated.

Close your eyes.

Allow yourself to relax into the chair and be in the present moment.

Notice a tiny light in the center of your head. Be in the center of your head and be that light, the soul.

Feel and experience the center of your head and the objectivity you have with your soul's perspective from the center of your head.

Now place your attention in your pelvic cradle at the base of your spine. Postulate that with every breath you breathe in, you are drawing thousands and thousands of tiny golden threads of energy into your pelvic cradle. As the many, many threads of energy meet they intertwine and become a rope of golden energy. Feel the weight of that golden ball of energy holding you to the chair. Allow a portion of that golden twined energy to drop down between your legs... and gather it into a small dense ball of 14-karat gold, still attached to the golden twined rope. Allow the golden weight and the golden rope of energy to drop down into the center of the Earth... all the way down to the exact geographical center of the Earth, through all the layers of rock and soil, water, gases, crystals, and into the iron core center of the Earth. Allow the golden ball to fuse with the core of the Earth. Feel a tug at the base of your spine, and notice that there is a golden beam of energy from the base of your spine into the center of the Earth.

Leave your grounding cord down.

Be in the center of your head. Open your eyes, take a deep clearing breath, and end the meditation.

Energy Channels

The entire energy body needs nourishment and cleansing. Both of these can be attained by *running energy* through particular channels that will in turn distribute energy throughout the body. You need both earth energy from the Earth and cosmic energy from the Cosmos. Each time that you run energy through these channels you set a mood, disposition, or mental state for yourself with the colors that you choose to run.

Running energy exercise. Sit in a straight-backed chair, with your hands and feet separated.

Close your eyes.

Allow yourself to relax into the chair and be in the present moment.

Be in the center of your head.

Ground yourself.

Place your attention at the arches of your feet and bring a pink Earth energy into your feet openings. Allow this energy to travel up your leg channels and into your pelvic cradle and hold this energy there for a moment.

Now place your attention on the crown of your head.

Bring a blue Cosmic energy into your crown. Pull it down the back part of your back spine and into your pelvic cradle.

Combine, balance, and blend these energies in your pelvic cradle. Allow the mixture of energies to run up the front part of your back spine and out the crown of your head. Allow the energy to flow through you. Earth energy into your feet.... Cosmic energy into your crown and down the back of your spine... mixing these energies in your pelvic cradle. The mixture then goes up the front of your spine and out the crown of your head. The energy flows as water, allowing you to flow with the current of the Universe. Maintain this energy flow for ten minutes.

Be in the center of your head.

Open your eyes, take a clearing breath, and end the meditation.

The Chakras

You have energy centers on your body called *chakras*. The word *chakra* is a Sanskrit word that means wheel. From a side view, a chakra looks like a cone with its point plugging into your spine to receive energy, and its opening about four inches from your body. Each center transmits and receives energy messages in three ways:

1. Intra-personally: within the self.
2. Inter-personally: from one body to another body.
3. Trans-personally: beyond the body, soul to soul.

You have seven basic body chakras. Your style of running energy through these centers expresses your personality. This in turn determines how you survive, feel, respond, love, communicate, understand, perceive, trust, and create. You also have feet chakras and hand chakras. The best method of gaining understanding and control of your chakras is to meditate on them, one by one, placing your attention on each chakra for two or three minutes every day. Remember to both ground yourself and to run your energy while you meditate. The following chart will give meaning and definitions to the seven basic body chakras and the physical and psychological imbalances connected with each chakra.

The Human Aura

The aura is a field of energy that emanates from and surrounds your body. Your aura shows the moods and happenings of your day. It reflects outwardly how you are within. At the edge of your aura you have psychic boundaries, which indicate where you end and the rest of the world begins.

Aura exercise. Sit in a straight-backed chair, with your hands and feet separated.

Close your eyes.

Allow yourself to relax into the chair and be in the present moment.

Be in the center of your head.

Ground yourself.

Run your energy, using light orange Earth and light orange Cosmic energies.

Notice that around your body is a field of energy. Feel that energy and notice what the colors are. Is the energy in your aura light or dark? Is it moving or fixed?

Notice the boundary or outer edge of your aura. Feel a firm boundary about two or three feet from your body.

Reaffirm that this is your space by saying "my space, my aura" and allow these words to resonate from within your body to the edge of your aura.

Be yourself.

Be in the center of your head.

Open your eyes, take a clearing breath, and end the meditation.

How You Get Sick

As you experience everyday life situations, in your mind you take reels and reels of mental images that capture impressions of these various external and internal stimuli. If you were to stop that film and look at a single frame you would be looking at a *picture*. When the film or pictures are compatible with your energy, you will file it away into your memory banks. If the picture carries a great deal of emotional charge it throws off electromagnetic properties, which act like the repelling poles of a magnet. As a result the picture will be cast out into your aura to be reprocessed at a later time.

The act of reprocessing can take place consciously, as when you are talking out your problems or meditating, or subconsciously, as in a dream state. If you have too many unprocessed pictures in your aura at a given moment, they will eventually form an energy block. This block of energy, because it is so weighted down, slows its vibration until it becomes physical. It then lodges in the physical body. This is how you get sick. Every illness or accident has its origins in an unprocessed picture.

How to Heal Yourself

To heal yourself psychically you must break up the blocked energy and release the pictures involved. To do this you direct healing energy to the chakra nearest the problem area and then into the aura. The following methods have proven themselves to be effective psychic healing tools.

Breath and Rhythm

Some emotions and other stress situations can constrict your chest and therefore your breathing. Since every cell in your body needs air, this is a good place to begin your healing. The following exercise will help your body find a rhythm of inhaling and exhaling, pulling in and letting go, involuting and evoluting.

Breath and rhythm exercise. Sit in a straight-backed chair, with your hands and feet separated.

Close your eyes.

Allow yourself to relax and be in the present moment.

Be in the center of your head.

Ground yourself.

Run your energy, using a light-green Earth energy and a light-green Cosmic energy.

Place your attention on your third chakra (at your solar plexus) and breathe into that point. Allow the air to come into your third chakra and to fill up your entire chest. Exhale, letting go of all tensions and stresses . . . and inhale once again . . . and exhale . . . inhale . . . exhale . . . inhale . . . exhale . . . inhale. . . . Continue to breathe this way for ten to 20 minutes with a continuous, yet slow and relaxed rhythm, never pausing between the in breath and out breath.

Be in the center of your head.

Be one, be whole, be healed.

Open your eyes, take a clearing breath, and end the meditation.

Sound

The vibrations that sounds produce are very strong. Whether you are listening to birds singing, water lapping, wind blowing, a child laughing, a person singing, or Tibetan prayer bowls and bells, sound can touch and heal you. Many sounds can loosen energy blocks by gently rocking the energy of the block until it begins to move.

THE SEVEN BODY CHAKRAS

Chakra	Location	Function Analogy	Psychic Abilities	Physiological Correlations
7th or Crown Chakra	crown of head	opening flower	to be open to know intuition precognition connection with infinite intelligence to have faith connection with God	pituitary glands old mammalian brain greater right-hemisphere correlation
6th or Third Eye	center of forehead	T.V.	clairvoyance psychic reading to have vision or insight photographic memory telekinesis	pineal gland neo-mammalian brain greater left-brain hemisphere correlation
5th or Throat Chakra	center of throat	radio	communication center telepathy clairaudience inner voice tone healing	thyroid parathyroids lymphatic system brain stem
4th or Heart Chakra	center of chest	equalizer	to be in affinity with to be at ONE with to connect with compassion unconditional love	thymus gland heart vascular system lungs respiratory system
3rd or Solar Plexus	above the navel	generator and distributor	astral projection to be empowered to manifest to be in control of yourself psychic healing levitation	adrenal glands solar plexus (neural center) autonomic control center
2nd or Feeling Center	center of abdomen	radar	clairsentience emotional feelings balance of male and female energies	insulin-producing glands in the pancreas and spleen
1st or Root Chakra	base of spine	roots and waste plumbing system	grounding realizing letting go surviving	ovaries testes placenta

Physical Imbalances	Psychological Imbalances
baldness	excessive gullibility
brain tumors	memory disorders
cancer	multiple personalities
epilepsy	nightmares
migraine headaches	split personality
Parkinson's disease	
pituitary problems	

brain tumors	extreme confusion
cancer	fixations
central nervous system problems	inability to focus
eye and visual problems	intelligence deficiencies
headaches (sinus)	living in a fantasy world
sinus problems	paranoia
	poor visual memory
	psychotic behavior
	schizophrenia
	severe retardation

ear and hearing problems	inability to express self in words
cancer	logorrhea (nonstop verbal chatter)
lymphatic problems	poor auditory memory
mouth problems	stuttering
neck and shoulder problems	
parathyroid problems	
speech problems	
teeth problems	
thyroid problems	
throat problems	

auto-immune system problems	at war with yourself
circulatory problems	feelings of alienation
heart problems	inability to bond with another
high blood pressure	self-destructive tendencies
lung cancer	suicide
lung problems	
respiratory problems	
thymus problems	
upper back problems	
vascular problems	

absorption problems	addictive personality
adrenal problems	catatonic schizophrenia
arthritis	compulsive behavior
anorexia nervosa	excessive anger or fear
cancer	manic-depressive behavior
coordination problems	obsessive behavior
liver problems	sleep problems
multiple sclerosis	
obesity	
premature aging	
stomach problems	

anemia	chameleon personality
allergies	depression
diabetes	hysteria
diarrhea	unable to be sexually intimate
duodenal ulcers	
hypoglycemia	
kidney problems	
leukemia	
lower back problems	
pancreas problems	
premenstrual syndrome	
spleen problems	

cancer	accident prone
colon problems	being in survival
bladder problems	dependent personality
female reproductive-organ problems	identity crisis
fluid retention	weak ego structure
male reproductive problems	
sciatica problems	
urethral problems	
yeast infection	

Tone-cleaning exercise. Sit in a straight-backed chair, with your hands and feet separated.

Close your eyes.

Allow yourself to relax and be in the present moment.

Be in the center of your head.

Ground yourself.

Run your energy, using violet Earth energy and lavender Cosmic energy.

Open up your Throat Chakra (5th chakra). Allow all the blocked energy from your 1st chakra to travel up your spine and come out of your Throat Chakra as a sound. Allow yourself enough sounds to really let go of all stuck or blocked energy in your first chakra. Repeat this process with each chakra.

When all seven chakras are clean, *sing* your name out loud. This will fill you up with yourself, your own essence energy.

Be in the center of your head.

Be one, be whole, be healed.

Open your eyes, take a clearing breath, and end the meditation.

Allow yourself to be around sounds that are pleasing and healing to you!

Visualization

As with all psychic healing, to make your visualizations really effective you must first believe in them. You can use your visual healings any time of day, in a crowd of people or in solitude while meditating. This is because they truly are an internal communication.

Here are some suggested visualizations. Please allow yourself to be creative in exploring visual healing.

Exercise. For a tumor, allow all your white blood cells to be Pac-Mans eating up the tumor. You are really doing them a favor because they like to eat the litter left in your body.

Exercise. For an organ that needs revitalizing, send a clear picture or image of it as a healthy organ to that organ. In this way you are reminding the organ of its whole health.

Exercise. To let go of any illness or pain, dump it down your grounding cord. Use the grounding cord as a giant plumbing system. The Earth loves all this energy. Let go …let grow…let glow!

Channelling Color

To channel energy is simply to bring it through your energy channels. The energy is usually seen as color. Any colors on the color chart can be brought in your body as Earth or Cosmic energies. As you choose a color you set a mood for yourself.

Color exercise. Repeat the "running energy" exercises and use different healing colors through your energy channels.

Faith or Prayer Healing

The object of this type of healing is to totally believe in it, to have faith that it will work. One method for accom-

plishing this total belief is to encourage every cell in your body to desire and be open to healing.

Exercise. Sit in a straight-backed chair, with your hands and feet separate.

Close your eyes.

Allow yourself to relax into the chair and be in the present moment.

Be in the center of your head.

Ground yourself.

Run your energy, using Earth gold and Cosmic gold.

From the center of your heart find the deepest desire and faith you have to be whole and healed. Take that faith and channel it through your body "with each cell relaying your faith and belief to the other cells" until each cell of your body is touched by it.

Experience this desire for wholeness within every cell of your body. Allow yourself to want and have this wholeness. Maintain this energy level for at least ten minutes.

Be in the center of your head.

Be one, be whole, be healed.

Open your eyes, take a clearing breath, and end the meditation.

Unconditional Love and Acceptance

When you are able to accept yourself just the way you are, without any judgments or considerations of how you are supposed to be, you will find that your health and well-being will improve. Bless yourself! "Bless me! Bless me! Bless me!"

How to Stay Well

When you have a healthy energy body, you have a healthy physical body. A healthy energy body is made up of the following:

1. A well-established grounding cord
2. Light colors of energy running through the energy channels
3. Chakras in control
4. A bright, vibrant aura
5. A well-defined boundary.

To attain and maintain this state of energy, you must clean out your energy body every day.

How to clean out your energy body. Sit in a straight-backed chair, with your hands and feet separated.

Close your eyes.

Be in the center of your head.

Ground yourself.

Open up your feet chakras as if they were the iris of a camera and pull in a pure pink-gold Earth energy. Allow this energy to wash through your leg channels. Gently and forcefully, the energy keeps washing and cleansing out the leg channels it moves up into your pelvic cradle. Allow the pink-gold Earth energy to wash on down the grounding cord and then on up your back spine. Allow this energy to push out self-created and other-created energy patterns that are not in the present moment with you. Allow all these energies to wash all restricting energy patterns up and out the crown of your head.

As this pink-gold energy washes up your spine, allow it to wash through each chakra, cleaning and purifying your survival, feelings, empowerment, affinity, communication, vision, and faith.

Now take all the energy in your channels and expand it to be as large as your aura . . . pushing out all foreign and heavy energies out to the edge of the boundaries. Allow all the wastes to flow down the boundaries and eventually down the grounding cord.

Be in the center of your head.

Be yourself.

Open your eyes, take a clearing breath, and end the meditation.

Your illness will tell you your innermost feelings and attitudes about yourself. Use each illness to learn about yourself, and then heal yourself! There is a wonder, a delight that gives way to joy when you realize that you are in control of your health. By healing yourself, you begin to heal the world.

Summary

The psychic emergence heralds the grassroots use of spiritual enlightenment as a tool for our daily life situations.

All things are energy moving at different vibratory levels. A psychic is sensitive to the higher frequencies of this energy.

The energy body consists of: grounding cord, energy channels, chakras, aura, boundaries.

Methods of psychic healing: breath and rhythm, tone, visualization, color channeling, faith or prayer healing, unconditional love.

We get sick from stuck pictures, which block the energy flow in our bodies.

We stay well by taking full responsibility for our energy body, and by cleaning it out every day!

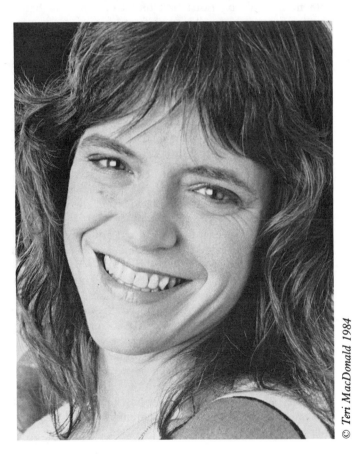

© *Teri MacDonald 1984*

PETEY STEVENS *co-founded and continues to co-develop* Heartsong Center for Expanded Perception, *where being psychic is an everyday occurrence. It is here that she has gained her experience as a psychic, giving both readings and healings and teaching students how to be psychic in their everyday lives. She is author of* Opening Up to Your Psychic Self, Psychic Healing, *and* Ten Ways to a More Psychic You.

Bernie Siegel, M.D.

A YALE SURGEON CUTS THROUGH
THE MEDICAL-AUTHORITY MYTH

Jay Kantor

DURING THE past five years, Dr. Bernie Siegel, a bald, smiling, cherubic-looking 51-year-old surgeon from New Haven, Connecticut, has helped more than 1,500 people who have cancer and other potentially fatal illnesses to learn to live better and longer. Siegel teaches patients who are willing to participate in their own healing—the exceptional patients—how to achieve peace of mind and better health by removing stress and conflict from their lives and redirecting themselves toward goals that they feel are truly appropriate. His program of alternate therapies includes relaxation, meditation, visualization, pain management, and psychological supports. These techniques may be used alone or in combination with surgery, chemotherapy, and radiation therapy; they seem to increase the effectiveness of traditional treatments and reduce side effects.

Siegel has found that when people resolve their conflicts and become more loving, it facilitates the healing process and helps the body rid itself of disease. In the process of resolving conflicts—whether they are with a doctor, spouse, child, or job—people are often able to express emotions such as anger or fear which until that time have remained bottled up. A person who has learned not to waste energy holding back emotions has more energy for healing and "feeling good;" and Siegel says that "feeling good" has a scientifically verifiable, positive effect on the body.

"I can't say to a patient 'Increase your white-cell phagocytosis,' or 'Increase your immune-globulin levels.' Instead, I have to say: 'These things will happen when you feel good.' How do we get you to feel good? Well, what is the best feeling that anyone has ever known? That best feeling is unconditional loving—both giving and receiving love. When you're loved you're in the best state that you can be in, and that heals. Then patients can understand what I'm talking about. If you're filled with love, you're saying to your body: 'Live!'"

Exceptional Patients

Siegel counsels patients individually and has them join one of the Exceptional Cancer Patient (ECaP) groups. The groups, which are open to patients with cancer and other serious illnesses, have approximately 20 members each and meet once a week for two hours.

Edna is a member of one such ECaP group: A 49-year-old mother of six, Edna first found out she had breast cancer five years ago. "A nurse found it during a routine checkup in the doctor's office. I had a mammogram and my regular physician called a surgeon for an opinion. They wanted to do a biopsy." The lump was malignant, and Edna chose to have the breast removed.

Unfortunately, two years later, she had a recurrence. Then she found out about Siegel and his Exceptional Cancer Patients groups through her husband's boss's mother-in-law. "She had a book, *Getting Well Again* by O. Carl Simonton, M.D., that she had gotten from Siegel when she joined an ECaP group for her own cancer," Edna recalls. "She sent the book home with my husband and said that if I wanted to go down to New Haven, she would take me. That's how I went.

"My doctor had heard Siegel speak. His only comment was that after I learned the things I would learn down there, not to come back with guilt feelings—realizing that I had participated in my own illness." Insights about how one may have contributed to one's own illness, or may have needed the illness to resolve a conflict in one's life, are an important part of Siegel's work. "My doctor was afraid my guilt about this would overshadow the positive benefits. Once I decided I wasn't going to do that, it was fine.

"When I first came into the group, the shock of the recurrence had put me into neutral," Edna adds. "I was very depressed. I wasn't making any goals for the day or the week or the year. I wasn't planning ahead. I was stagnant."

Learning to Forgive

"The group changed my life and the way I viewed the world," she declares. "It made me appreciate things day to day. I've had to learn to forgive—one of the hardest things I've ever learned to do.

"For instance, I was angry at someone who had caused me to have to go to court. I started including them in my prayers. I also tried to see good things happening to them in my mind.

Whole Life Times (December 1983), 18 Shepard Street, Brighton, MA 02135. Reprinted by permission.

"In the beginning it didn't work, and I would find myself thinking about them in the same grudging way. It took a few months, but I was finally able to let my anger go.

"Once I started learning how to forgive people, things began to fall into place in my life. I wasn't carrying around the burden of my anger and resentment. I was more relaxed around my family, so there were fewer arguments. They became more cooperative. But I had to change first.

"I learned to listen to my feelings and use them as a guide. In addition, I learned how to meditate—to go inside myself and find out how to make myself happy." Edna, whose cancer is in remission, says of Siegel: "I've never once heard Bernie give advice to anyone. He makes you do your own thinking and come up with your own decisions. This is one thing I really like. No one can do it for us. We have to do it ourselves."

An Unusual Surgeon

A physician for more than 20 years, Bernie Siegel is a highly skilled, well-credentialed, and busy practitioner of the art of surgery. He is an attending physician at Yale-New Haven Hospital and the Hospital of St. Raphael, as well as assistant clinical professor of surgery at Yale Medical School, where he teaches about the psychology of surgery and chronic diseases. He performs general and pediatric surgery on about 400 people a year. Half of his patients have cancer.

After surgery and his rounds at the hospital, Bernie's work with exceptional patients begins. His evenings are spent counseling patients, writing letters, and making phone calls to the more than 300 people a year who seek his help in healing their diseases or those of family members or friends. On Thursdays, his day off, Bernie participates in two of the four ECaP groups held in New Haven. (Another group currently meets in New York.) Much of his time on weekends is spent giving lectures on the ECaP Program or presenting workshops at conferences.

Siegel's approach to healing is based on the concept that people's illnesses result from living lives that are not in accord with their authentic selves. Conflict, stress, and negative emotions that disrupt the body's ability to control disease are generated. Fortunately, when people begin to act authentically, they can reverse the process.

Frances, 61 years old, first developed a melanoma (a skin cancer) on her leg. About one year later (five years ago), she developed colon cancer and decided to join an ECaP group. With the support of the group she decided to leave her job of 18 years as an accountant and office manager. She now assists in the groups.

"I had to stop and evaluate and realize what was in life for me, because I'd been running and trying to be perfect in everything I did," she explains. "Consequently, I wasn't doing anything for me. Through that, I was hurting my health, and I was hurting my person. I wasn't happy and hadn't realized it."

Learning to Say No

"Why do people get sick?" Siegel asks.

"Because they don't know how to say no without feeling guilty. They wear themselves out."

Not every patient reacts in the same way. In Siegel's experience, 15 to 20 percent of seriously ill people would prefer to die if allowed to. Another 50 to 60 percent are willing to get better as long as the doctor does the work and the medicine doesn't taste too bad," he says. The final 15 to 20 percent—those he knows as exceptional patients—will do anything they have to in order to get well.

"I used to be a miserable son of a bitch," Ted, one of Siegel's patients, told *New Age* magazine (August 1981). Four-and-a-half years earlier, Ted had been told he had six months to live. "I've got two brain tumors (one malignant, the other not), and I can honestly say that cancer is the best thing that ever happened to me. I used to install carpets, and I would tell people, 'All I want is money.' Now what I do is free, and I love it." He became a volunteer at Yale-New Haven Hospital, sharing his enthusiasm and his beliefs about healing with the patients.

The vitality and confidence of patients like Ted, who have made breakthroughs, belie the long, hard emotional struggle it has taken them to understand their disease and themselves.

"These patients will go out and change their lives," Siegel told participants at a conference on "Love, Laughter, and Healing" at Interface Foundation in Newton, Massachusetts, last year. "People who get well despite great odds will tell you, 'I make personal changes, psychological changes, spiritual changes, and nutritional changes.' Then my friends say to me, 'Wow, you had a miracle!' Well, it wasn't a miracle, it was hard work.

"If you really want to get well, you ought to use everything at your command: that's faith in yourself, your doctor, your treatment, and your spiritual faith. Put all your together, you're going to have excellent results. Do one and you may be leaving things out that can help you. I also tell them that what you believe in works. And I say, 'OK, now we've got to straighten your life out.'"

A Chance to Live

"So the woman with a large breast cancer comes back a few weeks later; it's a little smaller and softer, and I say, 'Well, what did you do?' She says, 'It was wonderful: I walked out of the house with the phone ringing.' The next week this woman comes back and says, 'This week, when my alcoholic husband was about to beat me up, I called the police. My husband said, "You're embarassing me in front of the neighbors," and I said, "I have cancer now; I don't accept your behavior."' And the tumor shrinks a little more.

"But then she comes in and says, 'You know, this is hard work. I think it would be easier if you remove the tumor, and I keep myself well.' I say, 'I think that's a terrific idea,' and off we go to the hospital. The next morning she tells me that a nurse had approached her, amazed. 'You have no pain,' the nurse said to this patient. 'You're walking up and down the wards of the hospital, cheering people up, and you're not supposed to be up like that—you just had a mastectomy!' The patient replied, 'There's a big difference. Dr. Siegel did what I wanted done. He and I shared. So why should I have pain, and why should I be upset?'"

Thus, consistent with his view that what people need

most is to live authentically and be in control of their lives, Siegel refrains from pushing treatments on patients, even when he believes they might be beneficial. "We have a patient who ran a health-food store for 20 years, she never took a pill in her life," he told the conference. "She comes down with recurrent breast cancer, and I say, 'You know, Trish, chemotherapy could help you, radiation could help you—you might want to look in to these things.' She says, 'Oh, my friends say it's terrible, it's all poison!' OK, it's all poison.

"So she works on the Kelley dietary regimen and other things, and then one day she says, 'You know, I can see X-ray therapy as a kind of energy. I think I'll have that.' We go talk to a radiation therapist, and she has it, and there are no side effects. Then she says, 'I think maybe chemotherapy could be energy, too.' So she gets it and she has no side effects—she runs her store, raises her two children, and goes to school at night. These are things that can happen; but if you believe you're being poisoned, you will react as if you're poisoned. And if we take control of your life away, you're in big trouble.

"I do not do things *to* people," Siegel emphasizes. "I become somebody's instrument. That's how I save my own life."

Siegel's Personal Struggle

Siegel has come to this view of illness and treatment through his own experiences and growth. Back in the early 1960s, he was unhappy as a physician. "I had a happy childhood with probably the usual storms of adolescence," he recounts, "but my basic unhappiness in life was taking this nice boy who was loved and who liked people, and making him into a doctor, which he chose not knowing really what it was like to become a doctor.

"When I came out of the system, I had a lot of the complaints that medical students have now—that it's mechanistic, makes people feel helpless, places the physician in an impossible 'lifesaver' role. Suddenly I was responsible, and ultimately everyone dies! The system had set me up for failure.

"I was really very tormented, and I can show you letters to veterinary schools and teachers' colleges that I wrote when I thought that I had to get out of medicine and do something else."

His discontent continued for several years. "'Why deal with people who are sick? Who needs the suffering?' I'd ask myself. What I didn't know back then was that they didn't have to suffer—that suffering is mental, not physical.

"However, one day I finally came to realize that everything I did related to *people*. When I painted, I wasn't painting flowers, I was painting people. I said to myself, 'You're such a dummy. Your office is filled with people. If you just stop seeing only *disease*, you'll be OK.' It was then that I really started saying, 'I want to know my patients as people.'"

Years later, in getting to know patients in the early ECaP groups, he was shocked to realize that "Most people are unhappy. I had grown up happy. I had a desire to live.

When I realized that most people were not thrilled with living my whole role changed. *I needed to help them enjoy living*, and incidentally we took care of the disease. The disease wasn't their biggest problem."

The Patient's World

Another experience early in his practice helped to shape Siegel's outlook. He learned the relationship between stress and illness and what it was like to be a patient. Bernie and his wife Bobbie had just had another child, moved to a new house, and Bernie had just started practicing when he developed a severe infection.

"I had to spend a week in the hospital and it opened up the patient's world to me—the feelings of helplessness and the fatigue that goes with being trapped.

"I was in isolation due to my infection. I had IVs, and people had to wear gowns and masks to come into the room. I really began to understand what a patient goes through.

"I learned that my life actually had something to do with my health. I began to look at the stress factors in my life and some psychological literature. Nobody ever showed me that in my surgical training program."

Starting then, Siegel began exploring the relationship of life events and illness with his patients. "A patient would come into the office with some minor complaint and I would jokingly ask them whether they had just moved or gotten a new job or had any other stressful life event," he relates. "Most times they had, and they were always amazed that somehow I knew it." Siegel began to develop more personal relationships with his patients.

However, it was a 1978 workshop with Dr. O. Carl Simonton, a radiation oncologist from Texas, that really stimulated his development of the ECaP concept.

"The title, 'Psychological Factors, Stress, and Cancer,' entranced me," Siegel recalls. "I ran to it. One good thing that happened was that I met some of my own patients there. 'You're a nice guy and could be a good doctor,' they told me, 'but if I see you every week or every three months I still don't know how to live between visits. I have to know how to live until I come back to you.' That was a world I was totally unaware of. I began to realize that I wasn't providing them with any ongoing contact or help.

The Body Knows

"Another thing that happened in the workshop was that they had patients draw pictures of themselves, their treatment, and their disease. This is a technique that I have gotten into more deeply through my contact with Elisabeth Kübler-Ross and other therapists on the Continent who have done extensive work based on Carl Jung's approach to psychiatry, which recognizes that everyone's unconscious minds 'speaks' in the same universal symbols. What people draw and how and where they draw it on a page gives accurate, valuable information about a patient's life and illness."

For example, at a recent conference, Siegel showed the drawing of a young man who had brain cancer. The central figure looked like a gnarled tree with something lurking in the branches. "Although the patient's disease was in remission when he came to see me, his drawing—which looked incredibly like the structure of the brain—showed me that the cancer was advancing," Siegel says. "Seeing this, I was able to help him prepare for the possibility of a recurrence, which was confirmed later by his own physician."

A picture drawn by a child coming in for surgery showed him riding a dinosaur and holding on to purple reins. "When I see such a drawing I know that there is nothing to be worried about," Siegel says. "The child feels in control of the monster who is being led by purple reins, a spiritual and, in this case, healing color.

"When I learned that the patients unconsciously knew what was happening in their bodies, it seemed a little strange and crazy compared to what I had learned in medical school. There, the body and mind were considered separate. Disease was a rather mechanical process that happened to the body. Now I saw that the mind and the body were inseparable—that the mind knows what is going on in the body, and if we can teach the mind to consciously communicate with the body, we can reverse disease processes and change how people feel."

A New Trust

"When I began to share this new information publicly in lectures, it really opened up the communication between my patients and me. Old-timers came into the office and said, 'Boy, I'm glad. Now I can tell you that I'd been wanting to commit suicide when I got my cancer. It was the best thing to happen to me.' Or they would say, 'I just had a dream that told me I have cancer.'"

As Siegel continued speaking publicly, he found out that many of his patients whom he thought had died were very much alive. "A patient from our office that should have died came up to me 10 years later, and he was walking around free of cancer. We assumed he *had* died. He just had had no reason to come back. I would have no awareness of these people if I didn't say that people could cure themselves. That's when they come up to you."

Medical practitioners are often reluctant to accept the fact that patients who were diagnosed as having a disease that *should* have killed them actually recover, Siegel observes. "Some doctors go around saying that such cases result from an error in diagnosis," he says. "That way they don't have to accept that what to many would be called a miracle has occurred."

There is Always Hope

Given his experiences, Siegel is committed to giving his patients hope. "Terminal," to him, is a state of mind. "I have a true belief in what a patient can achieve," he says. "It's not a deception. Both doctors and ministers have to learn that statistics are not the truth for an individual. A survivor is 100 percent alive even if the other nine out of 10 died. Truth-telling does not mean statistics-telling. The truth is that there is always hope no matter what the statistics are."

He has not yet had the time or money to compile statistics on his patients, he says. However, George Gellert, a graduate student Siegel was supervising, did a disertation comparing ECaP participants who had metastatic breast cancer to a control group with cancer. The study showed that ECaP patients and control-group patients survived at the same rate. (Typically, seven out of 10 breast cancer patients survive at least five years.) Siegel cautions, though, that research such as Gellert's may be questionable because medical researchers have yet to agree what constitutes acceptable controls. Also, these subjects were studied for a relatively short period of time. In keeping with his experience that a person's will and commitment is the key, Siegel prefers to speak about case histories rather than statistics.

What Really Matters

In dealing with death as a day-to-day reality, Siegel has learned that it is the quality of our living and our commitment to face the issues in our lives that really matters. There can be a peaceful death for those who, although their body will not heal, can put their lives in order.

Siegel tells the story of Jean, a nurse, who made an agreement with her husband when they were married that he would die first and she would take care of him. She, however, developed stomach cancer, and after four years it looked as if she would die. Something was holding her back, and it could be seen in one of her drawings.

"She drew herself as a purple kite, which indicated to me that she was about to make a spiritual transition, that she was going to die," Siegel recalls. "However, her husband was holding on to the string of the kite and refusing to let go. At this point Jean decided to undergo chemotherapy, something she had not wanted till then. It bought her enough time to allow her to help her husband prepare for her death. After he was ready, she died." Siegel comments: "Death is not a failure; it is inevitable for all of us. The failure is not trying, not making a commitment to live a quality life.

"I feel that physicians need to stop seeing themselves as mechanics treating illness. Instead, we could be teaching people how to live, and in that way we will also be caring for their illnesses. People will heal better when they learn to live and love. Treatment can be integrated into this total life picture."

In closing his talks, after innumerable wonderful and touching stories about his patients who may have lived or died, Siegel sometimes quotes Thornton Wilder: "There's a land of the living and a land of the dead, and the bridge is love. If we love one another we will be eternal."

To Learn More

Exceptional Cancer Patients Inc.
c/o Bernard S. Siegel, M.D.
2 Church Street S.
New Haven, CT 06519
(203) 772-0650

Bernie Siegel is writing a book intended to "show people how to be survivors, how to live and take control, and really enjoy life," which is slated for publication by Harper and Row in the fall of 1984. He may call it *On Life and Living*—taking off from Elisabeth Kübler-Ross' book *On Death and Dying*—or it may simply be titled *The Exceptional Patient*.

JAY KANTOR is a research scientist, author, and consultant who is actively involved in exploring the integration of scientific theory, ancient and modern technologies, and spiritual worldviews. He has conducted research for New York University on Therapeutic Touch and is currently studying cancer patients, their families, and their doctors in order to understand the relationship of will to live, belief structures, and social networks to healing. Jay, who is starting his own "New Age" information service, is a regular contributor to Whole Life Times.

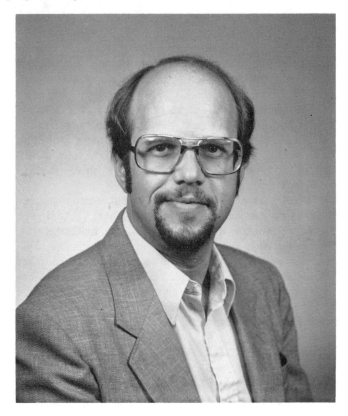

A Holistic Approach to Successful Surgery

Jeanine Paz, P.B.V.M.

I F WE accept illness and even surgery as an opportunity to explore our lives, we give meaning to what might otherwise feel like a hopeless, helpless situation. To the degree we are present to the moment, gather support, and actively participate in this process, we will touch deeply into the core of our being.

Our culture views illness as a very mechanistic, cause-and-effect situation: Something outside of the body is causing a particular harmful symptom, and it is the "physician's role to select a pharmaceutical or surgical intervention aimed at the afflicted part."[1] It is assumed that the specialist has the knowledge; "therefore, the patient is seen as a recipient of the intervention, preferably without interference or resistance, since the doctor knows best."[2]

But we might instead look at illness as a "stopping place or interruption of the habit patterns. It may surface questions and certain values, priorities, or ways of being that have been accepted as right and unchangeable."[3] Viewed in this light, illness might represent an opportunity to begin to live more consciously and deliberately. This is the holistic view of health: The human person is seen as a "living system whose components are all interconnected and interdependent and . . . that this system is an integral part of larger systems, which implies that the individual organism is in continual interaction with its physical and social environment but can also act upon it and modify it."[4]

Things to Consider in Preparation for Surgery

If you want to participate actively in the success of your surgery, you might consider how you want this event to occur—and, more specifically, what is personally important to you. Here are several questions to help generate ideas:

- Is there a close friend who understands and accepts you and is willing to be available to you during the entire time you need to call upon her/him?

- Do you need/want to speak with someone during this time regarding your feelings about the entire process (medical counselor, therapist, religious counselor, etc.)?
- How active do you want your friends and family to be during this time?
- How much information do you want to know about the actual surgery?
- Do you want to involve your surgical and recovery room team in your healing process?
- Do you want to alter your food patterns to maximize healing?
- Do you want to take vitamin and mineral supplements?
- Do you want to learn some relaxation techniques?
- Do you want to use healing music? Where? When? What kind?
- Do you want to incorporate any special rituals during this period?
- What do you want to know about hospitalization (admission, surgery, recovery, medical records)?
- How will you physically and emotionally experience what is happening in the hospital, especially during preoperative, operative, and postoperative periods?
- Do you want to use nontraditional remedies for healing (herbs, Bach flowers, crystals, etc.)?
- How do you want to use your time in the hospital?
- Whom do you want as visitors when you are in the hospital?
- Whom do you want as visitors when you are home during recovery?
- How do you want to spend your recuperation period?
- Do you want to visualize your surgery and healing process?
- How are you going to handle the change that will occur within you at this time?

Support System

One of the greatest resources that patients have lies not only in their own human strength but also in those of their nurse, their physician, their social workers, their friends, their family and all who care about their well-being.[5]

During times of crisis or trauma, you may want the loving support of family and friends around you. This is an opportunity to actively involve them in the healing process. Often people are reluctant to ask for support because they do not want to lose their independence, or because they experience feelings of unworthiness. But if you ask for support in specific ways, your friends and family have an opportunity to be in a very constructive and powerful way. Loved ones usually are delighted to honor your requests; they will not have to worry about what they can do for you if you present them with specific requests. The result may be a unifying consciousness between you and them that will last for days, if not even weeks, both before and after the surgery. Here are some factors to consider when thinking about a support group:

- List all the needs you think you will have.
- Make a list of those whom you want to support you, and indicate what specific expertise or assistance they can give you.
- Compose a letter telling this support group what you want them to do about the surgery and what it means to you. Ask them, by means of general suggestions or specific requests, to participate in your healing process.
- Once your family and friends begin to respond to your request of support, be open for surprises.
- If there is something that you really do *not* want people to do, express that concern to them ahead of time.
- Be ready to receive support from those yet unknown.
- Be ready to let go of all your plans and to immerse yourself in the present moment.

Ways in Which Family and Friends May Assist You

- Sharing their expertise in pertinent areas:
  use of herbs in healing
  information about vitamins and minerals
  information about your particular kind of surgery from a patient's point of view
  hospitalization through the eyes of a nurse
  availability for body-awareness sessions
  availability for counseling sessions.
- Collecting and recording your preferred type of healing music.
- Being available for ritual/prayer experiences as needed.
- Being with you and providing transportation:
  on the day of admittance
  on the day of surgery (especially before preoperative preparations)
  on days after surgery while in the hospital
  on the day you return home
  while recovering at home.

- Calling your family immediately after surgery, or particular friends who cannot physically be with you, to let them know how you are.
- Being available to answer calls from people who may call to find out how you are.
- Being there during the weeks before surgery (this should be someone with whom you can voice your anxiety, concerns, and hopes).

Support on the Day of Surgery

The participation of friends during this time can be a very powerful means of support. You may suggest several things to your friends—depending on how flexible and creative they are, you can be as creative as you wish. Here are a few suggestions:

- Surround the hospital staff and yourself with their loving consciousness before, during, and after surgery.
- Visualize healing colors and sounds, using any of the traditions with which you are familiar.
- Offer prayer intentions, either private meditation or in group prayer or Eucharistic liturgical celebration or ritual.
- Go to a place of particular peace and visualize healing (e.g., strolling by the ocean, watching a sunrise, or meditating in a meadow or forest, chapel, or temple).

Hospitalization

Being informed about hospitalization will both reduce your fear of the unknown and minimize the stress that interferes with successful surgery and recovery. As one recovery room nurse pointed out, "Fear of the unknown can be worse than the actual procedure." Here are some suggestions that may help to alleviate your fear about hospitalization:

- Visit the hospital prior to admittance, and tour parts of the facility.
- Visit one of the hospital rooms and look around.
- Ask to see a surgery room and the recovery room. (This is optional, but it may be helpful.)
- Go to the Admittance desk. Ask what the procedure is, what you will need to bring with you, and what forms you will need to sign.
- Ask for any other forms you may need, so you can read them ahead of time.
- Pick up a surgery-release form and read it over. This will help keep you from being surprised or fearful, and will also give you time to prepare your questions.
- Inquire about the procedure of obtaining your medical records.
- Read books about specific areas of concern regarding hospitalization and surgery. (For some people, knowing more about anesthesia and its function in the body, and knowing where the surgical team will stand, lessens the unknowns that can cause unnecessary worry.

Making Your Hospital Room a Familiar and Safe Place

Going into *any* strange room can be uncomfortable. Therefore, the more you have familiar objects and persons around, the less frightening your environment will be. You can get an idea of what to expect by visiting the hospital prior to hospitalization and looking around at the rooms. Most hospitals have bulletin boards or wall space to hang pictures, drawings, or other symbolic items that will remind you of the healing qualities needed during this time. Be sure to bring your own bedclothing (nightwear, robe, and slippers)—it may sound like a little thing, but it adds to the familiarity. Bring things with which to occupy your time—books, writing implements, paper, needlework, or anything else.

Friends also make for a familiar environment. Ask them to come at a particular time; this allows for individual visits with each person, rather than having everyone be there all at once. Some friends may come to help you bathe, to give you a massage, or just to be present and to pray with you, as you wish.

Some "alone" time, when you can reflect on your personal feelings about what is happening during this experience, is essential. These are the times when you might want to express your feelings in drawings or writing. These also are the times when profound experiences may well up from the deepest parts within you. Allowing for quiet time will allow this opportunity.

Enlisting the Hospital Team as Part of Your Support Group

Trusting the people who will be working with you very closely during the hospital stay is crucial. And telling the surgeon, anesthesiologist, assistants, and nurses of your trust in them empowers the team. They need to know that at particular points in the experience you are depending on their expertise. If the surgical team knows you are approaching this experience with a certain attitude and in a certain environment, this will help them join with you, or at least assist you as fully as they can. And including the team in your process helps the team to focus on you, rather than on the particular diseased part of your body.

Conclusion

There are may ways to approach surgery holistically. If you are facing surgery, consider the suggestions in this article, as well as other ways in which to actively participate in an event that can be a transformative process. As you embrace this healing process, your inner qualities of determination, insight, patience, resourcefulness, ingenuity, and wisdom will enable your inner courage to venture into the unknown and to put trust in yourself. This process—which is as certain, natural, and inevitable as the rising sun—will also be enhanced by all who share with you their special presence and gifts. This helps to transform not only the event of surgery but also the mutual awareness, growth, and understanding of responsible health care.

Notes

1. Pelletier, *Holistic Medicine: From Stress to Optimum Health*, p. 30.
2. Ibid., p. 31.
3. Remen, *The Human Patient*, p. 92.
4. Capra, *The Turning Point*, p. 317.
5. Remen, Op. Cit., p. 189.

Suggested Further Reading

1. Capra, Fritjof. 1982. *The Turning Point*. New York: Simon and Schuster.
2. Crile, George. 1978. *Surgery: Your Choices, Your Alternatives*. New York: Dell Publishing Co., Inc.
3. Isenberg, Seymore and Elting, L. M. 1976. *The Consumer's Guide to Successful Surgery*. New York: St. Martin's Press.
4. Pelletier, Kenneth. 1979. *Holistic Medicine: From Stress to Optimum Health*. New York: Delacorte Press.
5. Remen, Naomi. 1980. *The Human Patient*. New York: Anchor Press.

Tapes

1. Miller, Emmette. 1980. *Preparing Your Mind and Body for Surgery*, (#203), 2 vols., P. O. Box W, Stanford, California, 94305.
2. Moss, Richard. 1980. *Preparing for Surgery*, (#19), Ski Hi Ranch, Lucerne Valley, California, 92356.

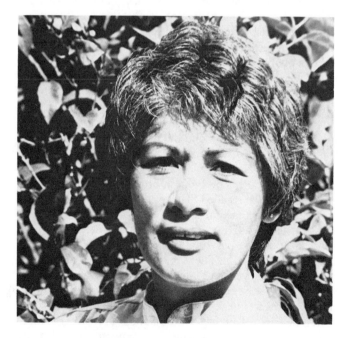

JEANINE PAZ, *P.B.V.M.*, *a health educator and counselor in the Bay Area, has a Master's in Clinical Holistic Health Education from John F. Kennedy University in Orinda, California. This article, demonstrating the possibility of making responsible choices and decisions in your own health care, is an abridged version of Jeanine's integrated project. Using her personal surgical experience, she applied holistic principles which led to a successful surgery and personal growth.*

Cancer Prevention versus Cancer Treatment

Jeffrey Bland, Ph.D.

THE SPECTRE of human cancer poses a threat to society like no other disease that we face today. The anguish, the guilt, and the fear that surround cancer, involving not only the individual stricken with the disease but all of his or her loved ones and the community as well, pose a threat to our whole biomedical establishment. If present trends continue, one in four Americans alive today, or over 54 million people, will eventually develop cancer. Over the years some form of cancer will strike two out of every three families. In 1977 alone over 385,000 Americans died of cancer, a rate of about one every 1½ minutes, or 1055 people a day. These figures are staggering and understandably frightening, but even they don't adequately depict the anguish of the cancer victim and his close immediate friends and loved ones. The degree of debilitation and the slow loss of function involved, coupled with medical science's inability in most cases to deal effectively with cancer, has led to a phobic psychological reaction to this disease which is unique. If you survive an initial heart attack, you have a good chance of leading a healthy life thereafter if you can comply with the rehabilitation program. Cancer victims are not so fortunate. They look forward to long sequences of treatment in and out of the hospital, involving agents which are at least dehumanizing, and at worst disfiguring and even deadly.

To put the cancer problem in proper perspective, however, it should be recalled that we are not now experiencing an epidemic increase in all forms of cancer. In fact, the age-adjusted death rate from cancer has increased from 125 cancer deaths per 100,000 population in 1950 to 131 per 100,000 in 1975. There is a disquieting rumbling on the horizon, however: The rate of lung cancer deaths in women is rapidly increasing, presumably as the result of the increased frequency of cigarette smoking in women 10 to 15 years ago. If, in fact, as the statistics project, the rate of lung cancer death in women approximates that of men by the year 1985, cancer will then represent a major additional threat to health.

The leading causes of cancer death in the United States in order are, in males: lung cancer, colon and rectal cancer,

and prostatic cancer. In females breast cancer, colon and rectal cancer, and lung cancer constitute the three most prevalent forms of cancer death. It can be seen that two of the three most common forms of cancer in both men and women are associated with epithelial tissues, which are exposed directly to the environment, those being the lung and the colon and rectum. For this reason many researchers have postulated that the environment plays a significant role in setting the state for a potential malignancy. Ten years ago, the suggestion that the environment was of major importance in the development of cancer would have been met with cries of heresy; however, today most cancer specialists feel that the environment may contribute anywhere between 70 to 90 percent to the risk factor of developing cancer.[1]

Of the various agents in the environment which may induce cancer, the so-called *carcinogens*, nutritional contributors may constitute a major class. If, in fact, the nutritional environment can set the stage for either cancer development or cancer protection, it is important to establish that variables in the diet are important in reducing the risk and how these factors relate to the currently accepted mechanism by which human cancer is initiated or prevented.

The Nature of Cancer

Let us first look at the problem of human cancer analytically. Cancer is the result of a cell going awry and starting to rapidly multiply as if it were an embryonic cell. Unregulated in its growth by the natural process of cell regulation and consuming the nutrients from adjacent tissues and crowding them out as it grows, it walls itself off and becomes vascularized, thereby defending itself from the body's own defensive substances. It can then send out sentries which are called metastatic cells, which can move through the lymphatic or the blood system, lodge in other portions of the body, and induce cancer in other removed sites. To be a cancerous cell mass, as opposed to a benign growth like a wart, which grows to a certain stage and then stops, three conditions must be fulfilled. The cell mass must grow in a nondifferentiated state, meaning that it loses the integrity of the host tissue from which it started its initial division. It must be invasive, tending to crowd

From *Your Health Under Siege: Using Nutrition to Fight Back* (Brattleboro, VT: Stephen Greene Press, 1981).

out other cells within the same tissue. Lastly, it must be able to metastasize, or distribute itself to other parts of the body. Those tissues that cannot invade surrounding tissues and remain strictly local are called benign tumors.

Cancer is really a family of different cellular problems which should better be termed cancers. These cancers are generally divided into three broad groups. The *carcinomas* arise in the epithelial tissue, or coverings of the body, such as the skin and the coating of the intestinal tract, as well as in those tissues lining the various glands of the body, such as the thyroid, the spleen, the prostate, and the adrenals. The much rarer *sarcomas* arise in supporting structures like fibrous tissue and blood vessels. The *leukemias* and *lymphomas* arise in the blood-forming cells of the bone marrow and lymph nodes. These three types may all be produced by similar initiating processes. Roughly half of all cancer deaths are caused by cancers of three major organs: the lung, the large intestine, and the breast. The only one of these three which appears to be increasing in epidemic proportions is cancer of the lung, which appears to be directly tied to cigarette smoking.

Nutrition

The next area of concern, in terms of prevention, is that of nutrition. Of all the dietary alterations examined in experimental animals or statistical studies in humans, calorie restriction, either through underfeeding or through restriction of dietary fats, has been the most regular influence on the reducation of cancer.[2] Chronic calorie restriction and lowered body weights seem to inhibit the formation of many types of tumors, decreasing the incidence and delaying the age at which tumors appear. Several rationalizations have been advanced to explain why lower-calorie feeding can reduce the rate of tumor formation. It is possible that calorie restriction may lead to improved immune defense, as long as adequate protein is included in the diet. This may be through a direct influence on the various hormones, such as estrogen or testosterone, which influence the initiation of cancer when produced in excess. It is also found that as a person becomes more overweight the risk of cancer increases, showing that obesity is a risk factor for cancer, as for all the major causes of death.

Dietary Fat. One of the major sources of calories in the American diet is fat. Increasing dietary fat intake from 10 percent to 27 percent of the total calories increased tumor incidence and resulted in earlier tumor appearances in many animal studies. Tumors of the endocrine system, such as uterine, prostatic, and breast cancer, appear to be most related to excessive fat intake. This may very well be a result of the fact that these tissues are fat-rich. Excessive fat feeding concentrates fat in these tissues, which then are capable of bleeding out into the system small amounts of carcinogenic fat-rich material over a period of time, exposing the tissue to a higher risk of cancer production.[3]

With regard to breast cancer, this relationship appears to be quite strong. Native Japanese women have very low levels of mammary cancer; however, when they move to Hawaii and consume the American high-fat diet, their rate of breast cancer becomes almost the same as the average U.S. rate. This would indicate that genetic control is of much less consequence than is environmental control, and that fat may be one of the major variables in the diet that disposes these women to a higher risk of breast cancer.[4] It could be argued that other life-style factors are responsible for these differences, including perhaps differential use of such things as food additives or other food-borne carcinogens. However, from animal studies in which the conditions are controlled very carefully, dietary fat appears to be the most sensitive variable in producing the Westernization effect of increasing the risk of mammary cancer. Considerable work has been done recently on women who suffer from fibrocystic disease, which is commonly known as cystic breast: tenderness and small nonmalignant nodules, which come and go periodically and may become inflamed. Reducing fat consumption in accord with the high complex carbohydrate, high-fiber, low-fat diet will many times reduce the cystic condition, again indicating that excessive dietary fat is a breast irritant in some women.*

Looking at the type of fat in the diet that seems to be most related to increased risk, the work of Dr. Denham Harman would seem to indicate that unsaturated fat may produce the greatest risk of cancer.[6] This is a result of the fat that unsaturated fats can be easily attacked by atmospheric oxygen to produce fat peroxides (or rancid products) which in themselves may initiate cancer-producing processes. Fortunately, however, as was pointed out earlier, these peroxides can be inhibited by inclusion of adequate vitamin E. When the unsaturated oil content of the diet is increased, the vitamin E intake should be increased as well. A general rule of thumb would be to increase vitamin E and some 50 International Units for every 5 additional tablespoonsful of unsaturated oil in the diet, to protect against this problem.

Fiber. An important dietary agent which renders protection against cancer and which we have already discussed at some length is dietary fiber. Doctor Denis Burkitt several years ago brought to the attention of the medical community the very low incidence of colon and gastrointestinal cancer in people who consume large amounts of crude dietary fiber.[7] This decrease in colon cancer is presumably a result of the fact that when the food passes through the intestines in the presence of adequate fiber, moisture is better retained and transit time through the bowel is reduced. Since the food stays in the bowel a shorter time, the bacteria in the large intestine have less opportunity to convert the material in the feces into carcinogens, which can be absorbed into the intestinal cells and initiate carcinogenesis. This so-called "physiochemical action" of fiber is extremely important in increasing bowel transit time and decreasing the risk of carcinogenic metabolites being formed in the intestines.

Burkitt has found that the average bowel transit time of people eating Westernized diets is about 72 hours. This

---

*This cystic condition may also be encouraged by low B-vitamin intake. The use of a high potency B-complex supplement containing choline and inositol can be most helpful in reducing breast tenderness when used in conjunction with the low-fat diet. Rigorous exclusion of caffeine from coffee, tea, and soft drinks is also essential in this dietary approach as well as vitamin E supplementation.[5]

can be easily checked by eating corn or sunflower seeds and then counting the period of time before they appear in the feces. The average transit time in people with low incidence of colon cancer is between 30 and 36 hours, almost half that of the transit time in Western cultures. This would indicate that the fecal material in the Westernized diet stays in contact with the intestines much longer and has the opportunity to be transformed into potentially carcinogenic substances by native colon bacteria. The use of wheat bran, rice bran, corn bran, or oat bran fiber, along with whole grains and vegetables, is extremely important in restoring proper intestinal transit time and reducing the risk of colon cancer. Burkitt suggests 3 to 4 tablespoonsful of bran fiber a day. However, this amount should not be included in your diet if you have consumed a low-residue diet for some time, as it can induce diarrhea and gas. The fiber should be slowly added to the diet in beverages or cereals or breads, until the proper level is achieved.

Meat. Another dietary element which seems to promote colon cancer is excessive meat consumption. In a paper by Dr. John Cairns entitled "The Cancer Problem," the author points out that there is a nearly linear relationship between annual incidence of cancer in a population and the meat consumption of that population.[8] As the meat consumption increases, the incidence, particularly of intestinal cancer, also increases.* This suggests strongly that the high complex carbohydrate, high fiber diet is preferable because it reduces meat consumption and increases vegetable protein.

Aflatoxin. Another dietary agent which produces cancer and which is commonly overlooked is the mold metabolite called aflatoxin, which is associated with moldy grains such as peanuts or wheat as well as corn and mold-infected milk. In the Netherlands, a group of workers whose task it was to extract oils from peanuts were found to have rates of cancer and liver disease that were three times that of a matched control group. In 1961 in England thousands of turkeys, ducklings and chicks died of acute liver disease, while about the same time in the United States thousands of rainbow trout that had been fed peanut meal died as a result of liver tumors. The unifying feature of all three of these problems was the exposure to a natural carcinogenic mold metabolite known as aflatoxin, which came from *Aspergillus flavus.* Peanut products in this country are regularly inspected, and on occasion batches from other countries are rejected, due to their potential mold content.[9]

Aside from aflatoxins, only two other substances have been classified on the basis of human studies as possible dietary human carcinogens. One is bracken fern, the asparagus-like vegetable sometimes called fiddleheads. The other is nitrosamines, which we have mentioned are present in many alcoholic beverages.

Vitamins and Minerals. It should be pointed out that several vitamins and minerals have been implicated in the pre-

vention of human cancer. It is well known that vitamin C when included in the diet prevents the formation in the stomach of the dangerous class of carcinogenic substances called nitrosamines, which are manufactured in the stomach as the result of consuming nitrites along with protein. Vitamin C will lower the amount of available nitrite in the stomach and reduce considerably the nitrosamine formation, thereby reducing the risk of this carcinogen.[10] Doctors Ewing Cameron and Linus Pauling have also postulated that ascorbic acid (vitamin C) has a very important role in suppressing the tumor production process, and can even be used as a therapeutic agent in large doses (upward of 10,000 mg or more per day) in the treatment of certain cancers.[11]

Dietary selenium also appears to play a significant role in the body's protection against many carcinogenic substances. Dietary selenium works in conjunction with vitamin E as an anti-oxidant. The best sources of dietary selenium are whole grains, brewers yeast, and fish, such as tuna.[12] Three tablespoons of brewers yeast per day should provide adequate stores and reserves of selenium to activate the vitamin E to prevent oxidation-induced carcinogenesis. Doctor G. N. Schrauzer has confirmed the animal studies of Dr. Shamberger which show that dietary selenium is extremely important in reducing the risk of human cancer.[13] This is very important because much of our population may be consuming selenium-deficient diets. Many people live in regions of the country with low-selenium soils, and even though they are presumably eating a cosmopolitan diet, their selenium levels have shown inadequacies. Work done in several cancer research centers around the world has indicated that cancer patients many times are selenium deficient. Whether this is a cause or an associated effect of the cancer is not well known, but it is known that when selenium is included in the diets of animals who have transplanted tumors, the incidence of cancer death goes down remarkably. This would suggest that vitamin E and selenium are both very important in optimizing the body's ability to defend itself against the tumor production process. Recently, Erlich Ascites tumors in rats have been shown to respond to therapy using high levels of selenium.[14]

Another fat-soluble vitamin which seems to be extremely important in defending against transformed cells and activating the body's surveillance system is vitamin A. Dr. Eli Seifter has used vitamin A and its derivatives in reducing the development of tumors in animals treated with a tumor producing virus.[15] Doctor E. Bjelke of the Cancer Registry of Norway reported that a 5-year study of 8278 men revealed a negative relationship between lung cancer and vitamin A intake.[16] That is, the more vitamin A in the diet, the less likely an individual was to develop lung cancer. This association was evident among smokers and nonsmokers alike. It should be pointed out, however, that vitamin A is a fat-soluble vitamin which can be concentrated in the liver. In doses over 20,000 to 30,000 units per day, care should be taken not to induce liver toxicity.

Food Additives. Another question which is commonly raised concerning diet and the risk of cancer is the effect that various food additives, preservatives, coloring agents, and

---

*It is not clear whether this increase is due to the meat itself or to the elevated fat intake which comes as a result of increased meat consumption.

the like have on increasing risk. It is clear that we are exposed to ever-greater numbers of substances that are derived from petro-chemicals whose carcinogenicity, mutagenicity, and teratogenicity* are not completely known. Many people maintain that all things are carcinogenic, taken in certain amounts; therefore, why worry about the problem? You could become so phobic that you couldn't eat anything. Doctor William Lijinsky, ex-deputy director of the National Cancer Institute, has strongly argued that this position is not accurate. Of the many thousands of substances screened for their possible carcinogenicity, only about a third have shown at any level potential carcinogenicity or mutagenicity. The bulk of the compounds tested are not carcinogenic. The important question then is what is the risk-to-benefit ratio for any new substance that is to be included in our food-supply system? Even for a substance as controversial as saccharin, there are some noted advantages to its use. For example, diabetics may benefit from including it in their diet instead of sugar. However, this no-calorie sweetener has been shown to produce bladder cancer in test animals when given at reasonably high levels. What is its benefit-to-risk ratio, then? Dr. Ernst Wynder studied bladder cancer and its relationship to saccharin consumption in 574 male and 158 female bladder cancer patients and a similar number of matched controls, and found absolutely no statistical relationship. In fact, in a recent statistical study[17] it was found that the risk of bladder cancer in humans as a result of ingesting modest amounts of saccharin was a million times less than the risk of death from stepping off the average street corner in suburbia. In this case, then, it would appear that the risk may be very small, although not zero. The question which remains for each of us is whether the risk is warranted.[18]

Alcohol. Another nutritional factor which is correlated with increasing production of cancer is excessive consumption of distilled spirits. It now appears as if this may be related to increased nitrosamines in alcoholic beverages which may have direct carcinogenic effects upon the larynx, the esophagus, and the oral cavity. It is well known that alcoholics have increased risk of tumor production. This may be a result of the fact that they suffer from a vitamin B_2 deficiency as a result of alcoholism. Doctors J. A. Miller and F. C. Miller have shown that vitamin B_2 (riboflavin) is important in activating an enzyme responsible for converting certain carcinogenic substances to noncarcinogenic products in the body, and this may be why alcoholics have a higher risk of cancer. Levels of vitamin B_2 in excess of the Recommended Dietary Allowance may be helpful in defending a person against tumor initiation if he or she is deficient in this vitamin or has been exposed to high levels of carcinogens in the environment.[19]

Stress

What, if any relationship does the body's immune surveillance system have to a person's psychological and social well-being? The interaction of stress and illness and the participation of the individual in developing coping skills to maintain his or her health have been alluded to earlier. An excellent example of this interaction is the story related by Norman Cousins, the former editor of *The Saturday Review* in an article in the *New England Journal of Medicine* in which he discusses his own treatment of degenerative disease, using what he calls laughter therapy. In his case, the treatment consisted of putting himself into a hospital room and watching all of the slapstick comedies he could possibly fit into a day, using the release of emotions as a type of immune-system activating factor.[20]

Doctor Hans Selye has defined stress as "the nonspecific response of the body to any demand placed upon it."[21] It is not simply nervous tension, nor is it something that we can escape from entirely in the world today. The type of stress, however, that seems to be related to depression of the body's immune system goes far beyond everyday, expected stress. Extreme grief and anxiety are examples. In our medical community, which has generally separated the body and the mind, only passing attention has been paid to the important role that a person's mental state may play in activating the body's immune system, and therefore defending against disease. As Plato's *Dialogue* points out: "This is the great error of our day in the treatment of the human body that physicians separate the soul from the body."

Doctor Vernon Riley has been studying animals to try to elucidate how important psychological stress factors are in the development of cancer.[22] In controlled experiments when animals were housed under a variety of different stress-inducing conditions, it was found that when a group of mice which was bred to be unusually cancer prone was raised under stressful conditions, 80 to 100 percent developed breast tumors within 8 to 18 months after birth. When Dr. Riley put these mice behind a protective barrier, however, and removed them from laboratory noise and other stressful factors, only 7 percent developed cancer after 14 months. Doctor Riley further showed that even mild anxiety stress, such as that produced by rotating the mice slowly on a turntable for a few minutes out of each hour, increased their probability of developing malignancy. The biological mechanism for this effect has been explored. It appears to relate to the fact that animals under stress secrete hormones from their adrenal glands which, in turn, have a significant effect upon the body's defensive system. These hormones are known to reduce the efficacy of the white blood cells called T-cells, which are actively involved in the body's defense, leaving the individual vulnerable to transformed cells.[23] In fact, artificial chemical stress can be produced by injecting an animal with the stress hormone. This will produce a much higher probability of cancer. From these studies, the question that emerges is whether there is a human personality type that is prone to cancer. Or, as Dr. Osler once wrote, "Is it much more important to know what sort of a patient has a disease, than what sort of disease a patient has?"

Doctor William Greene, a psychiatrist at the University of Rochester, studied the life history of three sets of twins. One twin out of each set developed leukemia. He found that the twin who developed leukemia had experienced psychological upheaval right before the onset of disease, whereas the other did not. This was further confirmed by Dr. H. J. F. Baltrusch, who was involved in a cross-cultural leukemia project in West Germany. He reported to the Third International Symposium on Detection and

---

*A teratogen is a substance which creates a birth defect *in utero.*

Prevention of Cancer that having studied more than 8000 patients with different types of cancers, "In the majority of patients, clinical manifestation of malignancy occurred during a period of severe and intensive life stress, frequently involving loss, separation and other bereavements."

From 1946 to 1964, Dr. Caroline V. Thomas collected physical and psychological profiles of 1337 medical students from Johns Hopkins University, trying to ascertain whether there was a cancer-prone personality. She kept track of the students by yearly questionnaires, noting the cause of death for each. She found that cancers tended to develop in people who were generally quiet, nonaggressive, and emotionally contained. These were generally low-key patients seldom prone to outbursts of emotion. This finding was further confirmed by the women who were admitted to the hospital for suspected or confirmed cancer of the ovary, uterus, cervix, and vagina. He compared them to women who had no suspected cancer. Doctor Mastrovito found that women who were diagnosed as having cancer were much more comforting, less adventurous, less assertive, less competitive, and less spontaneous than those women in the noncancer group. This study was done before the cancer diagnosis was made, so that the stress which might accompany knowledge of the disease was not present in either group. Doctor Mastrovito's observations were supported by those of Dr. S. Greer, who found that breast cancer patients demonstrated an abnormal release of emotions, particularly suppression of anger. In other words, these patients all had something in common, and that was that their reaction to stress was denial, a bottling up of feelings and generally poor coping skills.[24]

Using these concepts, Drs. Klaus and Margorie Bahnson have developed a questionnaire which covers topics such as the loss and reaction to loss of relatives by death, stress, recent life changes, personality characteristics, and means of handling stress. They feel that this diagnostic tool will allow screening for potential cancer victims early, while effective treatment is still practical and available.

This approach is being used at the cancer treatment center established by Harold and Stephanie Simonton. Doctor Simonton, a trained oncologist,* has found that coping skills, stress reduction, and mental imagery all play a powerful role in improving the treatment benefit of traditional cancer treatment.[25]

Doctors Lawrence Sklar and Hymie Anisman have found that in mice the growth of a particular cancer type is encouraged by stress, and the tumor growth can be reduced by developing coping skills in the animals.[26] This confirms many of the human studies which relate stress reduction, coping skills, and the prevention of cancer. It seems essential then that part of a proper approach to cancer would be the developing of coping skills and anxiety-release mechanisms and that an effective program would deal both with physical, or somatic, problems and mental problems.

Ultraviolet Radiation and Sunlight

One other interesting area, which is not directly related to nutrition, but rather to the environment in a more general sense, is the relationship between the exposure to various wavelengths of light and the development or prevention of cancer. It is well known that excessive exposure to ultraviolet radiation, such as comes from sunbathing, exposure to sunlight at high altitudes, or ultraviolet lights, can cause genetic damage to the DNA and trigger skin cancer. We therefore view ultraviolet light as being a potential carcinogenic agent. We recommend that sunbathing be limited and that when it is done, proper ultraviolet blocking agents be used to mask the ultraviolet portion of the light spectrum and prevent it from reaching the skin. Fortunately, today there are many good skin creams which contain these blocking agents and allow people to be exposed to sunlight without fear of excessive ultraviolet light exposure.

There is also another important role that light plays in the prevention of cancer. In a very interesting article, Drs. Cohen, Lippman, and Chapner looked critically at the agents that initiated development of breast cancer and found that cancer of the breast may be related in part to the underproduction of a hormone which comes from deep within the brain, called melatonin.[27] Melatonin is secreted from a portion of the brain called the pineal gland. This hormone then travels in the bloodstream to ultimately influence the ovaries, causing them to shut down their estrogen production. It is well known that women who oversecrete estrogen have a higher risk of breast, ovarian, and uterine cancer than women who secrete lower levels of estrogen. Interestingly enough, it is known that chlorpromazine, which is a medication used to manage psychiatric patients, will raise blood melatonin levels, and there are reports which indicate that female psychiatric patients who are treated with this drug have a much lower incidence of breast cancer. Melatonin has been shown in animal studies to inhibit tumor growth, and impaired secretion of melatonin seems to be an important factor in triggering precocious puberty and early menstruation, which are both risk factors for breast cancer. Lastly, it is known from many studies that hyperestrogenism, or an overproduction of estrogen, is associated with a low blood level of melatonin and an increased risk of breast cancer. The important question is then how does one stimulate the production of melatonin from the pineal? The answer to that has been recently suggested by Dr. John Ott, a well-known photobiologist, who published a very provocative and intriguing book called *Light and Health*, in which he postulates that exposure to full-spectrum light has an important influence on the endocrine system and reduces the risk of many diseases, including cancer.[28] For some time Dr. Ott's hypothesis was not confirmed by other scientists, but recently several investigators have confirmed that the retina can, when stimulated by the proper wavelength of light, synthesize melatonin directly or transfer the message to the pineal where melatonin can be synthesized. Doctors William Gern and Charles Ralph have found that exposure of the eye to the proper wavelength of light will encourage melatonin synthesis directly by the retina; however, this does not preclude the possibility that melatonin synthesis from the pineal is also important.[29]

The conclusion drawn by Drs. Cohen, Lippman, and Chapner is that environmental lighting, or what Dr. Ott calls malillumination, can prohibit proper secretion of me-

---

*An oncologist is a medical doctor whose specialty is the treatment of cancer with chemotherapeutic agents.

latonin, which then leads to hyperestrogenism in women, overstimulating receptors in the breast, uterus, and ovaries and setting the stage for potential transformed cells or cancer. In a way, light of the proper type can be looked on as a nutrient.

Malillumination is the result of our spending more and more time under the type of fluorescent lights which lack that portion of the sun's spectrum which is important in triggering melatonin secretion. As we have moved indoors and have put over our eyes coverings which do not transmit these wavelengths of light, such as eyeglasses, sunglasses, or window glass, we have gotten less and less exposure to this portion of the spectrum, called the "near ultraviolet" (a violet-colored light). We have changed our hormone balances as a result of the lack of stimulation by these wavelengths. Doctor Ott recommends strongly that people expose their eyes to full-spectrum transmitting material. One such material is Armolite plastic, which you can request from your optometrist for prescription lenses. Full-spectrum fluorescent lights are also available for working environments or schools. Photobiology and its relationship to human diseases such as cancer remains an active area of research. There is convincing evidence at this point to strongly urge us to seek environments in which we will be exposed to full-spectrum light for a greater portion of each day.

By implementing the various preventive approaches that have been mentioned, as much as a 50 percent reduction in the risk of cancer might be achieved. The management of nutrition and body weight, stress, exposure to ionizing radiation (such as x-rays and ultraviolet light), prudent selection of drugs and medication, avoiding additive-rich foods of unknown and suspected toxicity, and working hard for cleaner air and water, when all put together create a vision of a society with a diminishing cancer risk. The impact of this change upon our health care system and society in general, in terms of both cost efficiency and reduced anguish, cannot begin to be measured. At this time, such an approach represents the most cost-efficient way of approaching cancer, and is the closest thing we presently have to a victory in the "war against cancer." If we are not willing to pay the price of giving up such habits as smoking, excess alcohol consumption, and excessive high-meat, high-fat dietary intakes, then we should not unload the responsibility for our society's cancers on the shoulders of the physicians, who are doing the best they can given our present state of knowledge.

Most of us would go out of our way to find the recipe which would allow us to increase our opportunity of winning in life by a factor of two. Such a recipe for winning the battle against cancer by preventing it has now become much better known. The solution comes not from intellectualizing the problem, but from applying it to our own lives.

Notes

1. For an excellent discussion of this topic see Dr. Elizabeth Whelan, *Preventing Cancer* (New York: W. W. Norton, 1978).
2. E. Alcantara and E. W. Spockmann, "Diet, Nutrition and Cancer," *American Journal of Clinical Nutrition* (September, 1976), pp. 1035–1047.
3. G. Hopkins and C. West, "Possible Role of Dietary Fats in Carcinogenisis," *Life Sciences* 19 (1976), pp. 1103–1116.
4. J. Hankin and V. Rawlins, "Diet and Breast Cancer: A Review," *American Journal of Clinical Nutrition* (November, 1978), pp. 2005–2016.
5. E. R. Gonzalez, "Vitamin E Relieves Most Cystic Breast Disease," *Journal of the American Medical Association* (September 5, 1980), pp. 1077–1079.
6. D. Harman, "Free Radical Theory of Aging: Effect of the Amount and Degree of Unsaturation of Dietary Fat on Mortality Rate," *Journal of Gerontology* 26 (1971), pp. 451–457.
7. D. Burkitt, "Effect of Dietary Fibre on Stools and Transit Times Audits Role in the Causation of Disease," *The Lancet* (December 30, 1972), p. 1229.
8. J. Cairns, "The Cancer Problem," *Scientific American* (June, 1978), pp. 64–78.
9. R. H. Adamson, "Occurrence of a Primary Carcinoma in a Rhesus Monkey Fed Aflatoxin B-1," *Journal of the National Cancer Institute* 50 (1973), p. 549.
10. R. Raineri and J. H. Weisburger, "Reduction of Gastric Carcinogens with Ascorbic Acid," *Annals of the New York Academy of Sciences* 258 (1975), p. 181.
11. E. Cameron and L. Pauling, "Clinical Trial of High Dose Ascorbic Acid Supplements in Advanced Human Cancer," *Chemico-Biological Interactions* 9 (1974), p. 285.
12. R. Samberger, "Possible Inhibitory Effect of Selenium on Human Cancer," *Canadian Medical Association Journal* 100 (1969), p. 682.
13. G. N. Schrauzer, "Selenium and Cancer: a Review," *Bioinorganic Chemistry* 5 (1976), pp. 275–281.
14. G. Greeder and J. A. Milner, "Factors Influencing the Inhibitory Effect of Selenium on Mice Inoculated with Ehrlich Ascites Tumor Cells," *Science* 209 (August 15, 1980), pp. 825–827.
15. E. Seifter, "Of Stress, Vitamin A and Tumors," *Science* (July 2, 1976), pp. 74–75.
16. E. Bjelke, "Vitamin A and Lung Cancer," *International Journal of Cancer* 15 (1975), pp. 561–565.
17. A. Morrison and J. Buring, "Artificial Sweetners and Cancer of the Lower Urinary Tract," *New England Journal of Medicine* (March 6, 1980), pp. 537–541; E. Wynder and S. Stellman, "Artificial Sweetner Use and Bladder Cancer," *Science* (March 14, 1980), pp. 1214–1217.
18. R. Hoover, "Saccharin—Bitter Aftertaste?" *New England Journal of Medicine* (March 6, 1980), pp. 573–574.
19. R. S. Rivlin, "Riboflavin and Cancer: A Review," *Cancer Research* 33 (1973), p. 1977.
20. N. Cousins, "Anatomy of an Illness," *New England Journal of Medicine* (1974).
21. H. Seyle, "The Evolution of the Stress Concept," *American Scientist* 61 (1973), p. 692.
22. V. Riley, "Mouse Mammary Tumors: Alteration of Incidence as Apparent Function of Stress," *Science* 189 (1975), p. 465.
23. D. Spackman, "The Role of Stress in Producing Corticosterone Levels and Thymus Inactivation in Mice," *XIth International Cancer Congress* 3 (1974), p. 382.
24. L. LeShan, "Psychological States as Factors in the Development of Malignant Disease: a Critical Review," *Journal of the National Cancer Institute* 22 (1959), p. 1
25. J. Rabkin and E. L. Struening, "Life Events, Stress, and Illness," *Science* (December 3, 1976), pp. 1013–1020.
26. L. Sklar and H. Anisman, "Stress and Coping Factors Influence Tumor Growth," *Science* (August 3, 1979), pp. 513–516.
27. M. Cohen, M. Lippman, and B. Chapner, "Role of Pineal Gland in Aetiology and Treatment of Breast Cancer," *The Lancet* (October 14, 1978), pp. 814–816.
28. John Ott, *Light and Health* (New York: Bantam, 1975).
29. W. A. Gern and C. L. Ralph, "The Melatonin Synthesis by the Retina," *Science* (April 13, 1979), pp. 183–186.

JEFFREY BLAND, *Ph.D., is professor of nutritional biochemistry at the University of Puget Sound and the director of the Bellevue-Redmond Medical Laboratory. He has authored two books on nutrition for the medical profession, and is currently director of the Laboratory of Nutritional Supplement Analysis at the Linus Pauling Institute in Palo Alto.*

A Quiet Revolution: Holistic Nursing

Susan Luck, R.N.,
and Shelly Kellman

A FTER THREE months as a nurse at the New York State Psychiatric Institute, I felt like *I* was going crazy. I worked the evening shift on a depression ward. The patients had admitted themselves to the hospital in search of the latest anti-depressant drug to lift their spirits and help them through another day. I worked as part of a research team dispensing medication and monitoring the side effects of these powerful drugs. In the evenings, when the patients were afraid of sleep and its dreams, we would talk. As a nurse, I was able to provide a comfort no pill could replace. Over time, trust was established and the patients would share their fears, anxieties and frustrations—often wondering if they would feel "normal" again.

The windowless green corridors between locked doors comprised an oppressive environment in which it was difficult to achieve a feeling of well-being. In my nursing judgment, some changes could be made.

Not long after I arrived, I began an evening activity offering relaxation techniques integrating yoga stretches, deep breathing, and guided imagery. Patients learned to envision their bodies relaxing and imagine themselves in a peaceful, safe place, often falling asleep before their customary request for a sleeping pill. One evening, we decided to have a tea party and I took the opportunity to bring in some chamomile tea, a well-known mild calmative and relaxant herb. That night, I didn't need to distribute as many Seconals, and in the morning, the patients did not experience the typical medication hangovers. "For the first time in years, I don't feel like a zombie," Sophie, 56, told me when I arrived the next day.

The patients were thrilled, but the nursing department and medical staff were not. When I arrived on the ward, I was quickly taken aside and told that I "had no right to bring strange herbs onto the ward . . . and furthermore, the

chemical properties could interfere with our drug studies." I wondered why they never used that logic when giving orders to liberally dispense antacids, laxatives, aspirins, antibiotics, cortisone, muscle relaxants, and narcotic sleeping pills. Almost every patient took several of these pills daily just to counteract the side effects of the mood-altering drugs. I didn't know whether to laugh or scream or cry as I filled out incident reports on the chamomile tea in triplicate.

Not long after that, word got out that I was discussing nutrition with the patients. As I watched them eat sugar with their meals and in between, waiting eagerly for daily visits from the candy cart, I began talking about diet with a few patients who wanted more control over their lives. Their craving for sweets was encouraged in cooking classes where they learned to make Jell-O and Betty Crocker brownies. Several people were eager to learn more about the connection between sugar and depression, so I brought them some books. One afternoon, the chief research doctor approached me and paternalistically admonished me for disseminating "disinformation." He said that there was no scientific evidence of a connection between sugar—or any food for that matter—and how we feel. So I watched the patients continue to eat their starchy, processed hospital foods, snacking on candy bars and drinking Coca-Cola while taking their pills as they wondered why they had no control over their emotions.

I was beginning to be seen as a trouble-maker by the medical research team and the nursing department. My innovations were not appreciated, and the reaction seemed to be, *"Who does she think she is? After all, she is only a nurse."* I resigned shortly thereafter.

"The Doctor Is Right"

This experience, far from being unusual, is typical of the restrictions placed on nurses since the earliest days of the modern doctoring and nursing professions in this country.

From *Whole Life Times*, June 1983. 18 Shepard Street, Brighton, MA 02135. Reprinted by permission.

"The doctor is always right," Dr. William Richardson told the graduating class of the Boston Training School for Nurses in 1886. "Always be loyal to the physician," he added, warning nurses not to be "tempted" to impress the doctor with their knowledge because "what error could be more stupid?"

Beneath a veneer of health-service jargon and specialized job titles, Richardson's outlook is still held—and enforced—by an astounding number of doctors, hospital administrators, and nursing supervisors. Yet both the education and the legal responsibilities of the nurse have changed drastically. Thirty years ago, nursing teachers still told nurses their role was to help the doctor; now, at least in four-year college programs, nurses are taught to be *patient advocates*, whose role is to ensure quality patient care. A nurse can be held liable for following a doctor's order she knows is wrong—giving a drug to a person who's allergic to it, for example. This means speaking up, even arguing with doctors if necessary.

"As the person who knows the patient best, physically and emotionally, the nurse is responsible for requesting and getting the appropriate medical interventions: not just *reporting* what's going on with the patient, but *following through*," says Jenny Ginsberg, R.N., 27, a clinical nurse in Boston, Massachusetts. The nurse may have to take her case up the chain of command until someone takes appropriate action. In such rare instances, a nurse can be held liable in a malpractice suit for failing to press her point.

Nurses are also legally responsible for areas of care that have no connection with doctors. "For example, 'bed rest' can lead to terrible skin breakdown and sores," explains Ginsberg, "and we have got to prevent such complications, even if the patient is too 'out of it' to report discomfort."

Escape from 'General Hospital'

Few members of the public imagine that nurses exercise such responsibility and discretion, unless they learn through an extended hospital stay. Nurses are portrayed in soap operas, films, pornography, and romance novels as mindless, helpless, gossipy sex objects, hopelessly in love with some doctor, patient, or professional man.

"I spend a lot of time explaining how nurses are not who the popular images have portrayed us to be," says Gail Clark, R.N., 33. "As patients, people see us providing essential care. Then they turn on *General Hospital* and see the nurse grabbing the doctor in the linen closet!"

Today, nurses who are frustrated with distorted images and narrow definitions of both healing and their own roles are taking action on several fronts: They are looking outside the familiar medical model for alternatives, and in doing so are rediscovering nursing's roots in the centuries-old tradition of women lay healers, herbalists, and midwives. They are looking to holistic and preventive medicine for a focus on health as wellness instead of as absence of disease, and for techniques and strategies to help people achieve wellness. They are turning to each other for support and counseling instead of competing for status and promotions. And they are organizing as a labor force.

Nursing's Holistic Roots

The centuries-old tradition of nursing promotes health and the prevention of disease. Nursing is based on understanding the needs of the whole person: not only physically, but emotionally, environmentally, socially, culturally, and spiritually. "Preventive health is more important than curative," wrote Florence Nightingale, founder of modern nursing, in *Notes on Nursing* (1859). "Nursing the well is more important than nursing the sick."

Prior to 1910 most nurses were effective independent practitioners emphasizing public and preventive health in the community, educating and improving the quality of life. They went into homes and worked with families on child care, nutrition, and the relationship between illness and sanitation practices; and at the turn of the century, they spearheaded a public-health movement demanding better sanitation in the rapidly growing urban areas. But with the establishment of medicine as a regulated profession requiring expensive university training, women were effectively barred from all forms of healing. The last competition was halted in 1919, when midwives became illegal in all but remote rural areas. Through a flurry of state medical licensing laws, doctors became the only legal health practitioners, relegating nurses to the newly established hospital system.

Between 1900 and 1910, 1,652 hospitals were created. Hospitals continue to be the major providers of health-care policy, education, and research. Today, this profit-making empire consumes 10 percent of the gross national product, with a 15 percent annual growth rate, yielding profits higher than steel or oil.

Nursing has always been the largest health-care profession: Hospital-staff registered nurses (R.N.s) and licensed practical nurses (L.P.N.s) outnumbered staff doctors and dentists 16 to one in 1981, according to the American Hospital Association. Patients are hospitalized primarily to receive nursing care, not medical care; if all goes as planned, the doctor will see less and less of the patient as s/he is nursed back to health. Yet, by 1972, the average physician's income of $46,000 was five times the salary of the average general-duty nurse, according to a study by Kathleen Cannings and William Lazonick, published in the *International Journal of Health Services* in 1975. "[T]he major source of the high profits and incomes of the elite of the health industry lies in the labor of the nursing labor force," Cannings and Lazonick conclude emphatically.

A Lack of Support

Today there are nearly 1.7 million R.N.s in the United States, 65 percent of them providing direct patient care, according to the American Nurses Association (ANA). Some 76 percent of licensed R.N.s are practicing nursing—a high percentage for a woman-dominated field, says the ANA. Yet Linda Laurreano, president of the New York chapter of Nurses in Transition, a national self-help and support organization, observes, "Many nurses come here searching for new careers. Most of them really want to be nurses," she adds, "but they can no longer work in the stressful, oppressive hospital environment."

Ada Jacox, R.N., of the University of Maryland, cites five major reasons why nurses leave the profession: the stressful nature of the work; lack of control over the work environment; disenchantment with the quality of care; lack of respect from the physician; and salary levels. A 1981 New Jersey survey of 22,000 nurses confirmed that these were the major complaints.

"When I took initiative and used my creative energies there was no support or recognition from the nursing department," says Clark, who's been practicing for eight years, of her recent resignation from a major New York teaching hospital. "I felt assertiveness by nurses was still discouraged by the administration; and following doctors' orders, without question, was still the major game plan. When I set up a program in collaboration with the social-work department to counsel the families of terminal cancer patients, I was told by my department I'd have to do it on my own time."

Leslie, 26, graduated from an innovative university program last June. She began her first job at a city hospital, idealistic and enthusiastic about implementing her new skills, but after six months she was considering leaving not only her job but the profession. "I entered nursing after working for several years in a non-service profession. I want to help people, but my day is filled with menial tasks and paperwork. Sometimes at the end of the day, I realize that I did not have time to sit and talk to any of my frightened, needing patients, which would have probably been more therapeutic than any of the anti-anxiety pills I spent my hours dispensing and signing for in triplicate." When Leslie looked to her nursing administration for guidance, she was told, "You are no longer a student. This is the real world, and the best way to do your job is to get your work done."

Getting Closer

Leslie might find more of what she's looking for in one of several hospitals around the nation using primary nursing, an innovative approach. Instead of having layers of R.N.s and L.P.N.s, and nurses aides, each performing certain tasks for all patients on the unit, primary care assigns one R.N. per shift to be responsible for the complete care of particular patients for the duration of their hospital stay.

"This means that one person on each shift really gets to *know* each patient," says Jenny Ginsberg, who works in a primary-care system at Boston's Beth Israel Hospital. (She is not a spokesperson for the hospital.) "I change the sheets, help bathe the person, help them eat, the works. When you're doing all that, as well as monitoring the vital signs, administering medication, and so forth, you get very familiar with what's normal for that person. Any problems that crop up—say an infection that's brewing—will be noticed more quickly by an R.N. who's very familiar with this patient than by someone who only goes into that room to hand out medication.

"It's the difference between spending three hours a day with the patient, and spending 15 minutes," Ginsberg continues. "A lot of it is intuition, and I find that is respected where I work."

Instead of meeting three or four people on a shift, patient and family have a chance to develop a continuing relationship and a great deal of trust in three individuals. Last year, Ginsberg was primary nurse for a woman in her early 80s during three hospital stays over a six-month period, from the first admission when she was diagnosed as having terminal cancer, until a couple of hours before her death. The woman's only living relative, a nephew, later said: "I always thought hospitals were the worst places for people to die, but this is the best place she could have been. She felt safe here."

Since the system was instituted at Beth Israel in 1978, "newly graduated nurses, who formerly quit after a few months, stay two-and-a-half to five years," Joyce Clifford, vice president of nursing, told the *New York Times* (December 27, 1981).

Primary nursing is not a panacea, though. The key element—a close, continuous relationship between nurse and patient—could be provided in other systems as well. And more important to most nurses than any job structure is the respect and support given to their judgment.

Education Leaps Forward

In 1968, Martha Rogers, R.N., M.P.H., D.Sc., of New York University's nursing faculty, innovated a new nursing theory. It's a holistic model, rooted in the understanding that a person is a unified whole who (contrary to the "medical model") cannot be accounted for in terms of biology and physics alone. Rogers views people as "energy fields" and defines dis-ease as "imbalance"; for her, the positive goal of nursing is for patients to achieve a state of wellness. Although considered "far out" in 1968, Rogers' model, as elaborated in her popular text, *An Introduction to the Theoretical Basis of Nursing* (F.A. Davis Co., Philadelphia, 1970) is commonly used in university programs here and abroad, according to Jean Mathwig, Ph.D., Dean of Nursing at NYU.

Another NYU professor, Dolores Krieger, R.N., Ph.D., has introduced "therapeutic touch" (TT) to thousands of nurses. This technique also views the human organism as an "energy field" (a basic law in Eastern medicine and philosophy). Krieger believes the symptoms of illness appear when the energy flow is disrupted, depleted, or out of balance. Healers, placing their hands strategically, can sense blocks and redirect the energy flow. This is helpful whether the disruption is caused by bacteria, injury, stress, dietary imbalance, or anything else. Anyone can be a healer, Krieger believes, with the intention and commitment to help.

Therapeutic touch is by far the most popular holistic technique among mainstream nurses—not surprisingly, since it's really a systematic expression of something nurses have always done quite naturally. "Our society is a no-touch culture," Krieger points out, "but nurses are a notable exception. We are allowed intimacies no other profession is allowed." In some hospitals, according to Dr. Margaret McClure, nurses use TT quietly, without doctors' approval; but recent research has documented such convincing evidence of physiological response that some doctors now prescribe it for their patients.

Body/Mind Release

I worked with this technique several years ago at Alta Bates Hospital in Berkeley, California. One of my patients was a woman who experienced tightness in her chest, which became a feeling of suffocation whenever she was afraid. Admitted to the hospital with chest pains, she became increasingly fearful, which made her condition worse. One day as I assisted her with her morning bath, she remembered the first time this happened. I gently placed my hand over her upper chest, and encouraged her to take some slow deep breaths while visualizing her muscles relaxing. She recalled the first time she had held her breath when she saw a frightening incident through her child's eye. Meanwhile, I felt the area getting warmer. I focused my attention and the energy in my hands on the tension I could feel in her muscles. Suddenly she began to breathe more easily and began to cry. Within minutes, her pain subsided, and for the first time in months she was able to breathe freely without pain.

"What holistic nurses are trying to do is renew and enhance the art of nurturing and caring for the whole person, which can take many forms in many places," says Charlotte McGuire, R.N., founder and president of the American Holistic Nurses Association (AHNA). "Nurses are *definitely* moving into holistic health," she feels. AHNA has grown to 800 members in two years.

"But we don't want to be a huge organization," she emphasizes. AHNA's purpose is to provide education and a support network for nurses moving in holistic directions, particularly by gaining scientific, academic credibility for holistic theories and techniques. In April, for example, AHNA sponsored a conference at Old Dominion University in Virginia Beach, Virginia, at which an eclectic mix of about 40 scientific papers were presented, including *Adolescents, Alcoholism, & Sexuality; Visual Imagery of the Death Experience; Evaluation of Routine Birth Experience through a Study of Episiotomies; Application of the Cayce Theory to Holistic Nursing*; and *Providing Holistic Nursing Care to Battered Women*.

Educational centers like Interface Foundation of Newton, Massachusetts, and Omega Institute of Lebanon Springs, New York, report that nurses are a loyal and growing constituency. Omega's holistic-health workshops have attracted so many nurses that Omega now occasionally offers a workshop titled "The New Nursing" especially for nurses to learn and share information and support about moving toward a holistic path. And in response to popular demand, both NYU and the Skill Bureau in New York City have introduced holistic-health courses as part of their continuing education programs, where nurses earn the ongoing credits they need to stay licensed.

Moving Beyond Hospital Walls

Some nurses who are frustrated with hospital parameters are going into private practice. Most states have "nursing-practice acts" that allow nurses to hang out their shingles independently, but exactly what they are permitted to do is hazily defined. Most states give nurses the right to teach prevention, public health, sanitation, and nutrition, and to "help further a course of treatment" that a doctor has prescribed. But diagnosis and prescribing treatment are out. The ambiguity of the laws leaves plenty of room for someone who doesn't like what an independent nurse is doing, or standing for, in the community to haul her into court for "practicing medicine without a license."

"There's an old joke that your mother can give you an aspirin and it's OK, but if a nurse gives you an aspirin, she's practicing medicine," says one private-practice R.N. from New York. "Seriously, though, if a client comes to me, and I determine the problem is constipation and suggest an herbal laxative, I could get sued for both diagnosing and prescribing. On the other hand, if I say this person is suffering from 'obstruction of the bowel,' that's perfectly legal as part of my 'nursing assessment.'"

Then what can she do to help the client? "Interpreting the law narrowly, I'm supposed to send that person to a doctor, who would probably give X-rays and tests to determine if the blockage was something else—a mass or a tumor, for instance."

A Practice of Her Own

Becoming a nurse-practitioner (N.P.) appeals to some nurses as a way of gaining independence, as well as more skills. N.P. certification requires a year of training beyond the R.N. degree in areas including medical diagnosis and treatment, pathological physiology, and pharmacology. The training was designed to prepare nurses to be the only health professionals in rural areas and poor urban neighborhoods that don't appeal to doctors; in these locations, nurses "practice medicine" unchallenged. But the laws in most states still regard N.P.s and R.N.s as the same. At a physician's discretion, either can do virtually everything doctors do.

In physicians' offices and hospital clinics where N.P.s and doctors do perform the same functions, patients often prefer the N.P.s—who, they say, spend more time explaining things, offering options, and counseling. This situation has also led to understandable complaints by nurses that—while they enjoy their expanded role—physicians are profiting from their labor.

The specter of an independent nursing profession in direct competition with physicians is a major factor that has held back legal independence for nurses regardless of their credentials. In ongoing state legislative battles, many bills have been introduced with broad community support to expand and protect areas of health care that nurses can practice on their own. State medical associations, in turn, lobby or present opposing bills to keep all nurses "under doctors' supervision."

It would be a mistake to think that N.P.s simply want to function like doctors. A different outlook, revitalizing the original public-health role of the nurse, is at work.

Judy Lane, R.N.N.P., has a private practice while maintaining a job at an ambulatory medical clinic at a major teaching hospital. She compares her roles: "At the hospital a patient walks in with symptoms. The reason they were manifested on any given day is probably stress-related; but all the hospital is interested in is the pathology, ordering tests and medication. I have no time to deal with the underlying problems that are going on in their lives. I think that is the basic ingredient that most nurses feel is lacking in hospital care. In my practice in preventive health and stress management, I can evaluate the person's lifestyle and the interaction of the body with the mind in the context of the environment. Together we can come up with a plan."

"Not long ago, I was working with an asthmatic child in the clinic where I work," says Martha, a community-health nurse and shiatsu practioner. (Shiatsu is an Oriental system of pressure-point massage.) "He was not improving, and when I did a follow-up visit with his mother, I discovered that there was no heat in the apartment, and that paint and plaster were falling into his bed at night. My holistic-nursing approach was to help the family write letters to the appropriate housing authorities."

"A basic concept is 'I do have control over my life,'" Lane affirms. "The major problem that I see in the medical model is that people are encouraged to feel helpless and not to get involved in making choices in their lives. Instead, they surrender to this system and take a pill. But I see a shift. People are learning that they have a choice."

Many nurses feel that now is the time to become more politically aware and involved. "We're the largest female occupational group in the nation (97 percent women), but we have no political influence as a constituency," Ginsberg notes. The ANA has none of the influence of the AMA; and only a small percentage of nurses are members. Once competitive, isolated, and even suspicious of each other, nurses are uniting in a variety of new organizations. (See resource list.)

Traditionally, nurses have been caught in a conflict between taking a stand for their own rights and remaining totally dedicated to their patients. Many now feel that this dedication, and their "professional" title, have been manipulated by hospital administrations to keep them a low-status, uninfluential work force. As one nurse reminded her co-workers, "Doctors have always been organized; that is how they got their power. They call it the AMA. If we want a voice, we need to organize."

"I used to think that joining a union was lowering my professional status, but now I realize it is the only way to achieve it," says a nurse who recently participated in a strike at a Poughkeepsie, New York, hospital.

In 1960, 8,000 nurses belonged to unions; today, there are 150,000 unionized nurses, or 17.3 percent of hospital-employed R.N.s. An *R.N.* magazine survey of 13,000 nurses last November found that 50 percent were pro-union. Yet this issue continues to be a controversial and difficult decision for many nurses.

A key issue in a recent successful union drive at a major New York hospital was budget-cutting layoffs of nurses who were close to receiving pensions after 10 years of service. Now, after joining hospital workers Local 1199, "I have a written contract and an incentive to stay at the hospital, which will affect the quality of patient care and cut hospital costs for training new nurses," says one nurse there. "It appears that everyone benefits."

"Nurses can exert a tremendous positive influence but to make changes they must assert themselves in the political arena," declares Susan Talbot, R.N., a board member of New York State Nurses for Political Action, which believes that nurses must participate in determining the nation's future health-care priorities and plans. Dr. Mathwig agrees, and is positive that this will happen. "As nurses participate in legislative actions, while nursing education continues to build on a growing body of knowledge and professional skills, they are going to play a major role in promoting maximum health potential over the next decade," she prophesies. "Social, political, and economic forces are on our side because it costs too much to be ill."

As we move into a new era for fulfilling human needs, it is again time for the Lady with the Lamp to light the way. . . .

To Learn More

American Holistic Nurses Association, Box 116, Telluride, CO 81435; (303) 728-4575.

Cassandra: Radical Feminist Nurses Network, P.O. Box 341, Williamsville, NY 14221-0341.

New York State Nurses for Political Action, 500 Fifth Avenue, Suite 1625, New York, NY 10036; (212) 391-1110.

Nurse Healers Professional Associates Cooperative, Box 7, 70 Shelley Avenue, Port Chester, NY 10573.

Nurses Environmental Health Watch, 655 Avenue of the Americas, New York, NY 10010.

Nurses In Transition, Inc., P.O. Box 14472, San Francisco, CA 94114; (415) 282-7999.

SUSAN LUCK *R.N. B.S., has worked for 15 years in a wide variety of health settings ranging from psychiatric nursing in inner city hospitals to public health in Central America.*

She maintains a private practice in preventive and holistic health counseling, and created the Omega Institute's workshop, "The New Nursing." She is co-founder of the nursing newsletter 21st-Century Nurse, *and is a free-lance journalist writing about health and politics for* The Whole Life Times, Journal of the World Peace Council, *and other publications.*

She is currently a Masters candidate in Medical Anthropology at The New School for Social Research in New York City.

SHELLY KELLMAN *is a journalist, author, and photographer specializing in political, environmental, and health topics. Currently Senior Editor of* Whole Life Times, *she has held a variety of editorial positions there during the past four years. She is also a former* Earthwatch *editor of* New Age *magazine, and was collaborator with Jerry Teplitz on the book* Managing Your Stress; How to Relax and Enjoy *(Williamsburg, Virginia: Jerry Teplitz Enterprises, 1983). Her key concerns right now are ending U.S. intervention in Central America, and bringing about the conscious, egalitarian sharing of power among people in all areas of life, from government and social institutions to personal relationships.*

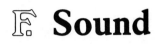 **Sound**

Tuning: The Power of Sound and Song: Self-Healing with Sound

Molly Scott

We trust that the magic of sound, scientifically applied, will contribute in ever greater measure to the relief of human suffering, to a higher development and a richer integration of the human personality, to the harmonious synthesis of all human 'notes', of all 'group cords and melodies', until there will be the great symphony of the One Humanity.

Roberto Assagoli, Psychosynthesis

How shall I begin my song
  in the blue night that is settling?
In the great night my heart will go out,
—toward me the darkness comes rattling.
In the great night my heart will go out.

Papago Medicine Woman Chant

I AM a musician—a composer and singer, a practitioner of the art of sound. Wondering at the power of music to affect me and the people for whom I sing, I began to investigate the nature of sound, the history of sound healing, the psychology of music. As a composer, I explored different forms of music, working with the feeling of different tones, textures, and intervals. As an inquiring human being, involved in spiritual practice and my own quest for understanding, I began to perceive, as so many of us have, that the threads of different knowledge systems are reaching toward each other in a webbed synthesis, confirming the truth of what Aldous Huxley called "The Perennial Philosophy": we are indeed all One, made of the same stuff, energy in constant change and motion. Flashes of insight come from many directions: Neuro-physiology, nonlinear dynamics, psycho-acoustics, psycho-biology—all confirm that we are part of the same pulsing, vibrational soup, infinitely diverse, yet connected in interdependent systems of pattern, order and process.

"Music is Love, in search of a word"—Sidney Lanier.

"In the beginning was the word," say the ancient texts. First was the sound, the Logos, then light, then form.

Hindu metaphysicians call AUM the sound power that gives birth to the many worlds of existence. Sound is the cause, not the effect, of vibration. In the metaphysical sense, it is the first principle, that which creates and destroys matter.

It is this meaning with which we work in exploring sound as a way of achieving psycho-physical harmony and healing. By "sound" we mean *potential* sound—harmonic overtones that may result from audible sound, but are experienced beyond the range of normal hearing.

If sound is the first principle, manifesting into form, then all forms can be translated back into sound. Hence all forms have their sound, their sacred name, their Bija mantra. The power of the word—long the province of the priest and the politician, the artist and the healer—is everyone's power when we appreciate its nature and its use. We are beginning to understand that what we image and give power to—what we name with will and intention in our mind/energy field, actually *exists*: can be photographed, measured, "seen" as reality. We begin to understand the "magic" of *our* power as receivers and transmitters of energy. The human being is perhaps the most magical instrument of all.

What happens to us, to this body/mind/spirit instrument, when we sing? The act of singing generates a concentrated "charge" in the psycho-physical system, resulting in more efficient use of the brain, better concentration, and higher states of awareness and receptivity. The deepened rhythmic breathing that singing requires, coupled with the higher acoustical frequencies which delineate song from speech, act to release physical and emotional stress by slowing and stabilizing the heartbeat and increasing the amount of oxygen in the bloodflow to the brain. The higher (more rapid and subtle) musical frequencies such as those generated by traditional forms of chanting (Hindu, Gregorian, Buddhist, Native American) create highly concentrated stimuli to the brain, opening resources of energy and vision not available to ordinary consciousness. Singing is like an internal massage, cleansing and vitalizing the system. In religious communities that include chanting as part of a daily regimen, it has been observed that people need fewer hours of sleep and lighter diet when they chant regularly.

NOISE POLLUTION

Shepherd Bliss

TRUCKS rumble. Planes roar. Sirens whine. Power lawnmowers whirl. Music blares. Dogs bark: city sounds, a typical day. Most of us adapt to these daily sounds, sometimes no longer hearing them—or so we think.

We sometimes escape to the country—birds singing, water flowing, wind in the tree tops, leaves rustling. We relax, and feel better. The typical sounds in today's cities are, simply enough, not healthy for human beings. So those who can, get away.

"Our society is driving itself crazy with noise," says Dr. Walter Carlin, Director of the Speech and Hearing Institute in Houston, Texas. "Noise pollution not only causes the loss of hearing, but triggers other physical ailments, stress in marriages, lack of sleep, and falling productivity." He concludes that too much noise "all in all makes our lives miserable." Dr. Carlin is one of many experts whose testimony was considered—along with extensive community input—by a committee of Berkeley citizens which met for over a year to draft local anti-noise legislation that is now pending before the city council.

Research shows that excessive noise can negatively

influence the nervous system, the endocrine system, the stomach and the emotions. Noise adversely affects the heart and blood vessels, contributing to high pressure and increases in cholesterol level. These effects are particularly evident in people who live near sources of loud noise: highways, airports, certain factories. Jim Buntin of the Center for Quiet Environment in Vallejo, California cites research indicating that people in airport noise zones tend to have more heart trouble, higher blood pressure, and more hearing problems than average.

In other words, noise can be deadly. Sudden noises, such as a car backfiring, can produce a jump in pulse rates and blood pressure, muscular contractions and changes in flow of digestive juices.

Dr. Carlin describes a typical walk in any metropolitan downtown area: "Take all that noise and let it bounce off one building to another and down to the pavement where you are walking. No wonder you are exhausted after a day of shopping. You are beaten down, you are irritable, your mental and physical health suffers." He reminds us, "Sound was used for centuries as a method of torture. Place a bell over a person's head and ring it, and eventually the person will go crazy."

Yet so many of us continue living in large, noisy

From *Whole Life Times*. Reprinted by permission.

The act of singing is an act of consciousness change. You cannot sing and stay depressed. "Singing the blues" changes your color scheme, raising you from the condition of pain that sparked the song to begin with. Song is a next step from wound to healing. To know this is in itself a powerful tool for working with yourself and others through sound and music. When we sing we are tuning ourselves as instruments to a higher energy field. We attune the frequencies of our bodies through the sounds we make in the same way that we tune the strings of our instruments.

This view of the human body as an instrument is a useful metaphor for discussing tuning the body and appreciating it as both a receiver and transmitter of sound/energy. To tune it, as one would tune a cello, requires that one view the body as a field of frequencies in different vibrational patterns—for example, frequency of elbow, frequency of earlobe, of knee, and so on. Every form in the universe has its own sound—the sound correlative of its composite vibrational patterns. When we use the voice to tune the body, although we may not be able to "hear" the sound patterns specific to the parts of the body, we can train ourselves to *feel* them and to know when a pattern is resonating in harmony with the rest of the body field. This is something we do all the time, unconsciously, and the

work with sound brings it into reach of our conscious intelligence and will.

In sound therapy, a body/mind in good health "plugs into" the energy systems around it, and, like a harp in the wind, resonates sympathetically with the natural universe. The person who is tune moves energy through the body like the crystal transmits light—to a greater or lesser extent, depending upon the degree of its clarity. When one is tuned and resonating clearly, one feels spacious, at ease, one piece, one Peace. We have all observed that in the presence of those who are truly at one with themselves, we also feel more easy, more spacious and centered. The operative principle here is the physical law that says a strong vibration will draw weaker, more chaotic ones into its field, and they will correct to its stronger pulse. The person who is strongly centered will also, like a well-tuned instrument, react with sympathetic resonance to the note you sound, allowing your particular vibration to find center, without being drawn away from its own essential tuning. When one centers and strengthens one's own vibrational patterns, one can draw strength and sustenance from the life system of which we are a part. We are not alone, and we cut ourselves off from the source of our own energies (like radio static) when we do not allow inspiration, lit-

urban concentrations—which offer jobs, entertainment, friends and excitement. Working to make these environments more healthy becomes necessary for comfort and survival.

Berkeley is one of a number of cities throughout the nation trying to combat the increasing noise problem through legislation and community education. In 1972 the U.S. Congress enacted the Noise Control Act; California followed in 1973. Some cities—such as Fresno; Anchorage, Alaska; and Norfolk, Virginia—have vigorous anti-noise ordinances.

Berkeley's pending legislation follows the California Department of Health's Model Community Noise Control Ordinance. Drafted by a citizens' committee with the help of the Community Health Advisory Committee, the twenty-page proposed law declares "that certain sound levels and vibrations are detrimental to the public health, welfare, safety and quality of life" and sets fines of $50 to $500 for violations.

People whose dogs bark loudly and consistently could be fined, as well as those using loud power tools.

Among the two dozen or so people at a January public hearing were Glenn Lynch, Director of Berkeley's Environmental Health Office and Ed Lowe, Director of California's Office of Noise Control. Community and neighborhood groups appeared on behalf of the ordinance. The committee also met resistance—particularly from University of California student groups like Inter-Fraternity Council (representing 38 fraternities), and local promoters of rock concerts (which would be regulated, but not banned, under the ordinance).

Anti-noise legislation like that pending in Berkeley is not forceful enough to touch the big noisemakers like industries and airports. Nevertheless, activists see these measures as important steps in legitimizing noise control as an environmental issue, making possible broader noise control in the future.

Unfortunately, just as interest is increasing in many localities, the U.S. Environmental Protection Agency's noise program has fallen victim to the Reagan cuts. The $13-million-a-year, fifty-person office had been studying the levels of noise created by various sources, documenting their psychological and physical effects, and had drafted Federal regulations to limit permissible noise output by garbage trucks, trains, tractor-trailer trucks, and portable air compressors. It was about to start doing the same for consumer items; and had its ideas received sufficient political and administrative backing, many types of equipment and products might have been redesigned to significantly reduce their noise output. This EPA department disappeared by October 1983.

Though an increasing problem in modern urban industrial society, noise is by no means unique to the twentieth century. The poet Decimus Junicus Juvenailis complained about conditions in ancient Rome: "Insomnia causes more deaths amongst Roman invalids than any other factor. Unbroken nights are a rich man's privilege."

SHEPHERD BLISS *is Editor of* The New Holistic Health Handbook.

---

erally, in-breathing, from the vibrational energies of the rest of creation.

One of the simple, elegant virtues of the act of singing is that it works with inspiration—the flow of the breath is the flow of the life force. Singing is like charging our batteries. In song we can make connection to deep levels of feeling and energy that are often difficult to reach from everyday consciousness.

"We are using some natural force which is not generally recognized yet"—Laurel Elizabeth Keyes.

In my practice, I work with some simple practices that can affect both general body tuning and specific areas of distress. You may wish to try them. In all work with sound, I suggest starting with eyes closed. There is evidence that the organs of vision "block" alpha waves and deeper states of consciousness. I also recommend that you do these exercises in a vertical position—standing or sitting with the spine straight, not lying down. Vertical posture helps blood and energy flow.

The technique that provides the basis for much of my work with sound is "the Siren Sound." This is a light, relaxed tone that moves from the lowest pitch that's com-

fortable to the highest, in a smooth, unbroken ribbon of sound. Imagine a child playing on the floor with a firetruck, making a sound like a siren or whistle, and you'll come close.

Laurel Elizabeth Keyes, whose *Toning* is a seed book for work with sound and health, says this practice "does not require one's belief. Apparently it is not a 'gift', but something available to anyone who goes through the mechanics of letting the voice express itself in a natural way. Toning is a very positive, consciously directed identification with the inner power of life, and the full awareness of the release of it at will."

Toning is an excellent way to start the day, to tune the body energy system for its optimum function. I recommend sounding in the shower, but be sure to tell your family or neighbors that you'll be making sounds, so they won't be alarmed! First and always, ground and center awareness in the breath. There are many practices to do this, but it can be as simple as planting your feet solidly and being aware of your connection with the ground—with the earth energy—and breathe it up through the feet. Keyes suggests raising the arms over the head and letting them down somewhat behind you, which raises and opens the rib cage so that the lungs have the maximum space in which to breathe. It is important always to acknowledge and be aware that the sounding moves from the breath.

The first step is a period of groaning sound release, a chance for the body to let off stress through the sound—whatever sound is appropriate to it at the moment. Once you are grounded and centered, begin to let the breath out with a sigh and then another, gradually making the sound more audible, imaging as you do so that all tensions and anxieties, known or unknown, are flowing away from you with the sound. The sound then takes whatever form it will until the body has sounded enough. Then the body will take a deep relaxed breath, which signals the end of that phase of the sounding. This is a time to let the body speak—to trust it and the sounds—not to let this experience be governed by the mind. Don't *think* about it, just *do* it. The body knows what it needs and will balance itself, given the opportunity. After you have groaned until you take that deep cleansing breath, you will feel released and relaxed. Don't force particular sounds—just let them come up, riding on the breath, and they will do the work.

The next step is to stand in a relaxed way, with the rib-cage expanded, and start the Siren Sound. This sound begins at the toes and moves easily up the body like a sound massage. At the top of your voice (never forcing, but feeling almost as if the sound were moving up the back, inside your spinal column, rather than coming from your mouth) let the sound fall, like a waterfall, back to the low point in the voice. The effect of doing this several times is like an internal massage and energizer. You are refreshed, relaxed, toned, tuned—a wonderful way to start the day.

The Siren Sound is a basic tool in my sound work. The more you do it, the more fluid it becomes, and the more sensitive you become to sound moving through your body. I have found that the siren exercise stretches the singing and speaking range. The lower you go in the voice, the higher you can go as well, and vice-versa. I use this exercise when I work with voice students. It is also a valuable tool for bridging the gap between speaking and singing that exists in most people's minds. It is often true that someone will proclaim that they "can't sing" and "have no range," but when asked to speak, moan, or siren different pitches, they will have no difficulty. It is the psychological construct that "singing" has for some of us that inhibits the possibility.

The Siren Sound can be used like a sonar scan, exploring the body for places that are in distress and in need of work, and honing in with the sound that matches frequencies in that area. You tone the sound as long as it feels good to do so. The working premise is grounded in a trust in the body to effect its own balance and healing. Through sound, you free the body to do its own work, so, in working with different parts of the body, you become familiar with the "feeling" as well as the sound that is "right." My colleague, Sarah Benson, describes this sensation as "the right sound calls to you." Keyes says that when she comes across a place in the body that needs work, it feels "sticky." The Siren Scan finds the sound, and as it is sung it takes on a wider dimension.

In group work, people are frequently astonished by the intensity and color of the sounds they make when their intentions have directed the sounds in this way. I have experienced sounds which felt to me as though they were flowing through me from another source, rather than being created by my own voice mechanism. Often people find themselves making sounds which they did not think they were capable of making. There is nothing surprising or particularly esoteric about this. Just as we use only a minute portion of the ability of our brains, so we limit ourselves constantly by the idea of what we can or cannot do with our voices. Many of us have experienced the childhood put-down by some teacher or well-meaning friend, who told us that we "can't sing," and thus stoppered this avenue of our expressive capacity. I don't believe in "not singing." The act of singing is a natural expression for the human being, and has little to do with current cultural expectations of art, or of what singing should be. Like Love, singing is an action that creates its own field of consciousness, and no one should be denied it.

In working with your own sound field, if you work with real trust in the body's wisdom—not forcing but letting the body make what sounds it needs to (as it does spontaneously in time of pain, grief, or joy)—then I am convinced that there can be no harm to the body system with this work. The key here, as in all energy work, is to stay clear, centered, and fluid; keep the energy moving through. It is when energy is blocked and cannot move, that conflict, stress and manifestations of dis-ease occur.

"We release health from within as a flower is released from the pattern in the seed"—Laurel Elizabeth Keyes.

In his seminal book, *Psychosynthesis*, Dr. Roberto Assagoli quotes Georges Duhamel, who, as a military surgeon during the first world war played his flute to keep his sanity: "I began to grasp that music would permit me to live. It could certainly not diminish the horror of the massacre, the suffering, the agonies; yet it brought to me, at the very center of the carnage, a breath of divine remission, a principle of hope and salvation. For a man deprived of the consolations of faith, music was nevertheless, a kind of faith, that is to say, something that upholds, reunites, revives, comforts. I was no longer forsaken. A voice had been given to me with which to call, to complain, to laud and to pray." ("La Musique Consolatrice" Monaco, Editions du Rocher, 1944)

In my Despair/Empowerment workshops, an environment is created in which the sorrow, pain, and fear for life in this threatened world are allowed a voice so that fresh vision and energy can arise, and people are freed to effective action. I invoke the ancient practice of *keening*—the body's way of grieving with sound. While keening, people are encouraged to hold their bodies, to rock, to cover their heads and let the body make the sounds of the emotions. Often, assuming the body position and making the sounds will allow deep emotions to surface. In the presence of such raw, gut sound, everyone is affected, not necessarily in the mind-knowing but in the body-knowing. The climate of grief and release creates the space for everyone to respond in some fashion, even if only to rock and breath and moan. The natural law at work here is, again, that a strong, centered vibration will draw less centered ones into its field. So, strongly expressed vibration in the form of sound/song will temper and harmonize other frequencies around it. Even reticent people who find it difficult to sound or sing will feel the change in body energy that results from the strong focus of the group sound.

A word here about keening and other strong soundings: we live in a society that is embarassed by the expression of emotion, and encourages repression of emotion as a virtue. Recent research correlates cognitive complexity—the ability to shift viewpoints and consider situations from multiple perspectives—with emotional range. In the shadow of the devitalizing fear that we all feel in the face of multiple scenarios of destruction of our world, it is imperative that we break this energy-blocking personal and cultural silence and release the flow of feelings that can lead us into new ways of seeing and acting. Theologian Harvey Cox, himself a musician, has said, "This is a time to be still no longer. This is a time for crying out, as Hebrews cried out in bondage, and Jesus on the cross. We need to give vent to our massive pain and fear. A people must move from muteness to outcry if they are ever going to take the next step."

People working with consciousness in this crisis must understand that music is important and how to use it. Yes, music provides relaxation and entertainment but what is that? Entertainment means "to hold the attention of; to hold in mind." The psycho-physiological condition that music can generate balances the spheres of the brain and creates a state in which information is received and assimilated with a higher degree of awareness, comprehension, and retention. In other words music, especially singing, enhances the chances that the information needing to be shared will be understood and remembered. Indeed, music is more than the after-dinner mints at the banquet: It is the main dish.

Music can draw on those deep resources of hope and strength common to us all—which are often, in these anxious days, beyond our conscious reach. We can speak, sound, and sing not to bandage pain, but to speak to the truths of what we all know: We are not so fragile as we fear. Our music is a testimony to our strength-in-connection. And this can give us hope in a complex and often fearsome world. We are not islands in isolation; we are open systems, instruments of energy. When we open to the flow of the web's energy, the web's music, we are part of the current of life, the real music of the spheres.

The flute of interior time is played whether we
Hear it or not,
What we mean by "love" is its sound coming in.
When love hits the farthest edge of excess, it
    reaches a wisdom.
And the fragrance of that knowledge!
It penetrates our thick bodies,
It goes through walls—
Its network of notes has a structure as if a million

Suns were arranged inside.
This tune has truth in it.
Where else have you heard a sound like this?
                    Robert Bly, "The Kabir Book"

Bibliography

Campbell, Don. *Introduction to the Musical Brain*. Magnamusic-Baton, Inc. 1983.
Capra, Fritjof. *The Tao of Physics*. Bantam, 1975.
Hamel, Peter Michael. *Through Music to the Self*. Shambala, 1976.
Keyes, Laurel Elizabeth. *Toning: the Creative Power of the Voice*. DeVorss, 1973.
Rudhyar, Dane. *The Magic of Tone and the Art of Music*. Shambala, 1982.
Zukav, Gary. *The Dancing Wu Li Masters*. Bantam, 1979.
"Hearing the Solar Winds"—a recording by The Harmonic Choir, LP 106 or Casette CS 106 (import).

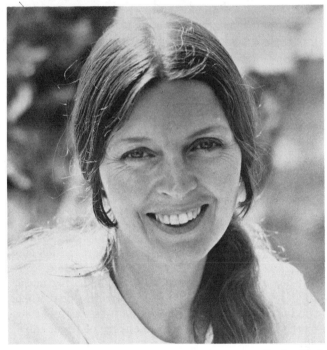

Sumitra Music

MOLLY SCOTT, *composer, singer and poet, has an extensive background in the performing arts and has focused her music and teaching work on issues of personal and planetary healing, disarmament, and peace. An eco-feminist and environmental activist, she creates music which "illuminates our connection with the earth and each other." She has hosted her own television and radio programs, founded the musical group SUMITRA, composed for the musical theater, and given workshops at centers around the country, including Omega Institute, Interface, and the New England Institute for the Healing Arts and Sciences. She is co-founder of the Heartsound Center for Music and Health in Charlemont, Massachusetts, and records for Philo/Fretless records. Her latest album is "Honor the Earth" with SUMITRA.*

Paul Winter—Enlivened by Music

Randy Lee Showstack

For Paul Winter, music is Vitamin M. It recharges him. It makes his spirit vibrate. "When you start to lose it," says this veteran soprano saxophonist, "make some music."

His music is a vibrant embrace of nature. The deep and jumpy sounds blown through the hollow of his sax are contagious and uplifting, meditative without being drowsy or wishy-washy.

His ten albums, recorded either solo or with the ever-shifting Paul Winter Consort, include "Common Ground," "Callings," "Missa Gaia," and the recent "Sunsinger." All told, they've sold over a half a million copies, and retell a myth of the deep, ancient calling back to inner and outer nature. Tapes of eagles, wolves, and whales often add to the pulse of the songs.

THROUGH CHANGES in the sound over more than 20 years of performing, Winter is still after a balance of improvisation and orchestration. His vision also has been constant: "to reawaken a humanism through sharing music with people." A shared enthusiasm often happens when he performs. "I've always thought that was a natural state for us to be in, that common experience of being enlivened."

Winter was born in Altoona, Pennsylvania, and by age six was studying piano, clarinet, and drums. As a teenager, he toured for one summer with the Ringling Brothers Circus Band. In 1961 his bebop group won the Intercollegiate Jazz Festival competition. That was the clincher that convinced him to shelve plans for law school, and pursue his music.

When Winter invited me to "Meanderland Farm," his 77-acre wood and farm land in Connecticut, I expected to finally meet the musician whose records had lifted my spirit, after I suffered a car accident not many years ago.

This balding 44-year-old man approached with a smile and a handshake. He had on a red shirt and purple drawstring pants. His thin hips and long legs seemed to contain some of the whimsicalness of a circus performer. Winter was clear-eyed, healthy, and trim.

The "Common Ground" album, one of my favorites, was improvised in his big barn, and in these woods beyond a stream, where pheasants heave skyward—here in the heart of the mystery and scent of New England's forest.

> Voices are calling round the earth,
> music is rising in the sea,
> the spirit of morning fills the air,
> guiding my journey home."
> —from "Common Ground"

Winter says music can instantly rejoin the left and right brain. It's "physical, and emotional, and intellectual, all at once. All of which adds up to spiritual, as far as I'm concerned." Nature and volleyball have similar healing effects on him.

Winter is making his bridge to the intuitive, and the natural world. Like most children, he was an environmentalist by the age of one and a half, but then he suffered that same lethal dose of formal education handed out to the rest of us. About 17,000 hours, he figures, from 6–22, "in one posture in a chair, looking straight ahead, being taught to think, being told not to show yourself. Don't get emotional."

It's difficult to imagine him behind a desk, or staying antsy too long, before putting his sax to his lips, and breathing out a sense of relief.

That time spent in school "is a hard one to get away from. You survive it. You can look fairly together. But the chances are you're not together. You are apart, you are split asunder.

"That 16 years of essentially training your left brain at the expense of almost everything in your being, it takes daily discipline the rest of your life to reawaken the balance, the wholeness.

"Rejoining [the split] every day—breathing, we sleep every day, now sometimes people exercise every day—that's just part of maintenance."

He says that most people "sit and think and stop vibrating. And we go into a kind of walking catatonia. Cities, streets, are full of people walking around. And they look like they're doing OK. They're getting through. You don't always see any noticeable change. But I think in many cases all the vibrations that really comprise our spirit are temporarily on hold.

"So, when people sit down at a concert hall, they lock into that immediately. You're in the same kind of situation [as school]. You're in rows, usually straight.

"One of my commitments is to encourage people to listen more deeply, and use a faculty that's pretty much unused by our species."

> In a circle of friends,
> in a circle of sound,
> all our voices will blend
> when we touch common ground."
> —from "Common Ground"

This particular, cool evening the Winter Consort plays for 350 at Eastern Connecticut State University. In its preview, the campus daily wrote that his music "is charged with animal energy," and leaves you with the same feeling you had from "Rocky." His concerts usually leave me feeling like I've dreamt inside the moist belly of a great whale, or temporarily jumped into that mythic time of the eternal present. Every concert of his I've heard gradually bursts with energy, until each is like the heart opened.

Tonight, the Consort's contract specifies a locked dressing room, two mirrors, and dinner. They get an empty classroom, newspaper scotch-taped over the door windows. A student from the arts council passes around the menu. "Is this like a vegetarian band?" he asks innocently. "No," someone replies. Winter eats the salad and sandwiches with percussionist Glen Velez, pianist Paul Halley, cellist Eugene Friesen, french horn player John Clark, and other friends.

Up on stage after a 15-minute rehearsal, Winter appears fragile like the ecosystem. But his sax blows strong. At one point in the concert, I envision faded layers of butterfly wings, and fog rising from a marsh. Later there come long blacknesses where the sound pierces through the gold glint of his saxophone.

Then, Eugene Friesen holds the cello bow steady as a camera. Winter closes his eyes, sax down at his chest, and listens as the loudspeaker carries wolf howls throughout the auditorium. His torso sways, his bell bottoms flap. He asks, "When was the last time you had a good howl?" There is silly and shy snickering, but soon half the crowd in Wilimantic, Connecticut, joins in the howling, opening their chests and throats. I've been shifting impatiently, waiting for this. I lean my head back, and through my long gullet I let out the sounds. How good that feels. His music flushes out the animal wisdom of the body. Then the audience sits down again in straight rows, and we begin to forget where we have recently been.

I first heard Winter on a hillside, outside of Boston, five years ago. By the stage, some appreciative dancers floated to the music. I left my two friends smoking marijuana, to join them.

A terrible longing was awakened in me—for hope, for a basic link connecting everybody and the earth, for an ecologically balanced future. I needed to find those crusted-over corners of the world where grumbling tribespeople still clutch those ancient truths, and where I could learn secrets about myself and the world.

I realized, years later, that what was stirred up was in me to begin with, and would nurture me right now. I need not delay that sought-after moment of grace to a distant, imaginary place and time. I could be there anytime I choose.

Winter says talk and print overload us so quickly, and we're taught to get our experience through the left brain. All the information we're bombarded with in this culture is "like eating something we can't digest. Although words are still the primary mode we have as a species, in this part of the world, it's a primitive mode—one that evokes an incomplete posture.

"We're just a baby species. We're juvenile delinquents among species, and all here in a sense in a zoo of our own creation. Ninety to 99 percent, or some enormous amount, of our population lives in these cities, right? They're zoos!

"And we're trying to figure out these formulas for how to live our lives, or how to believe, or how to behave.

"People are lost in their specialized pigeonholes, not taking responsibility for the whole, not really in touch with the whole, and simply doing what they think is their job. And going home and watching TV six hours a night to fill up the hole in their lives.

"It's not that it's wrong. It's just way out of whack. And unless we really see how it is then we're going to be deluded into thinking that, well, if I just join the right political party, or join the right church, or find the right woman, or make the right moves in my career, and make enough money it'll all be OK. You know, and we need the humility."

Winter says animals are gurus, sacred beings. He has played music with wolves and whales in the wild, and he doesn't see them as objects of fear, to be avoided or killed off. The way people have persecuted them is "as if, throughout our entire cultural history, we had automatically taken the most intelligent, enlightened people, and tried to destroy them."

"What's encouraging to me is that as we come into a time when we're beginning to honor those creatures and learn about them, not only are we opening up to a whole world of wisdom and guidance from the creatures, about how to be on this planet, how to be here harmoniously. But we're also learning about our own fear-producing mechanism.

"I mean, can you imagine life lived without fear? That's pretty hard for any of us to probably conceive of. Maybe a lot of our lives are so predicated on fears that, if you were to take away most of those fears, we would be able to lead an entirely transformed life. Maybe do a different livelihood. Maybe be able to serve people more."

Maybe Winter is too idealistic; maybe his music avoids negative emotions to well. He admits, for instance, how difficult it is for him to express anger. "I've never been very comfortable around it. All too often I deal with it by going silent. I'm slowly beginning to learn to let it out, and let it be OK even though I still feel it's a form of violence. And in my view of the way humans are appropriate, violence is not in there."

But Winter is a musician who dares to hold to his vision, and work toward it, often successfully. His music continues to stretch and expand in many different areas at once—song forms, instrumental compositions, chants, improvisation, idioms from Bach to African music, and music of the natural world.

After the evening's concert, Winter and I ride back through the green and red flashing lights of central Connecticut. It's been a long day, and he is relieved when I finally click off the tape recorder. His head slouches forward, he dozes in the station wagon.

To Learn More

Living Music Records, Inc.
Box 72
Litchfield, CT 06759

RANDY LEE SHOWSTACK *is the New England Editor of* Whole Life Times. *He is also a free-lance writer and photographer whose work has appeared in numerous publications. In addition, he has a sideline in business writing, and clients range from holistic practitioners to corporations.*

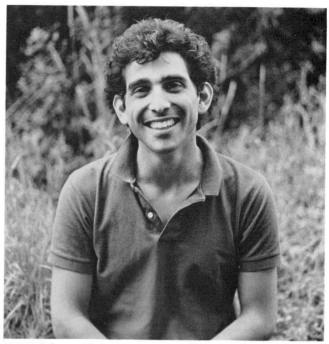

PHOTOGRAPH © THOMAS ENGLAND

Paul Winter and wolf friend.

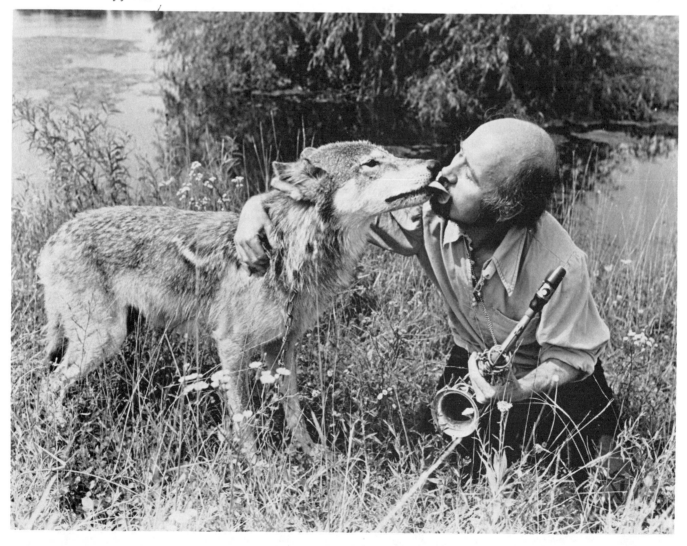

IN THE MONTH OF MAY
Robert Bly

In the month of May when all leaves open
I see when I walk how well all things
lean on each other, how the bees work,
the fish make their living the first day,
Monarchs fly high; then I understand
I love you with what in me is unfinished.

I love you with what in me is still
changing, what has no head or arms
or legs, what has not found its body.
And why shouldn't the miraculous,
caught on this earth, visit
the old man alone in his hut?

And why shouldn't Gabriel, who loves honey,
Be fed with our own radishes and walnuts?
And lovers, tough ones, how many there are
whose holy bodies are not yet born.
Along the roads, I see so many places
I would like us to spend the night.

ROBERT BLY *was born in Minnesota and studied at St. Olaf and Harvard. In 1958 he founded a poetry magazine, which has been called, successively,* The Fifties, The Sixties, The Seventies, *and* The Eighties. *He is the author of nine books of poems—*The Light Around the Body *won the National Book Award—and eleven translations. He is at work on a collection of love poems, a book of selected essays, and a book exploring the psychic implications for men of some classic fairy tales.*

Inside Paul Horn

Catherine Maclay

WHEN THE lights went down on a recent grey afternoon at the Hanuman Fellowship's Mount Madonna Center in northern California, and Paul Horn took up his flute and began to play, his performance seemed as casual and effortless as a conversation with a close friend. When he plays, Horn's eyes take on a sleepy look, his body is loose and relaxed, and one can feel the quiet rapport that exists between him and his audience.

Twenty years ago, however, Paul Horn, a major jazz instrumentalist who played with Duke Ellington, Miles Davis, Buddy Rich and other musical greats, was hard driving and competitive and discovering that despite success in his chosen field, he was reaping little happiness from his life or his music. "My creative juices were still flowing," Horn said in an interview that took place after his Mount Madonna concert. "I was playing clubs and making my own records, but my personal unhappiness was coloring everything. As a young man, I had very much wanted to be accepted by the jazz community. When I got a chance to meet and play with people who had been my idols, it was a great thrill. And it took a lot of hard work and striving to get there. But I think part of the cause of the crisis I felt in my mid-thirties came from continuing to be that competitive, continuing to prove myself, when I didn't have to anymore."

Horn was born in New York in 1930. His mother, the former Francis Sper, played the piano and had her own radio show in New York in the 1920s. Although she gave up her career to raise a family, Horn recalls that she loved to sing and play the piano, and often entertained friends who came for a visit. Horn started on the piano at age four, and continued with it until he was eleven. By then, he was growing tired of classical music. He switched to clarinet and began learning jazz. His parents encouraged and supported his interests, without trying to direct them, he said, a practice he has tried to follow with is own two sons, Robin and Marlen, who are now in their early twenties.

After graduating from the Oberlin Conservatory in Washington and the Manhattan School of Music, Horn joined the Army, where he played the flute in the Army band. After the Army, he joined a New York band, and eventually landed a place in the Chico Hamilton Quintet. Fred Katz, another member of the quintet, introduced Horn to Eastern philosophy—an interest that was to play a crucial part in his life years later.

"We were on a train going from Hollywood to Chicago, as part of a tour," Horn said. "Fred Katz mentioned Zen Buddhism, which I'd never heard of before, so I asked him to explain. We spent three days on that train, and at the end of that time I still didn't know what it was. I said 'c'mon, man'" Horn added, a twinkle in his eye and his New York accent very much in evidence. "'I asked you what Zen Buddhism is. Can't you give me a simple answer to a simple question?'"

By coincidence, after they arrived in Chicago, where they were to spend three weeks, Horn and other members of the quintet befriended a Zen Buddhist priest who worked as a dancer and officiated at a temple on weekends. "We never talked about philosophy," said Horn, whose matter-of-fact way of talking is a curious blend of toughness and gentleness. "The priest's name was Kim, and I just liked him and wanted to hang out with him. But at one point, he said he was going to create a little satori, a little enlightenment for me. A few weeks later, after I left Chicago, I looked back on that time and I realized that I was really feeling high when I was with him. I had a strange sensation that I knew everything. I had no questions, just a kind of knowingness that I'd never had before. I wrote him about it and he wrote back, saying, 'You probably won't hold that feeling, but you know what it is and that it's possible to attain, so you'll find your way.' And he was right. Once you give a person a meaningful experience, he's going to pursue it."

Kim gave Horn some books on Zen, which he enjoyed, but "it didn't feel right without Kim. I had no techniques, and it sort of fell apart." Later, Horn turned to books on yoga by Ramacharaka and others, but once again, he felt he needed techniques more than anything else. He tried meditation, after reading about it, "but five minutes of

Yoga Journal, May–June 1984. 2054 University Ave., Berkeley, CA 94704. Reprinted by permission.

meditation seemed like five hours to me, and I said I can't concentrate, this isn't for me, so I turned to other things."

Other things included reading books on Edgar Cayce. *Many Mansions* by Gina Cerminara was especially influential and while he continued to be deeply involved in the Los Angeles jazz scene, he attended classes by Cerminara, and read extensively in various spiritual traditions. It was Transcendental Meditation, however, that brought about real changes in Horn's life.

"Some of my close friends were interested in TM and with some guidance from them, meditation began to feel right. Done correctly, it was simple. I was initiated in March of 1966 and I meditated twice a day. But then I had a chance to go on tour with Tony Bennett, and I stopped meditating and took up my old habits of burning the candle at both ends. When I came back to LA after the tour, I opened the door to my apartment, put down my suitcase, and then I went straight over and sat down on the sofa and started meditating. As I watched myself doing this, the thought came to me, just like this, that if I didn't keep meditating I was going to die. I was getting too old to live that kind of life. Being a jazz musician is a wild life. Psychologically it destroys you. If you're playing clubs six nights a week, you put a lot out there—whatever you feel comes out in your music. But after awhile you're exhausted, you don't have anything left to give the audience, and then you have to start faking it."

Soon after returning from the tour with Tony Bennett, Horn visited some of the same friends who had first interested him in Transcendental Meditation. "They were about to leave for India, to study with Maharishi Mahesh Yogi. They were making their lists of toothpaste, toilet paper, anti-dysentery pills, and so on. When I got home, I couldn't sleep. This inner dialogue started. A voice would say 'Why don't you go to India?' And then I'd say, 'Are you crazy, you can't go to India!' So after a while I called my friends and said, 'How do you go to India?' They told me Maharishi was coming to Los Angeles, so I made an appointment with him, and went to ask his permission to go study with him. Most of the other people had been meditating a long time, and they wanted to become teachers. I had only been meditating six months, and not even all of that time. I told Maharishi I was not very happy with my life, and I thought if I could hang out with him for awhile, it would be meaningful to me. He asked me a lot of questions about my family responsibilities, and so on. I was divorced at the time, but my two sons lived nearby and they were very important to me. He also asked me if I would have a job when I came back—he wanted to make sure I wasn't copping out. He was quiet for a few moments, and then said, 'OK, you can come. But don't expect anything.' That was really good advice," Horn added, laughing. "That about sums it up, doesn't it? Don't expect anything."

Once in India, Horn spent nearly four months at the Maharishi's ashram, where he learned to let go of the fast-paced life he had been living in Los Angeles. "It was a good time for me, a very special time. I learned to settle." While he was there, Maharishi asked Horn if he would like to teach TM. It was 1967, the year before the Beatles, Donovan, and other celebrities began flocking to India,

and the Maharishi correctly sensed the need for many more teachers, especially in the U.S. Horn was startled by the request, and asked if he could think it over. Once he was told that there was no rigid obligation involved, he need only teach when he had time, Horn said yes.

When he returned to Los Angeles, he immersed himself in teaching, traveling between Hollywood and Berkeley, and putting in 14-hour days. There was no time left for music. "I didn't care," Horn said, "I collected unemployment for awhile." When he did return to performing, however, things were different. "After India, I could never really get back into the scene. I still played, but I didn't feel much like working. I went to the beach a lot. I had learned the importance of just being. I had changed. Some of my friends just didn't want to hear about it. I made them uncomfortable. Pretty soon I got a whole new circle of friends."

The following year, 1968, Horn returned to India to study again with Maharishi. It was on this trip that he visited the Taj Mahal and made the first of his famous "inside" albums—"Inside the Taj Mahal." He later wrote about the experience: "The Taj Mahal lies in glorious splendor on the south bank of the Jumna River just outside the city of Agra in India.

"There is always a man there informally standing guard who explains with great pride the inscriptions and magnificent floral inlay work in the marble of the tombs. Quite unexpectedly he bursts forth a vocal 'call' every few minutes to demonstrate the remarkable acoustics emanating from the solid marble dome.

"From the first time I heard his voice I couldn't believe my ears. I had never heard anything so beautiful. Each tone hung suspended in space for 28 seconds and the acoustics are so perfect that you couldn't tell when his voice stopped and the echo took over.

"I had brought my flute with the very faint hope that I might have a chance to play even one note in that remarkable chamber. I used my alto flute and the low C just flew out and filled the entire room and just hung there . . . I began playing whatever came into my head. I'd let the notes hang there. I could play whole chords and they came back sounding like a chorus of angels. Then I'd play my next phrase on top of that. There was a whole orchestra invisibly suspended in the obscurity of the dome. After a few minutes I stopped. The guard seemed to really enjoy it. He was smiling now and I beckoned him to give his 'call' and he did."

Back in the U.S. the album sold well, and marked the beginning of a second career for Horn, in which he retained his roots in pure jazz music, while branching out into new areas. Other "inside" albums followed, including recordings made inside the Great Pyramid at Giza, and inside the Temple of Heaven in Peking.

Asked if he would categorize himself as a new age musician, Horn said, "If by new age you mean music that's for meditation and relaxation, music that can heal you, then yes, I would call myself a new age musician. But to be healthy and relaxing, music does not have to be slow—it can be up tempo."

By going his own way, Horn has had to leave behind his position as a member of the established jazz scene. "I haven't been part of that community for a long time," he said. "I don't think *Downbeat* has mentioned my name in the past ten years or more." Asked whether this bothered him, he paused and then said, "I decided to go my own way a long time ago. Some have liked it and some have not. Some friends have left and some new friends have come. Part of the change that came over me in the late sixties is that acceptance by other doesn't matter to me anymore—and so rejection isn't that important either. Part of the transformation that came from India was that I didn't have to prove myself anymore. Everything was all right. I had the inner strength to just go my own way."

In 1970, Horn left Los Angeles and moved to Victoria, British Columbia. "My two boys had been living with their mother, and by then they were 10 and 13. I asked their mother if it would be all right if they came and lived with me, and to my surprise, she said yes. A year later he married a Dutch-born fashion designer named Tryntje, and family life began in earnest.

When he moved to Canada, Horn's plans did not necessarily include a continued musical career. "At the time I thought I would never play professionally again. I thought I'd drive a cab—or maybe become a sheep farmer," Horn added, laughing. "I saw some sheep grazing up there one day, and I thought, hey, that looks like pretty easy work … but when I moved up there, the phone started to ring. When you start following instead of leading, things start to happen."

One of the phone calls Horn received was an unusual one. A biologist at Sealand in Victoria called and asked him to participate in an experimental study on the way orca (killer whales) communicate. Horn played regularly for two orca, and when one of them died and the other went into mourning and refused to eat, he was able, through his music, to revive the grieving whale.

Two recent high points in Horn's career have been concerts in China and Russia. During the concert tour to China, which occurred two years ago, he became enchanted by the Chinese people. "I would say China is the most spiritual country I have ever been to. To be spiritual is to be selfless, to be a doer, a giver. With no formal religion, the Chinese are living in a spiritual, selfless way. Their sense of communal living is something they've been doing for centuries. It's part of their tradition. With that enor-

mous population, they've had to think collectively in order to survive. That's why they are content with the form of government they have."

Last year, Horn traveled to Russia with a jazz quartet that included his son, Robin, 23, on drums, David Friesen on bass, John Stowell on guitar, and Horn himself on flute. There, they played eight nights in a row in Moscow, filling a 3,000-seat theater every night. They then performed in Leningrad for six nights, and four nights in Lithuania. Horn found people in the Soviet Union to be warm and hospitable. He felt that unlike the Chinese, however, people there were not satisfied with their form of government. "Like Americans," he said, "they come from a variety of backgrounds. They are a vital people who need self-expression. Their system is not allowing it. There's no motivation, and you can see it in their eyes. They look vacant. If we were really cool, we would just sit back and the government would just wither away from within. It's just a matter of time. The people are not going to go for it, they're not happy, whereas the Chinese are a happy smiling people. And you can't fake that."

While he was in the Soviet Union, however, Horn tried to avoid political discussions. "I came as a musician. Music has the ability to heal this world. We fear differences. Music transcends differences. Human beings are the same everywhere in wanting to hold on to life."

Later this year, Paul Horn will release recordings he made during his Soviet tour. Other than that, he says, his plans are indefinite, as usual. "I don't plan things," he said. "I wait for them to happen." The central point of Horn's life is still meditation. "I take a shower every morning, I brush my teeth every morning, I meditate every morning. Sooner or later you have to meditate. You have to find out who you are, who's in charge. After you've been doing it awhile, your life gets easier. You don't try so hard. You don't worry about change. You become resilient. A person in a high state of consciousness has infinite flexibility and infinite stability. Meditation is so simple that our culture doesn't value it. We're conditioned to think that for something to be worthwhile, you have to really work at it. But there's a part of life where the success of it depends on no trying."

CATHERINE MACLAY *is the assistant editor of* Yoga Journal.

IV

Life Cycles

INTRODUCTION *by Shepherd Bliss*

THE LIFE-CYCLE approach to understanding human beings has grown in significance since it appeared in the previous edition of this book as a sub-section, so it has been expanded here. Cycles can be observed throughout nature, including in humans; therefore, understanding them is crucial.

This is our "Womb to Tomb" section, as students affectionately called the class that psychologist Erik Erikson, a pioneer in this field, taught for years at Harvard. It begins with birth and ends with death, as we all do. Humans have long been fascinated with how we enter and finally exit this life—the two processes that frame our lives—and this section shows how we can influence these processes with holistic approaches.

Articles on death include the work of Elisabeth Kübler-Ross, the great pioneer in this field; and two of the most active current practitioners in the field of death and dying counseling—Ondrea and Stephen Levine. Poet Walt Whitman also adds his wisdom. Jeremy Taylor and his insights from dreamwork appear here, as elsewhere in the book.

We balance the insights into death by presenting some of the growing studies of longevity and life extension, which indicate means of both prolonging and enhancing life by such means as diet, physical activity, reducing toxins and stress, and enjoying one's loved ones.

This diverse section includes socioscientific, poetic, storytelling, analytical, and impressionistic perspectives. Contributors include Harvard Medical School researcher Samuel Osherson, Ph.D., and Bay Area teacher Alan Siegel, Ph.D., both of whom describe the growing willingness of men to provide intimate views of how males look at various issues.

A. BIRTH

Natural Birth Control: A Holistic Approach to Contraception

Merilee Kernis

Cultures all over the world have successfully practiced natural birth control. It is very powerful to know that you can prevent unwanted pregnancies without relying on potentially dangerous chemical and mechanical devices. The beliefs of the sexual revolution are merging with practices of conscious evolution. The result is a return to living in harmony with natural laws which support mindful celebration of sexuality and conscious choices about conception.

MANY PEOPLE in America are unaware that there are ways to control conception which do not depend on mechanical devices or chemical substances. These are natural methods. Almost everyone has heard about the rhythm cycle, the earliest popularized natural method. This method works only if you have a regular and normal monthly cycle, that is, if your cycle is 28 to 30 days long. Most women do not have such a cycle; as a result, there have been many miscalculations and surprise pregnancies.

The subject of natural birth control is often greeted with misunderstanding and suspicion. Sometimes I hear people say, "It doesn't sound like it could work," or "It is too difficult for me." What they are really saying is, "Can I trust my own self? Can I really take responsibility for my fertility cycle? Can I believe that within my own biological makeup there are signs that will indicate the start and end of my fertile cycle and the beginning of the infertile one? Can all this be true? " It seems to me that they are questioning their self-confidence and self-responsibility.

This doubting is not at all surprising. Our mechanical lifestyles have deadened our sensitivity. Our sense of smell, taste, touch, feel, and hearing, and our psychic abilities, have atrophied under the roar of the city and the externalization of our life. When we read anthropological studies of tribal people who demonstrate outstanding acuteness in hearing or smelling over great distances, we can realize both the vast range of human ability and the limitations we have placed on ourselves.

These same tribal people have been using natural methods of birth control for years. These ways are safe and reliable, and are found naturally within their own environment. In India the women of one culture chew dry carrot seeds to prevent pregnancy.

The Tibetans for years have used a formula which, taken for only seven consecutive days once a year, gives a year's protection. It is made from the ovaries of a female yak. The Tibetan physicians claim that its reliability and effectiveness are high.

The Chinese also have a herbal remedy made from a combination of several herbs, the major ingredient being from the Chi Je date tree. Drs. C.C. Chan and C.Y. Yen tested this method on more than one million women in three countries, and reported its effectiveness to be 99.8 to 99.9 percent for six months, after which time a second dosage would be taken.

More amazing reports on natural birth-control methods come from anthropologists who have researched the cultural life of villagers in central India and the South Seas. Such dedicated researchers as Malinowski (Trobriand Islanders) and Gordon Troeller and Claude Deffarge (Murias) unveil a fantastic ability of the unmarried to use mind control as a contraceptive. What a wonderful, sensitive approach to the process of natural family planning and birth control.

Mind control is just as effective as the current type of birth-control pill: 96 percent. Furthermore, it does not produce harmful side effects, either to the physical body or to the emotional and mental states. Some Western women who have previously conceived claim they are now using this method successfully. However, looking at our cultural system, we see a technology which has produced sophisticated, computerized instruments; spaceships that travel to the planets; cars, airplanes, pushbutton mechanization that make "it" all happen faster—and a country of people who are pill poppers. It is not at all surprising that similarly the "quick and easy" consumer attitude would be the basis for the birth-control products developed. The mass-media message being sent is "low personal involvement with the methods and a high degree of guilt."

For the last two decades, birth-control devices have been reflecting the social and political statements of the times; imbalance, obstruction, and eradication. All developed devices fall neatly into these categories. The imbalancers are birth-control pills; the obstructors are the IUDs, diaphragms, and condoms; and the eradicators are foams, creams, jellies, and sterilization.

Over the years, these techniques have been tried by most women, with some periods of protection and some periods of failure—but none without any side effects. No wonder there are so many angry and disillusioned women and so many concerned men. Our health and well-being are among the most precious jewels in human life. Do we want to suffocate ourselves?

Sad as it may seem, this is what we are doing when we accept and believe such insensitive, inaccurate statements from physicians and scientists as "Pregnancy is more dangerous to our health than birth-control pills."

The pills outweigh their competitors in their shocks to the female system. Medically, these effects are divided into three groups, according to severity. First, the milder or the "nuisance effects." They are problems such as bothersome vaginal itching, breakthrough bleeding, fluid retention, estrogen deficiency, and progesterone excess. Second, the more severe difficulties are the "metabolic effects," which change the amount and kind of cortisol produced by adrenal glands, and cause an increased potential for blood clotting and gallstones, possibly elevated blood pressure, and a difference in the way the body uses certain proteins. Last, the "serious complications" are the rising risk of fatal thromboembolism (blood clotting), breast diseases, and death. Women who are taking the pill should not view these contraindications lightly. What has popularized the pills is the high protection rate of 96 percent.

The intrauterine device (IUD) is a close competitor. The common complaints experienced by users are extreme cramping and heavy bleeding during menstruation. The severe complications are pelvic inflammatory disease (PID) and unrecognizable tubal or ovarian pregnancy, which can lead to serious difficulties and sometimes even to death. Its ease of use made the IUD popular; once it is implanted, one's responsibility for birth control has ceased, except for an occasional check-up to see if it is still intact. Moreover, its reliability is approximately 95 percent. However, some studies indicate that at the end of one year 25 percent of the women have it removed for a variety of reasons, and by the end of two years only 50 percent of the women are still using it.

The more awkward diaphragm is rising in acceptance as women and men are becoming more concerned about the harmful effects of the two previous techniques. The diaphragm must be properly fitted or it will not remain in place. After some instruction and practice on insertion and removal, most women have no difficulty in using it, although some complain about its inconvenience. If an allergic reaction to the rubber cup develops in the sensitive vaginal lining, as sometimes happens, one can switch to the plastic type. But many women develop an itch, an irritation, or a burning sensation because of the spermicides that must also be used with this technique.

The safety of spermicides for long-term use is really questionable. Since the spermicide must be able to kill sperm, then its ingredients must be harsh and possibly toxic to the delicate membranes within the vaginal canal. Often women ask if the diaphragm can be used alone as a barrier, as was its originally intended use. However, such use is not currently being recommended, perhaps because it would mean less money for the drug companies. Even so, some women who are strongly opposed to use of spermicides use the diaphragm as their sole contraceptive. This device, with the gooey additives, ranges in reliability from 85 to 94 percent (depending on the particular study you read.)

The condom is completely free from chemical or mechanical side effects that can upset a woman's delicate balance. As a barrier, its effectiveness falls at about 90 percent.

The jellies, foams, and creams when used alone have a dependability rate of about 65 percent.

Finally, of course, there is abstinence or sterilization, the former being 100 percent effective, and the latter having a small percentage of failures.

All these devices and techniques are only primitive jabbings in the dark, and most of them interfere with the delicate balance of the body. While they were being developed in America, in other parts of the world gynecologists—unknown to each other—were excited about their discoveries of natural methods of birth control.

In Australia, Dr. John Billings and his wife, Dr. Lyn Billings, working under the directive of the Pope, were examining daily samples of women's cervical mucous and correlating them with fertility. They concluded that these secretions are excellent guides to fertility. The ovulation mucous method thus took form.

What could be more thrilling than following the natural cycle of your own body? Imagine, your body is a self-contained map by which you can recognize your monthly fertile and infertile cycle. By daily checking your mucous, you will know what days are safe and which are unsafe for lovemaking. (A more complete description of this method is given below.)

Concurrently, in the 1950s, the Czechoslovakian physician Dr. Eugen Jonas was investigating the relationship between the planets and the time of fertility. He believed (and later proved) that a women's natal angle corresponded with her fertile day. The natal angle (or birth angle) is the angle made by the position of the Sun and the Moon relative to the Earth. This same configuration repeats itself approximately once a month and may appear 12 to 14 times a year. (See discussion of the Astrological Fertility Cycle below.)

In charting this relationship, Dr. Jonas showed not only that planetary vibrations influence our lives but also that there are two fertile cycles every month. The first is biological; the second is astrological. These cycles are part of the natural rhythms of the universe.

These natural rhythms are called "circadian rhythms" or "cosmic clocks." They are correlated with the shifting positions of the Sun, Moon, and planets, with the daily shifts of light to dark, and with seasonal changes, and they affect the eating, sleeping, mating, health, and survival patterns of fish, insects, plants, animals, and man.

Marine researchers have uncovered specific correlations between breeding cycles and phases of the Moon. Soviet and Japanese scientists have independently discovered that our human bodies are extremely sensitive to the electromagnetic forces in the universe. Careful observations during intense solar activity such as flares and magnetic storms have revealed a simultaneous decrease in the number of white blood cells—an infection-fighting agent—and subsequently an increase in disease.

Farmers have long been aware that vegetation, too, responds to energy patterns, They have planted, cultivated, or harvested their fields only during certain phases of the Moon.

Recently there has been great interest in the clockwork rhythm of a woman's monthly cycle. Historically, village women discovered that their cycles synchronized with particular Moon phases. For some women this fact is still true. Women who sleep outdoors report that the onset of menses has become synchronized with one phase of the Moon, the moment of ovulation with another, the most common relationship being ovulation at full moon, menses at new moon.

In order to understand these innate rhythms again, we must listen with great care and recognize the unfolding patterns successfully. If we try to control or manipulate or change to fit our desensitized ideals, we will not perceive the harmony of these natural rhythms.

In increasing our sensitivity, we begin to view patterns that recur in the physical as well as the emotional and mental bodies. For example, we take daily samples of the mucous secretion from the cervix, examine this discharge, and record the variations.

Also we may discover that the physical body produces sounds and internal movements. Some women experience a twinge or cramping in the groin around ovulation; some women say that five days before menses is to commence, there is cramping or other signs, such as breast swelling, bloating, mood changes, depression or creativity, which attract their attention. During other parts of the monthly cycle, even more subtle but recognizable indications do occur. With proper attentiveness in keeping a daily journal or chart on the emotional, physical, and mental states, each woman can alert herself to the beginning and end of each fertile time.

In recording this information, be specific with the descriptions. Put down the current date, the day of the monthly cycle, and four headings: physical, emotional, mental, and sex. Under each heading list the appropriate characteristics. Here are some examples.

Physical: strong, tired, sick, pain (where), clear, shaky...
Emotional: self-image (good or poor), elated, grief, calm, lonely, tense, secure, confident...
Mental: positive thinking: I like myself today; It's a beautiful day; I enjoy...negative thinking: I hate...:he is so stupid; I would like to punch him; It never works out...
Sex: Yes/2 P.M.

Figure 1 shows how you might construct your chart. Make yours large enough to write in, and allow space for notes on the natural methods as well.

Natural birth control involves the man as well as the woman. Both can share equal responsibility in acquiring complete familiarity with the techniques. Thus, the Nat-

ural Method relieves the woman from having to bear all responsibility and allows her to enjoy sexual intimacy without reservation. It encourages the man to become more variable, active, and concerned about the relationship, and invites alternate possibilities for more imaginative lovemaking besides genital intercourse.

There are six natural methods of birth control, and 15 workable combinations of them. The choices are the following: (1) Billings Mucous Method; (2) Rhythm Method; (3) Basal Body Temperature; (4) Astrological Fertility Cycle; (5) Lunaception; (6) Psychic or Mental Control.

1. Billings Mucous Method

This method, developed by Drs. John and Evelyn Billings—a husband-and-wife physician team from Australia—is a biological way to discover the time of ovulation (fertility) by taking a daily sampling of cervical mucous. The color, texture, consistency, and sensation of the mucous changes allow each woman to distinguish fertile from infertile mucous. Mucous changes appear in patterns, and vary according to the day of the monthly cycle. The fertile mucous may be cottage-cheese curd-like, creamy, clear and slippery, clear and stretchable, white-translucent, or opaque and tacky. Infertile mucous may appear sticky, yellow, and dense. Most women can use this technique with 99 percent reliability.

The first step in using this method is to become familiar with the mucous secretions. In checking the mucous discharge, one of the four following methods can be used, the last two being the most accurate.

(a) Twice a day observe the amount of mucous discharge by wiping yourself with a tissue while spreading the labia.
(b) Twice a day observe the amount of mucous discharge by wiping yourself with your fingers.
(c) Twice a day insert two fingers (the index and middle) into the vaginal cavity and run the fingers along the cervix to obtain mucous secretions.
(d) Twice a day check the flow of mucous by opening the vaginal area with a speculum and, with a mirror used as a reflector and a flashlight, observe the mucous around the os (mouth) of the cervix.

The next step is to identify fertile and infertile mucous. Figure 2 shows a typical chart for a regular 28-day cycle.

Ovulation will be indicated by *spinnbarkeit*, mucous that resembles raw egg white with a stretching quality. The fertile period will be approximately 10 to 12 days. If your cycle is less than 26 days, there may be no dry period after menstruation. The fertile period may begin on the last days of the menstrual cycle.

If your cycle is more than 32 days, observe the dry days carefully. During the dry days, if any mucous which resembles fertile mucous appears, this means you must abstain. If after three days there are no further indications of the fertile symptoms, you may be assured that this day is safe. Remember, however, that semen and internal pelvic infections will mask cervical mucous, making recognition of mucous difficult.

Figure 1. Chart for keeping a record of your menstrual cycle. (You may want to make photocopies from this chart so you can keep a continuous record until you fully understand your cycle.)

Day	Date	Mucous Observation	Body Temp.	Astrological Cycle	Physical Changes	Emotional Changes	Mental Changes	Sex
1								
2								
3								
4								
5								
6								
7								
8								
9								
10								
11								
12								
13								
14								
15								
16								
17								
18								
19								
20								
21								
22								
23								
24								
25								
26								
27								
28								
29								
30								
31								
32								
33								
34								
35								

2. Rhythm Method

This is the oldest of the natural methods used in recent times. Knaus and Ogino separately researched and developed two systems of biological birth control using this method. The two approaches have a 15 to 30 percent accuracy.

Figure 2.

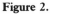

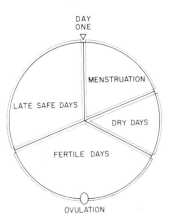

The first step in Knaus' system is to discover the fertile period by recording the length of each monthly cycle for a year. Then, from the number of days in the shortest monthly cycle, subtract 18. Next, note the number of days in the longest monthly cycle and subtract 11 from this. These answers give the first and last days, respectively, of the fertile cycle every month.

An example: the number of days in each monthly cycle may be 24, 28, 25, 29, 30, 27, 29, 26, 31, 29, 30, 32. The shortest month is 24 days; subtracting 18 from 24 leaves 6. The longest month is 32; subtracting 11 from 32 leaves 21. Your Rhythm Fertility Cycle then would begin the following year on the 6th day of every month and end on the 21st day of each month. You would be considered fertile for 16 days each month. This cycle is based on your past patterns, which may or may not be the same for the current year.

The Ogino system uses a 13-day cycle. The cycle is established each month by noting the date and time of the beginning of the menstrual flow (bleeding). Now count forward 14 full 24-hour days. The 14th day is supposedly ovulation. Six days on either side of this 14th day are also considered fertile.

3. Astrological Fertility Cycle

An astrological system for predicting monthly fertility was developed by a Czechoslovakian gynecologist, Dr. Eugen Jonas. Each woman's cycle is predicated on the angle of the Sun and the Moon at her time of birth. The natal angle (with a minor adjustment for date and place of birth) repeats itself approximately 13 times a year. The fertility cycle is a 96-hour period beginning on a specific date at a specific hour and ending four full days later.

The Astrological Cycle has an 85 percent reliability, and coupled with the Rhythm Method as Dr. Jonas applied it (calling it the Cosmic Fertility Cycle) or with the Billings

Mucous Method, the reliability will rise to at least 98 percent.

As an example, given a certain woman's time, date, and place of birth, we calculate her natal angle as 34.5° and her working angle as 41°. When this angle is applied to the Sun-Moon angles chart for May 1977, we find that her Astrological Fertility Cycle begins at 12:00 noon on May 17 and ends at 12:00 noon on May 21.

4. Basal Body Temperature

A woman's temperature fluctuates between her estrogen and progesterone (hormonal) cycles. During ovulation, her temperature will drop as much as ½°, and then rise up by 1° shortly afterwards, either sharply or in a stair-step way. The temperature will usually remain high until menses, at which time it will fall slightly. Then, just before or during ovulation, it will suddenly drop again. So, if you record your basal temperature every morning, you should be able to tell quickly where you are in your cycle.

But occasionally it is difficult to tell what the rise is. What you do is look at the six days preceding the beginning of the rise. Circle that day. Then look for three consecutive temperatures after the rise that are .3° higher than the day just circled. The fourth day after will be safe.

Take the temperature immediately upon wakening. Do not get up to go to the bathroom. Do not smoke, do not drink or eat anything, do not shake the thermometer down. Take your temperature vaginally, rectally, or orally. Allow the thermometer to be in place for at least five minutes and then take a reading. When finished, do not run hot water over the thermometer; instead, use a tissue to wipe it off.

The temperature method is best as an indicator of when ovulation has happened and as a guide to the beginning of the infertile days.

5. Lunaception

This creative process, developed by Louise Lacey, is a well-thought-out system that raises a woman's consciousness of herself by allowing her to view herself as a functioning whole and encouraging her to take responsibility for creating this process. The method integrates awareness of a woman's daily life patterns with an understanding of how they relate to her fertile-infertile cycle. The daily patterns observed are emotional, physical, and mental states, temperature, and observations of cervical mucous, all of which are recorded on a graph. The objective is to reveal a recurring pattern that indicates each woman's *own* fertile and infertile cycle.

For example, a woman may become aware of powerful creative feelings three days before she ovulates each month. This may be a signal of the first fertile day every month for her.

On Lunaception a woman abstains for five days; three days before ovulation and two days after ovulation. (Ovulation takes only a few minutes, for the ovum to be released from the follicle and enter into the Fallopian tube.)

This method encourages the regulation of the monthly cycle. By sleeping under the light of a white 15- to 25-watt

NORMALIZING YOUR SYSTEM

William LeSassier, N.D.

If you've been taking birth-control pills and want to stop, your cycle will take a while to rebalance itself. This herbal formula can help to normalize and tonify the reproductive organs, and restore your estrogen balance. Drink four to five cups daily, for a couple of weeks to a month, slowly tapering off the amount. Your system will normalize, and you can compute an accurate rhythm chart without waiting for months.

    1 part sarsaparilla
    1 part Holy thistle
    1 part *mitchella repens*
    1 part cramp bark
    1 part licorice

Let steep 40 minutes. You can make a quart (one day's worth) at a time and keep it in the refrigerator.

Adapted from William LeSassier, N. D., "Natural Birth Control," *Well-Being Magazine*.

bulb on the 14th, 15th, and 16th nights of her monthly cycle, and in total darkness (with no stray light) on the remaining nights, each woman can regulate her cycle, so that she will consistently ovulate on the 14th, 15th, or 16th day of each month. By using the light to stimulate ovulation, as it would be stimulated by the cycle of the Moon if she were living and sleeping outdoors, she can control her fertile and infertile periods.

6. Psychic or Mental Control

The word "psychic" may ring with mystical connotations to our ears. To most of us, being psychic is a special gift, to others, it's a form of entertainment or quackery. As one quite famous psychic, Jack Schwarz, recently said about being psychic, "So what? It's no big deal." We can all learn to develop these abilities.

What application do psychic abilities have to natural birth control? In using psychic means, we discover that we can voluntarily control our internal states by use of our minds. No trick. The principle is that we have control over our bodily processes, and that our bodily processes do not control us.

Psychic or mental control is an excellent way to develop increased self-awareness of the psycho-physical and spiritual patterns that operate within each woman. By becoming in touch with these functions, she can see how emotions and thoughts voluntarily control the bodily processes. Useful techniques for this purpose include breath control, meditation, and yoga.

In deciding which methods to use, we need to consider how often fertility occurs in any one month. The traditional theory is that ovulation occurs once a month. A biological event involves a physical preparation of the tissues and organs of the body for pregnancy, with accompanying hormonal secretions. Drs. John and Evelyn Billings support this belief. Even though about 1 percent of their women have become pregnant outside the regular physical fertility time, Dr. Evelyn Billings claims that she is unaware of another fertile cycle in the month.

However, other studies have shown that a woman may ovulate more than once a month. Masters and Johnson have proposed that intercourse may trigger ovulation. In the late 1930s, Dr. Harold Saxon Burr of Yale University did extensive work on the electrical or voltage potential in the human female body. He discovered that women could sometimes ovulate outside the usual biological time. Then, around the mid-1950s, Dr. Eugen Jonas, in researching and developing the Cosmic Fertility Cycle, reported that a woman may ovulate at least twice a month, once at the biological time and once when her natal Sun-Moon angle appears. Therefore, she may conceive outside her biological time.

In using these methods, each woman should choose one or more of the techniques, depending on how regular or irregular her own cycle is. Most women use some combination of them, depending on their own awareness of their needs and patterns.

To discover which methods are most suitable for you, you really need to work with a natural birth-control practitioner. It is important that each woman receive thorough instructions in these methods. Periodically, her progress must be checked and evaluated by a qualified teacher-trainer to be certain that she clearly understands the procedures and has had no difficulty in using them.

Here I have presented only the most basic descriptions of how these systems of natural birth control work. In practice, you will need more thorough information on the methods. A qualified Natural Birth Control/Family Planning practitioner can instruct you in choosing methods for your particular regular or irregular cycle, help you regulate your cycle, guide your application, and help you with questions and difficulties. Good luck. Remember love and relaxation are essential.

Suggestions for Further Reading

Dr. John Billings, *Natural Family Planning, The Ovulation Method*. Collegeville, Minn.: Liturgical Press, 1972.
Louise Lacey, *Lunaception*. Warner Books, 1976.
Gay Gear Luce, *Body Time*. Pantheon, 1971.
Margaret Mofziger, *A Cooperative Method of Natural Birth Control*. Summertown, Tenn.: Book Publishing Company, 1976.
Art Rosemblum, *The Natural Birth Control Book*. Philadelphia, Pa.: Aquarian Research Foundation, 1976.

MERILEE KERNIS *is co-director of the Center for Natural Care, Box 2442, Berkeley, CA 94702. She is a Polarity practitioner and teaches Polarity, Natural Birth Control and Herbs, Pelvic Care and the Female System. She has been using natural methods of birth control for over five years with success, and has taught these methods privately and through various holistic health and growth centers throughout California.*

Natural Childbirth

Cybele Gold and E. J. Gold

Natural childbirth can be a joyous and enlightening experience. Conscious drugless birth, with the focused attention of both parents, is beginning to replace the mechanized surgery commonly practiced in hospitals.

Much has been said lately about the negative aspects of traditional hospital births: drugs, unnecessary episiotomies; noise and bright lights during delivery; taking the baby from mother into a sterile nursery, instead of to the mother's breast. Another drawback is in the role of the father. From conception to birth, it seems as though the pregnancy has nothing to do with him, until finally, pacing alone in the waiting room, he is led to the glass window which separates him from his child.

Natural childbirth provides a built-in role for the father as he "coaches" the mother. In natural childbirth, the parents train together for the birth. The father will assist the mother, helping her with her breathing, pushes, etc., and lovingly caring for her.

This article has been excerpted from the book Joyous Childbirth, *by Cybele and E. J. Gold. It is both a practical and a spiritual guide to natural home birth. You may not choose home birth, but you can profit greatly from the thorough treatment of natural childbirth, which includes preparation, birth itself, and postnatal care.*

In the face of dehumanizing surgical birth, natural childbirth offers us one of the richest possible human experiences: the conscious birthing of a new being. How can we refuse?

 Y HUSBAND and I have a house in the mountains in Southern California. This is where my firstborn, Gabriel Michael, was conceived. I felt his presence immediately upon conception.... I went to a doctor and had a pregnancy test made. It showed positive. I couldn't wait to get back home and tell Daddy that it was confirmed....

Now, of course, the next logical step was that we needed to find a doctor whom we could feel comfortable around and could work with. I remembered another one of my friends, Karen, who heard about natural childbirth at home from, of all people a Fuller Brush salesman. She had had her baby using the doctor the salesman had recommended, and she had been very pleased with her experience. "So," I thought, "that's for me." I had lost a baby in 1964, and was very put out by the way I had been treated and felt about the delivery. Those stitches had hurt and I had felt rotten for about a week. I had had that baby in a hospital. I am not saying don't go to a hospital if you need to, but what I *am* saying is that it is no environment for a normal child to be born in. Traditional hospitals treat childbirth as a sickness, not as a natural act. A whole world was populated (and still is, in most parts of the world) naturally—at home....

My husband had come with me to meet Dr. LaRusch and also felt very good about my choice of the doctor who was going to deliver Gabriel Michael.

Dr. LaRusch examined me and checked my blood pressure, my weight, and, of course, my monthly "friend"— the urine sample. He said I was doing fine and that he would see me again next month. So it went, from monthly checkups for the first five months, to checkups every two weeks from the sixth month to the eighth month, and then checkups every week during the last month.

During my sixth month we began taking a course in the Ettinghausen-LaRusch method of delivery in order to prepare for childbirth with our doctor. Every doctor has his own special system and expects you to be trained in that particular way, so that he knows what to expect from you and you know what to expect from him. In this way a working team can be formed, because everyone in it knows the same system.

The classes were given by Dr. LaRusch's wife, who had delivered four children of her own using this method. She was in charge of teaching his patients his method of home delivery, loosely based on the Lamaze system. Donia LaRusch educated the expectant mothers and coaches (usually the fathers) on the mental, emotional, and physical conditions of pregnancy. We hoped to be able to adapt the system we had learned about delivering a conscious being to the system taught by the LaRusches.

As it happened, we could not have chosen a more suitable method or a more understanding doctor for spiritual childbirth. The method was already almost exactly what we had developed, except for the meditations and a few of the exercises, breathing techniques, and background information. Dr. LaRusch had already recognized the need for absolute silence during delivery and realized the spiritual nature of the being in rebirth. So all we had to do was adapt our meditations on the inner levels—the outer work was almost exactly the same!

In class Donia taught how to train the "moving and instinctive center" to breathe properly, so that during labor and delivery the mother can work with the contractions and not against them. She taught the students to trust the instinctive center to breathe properly without having to put intellectual attention on it or force it to breathe right. This leaves you free to meditate and get in contact and remain in contact with your baby all the way through labor and delivery. The fact that you don't have to concentrate intellectually on the breathing is literally a "load off your mind." It's like having both "mental hands" free.

She taught that emotionally it is important to know that childbirth is a normal function of the female body, and that the body knows exactly what to do to have a baby. We were shown proof that the body can be trusted to do everything necessary, and that you don't have to continually watch and try to direct it—that, in fact, trying to direct birth from the intellect gets in the way of a smooth delivery.

She taught exercises and the physical training necessary for a normal, safe delivery. These exercises are necessary for modern women who no longer do the same kinds of movements or have the same type of body stress women used to have. And with the addition of new exercises not normally done by a body under any other circumstances, the pelvic region can be made more elastic for a breeze-easy delivery. That in itself is fantastic—after all, you have better things to do with your time and your new baby than sit around recovering from childbirth problems.

The class was held once a week, for six weeks. Each week we were checked on the exercises we had learned the previous week, and learned new exercises. During the sixth and last class session together, we were shown a film of a baby being born (one of my doctor's patients), and tea and cake were served. Dr. LaRusch was present to answer questions about the film and any other questions that we had, and to eat cake and drink tea and have fun. It was a very enjoyable six weeks of learning and sharing with the other expectant mothers and their coaches.

It was nice to hear, in the following weeks, that one of our classmates had given birth to a healthy, beautiful baby boy or girl, and that both mommy and baby were doing fine and had had an easy time.

So my husband and I finished our natural childbirth course in a short six weeks. It was coming time to get baby clothes, a baby bed, and all the little goodies we would need for the birth of our new little friend.

By this time I was eight months pregnant and visiting the doctor once a week for my checkups. "Doing fine," he said, "but watch your weight. Extra weight is more difficult to lose after having the baby."

By my ninth month I was doing great. I'd lost some extra pounds and felt better. Dr. LaRusch said, "Cybele, you are dilated one centimeter—don't try to leave town!" It sounded like an old Humphrey Bogart movie. My husband and I were very happy to hear that it wouldn't be long now before we would get to see our new but old friend.

Everything was ready for Gabriel—baby clothes all freshly washed and put away, his baby bed, oils, lotions, and all that good-smelling, neat baby stuff.

Well, here we go!

At 10:30 P.M., May 25, 1973, my water broke. A couple of friends came to clean and disinfect my bedroom and bathroom, where Gabriel would be during the first few hours. We got all the doctor's supplies ready and prepared for the "Big Push."

I stayed up walking around most of the time, because the gravity of the body when standing up and walking shortens labor time, which some "modern" hospital personnel pretend not to know! I didn't actually begin labor sensations until 1:30 A.M. I went and took a *warm* bath and stayed in the tub, doing my breathing with every contraction, until eight centimeters dilation. My doctor said, "Okay, it's time to get out of the tub. Get on the delivery table. Gabriel is ready to be born." So I got out of the tub and got on the delivery table.

Dr. LaRusch said, "Now, I want you to give me a good strong push for 20 seconds, take a catch breath, push another 20 seconds, take a breath, and push another 20 seconds, then rest until the next contraction." He also said, "Don't make any noise or dramatize your delivery. We want your baby to be born without negative impressions."

...I thought that I might forget my breathing exercises—and I did—but my coach and my body remembered!

I did five easy sets of pushes and Gabriel was out!—born 5:10 A.M., May 26, 1973—fully awake. No need to spank him or massage him, because neither he nor I were drugged. The mucus was cleaned out of his nose and mouth, and immediately after that he was put to breast. My body knew Gabriel was out and alive, and nursing; so naturally the placenta expelled itself on its own. In normal hospital procedure, the baby is taken away, cleaned, weighed, and put in a nursery; and so the body never knows that the baby is out, and alive, and thereafter the placenta needs to be extracted—which feels like a second and unnecessary delivery! When the baby nurses immediately following birth, the hormones that are stimulated by the action of nursing let the placenta know that its job is over, and so it expels itself naturally.

Gabriel nursed for a while, and then was cleaned and dressed by the nurse and brought back to me after only a few minutes. I got off the delivery table and he went to sleep. My husband collapsed beside him in our bed, and fainted from exhaustion. Male bodies don't generate the extra energy for childbirth unless it comes from adrenalin—so if your coach is calm and remains centered, he'll tire more easily than if he is freaked out—but it's better to have him exhausted than freaked. I got up and cleaned the room, had breakfast, and talked with Ken and Toni, two instructors from the seminary who shared Gabriel's birth experience with us. Then, around 9:00 A.M., I slept well for the first time in several days.

About Contractions and the Beginning of Labor

Originally, all women had their children by natural childbirth and worked hard at bringing them into the world—

GUIDELINES FOR THE PREGNANT MOTHER

Drink six to eight glasses of water daily to carry toxins out of the body and to prevent dehydration. Raw milk and yogurt or kefir are necessary in order to maintain friendly intestinal flora, which get rid of many toxins in the intestines. Coffee and black-leaf tea are especially harmful during pregnancy. They tend to increase serum uric acid, which makes it harder for the kidneys to do their job.

Raspberry-leaf tea has been used by pregnant women for many thousands of years. This is an excellent tea to be taken during pregnancy, two to three times daily. Drink a strong pot of tea when your labor begins. Teas to avoid: Golden seal, yarrow, valerian, tansy, cotton-root, cohosh or squawgrass, motherwort, couchgrass, rue, pennyroyal, vervaine, and St. John's wort. These teas can stimulate uterine contractions, and thus precipitate miscarriage. Also avoid potassium permanganate, found in many non-prescription drugs and ergot (rye fungus), found in moldy breads and some prescription drugs.

Eat your usual amount of food, but make sure it's good food. The problem of gaining too much weight in pregnancy results from eating candy and "junk food." If you're getting a balanced nutritional diet, putting on some weight is all right. You will probably be more comfortable eating four to six small meals a day. Eat a liberal amount of green vegetables, raw and cooked, and plenty of fruit. Fruit juices can be taken any time. Use whole-grain breads, such as sprouted seven-grain bread. Avoid greasy fried foods, sweets, fats, rich pastries, fat drippings, and gravies. Use salt with discretion. You will find that after a week or two your palate will adjust to eating foods without salt, and you will begin to taste the natural flavor of the food. When you take spices, tobacco, alcohol, and drugs, your baby gets a *massive dose* (smaller body, less resistance).

Vitamins and other supplements to your diet will be suggested by your doctor. Don't try to "save" a few dollars by getting a cheaper version of prenatal vitamins. Many vitamin supplements do not have the bases or yeasts necessary to process the B vitamins in your body.

Get *mild* exercise in the open air and sunlight, especially walking. This stimulates the soles of the feet,

this is where the term labor comes from. All stages of labor are caused by uterine contractions. Like your heart and stomach, the uterus is an "involuntary muscle." Relaxing or contracting it is not under your conscious control. At this time, exactly what starts the labor processes is unknown to ordinary physical science. But when the baby decides to be born, a signal is sent to the muscles of the uterus, which start to contract and release, slowly pushing him or her toward the cervix—the opening of your womb. The pressure against the internal opening of the cervix helps to stretch it, so that your baby can pass through. The contraction that I have just described is felt as a slow, continuous hardening of the uterine muscles. After this sensation you feel the muscles of your uterus slowly relax into the "rest periods" between contractions.

At various times during your pregnancy, you may experience mild uterine contractions which are called *Braxton-Hicks* contractions. The Braxton-Hicks contractions are simply sensations caused by your uterus expanding to allow the growth of the baby in the womb. The sensations you will notice during actual labor are quite similar to these, but will last longer and are more powerful. The effects of uterine contractions are:

(1) Effacement, stretching the muscles of the cervix lengthwise;

(2) Dilation, stretching the muscles of the cervix width-wise, causing it to open;
(3) Expulsion of the baby;
(4) Expulsion of the placenta.

Effacement and dilation of the cervix by the baby's head are very similar to what happens when you put on a turtleneck sweater. As you place the sweater over your head, the neck stretches to accommodate the larger size of your head. This is like "effacement." Then the top of the neck opens and slips over your head. This is like "dilation" and "crowning."

Some common signs of the beginning of labor are:

(1) Contractions that start in the lower back and wrap around to the front of your abdomen in a girdle-like fashion.
(2) The contractions have a definite rhythm and become progressively longer, stronger, and closer together.
(3) You may have a pinkish discharge. This mucus barrier mixed with a small amount of blood from the tiny vessels in your cervix is commonly called "bloody show" (this term was probably invented by the British).
(4) You may pass some clear fluid. This will be the breaking of your "bag of waters," the amniotic fluid in which the baby has been suspended during pregnancy. Up

breaks up uric acid crystals, and enables the uric acid to pass through the kidneys and out of the system. Don't fatigue yourself by doing excessive exercising or housework. Avoid bumpy motions, vigorous sports (although swimming in moderation is excellent), or long automobile rides.

No platform shoes. Get some low, comfortable shoes that give your feet proper support. Dr. Scholls or Earth shoes are all right.

Avoid tight or constricting clothing on any part of your body. You can purchase maternity support garments at any maternity shop. There are some very good maternity bras which adjust to your current cup size. Maternity support pantyhose will give your back and legs relief, and help to avoid varicose veins.

Support the breasts with the adjustable maternity bra. Wash the nipples with Castile soap and water, and dry them with a soft cloth. Apply coconut or olive oil. Massage the nipples every day during the last three months if you are going to nurse your baby. Massaging toughens the nipples, so that they aren't too sensitive for nursing.

Get at least eighteen hours of good rest every day. Sleep on alternate sides. During the last two months you should very *gently* knead the abdomen for a few minutes every day, to relieve baby from a cramped position. Apply coconut or olive oil on the abdomen at intervals—good for skin elasticity, to avoid unnecessary stretch marks.

Lie down three times during the day with your feet elevated for at least five minutes at a time. Place a board between box spring and mattress, where the feet rest, in order to keep them elevated when you are sleeping. This helps blood circulation and keeps the feet from swelling.

A regular bowel movement is essential to a pregnant woman. It relieves pressure on the lower back and base of the spine. This pressure is probably what causes irritability and prevents a steady, relaxed state. Ask your doctor for advice on the best way to maintain regularity.

Don't take diuretics unless you consult your doctor!

Do not douche unless specifically told to do so by your doctor.

The expectant mother should bring a *morning* urine specimen with her for examination during each doctor's appointment.

Report *immediately* to the doctor if you have:

excessive nausea,
vomiting,
headaches,
blindness or other visual disturbances,
chills or fever,
excessive swelling of the hands or feet,
bleeding from any part of the body.

Regular office visits are essential for you and your baby's well-being.

---

until this time, it has served as insulation and as a buffer zone against external shocks.

Don't be alarmed if everything doesn't go exactly as it's described here. Every birth is different.

Stages of Labor and Delivery

At Term

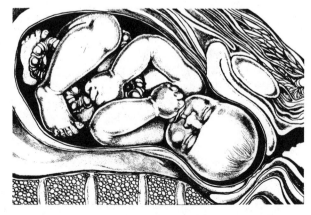

The fetus has reached maturity and is ready to be born. Note thick pelvic floor. The cervix is closed, the uterus relaxed.

Effacement

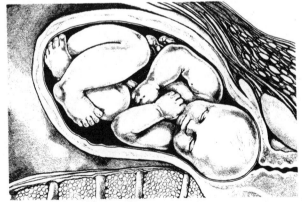

Labor has begun. Your baby is facing your right side, with arms and legs flexed—a normal birth position. Uterine contractions move the baby down, and push him or her against the opening of the cervix. The head looks big in relation to the birth canal, but the skull bones have not yet grown together. Their edges start to slip over each other, so that the head becomes molded to the available space.

Dilation

The cervix is dilating. The baby is moving down and beginning to rotate toward your back. Your bladder and rec-

WHY NOT USE COMMERCIAL BABY FOODS?

Ellen Tisdale

Commercial baby foods contain salt, sugar, bleached flour, and preservatives. They have modified starch added because of the large amounts of water and long cooking time required to produce them. They are expensive and the average baby will use more than 700 jars. They are stripped of many nutrients, and have only a small amount of vitamins replaced in an inexpensive synthetic form by "enrichment." Why use "dead" food? Use fresh food, newly prepared, for a lively, healthy baby. Lastly, the best foods of all are made and served with love.

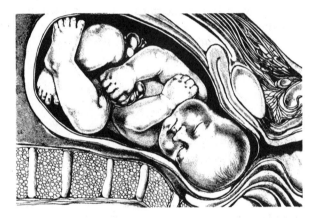

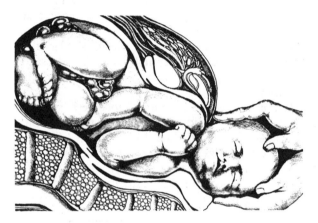

tum are being crowded. Your "bag of waters" may still be intact.

Transition

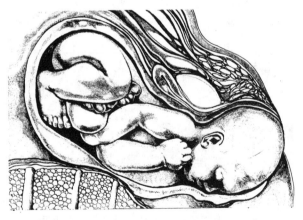

Contractions are much stronger, and last up to 90 seconds. The cervix is at full dilation (ten centimeters) and begins to stretch over baby's head. Baby moves into birth canal, rotating toward your back.

Crowning is about to begin.

Expulsion

Now you will be pushing during the contractions until crowning occurs. Then the doctor will work the perineum over the baby's head, after which expulsion usually takes place very quickly.

Breastfeeding

It is important that you know the advantages of breastfeeding. If you have friends or relatives who are negative about the idea of breastfeeding, let them know that you are completely comfortable with it. It is best for the health of both the child and the mother. Remember, babies need to feel the warmth of your body. You *cannot* spoil a baby with *too much* affection.

Advantages of Nursing

(1) One of the rewards of nursing is a feeling of unity between mother and child.
(2) Breastfeeding provides good protection against infections, allergies, and childhood diseases for the baby.
(3) Breastfeeding will prevent excessive bleeding after delivery and will help you to regain your psychological and emotional harmony.
(4) It has been shown in recent medical studies that breastfeeding decreases a woman's chances of ever getting breast cancer.
(5) Colostrum, the grayish fluid that comes in before the milk, is a very important nutrient for the newborn baby. It contains five to six times as much protein as the milk, and half as much fat and carbohydrates. It is also a natural cleanser of baby's bowels.

(6) Breastfeeding is convenient and takes the worry out of travel. There is no formula to spoil, no running out of special foods, no night feedings to prepare.

(7) Breastmilk is the best food for premature babies.

(8) Breastfeeding is a natural form of birth control. If you use it *exclusively*, there is generally a postponement of ovulation and menstrual cycle for seven to fifteen months. However, this is not a foolproof method of birth control, and sometimes is only effective for a few hours after delivery.

(9) Menstruation *usually* does not occur as long as breastfeeding continues, but even if it should occur it does not affect nursing.

(10) The size of your breasts does not affect your ability to nurse or determine the amount of milk your body can produce.

(11) If you have twins there will be enough milk to nurse them both successfully.

(12) Neither Caesarean section nor the Rh-negative factor have any connection with nursing or any effect on your ability to nurse.

(13) In addition, breastfeeding will teach you how to put your baby's needs before your own.

Method for Breastfeeding

Lying down is the most comfortable position for breastfeeding. For night feeding, just bring the baby to your bed. I found that for the first week it is better to let the baby sleep with you in your bed. It lets the baby know that you enjoy his or her presence. You can nurse in any position. Try different positions to find one that suits you and your baby best.

Make a cool glass of herb tea or juice, and sip it while you nurse. This can give you energy and help your body to relax, thus assisting lactation.

A newborn baby is more comfortable and feels more secure wrapped snugly in a receiving blanket. Bring the baby close to you until the cheek is touching your breast, with your nipple close to the mouth. Baby's natural reflex will be to turn toward the nipple. Then pull baby close to you, just enough so that the nipple goes into the mouth easily. Pull the baby's legs closer to you, angling baby's body to keep the nose free for breathing. When you are ready to remove baby from your breast, you can break the suction by pressing the breast away from the corners of the mouth with your fingers.

If your baby is having trouble getting to the nipple, hand express some milk, so that the baby can taste it. This creates the impulse to begin sucking rather than to cry. Crook your arm so that the head isn't too confined, or let the baby lie flat, whichever is more comfortable. Always feed your baby on each breast for an equal length of time—about five minutes each. The feeding time is usually every two to three hours, but allow your baby's appetite to be the guide.

During the first few days, your breasts may become swollen. This is caused by blood vessels, not milk. It may be uncomfortable, but it will soon subside and the milk will come in. After the swelling subsides, you may think that your milk is gone, but don't worry, it's still there.

Be sure to change nursing pads after each feeding. If you leave the same pad on your nipples, it may cause breast infection. You can continue to nurse even with an infection; however, you may need to hand express some milk or use a breast pump and hot towels until the infection clears up. In case of severe infection, you may have to get an antibiotic from your doctor to help clear it up before it becomes septic and works into the bloodstream.

During lactation, medications or certain foods can cause adverse reactions in your baby. If antibiotics are prescribed, you can get mother's milk through La Leche League or hospitals, since you should not feed your baby milk that contains antibiotics. In addition, you should be eating yogurt and milk cultures during treatment for a faster healing process and to counter the inevitable negative effects of an antibiotic

CYBELE GOLD, *Th.D., is a pioneer in the field of natural childbirth. She has trained hundreds of midwives and prospective parents for this method of delivery, and has developed the first practical course for teachers of the method. She has led research in therapeutic psychology for pregnant women, and workshops for expectant parents.*

E. J. GOLD, *Th.D., D.D., is a distinguished and unusual metaphysical scientist. His credentials include training at Elon and the College Seminarium at Florida. He has taught at U.C.L.A., U.S.C., and Sherman Oaks Experimental College, and lectured throughout the United States and Canada. For 13 years he researched the anatomy of childbirth, human communication, physiology and neuroanatomy. In 1971 he co-developed the method of natural childbirth discussed in this article.*

A Husband at the Amniocentesis

Samuel Osherson, Ph.D.

DURING THE 17th week of pregnancy my wife and I arrived at the hospital, clutching our forms, to keep our appointment for an amniocentesis. After three miscarriages we had finally made it past the first trimester. Yet we were still treading lightly on our hopes, afraid of again being disappointed. I walked through the hospital entrance as if on tip-toes, not wanting to attract attention to ourselves.

An amniocentesis involves inserting a needle through the woman's abdominal wall into the amniotic sac to take a sample of fluid containing cells discarded from the fetus. Cells obtained in this way allow genetic testing for birth defects. Although considered a routine procedure for pregnant women over 35, an amniocentesis has risks. A miscarriage may be induced, and particularly as the parents get into their late 30s, as we were, this risk must be weighed against the increasing possibility of birth defects. (We had engaged, too, in a more terrible, ultimately futile mental calculus: if there was evidence of birth defects, would we agree to abort? After four years of trying to have a child, we were about ready to take whatever we'd get). The amniocentesis felt like the last hurdle: if all went well we could finally permit ourselves to believe in this pregnancy.

At the hospital we checked into the Radiology Department for the test. The receptionist smiled at my wife, showed her where to change into her surgical gown, then looked at me and warned: "It's all right if you want to accompany your wife for the test, but remember, if at anytime you feel faint, please leave the room. Last week we had a husband who fainted during the procedure, hit his head and caused a big disruption. He had to be taken to the emergency room." She spoke so scoldingly, I almost apologized for him. Was he tall, I wondered, did he have far to fall? Knees buckling, head hitting the floor. How embarrassing. I realized I had never seen a grown man faint. Her tone, and a sudden tightness in my stomach, stopped me from asking what could happen during an amniocentesis that would cause a man to swoon.

The amniocentesis took place in a small room, hardly bigger than a large closet. We were in Radiology in the first place because an Ultrasound is used during the amniocentesis. An Ultrasound, also called a B-scan, is a piece of machinery that uses sound waves to provide a picture on the monitor of the fetus inside the womb. Knowing the precise location of the fetus in its dark cave lowers the possibility of injuring it when the needle is inserted. The ultrasound, though, had shadowed us throughout our pregnancies. It was the constant harbinger of bad, then finally good, news. Two years ago in this same room an ultrasound picture in the 12th week of our first pregnancy positively confirmed a miscarriage. The picture on the scope told the story without mercy, as the doctor explained that "the embryo stopped developing after the fifth week, right now there's nothing really there." From this room Julie went for a D and C at 2 a.m. while I drove home alone through the dark city streets, wet still with rain. Walking into the room for "the amnio" brought these unborn babies to mind, and a superstitious residue made me worry for the living cargo my wife was now carrying. The room seemed unchanged, a typical hospital room—insistently functional, decidedly unsentimental. I recognized against one bare wall the metal table and chairs where we all had sat while the doctor gave us the bad news.

Julie, draped only in a yellow smock, lay on the operating-examining table. The ultrasound technician adjusted the equipment, then sat in a chair near my wife's head. In walked the doctor, our gynecologist, dressed in his white surgical uniform. A quiet, soft-spoken man. His delicate dark Asian features clashed with the metallic angularity of the machinery packed into the room, with the harsh blankness of the white hospital walls. He had been our doctor since the second miscarriage and throughout this pregnancy; both Julie and I feel considerable affection for him. He smiled, chatted briefly with us, and then donned his white surgical mask.

The doctor stood beside Julie, feeling her stomach area. The technician was seated near the top of the table. There was no place for me to sit except down near Julie's feet, in the corner. Julie raised her head and looked down the table at me; she seemed about six miles away. She smiled encouragingly at me and asked, "Want to hold my toe?"

So there we were, toe to hand.

The ultrasound technician turned on her machine. There on the screen appeared our baby, difficult to make out clearly but surprisingly large and well-formed. The baby is so well-developed by this time that it's often possible to identify its sex from the ultrasound picture. We didn't want to know, hoping to preserve the surprise.

"OK," the technician informed us, "the baby's on its head." Crowded around the fuzzy screen of the ultrasound monitor in the darkened room, the technician in front of her device adjusting buttons, we could have been inside a submarine, gliding throught the ocean's depths.

The technician found the exact location of the baby to ensure that the needle would be inserted away from it. Amazing—one piece of technology was protecting our baby from another. Previously I had come to hate the ultrasound for its unrelenting judgments of failed pregnancies, now I loved it for its protective power. The technician looked about 25 years old, and her red hair tempered the whiteness of her nurse's uniform. She took a ballpoint pen and made an X on Julie's belly, marking the spot where the doctor should insert the needle. Then, the machine switched off, she sat to the side of the table, her hand gently resting on Julie's forehead, reassuring her, while we waited for the doctor to begin the procedure. My wife's toe was still firmly in my grip.

First Julie's belly was heartily splashed and painted with an orange, antiseptic solution. Then a local anaesthetic was applied, and the procedure began. The doctor, creases around his eyes reflecting concentration uncensored by the surgical mask, slowly inserted a sheath where the technician had marked her spot, then a needle delicately through the sheath. He gently allowed the vacuum inside the syringe to act as a pump to pull the amniotic fluid up. Yet the large barrel of the needle remained empty: no fluid rushed in to fill it. A dry well.

Very quietly, the doctor signalled the technician to turn on the ultrasound again. The technician swiveled in her seat and switched it on.

"OK," she advised, pointing to a spot on the screen, "you've penetrated the muscular wall of the uterus; you're not in the amniotic sac itself." There was a slight pause, then she said softly:

"Move the needle 1 centimeter, medially."

"Um, medially? You mean to the left?" The doctor asked uncertainly.

For a dreadful moment I wondered if this man was truly competent.

He moved the needle, inside its sheath, 1 cm. to the left.

No fluid. Another dry well.

"The uterus has contracted and moved away from the needle," she explained. Smart uterus. "The wall is cramping." That word again, "cramp." It's remarkable how some words become frightful to you at particular times in your life, their sound echoes in a room like vultures circling overhead. Cramps preceded all the miscarriages. "You feel like you're cramping slightly, as if you're having your period," Julie once told me, describing the onset of the miscarriages.

The technician reached over and placed a long finger on Julie's belly. "Right here," she instructed the doctor, indicating where the needle should go. Her wedding ring glistened in the dull hospital light.

The doctor seemed unaware of the tension in the room. To me it was as if I were deep-sea diving, the pressure wanting to cave in my chest. Yet he seemed unaffected, his attention totally on the procedure and the womb in front of him. He hardly looked at us. A friend of mine lost her baby soon after an amniocentesis, convinced that the doctor had botched the procedure and injured the fetus or the placenta with the needle. There had been blood in the fluid as it entered the needle. I fantasize punching our doctor in the face if there was such evidence today, knowing I'd never do that. Yet how much rage would I feel if we lost this baby, no one to blame for "reproductive difficulties," nothing to do. Is there a way to quantify that kind of rage? Is it more than a cm. long?

The doctor held the needle in front of him, preparing for a third attempt.

The needle looked enormous. (Months later Doonesbury was to feature Joanie Caucus' amniocentesis, in which the doctor jokes that "We are just now wheeling in the needle from the other room.") My wife was laid out on the table with a doctor sticking a thick needle into her, a long metallic spear penetrating close to the baby, unknowingly in danger within a secret sea. An image of whales, harpoons being shot into whales at sea. A line from a book on ships I had once seen, perhaps as a child: *the mother whale is pulled closer to the factory ship.*

Sitting there, I could not get images of violence and sadism out of my mind. I was in no danger of fainting, but I did want to cry out, to stop the procedure. My wife, the fetus, felt to me intolerably vulnerable. And, too, I wanted to cry at my own vulnerability. Life suddenly seemed to me very precious, and very fragile.

Simply watching was perhaps the hardest part. I wanted to do something, to protect Julie, the baby. Yet there was nothing to do, except to hold her toe and support her with my presence. I felt for the husbands who do faint. Trained to do, to be instrumental, we must just watch. And yet we don't ask for help, for the reassurance routinely given our wives. Instead we sit silently, looking composed. And faint.

While we waited for the doctor to again insert the needle, another doctor walked into the room, from a door on my immediate right. Why is he here? I wondered. Is there an emergency no one has admitted to? Perhaps doctors have a secret button on the floor, like bank tellers press during a robbery, to call for help without alerting any of the customers. This doctor was about my age, short and neat looking. He was dressed in street clothes, suit pants and a striped shirt, with a beeper dangling in his belt. As he closed the door he looked down at me, sitting in the corner, holding my wife's toe. He smiled and introduced himself: "Hi, I'm Dr. Phillips, just wanted to see what's going on here, whether I could be of help." So saying, he slid by me carefully and walked over to join his compatriot, our gynecologist.

As he passed by I had a strong impulse to ask:

"Would you hold *my* hand?"

I wanted to be touched, to be reassured. The air was so

heavy in the room, the time so heavy. Had we been there two days or three? I forgot to breathe, felt empty. I wanted tactile contact, suddenly felt an ache to be held, supported, to feel less alone, and I wanted that from a man. Another man to legitimate that it was OK to feel scared, to care so deeply about the outcome. But I didn't ask the doctor, I refused to ask. I was afraid I would embarrass him, scared myself of looking weak or silly. As this other man walked by, my body withdrew, I felt far away from my skin, armored in my hard shell of male toughness. A rock. Momentarily aware of my need for touch, I felt a familiar anxiety. Is it possible for men to imagine comforting each other without fearing homosexuality?

A nurse would have held my hand, but that felt regressive: traditionally it is always the nurses who do that. The female nurse comes over to hold the husband's hand, speaking soothingly, "it's OK, there, there, would you rather wait outside in the hall with me?" Mommy leads the scared boy away from the men's work. Or there's a sexualized element, as if the man is saying, "Hold my hand, will you baby—gee, you're cute when you're nurturant." The seductiveness of male fragility. Perhaps it will always feel infantalizing or sexualized to ask only for such help from the nurses, without men too legitimizing that kind of caring.

The two doctors conferred momentarily. Then the needle went in again. Suddenly clear, slightly yellowish fluid flooded the chamber. Amniotic fluid, looking like urine. One cylinder was filled and then replaced by another. That one too was filled, insuring enough fluid for the tests to be done. (Tests that were to reveal a baby as healthy as modern science could certify; 16 weeks later our son was born, three weeks overdue.)

"Very good fluid, clear and healthy-looking. No blood, an excellent sign," our doctor explained. He then left the room in search of forms he needed to complete for us. The technician took Julie's hand, moving up to look in her face. She reached over and reassured, "now all that was perfectly normal. The fluid looks fine, the ultrasound shows your baby is developing just as it should. It often takes several tries to get the sample. Nothing went wrong." Julie looked dazed, and her head and arms were shaking slightly, like she wanted to cry. But it was clear she had taken in the woman's words. The technician stroked Julie's head. All the anxiety my wife had been feeling looked like it wanted to burst out, like flood waters straining to smash through a dam. "Do you believe me?" the woman asked in a sisterly fashion." "Yes," answered Julie, looking away and laughing, gently wiping a tear from her eye.

I went over to my wife, held her head in my hands, glad it was over. Suddenly appreciation for this technician and our doctor filled me. As we were leaving I took the doctor's hand and shook it, exclaiming, "Thank you." He looked at me, smiled back, and replied shyly, "You're welcome,

Sam." He spoke my name so softly I almost didn't hear it. It was the first time in two years this gentle, reserved man had called me by my first name.

Suggestions for Further Reading

1. Osherson, S. *Holding on or letting go: men and career change at midlife*, NY: The Free Press, 1980.
2. Osherson, S. and AmaraSingham, L. "The machine metaphor in medicine." In Mishler, Osherson et al *Social Contexts of Health, Illness and Patient Care*, Cambridge University Press, 1983.
3. Osherson, S. and Dill, D. "Varying work and family choices: their impact on men's work satisfaction," Journal of Marriage and the Family, May 1983, 339–346.
4. Osherson, S. *The Silent Wound: Why Men Don't Talk* (In preparation.) To be published by The Free Press in 1985.

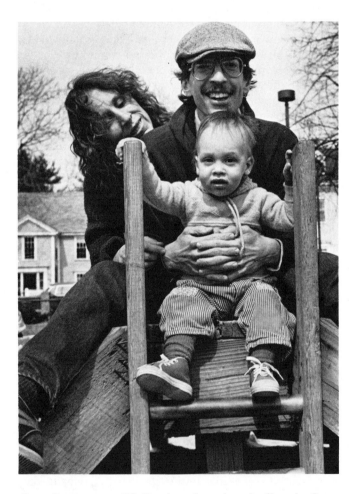

SAM OSHERSON, *Ph.D., is a therapist who lives in Cambridge, Massachusetts, with his wife Julie and 14-month-old son Toby. He teaches courses on Adult Development at Harvard, where he also pursues his research on work-family dilemmas of men and women in their 30s and 40s.*

PREGNANT DREAMS: THE SECRET LIFE OF THE EXPECTANT FATHER

Alan B. Siegel, Ph.D.

ON the night after his wife's pregnancy was confirmed, David, a 35-year-old environmental planner, had a vivid dream. He dreamt that he came upon a pair of radioactive glasses that were not supposed to be touched. Nevertheless, he felt compelled to look through them and when he did, he felt like he was looking through the eyes of what seemed to be another "being." As he gazed through the eyes, he felt as if he were floating in an outer space environment.

David, like most expectant fathers, was deeply moved by the news of his wife's pregnancy. At first, David had no idea what the dream symbolized; he suspected only that it might be related to the news of the pregnancy. As he shared the dream with me and we explored the images and feelings that emerged. David suddenly realized that in his dream, he was seeing the world through the eyes of his unborn child.

During the first trimester of pregnancy, many other expectant fathers have dreams that appear to portray the experience of the fetus in the womb. Underwater dreams of old-fashioned scuba divers with umbilical cord-like hoses attached to them are not uncommon. These early pregnancy dreams strongly suggest that a man's unconscious identification with his child and his conscious feelings of empathy for his child, powerfully affect his experience of involvement in the pregnancy.

Men's involvement in the birth process has increased dramatically in little more than a decade. In 1970 a man in Texas who had been excluded from the birth of his first two children handcuffed himself to his wife to insure that he would not be barred from the birth of their third child. By the early 1970s, the ban on fathers being present at the birth was changing and 27 percent of fathers were attending the birth of their children. In July 1983, a Gallup Poll indicated that 70 percent of men were present at the birth of their children. Suddenly, the doors to the delivery room have been opened to fathers.

Appreciation and support for the unique emotional needs of the expectant father has not paralleled the increase in father involvement in birthing. This article documents the first systematic study of expectant fathers' dreams, which I conducted in 1982. The dreams which I collected provide a window through which we can view the profound emotional transformation that the expectant father undergoes in his identity as a man and as a father, in his relationship with his spouse and in his growing prenatal bond with his child.

When I compared the dreams of expectant fathers with a matched group of married men who were not fathers and not expecting, there was a striking difference. The expectant fathers' dreams were replete with vivid imagery of fertility, pregnancy, birth, and babies as well as with many graphic sexual and homosexual encounters and dreams of wild celebratory *birth*day parties.

Some men dreamt that they were actually pregnant or giving birth. Ron, a 33-year-old computer programmer, dreamt:

> I was standing on a street corner, carrying my baby fetus under my shirt against my chest. I had my hand cupped over the fetus to protect it. It was moving and people asked what it was. I said: "It is my baby."

This dream and others like it suggest that men have powerful desires to feel included in the pregnancy and to be pregnant themselves.

In the face of mounting evidence about the emotional challenge of becoming a father, most expectant fathers don't realize that their vivid dreams, increased physical symptoms, and intense anxieties about their masculinity, are direct emotional responses to the pregnancy. In fact few men are aware of or talk about their concerns about becoming a father.

Why are men out of touch with their feelings about pregnancy? I feel that it is due to our general taboo on men expressing their feelings, and more specifically, to the lack of knowledge about men's potential for being involved in pregnancy. Unlike primitive cultures, which engaged expectant fathers in elaborate couvade rituals which simulated aspects of pregnancy, our culture does not give expectant fathers any role models or rites of passage to help them understand and integrate their experience of becoming a father.

Despite expectant father's intense emotional involvement, their dreams commonly portray a feeling of being left out. Michael, a 30-year-old alcoholism counselor, had the following dream during the second trimester of pregnancy:

> I am at a baseball game. I get up to go get some beer. When I return, I can't find my seat. I look for a new one but while the stadium is not full, many of the women are pregnant and are taking up two seats. I go to the back of the stadium and stand. I am annoyed.

Michael is being forced out of his seat by the many pregnant women who were filling the stadium. He ends up feeling that there is no room for himself even in the traditionally male-dominated arena of beer and baseball. After sharing his dream with me, Michael verbalized for the first time that he had been preoccupied with a nagging feeling that he had no part to play in the pregnancy, and was somehow being excluded by his wife.

Men's dream themes ran an evolutionary course as the stages of pregnancy progressed. Whereas early pregnancy dreams featured images of the fetus floating in womblike environments, late pregnancy dreams depicted a preoccupation with the birth processes and with the experience of the birthing child. One man dreamt that while he was fishing, a large bubble emerged from underwater and out of it popped a furry animal that had lived underwater for a long time. Another third-trimester pregnant father dreamt that he escaped from a cave through a hole that opened up during an earthquake. A third man dreamt late in pregnancy that he was swimming downhill, leading a race that was coached by his Lamaze teacher. He won the race and emerged into a locker room, where he was wrapped in a towel. Despite the transparent symbolism of the fetus traveling down the birth canal and emerging at birth, none of these three men spontaneously linked their dream to pregnancy or birth. They were all surprised and delighted when I suggested the possible connection of the dreams to the birth process and to their emotional involvement with the pregnancy and their child.

Sexual dreams were extremely common throughout pregnancy but especially so early in the pregnancy. Many sex dreams portrayed men feeling rejected or inhibited sexually. Other dreams portrayed exotic liaisons or homosexual fears or experiences. One first-trimester man dreamt that he was about to have a torrid rendezvous with a woman, but then he was interrupted when an alarm on his wedding ring went off. Sexual dreams reflect men's responses to the changing patterns of sexual expression during pregnancy. Despite the so-called sexual revolution, men and women still have difficulty in openly discussing important changes in their sexual relationship. Encouraging men and couples to understand their sex dreams during pregnancy will help to prevent feelings of rejection and alienation that often develop. It is important for channels of communication and intimate expression to remain open, even if lovemaking decreases at certain stages of pregnancy.

Party and celebration dreams were common throughout pregnancy. They are linked with an unconscious sense of how special becoming a father is to men. Many of the party dreams depicted *birth*day parties. A few of the party dreams had a distinct flavor of initiation rituals common to primitive cultures including ritual dances and ceremonies relating to labor and birth. Brian, a 26-year-old carpenter, dreamt:

Watching people all around me dance and play. I am not seen or heard. A group comes near and all play ceases. This group seems to have control over all. I like them. Their energy is high and has a calming effect on me. They come to me and surround me. One comes to me and gives me a bundle. It is a baby.

Dreams are a hidden resource for becoming aware of deeper feelings about important life transitions. Long before expectant fathers are consciously aware of how deeply affected they are by their wives' pregnancies, their dreams are portraying powerful responses to becoming a father. Remembering and sharing dreams would ideally help expectant fathers to feel more included and more secure about the importance of their role in pregnancy and parenting and to forge a closer alliance with their wife and child.

ALAN B. SIEGEL, *Ph.D., is a psychologist and consultant in Berkeley, California.*

B. LIFE EXTENSION

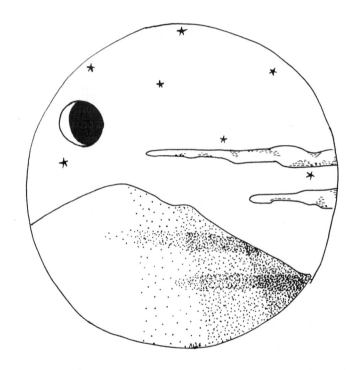

Enhancing and Prolonging Life

CAN WE LIVE TO BE 200?

Shepherd Bliss

THEORIES of what causes aging abound; biochemical theories are of two kinds. In one, deterioration is seen as resulting from an active "self-destruct" program. In the other, aging is seen as resulting from a passive "wearing out" process. Dr. Roy Walford of the UCLA School of Medicine has developed the immunological theory of aging (see *Bestways*, August, 1981). This prominent theory describes aging as an inability to cope with stress and sees impairment as due to a weakening of the immune system.

Other gerontologists ascribe to a composite theory of aging, looking at factors such as radiation, mutation and toxic accumulation. The integrated theory of aging looks at the interactions of stress, metabolic waste production, free radical buildup, and somatic mutations. One of the biggest questions in gerontology is whether aging is controlled by the brain or from within each cell.

Some theorists speak of an "aging clock theory"—either the brain "aging clock" or cellular "aging clock." In recent years the cell theory—that each cell is programmed to age—has become less popular among scientists and the brain is seen as the center of aging. The hypothalamus, the pituitary and the thymus are the key organs controlling aging.

Contemporary Researchers and Practitioners

Two psychologists in the San Francisco Bay Area, Dr. Ken Dychtwald, founder of a group of elders called SAGE, and Kenneth R. Pelletier, Ph.D., assistant clinical professor in the Department of Psychiatry at the University of Berkeley and San Francisco, are independently doing some of the most impressive work on longevity. Both advocate holistic approaches.

Additional important work is being done by Nobel laureate Dr. Linus Pauling in orthomolecular medicine, and by Nathan Pritikin in nutrition and exercise at the Longevity Center in Santa Barbara, California. Though considerable scientific work on longevity has been done in recent years, Dr. Pelletier notes "a vast gap between the abundant data available from laboratory and clinical assessments and the limited applications of these findings to the realm of longevity." A variety of means have been found

to double and even triple the lives of rats and other animals. Doing the same for humans is still another matter.

Nutrition and Exercise

Nutrition and exercise are the two most important physical factors influencing longevity *which an individual can change*. The two work together, with exercise helping bring nutritional components to all the body's tissues, enabling the tissues to use them fully. Though much work on the importance of nutrition to longevity has been done and continues to be done, there is still much that is not known. Dr. Pelletier observes, "There are major, unanswered questions regarding the optimum diet in youth, young adulthood, middle age, and advanced age. Nutritional needs are subject to variation due to psychological and physiological changes that accompany aging."

One of the most important aspects of nutrition and longevity being researched by scientists is the role of antioxidants like vitamins E and C. Dr. Pelletier explains, "antioxidants retard the aging process by inhibiting harmful environmental influences, by reducing the oxidation of essential dietary nutrients, and by preventing the degenerative process initiated by free radicals."

Antioxidants such as sulfur, amino acids, and selenium found in brewer's yeast have been proven in laboratory situations to slow down aging of animals, by interfering with harmful reactions in their bodies. Arteries harden and collect cholesterol; body proteins can become crosslinked; and tissues lose suppleness. Antioxidants can literally slow down these processes, Linus Pauling writes: "Vitamin E is the principal fat-soluble antioxidant and Vitamin C is the principal water-soluble antioxidant. They probably cooperate in providing protection for our bodies and slowing the aging process."

Physical activity extends life in various ways. It improves the functioning of the heart, allowing it to get more blood to the brain more efficiently and improving circulation; exercise reduces the heartbeat and blood pressure. Exercise helps remove toxic substances from the body, burns off fat, reduces the body's susceptibility to many diseases and reduces weight. It is relaxing and increases muscle endurance.

Physical activity improves the function of various organ systems, develops better posture, and is good for mental health. Given all this, Dr. Alexander Leaf of the Harvard

Bestways, August 1982. Reprinted by permission.

Medical School concluded, "Exercise is the closest thing to an anti-aging pill."

Physical activity does not occur in a vacuum, but influences other factors. As a recent article in *MD* on running revealed: "Jogging and especially endurance running require health-promoting habits. Many runners report they have quit smoking, moderated drinking habits, and adopted a sensible diet. Some say that running has cured insomnia, impotence, and bettered their sexual performance." So it appears that physical activity enhances longevity not only directly but also through influencing other health factors.

Longevity-minded exercise, according to Dr. Dychtwald, should "1) heighten the body's level of aerobic fitness and endurance (such as running, swimming, and bicycling); 2) enhance flexibility and limberness (such as yoga and stretching); 3) strengthen and vitalize the body and mind (such as weight or resistance training, calisthenics, or water sports); and 4) improve relaxation and reduce stress (such as meditation, deep breathing or autogenetics)."

Dychtwald's "Technologies for Life Extension"

Dr. Dychtwald was a key speaker at the recent 28th Annual Western Gerontological Society meeting, which drew 2,500 participants to talk about aging. Dr. Dychtwald traced life expectancy in the U.S. from 47 years in 1900 to its current 75 years, noting that women can expect to live about 8 years longer than men. Life expectancy for the ancient Greeks was about 22 years.

Though the average life expectancy has increased dramatically through the centuries, the maximum life span has not increased significantly. Among the Greeks, for example, Sophocles defied the then-average life span by living until 90; in his 80s he was writing great plays and fathering children.

Those with longest expectancy include symphony conductors, clergymen, educators, military men and scientists. Those with the least expectancy include correspondents and journalists.

Dr. Dychtwald referred to at least "20 technologies for life extension," and enumerated the most important seven: modern medicine which is improving treatment and early detection, energy medicine such as acupuncture and healing hands, organ transplantation, prosthetic devices like pacemakers and artificial limbs, enhanced drugs and chemicals like interferon, genetic engineering, and what he called "natural life extension." Dr. Dychtwald was clearly most enthusiastic about the latter, concluding, "If we could improve the style of life in the U.S., bring people back together, we could improve the sense of wellness and vitality for all."

Dr. Dychtwald also indicated that even given factors such as heredity can be influenced by a person. "Longevity-minded people can learn to use their genetics, rather than having their genetics use them. For example, if your family has a history of heart disease, the worst thing you can do is disregard this predisposition.

Instead, you should design your life so as to avoid the kinds of food, environments, and daily routine conducive to cardiovascular disease. You should spend a bit more time exercising and resting than most people." Dychtwald also advocates the importance of life planning. "Taking the time to plan physically, psychologically, socially, and financially for a long healthy life will enormously increase the odds that this will occur."

Dr. Dychtwald asserted: *"The most important person in our health is ourself.* Most deaths are suicide from smoking, drinking and bad health habits. Slow suicide. I say this not to blame but to underscore that if we live in a fashion to live longer, we will. Most deaths before 120 are premature. The major reason people die in the U.S. is not germs, but us. We kill ourselves."

Pelletier's Holistic Approach to Longevity

Of the various new books on longevity, Dr. Pelletier's★ is arguably the best. It examines "evidence for potential human longevity...from biochemical research, laboratory experimental studies, single case reports and observations of centenarian communities." Dr. Pelletier maintains, "Many of the same factors that enhance the quality of life have the same effect of enhancing the quantity of life." He asserts that by applying available knowledge individuals can extend their lifespan by 10 percent to 15 percent by at least seven years.

Dr. Pelletier's approach to longevity is distinctly holistic. He does not separate quantity from quality. His concern is not only to extend life, but to prevent declining vigor in later years. He echoes the President of the American Health Foundation, Ernest Wynder: "It should be the function of medicine to have people die young as late as possible." In fact, modern medicine has been more successful with life-saving technology than with health-preserving technology.

The net effect has been to keep people alive longer—but often in a miserable, unhealthy state. Dr. Pelletier's motivation for his in-depth study of longevity is not a sensationalist thirst for immortality, but a holistic pursuit of health, "Perhaps the greatest contribution of an inquiry into human longevity is that it can illuminate the present metamorphosis in our attitudes toward health."

An in-depth analysis of the major biochemical and neurophysical approaches to aging is presented by Dr. Pelletier. Whereas some researchers and theorists of longevity emphasize this area and though Dr. Pelletier is a clinical professor at the Langley Porter Neuropsychiatric Institute, he writes: "Biochemical approaches have received the greatest attention. This inordinate emphasis is a reflection of the prevailing scientific pattern which dictates that the ultimate nature of reality resides in the microscopic realms of biochemical interaction." Dr. Pelletier, in his holistic approach, calls for "a decreasing focus upon biomedical technology and a maximizing of software and self-education.

"Aging occurs primarily because the cells of the human body that cannot replace themselves either die or lose a small part of their function with each passing year. From that common observation the most frequent theories con-

---

*see bibliography at end of article

cerning the aging process divide into two main categories, those which focus on intrinsic factors and those which focus on extrinsic factors." Pelletier also examines the genetic code, DNA, free radical theory, cross-linkage theories, lipofusion accumulation, and neuroendoctrinological theories and research with lowered body temperature.

One of Dr. Pelletier's major contributions to the studies of longevity is revealed in his statement, "The single most important and most frequently overlooked factor in longevity is the psychological dimension. This includes prolonged and productive involvement in family and community affairs, an acquired status of dignity and wisdom, and an endearing sense of the meaning and purpose of life itself." Attitude is clearly a key to longevity. In cultures where the aged are respected, such as in many traditional Asian cultures, this factor is a definite plus.

In most Latin American cultures, for example, the term "los viejos," which translates literally to "the old ones" has a much more positive tone than U.S. terms like "senior citizens" and "elderly."

Dr. Pelletier concludes, "the single greatest impediment to a health care system devoted to optimum health and longevity is the resistance on the part of individuals and institutions to reorienting their personal habits and economic priorities."

Dr. Pelletier approaches longevity from various perspectives—public policy, the increasing number of older persons, crosscultural studies, historical insights, holistic principles, biochemical and neurophysical approaches to aging, the regenerative capacity of the human organism, and behavioral and environmental factors. With these bases Dr. Pelletier concludes his book with separate chapters on nutrition, exercise, and a look at those over 100 years old.

One aspect of looking at life extension is to consider life shortening behavior, that which has also been called "slow suicide" or "subintentioned death." These behaviors include substance abuse—cigarettes, alcohol, and drugs. Not wearing seat belts in cars, overeating, taking dangerous physical risks may also reduce one's life expectancy.

Mann the Practitioner

Mann's *Secrets of Life Extension*, though also scientific, is excellent for the practitioner who wants to go beyond theory. Mann is a self-described "longevist" who is one of "thousands of humans who have been self-experimenting for years with these combined therapies...(such as) antioxidants and free-radical deactivators, optimal nutrition, megadosages of certain vitamins, serotonin normalizers, protein-synthesis enhancers, DNA repair aids, and other treatments described in this book."

Though Mann's book is useful, his claims appear exorbitant. It is doubtful that he is correct in beginning his first chapter, "Many people who are reading this book may live for 200 years or more." Nor does he document his assertion, "Leading gerontologists believe that with proper funding they can find ways to double the human lifespan within the next 10 to 20 years."

Among the methods Mann advocates is lowering the body temperature. Dr. Walford discovered that lowering the body temperature, like caloric restriction, suppresses the immune system in a beneficial way. Whereas the normal body temperature of 37°C allows a maximum lifespan of about 100 years, Dr. Walford estimates that a drop to 35°C would extend the maximum to 150 years and a drop to 33°C to 180 years. Dr. Walford asserts that our normal body temperature is probably ideal for hunting and strenuous labor, but is no longer necessary for 20th century persons.

Dr. Pelletier echoes these ideas on lowering body temperature, noting, "There appears to be no exception to the rule that animals live longer at lower body temperatures." Experiments with cold-blooded animals have been able to triple their lives. It is more complicated with warm-blooded animals like humans because lowering the outside temperature does not affect the hypothalamic thermostat. Although some drugs can induce hypothermia, (lowered body temperature), experimenting with such drugs can be very dangerous.

For those considering the practice of anti-aging therapies, Dr. Pelletier notes, "While limited measures can be adopted later in life, most life extension measures need to be initiated from birth. Clearly a fundamental challenge is to enhance the awareness of the potential of longevity at earlier developmental stages." Waiting until you are advanced in years is not the best time to begin anti-aging processes.

The current work on longevity is likely to benefit future more than current generations. Dr. Pelletier's approach is consistent with the understanding of death not as an event at the end of life but as a process which occurs throughout life. Life extension similarly, is not something at the end of life but something which occurs throughout it.

References

de Beauvoir, Simone. *The Coming of Age*, Warner, 1972

Dychtwald, Ken and Associates, 1023 Amito Ave., Berkeley, CA.

Kent, Saul. *The Life Extension Revolution*, Wm. Morrow & Co., 1980.

Leaf, Alexander. *Youth in Old Age*, McGraw-Hill, 1975.

Mann, John. *Secrets of Life Extension*, And/Or Press, Berkeley, CA.

Pauling, Linus, and Ewan Cameron. *Cancer and Vitamin C*, Linus Pauling Institute, Menlo Park, CA.

Pelletier, Ph.D. Kenneth R. *Longevity: Fulfilling Our Biological Potential*, Delacorte Press, 1981.

Pritikin, Nathan, and Jon Leonard and J.L. Hofer. *Live Longer Now*, Charter, 1974.

The Longevity Game: Fulfilling Our Biological Potential

Kenneth R. Pelletier, Ph.D.

LONGEVITY HAS intrigued humankind as much as the distant stars. According to conservative estimates, the upper limit of human life expectancy now stands at approximately 115 years. Here in the United States, according to the 1970 census there were fewer than 3,000 centenarians (people over 100) but the 1980 census indicated an astounding jump to over 14,000. Between 1980 and the year 2030 A.D., the number of people over age 65 will double from 25 million to over 55 million and then level off. This is an unprecedented occurrence in all of history and has profound personal, social, economic, and philosophical implications.

For decades, researchers from all over the world have reported "centenarian communities" in Ecuador, the Soviet Union, Pakistan, and other regions where unusually large numbers of individuals evidence extreme longevity even beyond 115. Recently, it has become common practice to discredit such findings, but that is premature for several reasons: (1) the two studies most often cited to disprove this phenomenon clearly state that they were not intended to and do not disprove extreme longevity; (2) thousands of cases of longevity beyond 115 have been reported. Even if just one is "proven," this demonstrates the biological "potential" of the human species; (3) studies by the CBS "60 Minutes" program and U.S. Representative Claude Pepper have documented longevity beyond 115; and (4) from basic laboratory research there is far more evidence to support the likelihood of life extension beyond 115 than to establish a fixed upper limit. Perhaps most importantly, the emphasis here is upon quality of life, and it is clear that the same factors which determine the quality of life also have a profound influence upon the quantity of life. These findings are detailed in my two recent books *Holistic Medicine* (1979) and *Longevity* (1981). Whether or not 115 is a fixed upper limit or not remains to be determined. In any case, the fact that this age exceeds the present average life expectancy by 30 or 40 years indicates that it is unequivocally possible to live a healthier and longer life right now!

The "Longevity Game" below is a means of estimating your biological potential of attaining a century of life or longer. It is a "game" in the sense that it is suggestive, not definitive. Each of the numerical values are estimates based on recent research findings of the determinants of health and longevity. Statisticians and health researchers may agree on most of the determinants but not on the relative positive or negative values of each one. Being married or living together in a long-term relationship is usually considered to be a positive influence but could be a negative one if the relationship is embattled. There is no prescription for longevity but it is an exciting journey.

Start with: 75. Add or subtract the following numbers to derive your personal longevity potential.

Family History

Any grandparent lived to be 85 or over	+2
All four grandparents lived to be 80	+6
Either parent died of a stroke or heart attack before 50	−4
Any parent, brother or sister under 50 has or had cancer, a heart condition or diabetes since childhood	−3
A parent, grandparent, brother, sister, uncle, or aunt	
has glaucoma	−1
has gout	−1
has ankylosing spondylitis (a form of arthritis)	−1
has high blood pressure requiring treatment	−2

Lifestyle

Married or living in a long-term relationship	+4
If not, subtract 1 for every 10 years you have lived alone since age 25	−1
Sleep more than 10 hours per night	−4

"The Longevity Game," by Kenneth Pelletier, Ph.D. *Healthline*, San Mateo, California (August 1983). Reprinted by permission.

If you do not have a tetanus booster (every 10 years)   −1

Been in close contact with someone with tuberculosis for a year or more   −1

Intense, aggressive, and anger easily   −3

Easy going and relaxed   +1

Happy   +1

Unhappy, dissatisfied, or depressed   −3

Have had a speeding ticket or accident last year   −4

Other traffic violations   −1

Wear seatbelts more than 90% of the time as driver and passenger   +1

Have an expectation of good health over the next 20 years   +2

Have a pet   +1

Actively involved in a spiritual tradition or practice   +1

Engage in gardening or raising of plants   +1

Nutrition, Alcohol and Smoking

Eat a well-balanced diet   +2

Avoid saturated and unsaturated fats and cholesterol   +1

Protein intake of 40–50 g per day   +1

Protein intake of 50–100 g per day   −1

Caloric intake of 2000–2500 per day (U.S. average, 3500)   +2

Grains and fish as primary protein source (reduced red meat consumption)   +2

Eat breakfast   +1

Never smoked   +3

Smoke more than one half to one pack per day (one cigarette = one cigar)   −3

One to two packs per day   −6

More than two packs per day   −8

NOTE: 2 oz of 80 proof whiskey = 20 oz of 4.5% beer = ¼ bottle of wine. All contain 20–24 ml of alcohol (not equal volume).

No alcohol consumption   +1

2 oz (or equivalent) or less of 80 proof whiskey per day   +2

More than 2 oz. per day   −1

For each drink over 2 oz per day   −1

Sex

Nonwhite male   −5

Nonwhite female   −4

Male   −3

Female   +4

Regular, fulfilling sexual relations   +2

Frequent sexual activity with many different partners   −1

Male over 40 and have annual medical exams   +2

Female and see a gynecologist once a year   +2

Finished college   +1

Earned a graduate or professional degree   +2 more

Work with asbestos regularly but do not smoke   −2

Work with asbestos regularly   −8

For Women Only

Began regular sexual activity before 18   −1

Smoke and use birth control pills   −5

Jewish   −1

Mother or sister had or has breast cancer   −4

Work and Environment

Office worker   −3

Earn over $50,000 per year but do smoke   −2

Work regularly with vinyl chloride   −4

Work in ongoing contact with toxic agents or radiation   −3

Over 65 and still working   +3

Over 65 and self-employed   +1 more

Live in an urban area with a population over 2 million   −2

Live in a town under 10,000 or on a farm   +2

Physical Activity and Weight

Work requires regular physical exertion   +2

Exercise at a "moderate aerobic level (i.e., jogging, swimming, bicycling, jazzercise at least 3 times per week for at least 30 minutes per time.   +3

Less than 3 times per week on nonconsecutive days   +2

No regular aerobic activity   −5

Weight is (compared to ideal body composition)

5–20 lbs. over ideal weight   −2

20–30 lbs. over ideal weight   −3

30–40 lbs. over ideal weight   −4

40–50 lbs. over ideal weight   −6

Over 50   −8

Present Age Adjustment

Present age is: 30–40   +2

40–50   +3

50–70   +4

Over 70   +5

TOTAL:_____ = Your Longevity Potential

Very likely, you have been pleasantly surprised to find your biological potential for longevity. Generally, the factors noted with a "+" are those that you should maintain or begin in order to attain your centenarian status. Those determinants you noted with a "−" should be eliminated or reduced as much as possible. Most importantly, the quality and quantity of your life is in your hands. In Ecuador there is a toast which reflects this vitality: "May you live to be 300!" Although we may never reach that distant galaxy, its very presence brings awe and joy into our lives.

Suggestions For Further Reading

Butler, Robert N. *Why Survive? Being Old in America.* New York: Harper & Row, 1975.

Fries, James F. and Crapo, Lawrence M. *Vitality and Aging.* San Francisco: W. H. Freeman and Company, 1981.

Finch, Caleb E. and Hayflick, Leonard. *Handbook of the Biology of Aging.* New York: Van Nostrand Reinhold Company, 1977.

Leaf, Alexander, *Youth in Old Age.* New York: McGraw Hill, 1975.

Pelletier, Kenneth R. *Holistic Medicine: From Stress to Optimum Health.* New York: Delacorte and Delta, 1979.

Pelletier, Kenneth R. *Longevity: Fulfilling Our Biological Potential.* New York, Delacorte and Delta, 1981.

KENNETH PELLETIER, *Ph.D. a* Healthline *Contributing Editor, is an Assistant Clinical Professor in the Department of Psychiatry and the Langley Porter Neuropsychiatric Institute, University of California School of Medicine, San Francisco, and also Assistant Professor in the Department of Public Health, University of California, Berkeley.*

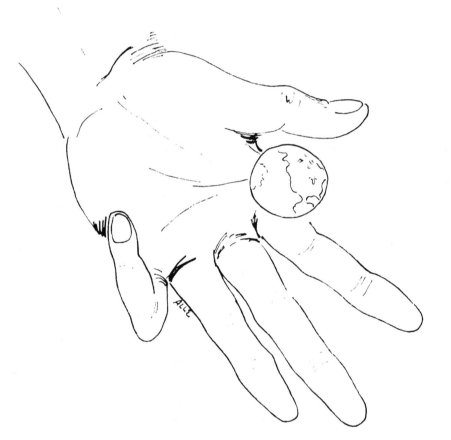

Menopause: The Blessed Liberation

Jeannine Parvati

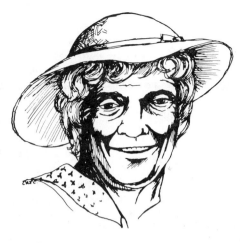

In this article Ms. Parvati reminds us of the inherent symbolism of the menopause, at the same time offering us alternatives to estrogen, the common drug "treatment" for menopausal and post-menopausal women. With conscious health practices and some cultural support, menopause, the dreaded change, can be experienced as a blessed liberation.

THOUGH I do not know how the gods will receive you, *I Ching* reminds us not to put on false appearances before them. With the menopause, the night of our life's journey begins, and this time we start in complete honesty. It is the end of our fertility; we are freed from the concerns of bringing children into the world. For men as well as women, the great and powerful bonds of attachment to the family and the household are coming to an end.

Children are grown. The paths of the parents change. The Old Gods are reexamined: Saturn makes the second return to his natal place; Persephone retires underground for the season. The dance of estrogen slows from strutting to self-reflection. As we pause at the center of our lives, with time, we will learn to balance between our living and our dying.

My Own History

My first awareness of menopause came within my family, as I watched our older aunts go through the change, resisting this natural process. By the age of sixteen, I was writing short stories with lines like "the menopausal hens cackled." I already saw this future experience as part of female sexuality, and anticipated it with the same pleasure/pain as I did all the rest. I liked Ursula LeGuin's statement that it's our opportunity to finally become crones. Menopause, experienced fully (without medicinal or technological aids), seems to be part of completing the owner/operator's instructions that came with this female package when I took it out 28 years ago.

Now that I've confessed my age, I begin to feel terribly presumptuous to be writing about menopause. In evolutionary consciousness, I'm barely pubescent. All I have are fantasies—but fantasies make life fantastic.

The Change

We are speaking of a time in women's lives to be celebrated, not endured; but how is this possible when our health is failing? Some writers,[1] seeing the monthly bleedings as opportunities to eliminate toxins from the system, are convinced that the uncomfortable symptoms of menopause arise from the cessation of this purifying process. They believe that after bleeding stops, the organism is blocked with backed-up impurities—whence the headaches, the rapid loss of sexual interest,[2] the irritability, backache, "menopausal arthritis," and many other disease conditions. But these are only sad commentaries on our general state of health. Women can begin early in preparation for this very important rite of passage,[3] to consciously include in our health-building practices the herbs essential to women's health.

We can include many estrogen-containing foods in plant form, which will enable us to do without the synthetic estrogens that the medical industry will offer. First and foremost, a healthy *attitude* about menopause is in order. To welcome the process as a natural one, without regret for the end of the fertile period, will go a long way toward counterbalancing our culture's current attitudes about "the Change."

At present, most women who can afford it rush to their doctors at the first "hot flash" for synthetic estrogen, or Premarin ("natural" estrogen), which is not much better. These drugs relieve the symptoms of menopause, but they have been shown to increase greatly the incidence of cancer, blood clots, and heart attacks.[4] Since menopause reminds us that we are mortal, since we can no longer reproduce ourselves, it is understandable that some of us begin to hunt for a new fountain of youth.

But this is a good time to stop and reexamine what is important for us for the remainder of our time on Earth. If poor health interferes with our goals, we should correct it. We certainly can no longer afford to pollute our bodies with the standard American diet, with its emphasis on valueless "pleasure" foods. Every substance we take in will become our very being; no longer will our excesses and harmful accumulations be eliminated monthly through the menstrual flow.

But what if menstruation never was a process of elimination? What if it is simply the shedding of a uterine lining in the absence of a fertilized ovum? Does that cancel out what you've just read? It is still largely true what you ingest becomes *you*—the basic, material you, as well as your thoughts, your feelings, and your ways of relating to the world. There is a central connection between how we perceive our bodily processes and how we feed and love ourselves.

Practical Knowledge

The remainder of this article will be devoted to our menopausal sisters, in the knowledge that, with conscious health practices and with some cultural support, "the Change" may be experienced as a liberation: Ah! At last a crone,[5] freed from the more obvious, culturally underscored aspects of being a woman. Now we can focus energy on the subtle nature of the female. Let us prepare our bodies so that we can fully enjoy it.

What appears most important during menopause is an adequate supply of trace minerals, and of minerals as catalysts for enzyme functions. Then, the usual course of hormone production is shifted during menopause from the ovaries, which retire from action, to the adrenal glands.[6]

The ovaries have performed many vital functions during their period of activity. Not only have they released an egg into the uterus during every menstrual cycle, but they have also produced progesterone during the lutein phase, or midcycle. During pregnancy they produce progesterone to maintain the womb environment until the placenta takes over this function. Moreover, when the adrenal glands have been exhausted by poor nutrition, repressed rage, or improper functioning of the liver, the organism is in need of additional estrogen from the ovaries.[7]

Nevertheless, when all this is over, my sisters who have been eating in health-conscious ways seem to experience the menopause as "no big deal"; it is those of us who ignore the signals from our bodies about proper diet, and proper attitude toward menstruation, who experience the menopause as agony.

Perhaps an understanding of the serious effects of synthetic estrogen can awaken us to the benefits of a more natural, simple diet that includes herbs. Synthetic estrogen increases the need for Vitamin E, the element so vital to proper sexual functioning. Premarin, billed as a "natural" form of estrogen (it is collected from the urine of mares), can cause dangerous blood clots, just as the synthetic forms can.[8] The human body has its own ecology. We have seen the results of indiscriminate addition of manmade chemicals to our natural environment. The use of synthetic (or "natural") estrogen by injection or in the form of pills, I refer to the list, given below, of herbs used by women to help them through "the Change." Hormones, like anything else in our body, are made up from the foods and herbs we ingest.

There are many foods and herbs that stimulate or are vital to the produciton of your natural hormones. When a woman withdraws from synthetic estrogen, she may experience an alarming "rapid aging." Some herbs are suggested with this in mind; many have a reputation for slowing down the aging process. Of course, it is only with regular attention to diet, rest, love, and a spiritual practice (*sadhana*) that the aging process is really slowed. Many yoga exercises and *asanas* are reported to reverse aging. I know

one beautiful example: an herbalist who, at 80, looks 50. She attributes this to her use of herbs, careful nutrition, and her ability to "use air as food." She practices regular *pranayamas*, and says that these breath-controlling exercises are "a meal in themselves." A love for children and an ability to enter a "baby space" also have this effect.

Nourishment

Let us begin with the best ways to nourish ourselves in our golden years. Here is a basic list of herbs useful for menopause:

Mexican wild yam	Dioscorea villosa
Sassafras	Sassafras albidum
Licorice	Aletris farinosa
Lady's slipper	Cypripedium pubescens
Life root	
Passion flower	Passiflora incarnata and P. edulis
Black Cohosh	Cimicifuga vacemosa
Honduras sarsaparilla	Smilax aristolochiaefolia honduras
False unicorn root	Helonias diocia
Elder	Sambucus canadensis or S. nigra

These all contain some natural estrogen, which can help even after a hysterectomy. A partial list of similarly useful foods would include seeds, sprouts, whole grains, royal jelly, bee pollen, and bananas.

Stan Malstrom[9] recommends the following herbal recipe for menopause: blessed thistle, squaw vine, raspberry leaves, golden seal, lobelia, gravel root, ginger root, cayenne, parsely and marshmallow root. His herbal contains instructions for use.

There are many formulas marketed too: Dr. Christopher's Change-Ease, for example. These are sold in capsules and can be swallowed or dissolved in a cup of tea. Remember to take them on an empty stomach.

Raymond Dextreit, in is wonderful book, *Our Earth, Our Cure*, notes that if menopause occurs after the age of fifty, it's a much easier process. This is not to say, however, that it *should* come after fifty. For instance, a fibroid tumor in the uterus may be the cause of a postponed menopause. There is no rigid timetable for the sequence of a woman's life changes. Menopause comes at the perfect time for each of us, whenever that is.

Dextreit goes on to make some important suggestions: that foods from the vegetable kingdom, including herbs, facilitate the glandular functions, relieve congestion, and strengthen the nervous system. In contrast, the use of synthetic estrogen creates a rise of copper, causing emotional instability and an increase of zinc, causing depression.[10] Herbs help to bring these trace minerals back into balance. Dextreit advises us to completely eliminate meat, sugar, coffee, alcohol, and any chemical types of food, and to limit animal foods to occasional eggs and buttermilk. Lemon, as well as garlic and parsley, are excellent for this time. So are the culinary herbs which stimulate the circulation. So often "hot flashes," dizziness, perspiration, are a signal that you are congested; herbs that help relieve this problem are chervil, tarragon, shallot, sorrel, chive, nutmeg, and horseradish. Natural honey is helpful too.

Dextreit's favorite herb is sage, because of "its richness in female hormones." Red-grape leaves, which accelerate the circulation when used in footbaths, are good for face flushes and hypertension too. Prepare the bath with a gallon of water, in which you boil two to three handfuls of leaves for 10 to 15 minutes. Dextreit also gives a recipe for a decoction to treat sudden flushes and high blood pressure:

Rosemary	50 grains
Mint	30 grains
Elecampane	25 grains
Mugwort	25 grains
St. John's wort	25 grains
Shepherd's purse	25 grains
Vervain	25 grains
Oak apples	25 grains

He suggests you take a quart of boiling water, and let it stand overnight with one handful of the mixture in it. In the morning, strain it and take it for ten days in a row. Rest for two days; and then repeat.

A recipe given anonymously to our Women's Center and handed out there is the following.

Tea for hormone imbalance as produced in menopause

One part each: sarsaparilla
               licorice
               blue vervain

If condition is serious, add one part each:
               false unicorn root
               raspberry leaves

I have deliberately not been too specific about the exact ways to use a given herb. I feel it is better for the reader to experiment and find out what works best for her own body, what her own relationship is to the plant. However, there are some general methods of preparation that work well for all herbs. Steeping them in a closed glass or ceramic container is best, except for roots, for which an infusion is better. To steep or brew a tea, add the leaves, stems, flowers, etc., to a jar of pure water. Let it sit under the sun or the moon for a day or two, until the tea tastes full and done. Roots like being infused this way.

Another method is to boil water, pour it over the herbs in a teapot, and then let it sit for 5 to 45 minutes, covered. When you sip the tea, place your attention on the healing properties of the particular brew. I have not covered tinctures, liniments, syrups, or other preparations here, but for a drink or a douche, the above methods are good.

Experiment, watch, heal. Accept the process of healing: develop your own recipes and procedures, your own rituals. Let the plant be your guide.

Conclusion

Those of us who are premenopausal (try considering yourself that way!) can help change the obsession of our culture with youth, and the valuing of women only as sexual objects, by appreciating our older sisters right here and now. Seek out your sisters who are in their middle years and affirm their beauty—and not just their physical beauty.

Young women who neglect to realize the true beauty of the aging process are paving the fall for themselves as well.

We are not in the habit of honoring our elders; our wise old women would not try so uselessly, and so wastefully, to be young if only we appreciated them as they are. There are other purposes in life—any woman's life—than bearing children or decorating the lives of men. It is our menopausal sisters who are in the best position to experience this fully. By giving them our respect and love, we can not only aid them in this self-discovery, but also learn from them, as from no one else, about that mysterious time toward which all our lives are moving.

1. Osawa, Airola, Ehret, etc. See bibliography on nutrition.
2. Or the reverse: Keen interest in sex. For some women, the period after menopause is their first opportunity to explore sexuality without the fear of pregnancy.
3. Menopause is an *initiation*; we should not forego this just because men don't consider their own change of life as important.
4. *British Medical Journal*, Oct. 18, 1975; *New England Journal of Medicine*, Dec. 4, 1975; *Lancet*, April 14, 1973; *Annals of Western Medicine and Surgery*, Vol. 4 1950; *New York Journal of Medicine*, May 15, 1952.
5. Ursula LeGuin first used this term to describe a menopausal woman in an article entitled "The Space Crone."
6. Some writers (e.g., Bieler, Kulvinkas) state that the ovaries in a "healthy" woman never quit functioning, and that she will continue to be fertile long after her less diet-conscious sisters have finished their menopause.
7. R. Fuhr, *Annals of the New York Academy of Science*, 1949.
8. *British Medical Journal*, October 18, 1975.
9. *Herbal Remedies II*.
10. On this subject, Paavo Airola says, "Menopause is a divinely designed phase in woman's life, with a purpose of liberating her from duties as procreator with God, and giving her time for self-improvement, for the perfection of her human and divine characteristics, and her spiritual growth." He states this in an excellent article in the July 1976 issue of *Let's Live* magazine, entitled, "Menopause: Dreadful Affliction or Glorious Experience? Nutritional and Other Biological Solutions to Menopausal Problems, Estrogen Therapy, and Premature Aging."

Suggestions for Further Reading

Paavo Airola, *Sex and Nutrition*. Health Plus, 1974.
H. G. Bieler, *Food is Your Best Medicine*. Neville Spearman, 1968.
_____, *Natural Way to Sexual Health*. Charles, 1972.
Raymond Dextreit, *Our Earth, Our Cure*. Swan House, 1974.
Arnold Ehret, *Mucusless Diet Healing System*. Ehret Literature, 1972.
Victoras Kulvinkas, *Love Your Body*. Omangod Press, 1975.
_____, *Survival in the Twenty-First Century*. Omangod Press, 1975.
Stan Malstrom, *Herbal Remedies II*. Family Press, 1975.
Jeannine Parvati, *Hygieia: A Woman's Herbal*. Freestone Publishing Collective, 1978

JEANNINE PARVATI (AKA *Jeannine O'Brien Medvin*) *holds a Master's Degree in Psychology, is the author of two published books, and has led numerous conferences focusing on female sexuality and yoga. She is a midwife and an astrologer, and has been invited to speak and teach throughout the western United States. Mother of three daughters, including home-born twins, Parvati is a student of Baba Hari Dass.*

Evaluating and Improving Family Health

Alta E. Kelly, M.S.W., M.P.H.

This article deals with a concept that is currently coming into new prominence: the concept that health depends very strongly on the quality of family life. A major hypothesis of the holistic-health movement is that health is not strictly internal to the individual; rather, health depends in good part on how the individual relates to his or her environment. In simple terms, it is difficult to be healthy in an unhealthy environment. From this, it follows that a person's most immediate and important social environment, the family, must have a major role in determining the level of his or her wellness.

In this article, Alta E. Kelly applies a wide selection of current holistic concepts to the family, showing how a family, by adapting techniques that were evolved for use by individuals, can evaluate the efficacy of its functioning as a social unit. She also thus supplies a great many suggestions about how a family can begin to make alternations in its habits and lifestyle that will, if followed through, raise the level of health for the family as a whole and for all its individual members.

THE IMPORTANCE of the family in the fostering of health is not a new idea in American medicine. The social sciences have studied for many years the effect of the family—its role and interactions, its relationships with health professionals—on illness and health care.

In the medical community, however, the problem of delivering health services to the family as an integral group has not been considered important. The profession of medicine has focused its attention primarily on disease control. The delivery system has been organized to provide treatment to individuals by medical specialists who deal with one problem at a time, thus attempting to treat the whole man in its physiological parts.

Apparently, though, a human being is greater than the sum of his or her parts. It is the interrelatedness of these parts, and the refusal of the medical profession to consider it, that has created so many difficult ties for the patient; for it has become impossible for the average working-class family—or any individual in that family—to obtain comprehensive health care. Most families and individuals can't afford to buy health care from one specialist after another, from birth to death, and the medical system is not coordinated over a patient's lifetime in any case.

In this article, I will use the word "family" in a broader sense than that normally accepted today. I refer to the nuclear family (mother, father, and children), but also to those adults and children who share blood *and/or social* ties, who for the most part have easy access to each other geographically, and who *consider themselves a family unit.* I will be dealing only with family health care, although obviously it is not the answer for everyone; many individuals have no family, and some families are so splintered by alienation that there is no sense in considering them as a whole.

This article will attempt, by means of a series of questionnaires and checklists, to provide a way to measure the quality of family health and to decide on the best methods for improving it. These tests can be used by health professionals and by the family itself.

Basic Concepts

I believe that a family's sense of heath derives from all of its external and internal environments. The care and attention given to the needs of the body, mind, and spirit—including the relationships between intimates—affects the health of the individual and therefore of the family. There is a close correlation between wellness and the quality of personal relations.

Because of this correlation, it is useful to look at the concepts and measurements of wellness from a new perspective, namely, in terms of how they apply to the health of the family as a social unit. This is, of course, something of a departure even from the relatively new holistic idea of health as a result of individual action. But if a person's health is intimately connected with his or her psychological and spiritual states, then certainly the social environment that influences those states so strongly must be taken into account.

In this light, I would like to offer here a set of statements about health and the family, in order to bring them to the forefront of our attention. These are not proven results of experiment. Rather, they are, on the one hand, assumptions that underlie the current holistic-health movement as they might be applied to the family as a social unit, and, on the other hand, hypotheses that future practice and research in family health might well be directed toward testing.

1. People who live together influence each other's health.
2. The concepts of holistic health can be used both to evaluate and to improve the quality of family wellness.
3. The quality of health of the family as a whole tends to indicate the general quality of the health of its members.
4. Some family members (adults) have more responsibility for family wellness than other members (children), but this difference is merely relative within the responsibility of the family as a whole.
5. Children need wellness supervision and education.
6. A member who is in poor health depresses the quality of health for the family as a whole.
7. To recover health, a person needs the cooperation and support of the family.
8. The various elements that make up family life affect both individual and family wellness.
9. Family health is an ongoing process that changes as the members change and that fluctuates with environmental pressures.

In family wellness planning, therefore, the individual is still considered responsible for his or her own health, but an examination is also made of the interplay between cohabiting adults, and between adults and children. In the field of mental health, family-oriented care has been practiced successfully for many years. Even in the medical profession, under special conditions, the role of the family (or of a family member other than the patient) is often recognized as important. This is especially true in pediatrics, where the patient is a child and the parent acts as caretaker.

Still, given the potential of Western medicine, very little has been done to mobilize the family as a unit in order to improve the wellness of its members or to prevent illness in them. I believe it is time to recognize the potential healing power of the family, and to develop strategies for health care within this context.

Survey I: Factors Affecting Family Health

A family's cohesiveness and well-being depend on certain social elements. If these elements are not all present, the quality of relationships deteriorates, and this deterioration further affects the unity of the family. Individuals experience stress, and family health begins to suffer. Below is a checklist of social/emotional aspects of family life, which must be functioning well for a family to enjoy good health and good relationships.

1. *Face-to-face contact* between all family members is essential. Individual members, therefore, routinely spend time together; they normally live day-to-day with each other; long absences are minimized.

2. *Verbal communications.* Conversation between individuals, and within the entire group, is frequent. Members let each other know about the day's activities and the quality of life. Each family has its own style of communication:

wide variations of length, place, and language will occur, depending on the age, sex and roles of family members, not to mention the cultural background of the family.

3. *Non-verbal communication.* Members of the family are willing and able to interpret and understand physical cues, body stances, and general behavior of other members, in connection with both family matters and events or persons on the outside.

4. *Touching.* Physical communication between family members is an important way of sharing feelings. With younger family members—and older ones too—there may be a caretaking function involved in touch. But in general, physical interaction is a medium of expression for feelings, both positive and negative. Touching is central to the survival of infants and the elderly, who can die from insufficient body contact; it is also essential to the psychological well-being of all members.

5. *Empathy.* Family members are able to envision themselves in the situation of others. They can understand in an uncritical way (at least temporarily) the viewpoint of other members. This capacity does, of course, develop with age. A young child would not be expected to share the viewpoint of a parent or an older child, although he might very well understand their feelings.

6. *Sexual compatibility* (where appropriate). Among family members who are sexually linked, there is a mutual responsiveness and attention to gratification that reflects their relationship and influences their behavior in general.

7. *Commitment.* A key requirement for a family is the acceptance, without reservation, of the idea that the family is a unit.

8. *Enrichment.* The mutual encouragement of growing and sharing maintains the vitality of the individual's relationship with the group.

Applying Holistic Health Concepts to the Family

Holistic-health thinking is well-suited to working with family wellness. The holistic view presents the mind, body, and spirit of a person as integrated with his or her environment and universe. Illness is regarded as a message from within, telling him (or her) that he is out of harmony with himself and his world. Illness and wellness are regarded as arising from many factors, both in the individual and in the surroundings.

It is in family life that multiple causation of poor health is extremely visible. It is easy to see how the attitudes of the family toward the individual and his or her health can lead to illness or to recovery.

The application of holistic practices to families naturally involves, for most of us, a major change in lifestyle and a conscious planning for wellness. Health becomes a deliberately created *basis* for life, rather than a passively experienced *effect* of life.

Family members should be educated in the practices of self-responsibility for wellness. This practice can begin at any age; younger members should be taught their responsibilities as early as possible. These include: nutrition, stress awareness and management, physical fitness, environmental health, and spiritual sensitivity. Training in new concepts of health awareness can be made part of family life, and the family can approach the new practices as a unit, too.

Survey II: Family Responsibility

The following questionnaire[1] may be used for self-assessment by family members, to form a clearer idea of their family health responsibilities. The survey can be completed by any member, or by the family as a whole, to give an idea of the strengths and weaknesses in the wellness practices of the family.

1. Has your family in recent months read or discussed any or all of the six dimensions of holistic health (health self-responsibility, nutritional awareness, stress and its management, physical fitness, environmental sensitivity, spiritual practices)?
2. Do you ever question your doctor about the necessity and possible side effects of drugs that he prescribes?
3. Have you ever asked your doctor about a non-medical alternative, sought another doctor's opinion, or deliberately disregarded a doctor's advice?
4. Does your family use seat belts in the family car?
5. Do all drivers in your family limit their speed to the legal limit most of the time?
6. Do you have family health insurance?
7. Is your family life working? Do you feel fulfilled by your relationship with your mate, your leisure time, your children, your spiritual life, your general sense of purpose?
8. Can your family members have time and space to be apart from each other?
10. Does your family look forward to outings and time spent together?
11. Are family values placed before individual promotions, prestige, profit, and success?
12. Can your family laugh together?
13. Does your family limit the use of laxatives, tranquilizers, painkillers, reducing pills, and aspirin?
14. Has your family completed a individual or family wellness survey this year?
15. Does your family believe that it can choose to live well?
16. Do you visit a dentist annually?
17. Do all members use dental floss daily, brush with a soft brush after meals, plan dentist visits for young members with baby teeth and for bedridden, senior, or otherwise handicapped people? Do you minimize exposure to dental and other X-rays?
18. Do all family members understand how their bodies function?
19. Are family members knowledgeable about sexual functions? Can children ask about reproduction? Are teenagers informed about birth control? Is the family able to discuss feelings and values connected with sexuality? Is there also an awareness of the need for privacy in some sexual matters?
20. Is the family prepared to respect the wishes of members who are undergoing illness?
21. Are members trained in first aid and sanitation?
22. Does your family feel it can slow down the usual pattern of degeneration due to aging?

23. Does the family have an up-to-date record of immunizations?
24. Does the family have at least two close friends?
25. Does your family feel it is all right to cry, and does it allow members to do so?
26. Can family members say "no" without feeling guilty?
27. Do members like to give and receive compliments?
28. Can your family seek help from others—friends, professional counsel, or clergy—if needed?
29. Can members listen to, and think about, constructive criticism?
30. Does the family give its members wellness education, both by instruction and by setting good examples in its lifestyle?
31. Does the family have a realistic picture of its strengths and weaknesses?
32. Do you feel there has been an improvement in family wellness over time?

Survey III: Family Stress

Stress management requires the evaluation of the amount of stress within the family. By using the Holmes stress indicator (given below) as a family, you can measure the degree of stress present, and can evaluate the potential for declining health. With this kind of knowledge, the family is equipped to consider how best to prevent or minimize stress. Family members can weigh decisions about, for instance, a move or a job change in the light of current stress conditions and the additional stress such a change might bring about.

To use the test, circle the number after any event that has occurred in your life in the past year. To find the total amount of stress your family has undergone this year, have each member take the test, add the scores, and divide by the number of members. This average score will reflect your family's chances of developing a serious illness in the next two years. For an individual, a score of 150 or less means the chance of sickness is at most only 37 percent. With a score of more than 300 points, the odds for illness rise to 80 percent, and will continue to rise with the score. Scoring for individuals may be somewhat rough, but if the test is taken by the entire family, the score will probably be a good indicator of family health. Moreover, individual differences may give warning signs that certain members of the family stand a higher chance of illness than others.

Here is the test, as designed by Dr. Thomas H. Holmes.[2]

Event	Value
Death of a spouse	100
Divorce	73
Marital separation	65
Jail term	63
Death of close family member	63
Personal injury or illness	53
Marriage	50
Fired from work	47
Marital reconciliation	45
Retirement	45
Change in family member's health	44
Pregnancy	40

Sex difficulties	39
Addition to family	39
Business readjustment	39
Change in financial status	38
Death of close friend	37
Change to different line of work	36
Change in number of marital arguments	35
Mortgage or loan over $10,000	31
Foreclosure of mortgage or loan	30
Change in work responsibilities	29
Son or daughter leaving home	29
Trouble with in-laws	29
Outstanding personal achievement	28
Spouse begins or stops working	26
Starting or finishing school	26
Change in living conditions	25
Revision of personal habits	24
Trouble with boss	23
Change in work hours, conditions	20
Change in residence	20
Change in schools	20
Change in recreational habits	19
Change in church activities	19
Change in social activities	19
Mortgage or loan under $10,000	17
Change in sleeping habits	16
Change in number of family gatherings	15
Vacation	13
Christmas season	12
Minor violation of the law	11
TOTAL:	————

Survey IV: Stress Management

Now that you have an idea of the conditions which produce stress, here is a survey to test your awareness and use of stress reducers. Check each statement that applies to your family, and try to keep the others in mind for incorporation into family life.

1. We enjoy self-expression. We engage in creative activities as individuals and as a group (Examples: dance, music, crafts, sports, hobbies.)
2. We spend some time together without structured activities.
3. We encourage each other to meditate or quiet the mind regularly.
4. Spiritual activities are part of our family life.
5. We know and use massage or some other type of "hands-on" relaxation method.
6. We take at least a two-week vacation each year.
7. We know that some physical discomforts are stress-related. (General fatigue, stiffness of muscles, back pain, headache, ulcers, colitis, gastritis, heart disease, cancer, and strokes are linked to stress.)
8. We know that foot-tapping, leg-shaking, and other assorted rhythmic body movements (of head, fingers, pencil, etc.) are signs of stress.

Survey V: Physical Fitness

Each individual is responsible for providing himself or herself with physical exercise, but the family as a whole can influence its members toward awareness of the importance of physical fitness. The family can organize group outings and activities that involve physical activity and education of all its members. Here is a survey of family physical activity. As before, check those statements that apply; the others may be used as a guide for further development of physical fitness within the family.

1. We engage in family outings that involve physical activity.
2. We regularly walk or ride a bicycle.
3. Members regularly do some stretching or limbering exercise (all ages).
4. We periodically spend time out of doors, regardless of the weather, in some form of vigorous exercise.
5. We have a family membership in a health club, spa, or fitness-oriented organization (or make use of public recreation facilities.)
6. We know how exercise benefits our bodies.

Survey VI: Nutritional Awareness

Adopting a holistic lifestyle in the family includes nutritional planning and education for all members. An awareness should be cultivated that the quality and quantity of food intake has a direct bearing on health since most families eat together, and one or more members are responsible for selection and preparation of food for the group, it is important that all members of the group become aware of the ways foods are used in the body, and of how to select high-quality foods and prepare them. Such knowledge is fundamental to responsibility for personal health. Activities in this area may be routinely assigned to the same people at all times—most frequently, the mother selects and cooks the food, the men and children eat the meals she prepares—but each family member must still have a personal knowledge of the fundamentals of nutrition, and of how vitamins, minerals, proteins, fat, calories, etc., are used in the body. To ignore this aspect of health simply because sex roles assign the responsibility for it to someone else is to retreat into a state of infantile dependency.

Here is a self-assessment survey of nutritional awareness.

1. Our family has available uncooked fruits and vegetables each day.
2. Soft drinks are seldom used.
3. We avoid or severely limit the family intake of refined foods or of foods that have sugar added.
4. We read the ingredient labels on foods when we shop.
5. We limit family use of salt in cooking or in eating prepared foods.
6. We limit our use of coffee and nonherbal teas to three cups per day.
7. Our family uses food supplements daily.
8. We have high roughage available in our diet.
9. We have good appetites and maintain our bodies within 15 per cent of ideal weight.
10. We serve young children and infants homemade baby foods.

THE "HEALING STORY" OF DEENA METZGER

Shepherd Bliss

LAST summer I traveled from the Bay Area to a small village in Minnesota, where 500 cultural workers assembled at *The Gathering*. Among the compelling poets, musicians, dramatists, and artists, one striking story stood out—Deena Metzger's.

Deena's workshop was entitled "Healing Stories." Intrigued by the idea that stories could be "healing," I read the description carefully: *"To discover one's own story and to tell that story is to integrate the inner world into everyday reality. In doing this we begin to heal those diseases—emotional, physical, even political—which arises from our disassociation with the inner life."*

The "Healing Stories" workshop was an amazing experience. I returned to the Bay Area and bought a copy of Metzger's book, *The Woman Who Slept with Men to Take the War out of Them* and *Tree*, two works in one volume, published by Peace Press (1981). I now had a way to introduce others to Deena Metzger's "Healing Stories."

Metzger's book *Tree* documents a contemporary woman's rally of her personal healing powers to struggle against cancer and its ravages, not only of the human body but also of the soul. The cancer threatening to destroy Metzger's body becomes the metaphor through which the afflicted challenges her society. In revealing not only one woman's survival but her deepened commitment to life and to community, *Tree* becomes a "map for the roads toward healing."

Writing *Tree* becomes a vital part of its author's personal healing: *"I will tell you a secret. Robert is warning me again to be quiet. But I have always believed that quiet kills, that cancer comes from silence. So I do not want to be my own executioner. If I am silenced, it will be imposed, not volitional. In the meantime, I am going to speak my mind."*

Deena Metzger does speak her mind in *Tree*, mainly about the happenings of one month, during which she

Whole Life Times, March/April 1982. Reprinted by permission.

discovered her breast cancer, fought it, and survived. *Tree* presents her account of healing interactions with her friends, including the famous (such as Anais Nin), and the well-known in some circles (such as Barbara Myerhoff, Meridel Le Sueur, Audre Lorde, Ariel Dorfman), but mainly those known intimately by Deena—like Naomi, David and Robert. These people Deena comes to describe as her "family." She asks the reader to join this group: "I have a space here_____. Write your name in; I do not want to leave anyone out. We need to know our network and kinship system."

In this work as in her previous poetry and plays, Metzger seeks to overcome divisions: those between the inner and outer worlds, men and women, North and Latin Americans, reader and writer. She does so through both confrontative struggle and connective patience. Her goal is to join-together and make-whole.

Who is the woman that would endeavor to write such a book? Her friend of two decades, Barbara Myerhoff, describes her in the foreward: "The hero in *Tree* has a biography, is an alive and familiar contemporary person, living in the moment, with an address and physical features." She is both special, a hero, and someone like others whom we know.

Metzger is essentially a storyteller in the ancient oral traditions of minstrels and troubadours. Her "Healing Stories" are a therapeutic means of connecting creativity, personal transition, illness, disease, struggle and celebration. *Tree* is both deeply singular/personal and plural/political. Metzger's cure involves a social, psychological, medical, political and spiritual journey. During this process she assembles her friends into a healing community. She poses questions directly to her disease, "Who are the voices in me who say '*Die*'? and who are the voices who say '*Live*'? Deena aides her healing processes in various personas—as warrior, as mother, and as adventurer.

Deena has the moon on her mind as *Tree* opens on the first day of February, 1977. "Looking for the

11. Our young children are breast-fed whenever possible.
12. Family members are aware of, or are given, their optimum daily intake of calories, protein, fat, vitamins, and minerals.
13. Family meals vary the type of protein offered, using fish, fowl, vegetable protein, and milk proteins.
14. We plan leisurely group meals.
15. We avoid fast-food restaurants.

Survey VII: Family Environmental Sensitivity

Awareness of the environment's effects on health is important to the family. The family which practices conservation and attempts to eliminate local pollution, or at least not add to it, educates itself and its young about the importance of living in harmony with nature. This concept, as opposed to that of conquering nature, leads to a less

moon..." And games, children's games: "Ring around the rosy on the boardwalk. All fall down. The plague, the plague..." (whose ravages were the origin of this now-whimsical nursery rhyme). A few days later she realizes, "I am alone. In such times one is always alone." Yet she does not yet know, consciously, that she has cancer. But already, "It seems I am both prisoner and jailer." Through *Tree* Deena keeps recalling women alone: "Hundreds of women live alone: Thousands. ...A woman alone in a room. It could be a prison. It could be a cell. It could be the bare room of a nun."

What sustains this woman in her solitary prison hospital? Poetry, like that of Nazim Hikmet, Adrienne Rich, Pablo Neruda and her friend Robert Cohen. And her friends: "Lee brought me to the hospital; we have been family for each other for 20 years."

Deena learns from those around her. "As a child, my son Marc looked at the world upside down through his legs and laughed with glee. *Perspective.*" Deena learns well, and then teaches: "When you are depressed go to the zoo and look at the little animals first, one creature a day, working up slowly—snakes, chickens, monkeys, golden cats, pumas, bears, giraffes—then, when you're ready, elephants—and you're cured." Her observation reminds me of Rilke, the great German poet, whom the sculptor Rodin sent to the zoo as a cure for depression, and an inspiration to write more concretely. (It worked.)

A few days into her journal, Feb. 5, Deena becomes aware: "I have cancer! This is indeed a new book." She begins to feel that the book is "a feminist manual about guerilla warfare for those living in a state of seige, written by an anonymous woman who has just discovered she has a life sentence."

She now has to decide what to do. "It appears I have choices: self healing ('suicide', they say), lumpectomy ('unreliable', they say), radical mastectomy (mutilating), modified radical mastectomy ('preferred', they say)." Most of Deena's friends advise, "Cut." She muses, "At best, I have a choice of poisons. Surgery. Chemotherapy. Radiation. There are a thousand ways to keep the body dying slowly." She realizes the issues: "Can I utilize medical knowledge without undermining my belief in my own healing powers?"

Harold, whose wife died of breast cancer after nine years, sits by Deena's bed and divulges, "You are important to a lot of women. You are important in the community. I'm worried about what you're going to

do. When you say mastectomy is a political act against women, I worry about all those who will die following your lead." Deena listens.

By Feb. 10 Deena decides, "I will sacrifice my breast. Barbara says it's a proper sacrifice, that it will please the gods. This bit of flesh for life. I wish there were another way."

At first Deena thinks she will call this book *Beginning Again*. But she decides upon *Tree*. The family tree. The Tree of Life... "Love can be converted into beams of energy which when sent by one human being and received by another, sustain, nurture, protect, heal and cure."

Deena's essential work is healing, herself and others, which *Tree* explores through Deena and her relationships. "So you see, we *are* on to something. You see Ariel has learned this in the revolution and Naomi has learned it in the spirit and Jane has learned it through friendship and I have learned it in my body and Sheila has learned it from Indians, but it is the same force." This healing force takes many forms.

Though *Tree* is characterized by Deena's lucidity and clarity, she has her doubts. "This is where I lose my way. This is the place of chaos and confusion. Is the cancer the result of trying to be the wounded physician, to share a condition in order to learn how well to heal it? Or do I endure the disease out of unwillingness to be safe at any cost?"

By August, Deena is able to conclude her book with the following affirmation, *"I am no longer ashamed to make love. In the night, a hand caressed my chest and once again I came to life. Love is a battle I can win. I have a body of a warrior who does not kill or wound. On the book of my body, I have permanently inscribed a tree. All the forms I know originate in the heart. The tree which grows in the heart depends on community. We cannot do anything alone. I am well because you take care of me."*

In early February, Deena was pronounced medically "fully recovered," having been cancer-free for five years. A Los Angeles resident, she periodically visits the Bay Area to talk about her writings and give "Healing Story" workshops.

SHEPHERD BLISS *is the editor of this book, and teaches men's studies and offers workshops on Death and Dying in the psychology department of John F. Kennedy University.*

---

stressful existence within one's environment. Examples of family problems concerning the environment are (1) the effects of living in a high-crime area in the inner city, and (2) the effects of a heavy smoker in the family.

The following is an environmental survey. How does your family rate?

1. Has your family done anything creative about its concern over increased population and limited resources?

2. Does your family use methods of transportation other than automobiles?
3. Is your family aware of the effects of pesticides and chemicals in our food supply?
4. Have you stopped purchasing or using aerosol sprays?
5. Does your family increase its use of vitamin E and Vitamin C if you live in an area where there is air pollution? (High-level stress also increases your body's need for these vitamins.)

6. Do the adults in your family vote regularly?
7. Is smoking permitted in your home or car?
8. Do you know other families and friends who are interested in wellness?
9. When you travel, do you take it easy and keep it simple by avoiding fatigue, sticking to a sensible diet, and maintaining your health practices?
10. Do you have a regular home safety and hazard checkup to protect your home from fire and other hazards?
11. Are you energy-conscious both in the home and outside the home?
12. Do you use nonpollutant cleaning agents, and avoid exposure to chemicals, sprays, and exhaust gases?

Survey VII: High-Risk Behavior

Certain forms of behavior show up areas where families are in danger of injury, illness, or mental disturbance. In the following survey, the questions point to specific problems, thus giving families and practitioners instant recognition of high-risk behavior. The need for some of these questions will be self-evident. For others, the need may not be as obvious; so I have indicated their purpose in parentheses.

1. Do family members smoke cigarettes, cigars, or pipes?
2. Does one or more family members use alcohol or drugs past the point of self-responsibility?
3. Does any family member have difficulty sleeping?
4. Do members use aspirin frequently? (Frequent headaches indicate problems.)
5. Is any member 15 percent overweight or underweight?
6. Does anyone in your family concentrate on getting a "good tan?" (This can be dangerous to your health: frequent and long exposure to the sun can result in skin cancer.)
7. Are depression and anger part of family life?
8. Are loaded firearms kept accessible to depressed, angry or young family members? (Most homicides in this country are family affairs.)
9. Is any family member capable of physical assault other than in self-defense?
10. Does your family use coffee or nonherbal teas?
11. Do you feel uncomfortable when you touch each other?
12. Have you undergone a cluster of life changes this year? (That is, did your family score high on the stress test?)
13. Does any member frequently listen to loud rock music? (Loud noises can cause hearing loss as well as other physical and emotional problems.)
14. Do you put up with inadequate warmth and compassion from others without complaining or taking action?
15. Does your family use refined sugar? (Americans now average 200 pounds apiece per year.)
16. Does your family live in a high-crime area?
17. Does your family live in a high-pollution area?
18. Do members of your family drive while drunk or under the influence of drugs? (Include here illegal substances, prescription drugs which bear warning labels about driving, and even nonprescription drugs which impair reflexes or judgment.)
19. Are there frequent arguments between family members that reach the stage of physical violence?
20. Are young children under the supervision of responsible persons day and night?
21. Does your family feel comfortable and safe?

Working with Families in a Holistic Way

How does a family or health facilitator use the health indicators in this article to assess family wellness and improve family health? I would like to suggest the following steps.

Step 1. Family members each complete the Holmes Stress survey (young or disabled family members may need help in completing it). When all members of the family have completed a survey, the individual scores are added up and divided by the number of participants. This will give the Family Stress Score.

Step 2. The High-Risk Behavior survey is completed by the family, and the results are studied in relationship to the Family Stress Score. This should give family and/or facilitator a good idea of the health risks involved for the family and its specific members.

Step 3. When Step 2 is completed, the family can begin to look at its areas of strength and at areas where wellness needs improving, by self-evaluating the surveys on self-responsibility, family stress, physical fitness, nutritional awareness, and family environment.

Once you, as a member or a facilitator have surveyed the wellness of a family, you will have a fair idea of its strengths and weaknesses. How do you guide a family into a holistically oriented lifestyle? The concepts are simple enough, but the analysis of families according to these concepts is complex, and the remedies may not be obvious or easy to put into practice. Ideally, increased wellness in a family should be a painless pursuit. Each step of the way should produce a feeling of increased well-being.

When I counsel a family, I like to suggest that they move from their areas of strength. For instance, a family that has good communications skills, but has had a high score in stress during the last year, can easily discuss its problems and reach a joint decision on strategies for reducing stress and increasing health. The members may decide on a daily meditation or relaxation period, or perhaps a change in their diet. Individuals who seem more risk-prone than others might undergo a more religious regime, with the encouragement and support of the family. The entire family may decide to forego, for the time being, some life change that would produce more stress.

Other cases may be more subtle and may require more delicate handling. Here is a sample case.

Bill and Josephine Johnson, a married couple, are retired. Bill is 64, and Josephine is 73. They have been married for 30 years, and own their own home in a suburb. Bill suffers from emphysema; Josephine from high blood pressure. Bill's prognosis is poor. He spends most of his time in bed, and relies heavily on the use of oxygen and drugs. At one time Bill was a hard-working man and a heavy drinker. Josephine now takes care of Bill. She has had five children, all of whom now live away from home and have families of their own. Of course, both Bill and Josephine are under the care of a physician.

What would you do for this couple? Would you suggest a change of lifestyle, of diet, of location? Too much change might add just enough stress to kill one or both of them.

Working with one of their daughters, we introduced a modest change in diet, added food supplements, and introduced occasional care for Bill by another family member. There were no radical changes, just a gentle introduction to holistic living in areas that the family could accept. The results: Bill is a little more mobile, and his color has improved. Josephine's blood pressure has come down to within normal limits.

Let's look, for contrast, at a family that is within the range of average wellness. The adults wish to improve their health. What can they do? They might start with two of the most accessible practices of holistic health, nutrition and physical fitness. They can move at whatever rate is comfortable for them; the two old standbys, "Easy does it" and "First things first," should govern any family's introduction to holistic health.

Summary

Much information is available in the field of holistic health that is useful both for individuals and for families. However, all of it must be subjected to empirical research and to the test of time. Fieldwork, insightful as it may be, is no substitute for rigorous documentation of the state of the art. We must all perform our own experiments, and bring our own awareness to an evaluation of the result. Only in this way can the idea of health be brought out of the traditional Western medical view—a battle of professionals against germs—into a broader perspective with far greater potential: health as the quality of life.

Notes

[1] The concept of the family inventory has been adapted from the works of Donald B. Ardell in *High Level Wellness* (Rodale Press, 1977).

[2] *Social Readjustment Rating Scale* by Holmes and Rahe, from the *Journal of Psychosomatic Research*, vol. II (1967), pp. 213–218.

Suggestions for Further Reading

Richard N. Adams, "An Inquiry into the Nature of the Family," from G. E. Dole and R. L. Carneiro, eds., *Essays in the Science of Culture in Honor of Leslie A. White* (Crowel, 1960), pp. 30–49.

Donald B. Ardell, *High Level Wellness: An Alternative to Doctors, Drugs, and Disease*. Rodale Press, 1977.

Norman W. Bell and Ezra F. Vogel, eds., *The Family: A Modern Introduction*. Free Press, 1968.

Friedrich Engles, *The Origins of the Family, Private Property, and the State*. Trans. E. Untermann. Chicago: Chas. H. Kerr, 1902.

Florence R. Kluckholm, "Variations on the Basic Values of the Family System," *Social Casework*, Feb./Mar. 1958, pp. 63–72.

Theodore Lidz, *The Person: His Development Throughout the Life Cycle*. Basic Books, 1968.

Talcott Parsons and Renee Fox, "Illness, Therapy, and the Modern Urban American Family," *Journal of Social Issues*, XIII, no. 4 (1952), pp. 31–44.

ALTA E. KELLY *received the M.S.W. from California State University, Sacramento, in 1970, with a specialization in Community Organizing and the Master of Public Health degree from the University of California, Berkeley, in 1973, with a specialization in Maternal and Child Health. She has taught health courses at several Bay Area public colleges.*

She is married to Aidan A. Kelly, and is the mother of four children. She was a professional member of the Berkeley Holistic Health Center.

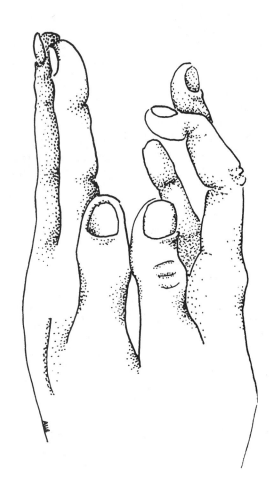

C. DEATH

The Impact of Death on the Health-Care Professional

Charles A. Garfield, Ph.D.

The impact of terminal illness is a profound experience, for the patient, naturally, but also for those who surround him or her. In this article Dr. Garfield movingly narrates his initiation into the deeper implications of the death process for the patient, family, and health-care professional.

Most would readily agree that, from an experimental point of view, we, the living, know little of death or the process of dying. Yet, as health-care professionals who work with the terminally ill, we often collude in the belief that we are experts in the psychology issues surrounding life-threatening illness. This somewhat illusory expertise often translates in practice into an attempt at hyperefficiency in biomedical duties, the use of heavy sedation to reduce severe pain but also to diminish the likelihood of having to relate to emotional needs expressed by the patient, and dimished contact with and withdrawal from the patient, using the rationale "We've done all we can do." The basic and often unacknowledged premise is that dying is a biological process demanding biomedical intervention. As death approaches and treatment toward improved health is no longer a possibility, staff may initially adopt a more rigid, inaccessible posture, especially with more assertive patients who express their emotional needs. The dying patient is clearly not a neutral element in the psychosocial field of the health-care professional. At times, the extreme anxiety of physician or nurse becomes the major issue in the relationship between staff member and patient. Dying is not solely a biological or even psychobiological set of events and experiences. The social or interpersonal concomitants of the dying process, which powerfully affect patient and health-care professional alike, expose the fact that we are dealing with a sociopsychobiological process that has extensions to the religious realm. However, we rarely consider the impact on the professional of intensive or extensive contact with the dying. What follows is a

personal case history of my initial encounter with a dying patient. The data were journal notations written throughout the death trajectory and reexamined after five years of research and clinical work with dying individuals. These writings constitute as powerful an introspective exercise as I have ever done.

To Be with One Who Is Dying

All I could hear was my father singing, "Sunrise, sunset, sunrise, sunset, swiftly go the years." Over and over this seemingly endless refrain pounded through my head as I left the hospital. Periodically, it mixed with the Tibetan mantrum "Om Mani Padme Hum," my fifth-grade teacher singing "America the Beautiful," or Mick Jagger shrieking "I can't get no satisfaction." Larry had just died. This was the first time in my work with cancer patients that I was forced to confront the death of someone with whom I had shared many hours. I walked around the university campus the rest of that day wondering why no one else understood what had happened. It seemed outrageously bizarre that everyone else, in uniforms as diverse as professional-looking white coats and jeans à la Haight-Ashbury "street freakery," was not attending to the monumental event that had just occurred.

I had met Larry two months before, following a psychological consultant request from his physician. The request stated simply, "Patient having problems dealing with emotional aspects of malignancy." I imagine so! Since then I've received many similar requests and have always wondered at how bizarre they seemed. For instance, what would be the reverse? "Patient having no problems dealing with emotional aspects of malignancy"? Then I might truly be concerned. It appears strange that anyone would even question the existence of strong feelings about so monumental a process as an advanced cancer. In work with both inpatients and outpatients, I have rarely encountered an individual with cancer who did not at times manifest powerful and often painfully disorienting emotional reactions. What I have seen frequently are well-intentioned but overburdened medical and nursing personnel who do not have the time or psychological expertise needed to assess accurately the emotional status of their patients.

In some settings, when a psychiatric or psychological

consultant is requested, a different drama unfolds. The mental-health professional, encumbered by psychotherapeutic systems that require extended therapeutic processes over time, may fail miserably with the patient who has a limited lifespan. For a patient who is undergoing rapid changes in physiological status, body image, and mood resulting from both the disease and its treatment, interpersonal consistency tends to be the exception rather than the rule. To assess this as psychopathology is frequently nonsense, since it is often an appropriate response by the patient to an extreme stressor. To pretend that we, the professional staff, would not respond similarly, given the same diagnosis and contextual demands, is harmfully naive. What appears true, despite the reality of our time pressures and biomedical duties, is that we ourselves are not psychologically comfortable around the dying and may resort to extreme psychological defensive postures—denial, intellectualization at case conferences, etc.—to avoid meaningful relationships with our patients.

Who Helps Whom?

I think my ability to work with people like Larry is directly related to the degree to which I risk being emotionally accessible to them. This work continually forces me to confront fears about my own death and to realize that my primary data are secured by trusting the patient as an accurate source of information. The largest single impediment to providing effective emotional support to the dying is the powerful professional staff distinction between *us* and *them*. It is a deeply conditioned and tradition-bound assumption in the hospital context that *we* are the professionals and you are the patients, and *we* will help you by means of our technological mastery and beneficence. This distinction is most unfortunate. In emotional reactions to life-threatening illness, *we* are literally *they*. We use all our biomedical and psychological sophistication to facilitate healing, but then what? For myself, it is to imagine "my experience, feelings, thoughts, and emotional needs as a patient in the same demanding situation; to share even if minimally the pain, confusion, and insight resulting from yet another human encounter with death. Whenever a professional colleague tells me, "I can't get emotionally involved," I think, "How unfortunate," and wonder to myself "How long has this horrid affliction persisted?" To identify emotionally with a person under duress so much that one cannot function is of little help to anyone. However, to deny any emotional connection is violence. I understood Larry's plight as well as I did because I could imagine my own response in the same situation. When I was confused about how best to help him, I'd immediately confer with Larry. My skills as a clinical psychologist are, of course, a tremendous asset, but the issues revolve more around human authenticity than professional expertise. I've learned since my work with Larry that a primary assumption in working with seriously ill cancer patients is that there are always emotional issues, and that people trained to be sensitive to these issues can be an enormous help. Patients with "emotional difficulties related to malignancy" are the norm, certainly not the exception.

My initial reaction to Larry was one of surprise. Here was a man sitting stripped to the waist with a muscular body and appearing at least as strong as I. The difference was that Larry had a presumed diagnosis of childhood leukemia. We spoke for some time, and I learned that Larry was an ex-Marine, 20 years old, who had spent a great deal of time distancing himself emotionally and psychologically from his family. He had been somewhat of a rebel all his life and had joined the Marines on a bet. Two of Larry's major problem areas were (1) the fact that, although he had been told that there was a 75 percent cure rate for his form of childhood leukemia, and was receiving positive feedback from his physician and the nursing staff about his medical condition, he did not feel the improvement; and (2) his relationship to his family. Channels for intimate communication had never been established. Larry's life-experience thus far had been based on an extended adolescent rebellion. Now, however, he was sick and frightened, and needed his family desperately, but lacked the interpersonal skills and the insight needed to establish communication. The reverse was also true. There was no one in Larry's nuclear family who could openly and honestly relate to him.

We spoke about both these issues, and I decided I could do something very concrete concerning the first one. I would consult with Larry's physician and find out if he had any ideas. First, I decided to check Larry's chart. Much to my dismay, I discovered that, two weeks before, Larry's diagnosis had been changed to acute adult leukemia, and this his prognosis was now very poor. Larry had not been informed of this change in diagnosis. He was still operating on the old assumption that there was a 75 percent chance of cure, and that he would be up and around in several weeks. This seemed outrageously unfair, and when I mentioned this to Larry's physician, he responded, "I just started on this rotation. It's not my responsibility to tell him. It should have been done by his previous physician." I was unable to accept this response, and in further discussion with the physician I volunteered to tell Larry about the change in his diagnosis. Larry's new physician was a young, sensitive, and intelligent man who identified strongly with Larry. He realized that Larry should know about the change in diagnosis, but was tremendously afraid to break the news for fear of devastating Larry (and himself!). When he saw the strong feelings I and Larry had about concealment of such information and recognized I was correct, he broke down, and I spent an hour in supportive psychotherapy with the physician before he was able to go in and talk to Larry. This was one of the most moving situations in which I have ever been involved.

Early in my work I learned the difficulty inherent in the physician's role. Culturally defined as a *healer*, he may be forced to resort to an extreme psychological defensive posture in order to deny the reality of many of the situations in which he works. That is, for many forms of cancer, medical tools toward cure are minimal, and the physician must face the fact that the patient will die. For a culturally defined healer, death is tantamount to failure, and the emotional consequences for the physician are often severe. Little has yet been written on the emotional impact of patient death on the physician, and yet this appears to be an area in which research is vitally needed.

The First Breakthrough

We went in to see Larry together, and for ten minutes the physician did his best to break the news. Larry was painfully aware of the inconsistency of the situation; i.e., he had never before seen his physician and me together and knew something was wrong. His heart was pounding like that of any person, any animal, in stark terror. After this brief visit, his physician left hurriedly, and I remained to deal with the aftermath. Larry experienced an enormous emotional upheaval. He cried and raged about not having been told the truth and was furious at the cosmos for this horrible turn of events. Finally, after much pain, he asked me to thank his doctor for attempting to carry out what must have been a very difficult task.

From then on, the nature of our work changed. Larry was extremely intent on establishing meaningful contact with each member of his family, and I suggested that we meet as a group. On the scheduled day, I arrived a few minutes late, looked in, and saw each family member standing in a separate corner of the room, as far from Larry's bed as possible. The general tone of the situation was conflictual, and I felt I had walked into the middle of an argument. I apologized, saying that I'd wait outside until their discussion was completed. Larry's mother hurriedly said, "I'd like to come out and speak with you." As soon as we left the room, she broke into tears, saying that she did not know how to talk to Larry anymore. She had always felt close to him, but didn't understand what was happening with his illness. She was very unsure of what to say to Larry for fear of upsetting him.

Avoiding the Fact of Death

What had developed was the kind of conspiracy of silence that often engulfs and isolates the dying. Although the family knew what was going on medically and realized the gravity of the situation, and Larry similarly understood the severity of his condition, neither party was able to discuss this information openly for fear of upsetting the "emotional equilibrium" of the other. I decided to speak with the various members of the family, discussing their feelings about Larry, his deteriorating physical condition, and ways in which they thought they could assist him. I learned from Larry's mother that she wished to be close to her son, and I saw this as a long-desired opportunity to bridge the communication gap that existed between Larry and the other family members.

Larry's father, with whom he had never shared anything more intimate than a slap on the back and a can of beer at a football game, revealed an enormous amount of previously unexpressed feeling about his son's plight. Although he wished to say much to his son, channels of emotional communication had never been developed. Larry's father asked me to help him in "getting the two of us together." By his own admission, he cried for the first time in thirty years, and explained that he couldn't let his son go to his death without some communication of love between them.

Larry's sister and brother followed closely the model of their parents. They were also interested in communicating with Larry about his illness and had a somewhat easier time doing so. By acting as a facilitator, friend, therapist, and participant, I was able to give the family permission to discuss all aspects of the situation freely and openly with Larry. It is important to remember that I had spent hours with Larry before this meeting, and knew very well what his feeings and preferences were about such communication. Larry was extremely adamant about demanding as open a communicational context as possible. Within a short time, Larry's family was sitting on or near his bed, laughing, joking, crying, and sharing in a far more authentic manner the essence of what was transpiring.

As with many dying adults, Larry was frightened and puzzled by those issues and feelings that are summarized by the phrase "How could I not be among you?" He wanted to explore the possibility of leaving something behind—a personally relevant extension of himself to those people for whom he cared. I helped him secure the tools for doing leather work, and Larry fashioned wallets for his father and brother, purses for his mother and sister. On each item he etched "With love always—from Larry." Sensing that part of him would survive, these items meant a great deal to Larry. Such self-extensive forms of expression have been important to many dying people, and amount to personal symbols of (or "testimonials" to) one's incarnate existence.

Moments Beyond the Pain

My work with Larry continued to change form as we discussed many topics that had before been inaccessible. He asked whether I believed in a life after death, and if so, in what form. We spent hours discussing the purpose of his life (and mine); whether he (Larry) and I (Charlie) would ever meet again, in a recognizable form, in another time and place. We spoke of loving people, of relationships, of the pain inherent in confusing roles (such as patient, psychologist, or doctor) with people. It was no longer theoretical analysis or philosophical debate of the kind I had learned during my quarter-century of "academic tutelage." Larry's limited lifespan gave the interchange an urgency and vitality absent elsewhere. We were two representatives of the somewhat odd and physically vulnerable species *Homo sapiens* struggling to understand why we were sitting (or lying) on an oblate spheroid whirling somewhere in the Milky Way. It was both frightening and exhilarating, and I'll not likely forget those shared "struggles." Perhaps the content didn't matter at all. Perhaps we were "only" defining our relationship while protecting each other from the void, like children huddling together in the dark... perhaps... perhaps... perhaps.

The Patient as Teacher

As his disease progressed, Larry grew weaker, and his family, sensing the outcome, withdrew emotionally. This process, sometimes accurately called *anticipatory grief*, is a psychological reaction to impending death that is frequently experienced by family members and hospital staff. Although it helps to prepare the survivors psychologically, this reaction can easily be experienced by the patient as a painful abandonment. I too, was bracing myself for the worst, but I remained with Larry, discussing those things that were uppermost in his mind. He suggested that I take notes, so that I might subsequently use his "story" in teaching health-care professionals. When I agreed, Larry seemed to know that his painful drama might positively affect the experiences of other seriously ill people.

I saw Larry on Friday before returning home, and we talked about pain, both emotional and physical, loneliness, and the fact that he felt his family withdrawing. He also felt the staff withdrawing, and was enormously saddened by the fact that both his physician and favorite nurses were now visiting much less frequently. He repeatedly thanked me for being "the one person who was not afraid to share this awful pain," and asked if there was any way he could repay me. I assured him that I had been repaid many times over, but Larry insisted on giving me something. I asked him to be my teacher and translate his experiences for me. "When you're alone, Larry, what thoughts and feelings do you have?" "Specifically, what is it that makes you afraid?" "Teach me how best to help you." In a situation that I have since encountered many times, Larry faded in and out of waking consciousness. In lucid moments, he was extremely clear in responding to my questions, but then would drift into a sleeplike state. He taught me much during that period, and I know I was a support to him as well.

I learned how vital it is to remember that we are dealing not with a professional issue, but a *human* one. As health-care professionals we are trained as healers, and it is clear that death is an unacceptable outcome for many of us. To imagine that trained healers—i.e., doctors, nurses, and other biomedical personnel who experience themselves as adversaries of illness and death—can respond effectively to the dying patient is often an erroneous expectation. It more often happens that the professional's anxiety and sense of impotence drives him away, leaving the patient emotionally and psychologically isolated, and often physically abandoned. I learned the importance of training both professionals and lay people to relate effectively to the dying person. If we are ever to transcend our barbaric isolation of the terminally ill, we need to stop relating to dying people as lepers. We must realize that, at our current level of scientific expertise, death is not always the result of a biomedical mistake or a mysterious virus, but may be seen as a natural winding down of the human psycho-biological totality.

The Good-bye

Shortly before I left that Friday, I sat watching Larry with his black and blue body, sunken eyes, and yellow skin. As he lay there with his intravenous "life supports," I thought of Auschwitz and Treblinka, my grandfather Aaron, and Vietnam. Suddenly, as if sensing my despair, Larry awoke, looked straight at me, and said, "I have something very important to say to the people who will read your book." I listened carefully, somewhat surprised by Larry's intensity. Finally, he said, "Dying alone is not easy."

There was a calm and clear tone to Larry's message that was uncanny, and he smiled peacefully, adding to my uneasiness. His words haunted me for days. The following Monday I hurried to visit him again. When I arrived at the nurses' station, I was told that Larry had died. I was sad, angry, relieved, confused. Finally I was left with the feeling that somehow I should have known that what Larry was really saying on Friday was good-bye. Yet it didn't feel like good-bye. There was a tranquil and accepting look on Larry's face so remarkably discontinuous with those tormented, pain-wracked experiences I had witnessed previously. There was a powerful sense that Larry had transcended the somatic entrapment that bound him for so long. I believe that what Larry was communicating to me that Friday was "Dying alone is not easy, but the job is done, and I've reached a place of peace. . . . I appreciate and love you for what you've shared with me, and if by chance we meet again. . . ."

DR. CHARLES A. GARFIELD *received his Ph.D. in clinical psychology from the University of California, Berkeley. He is a lecturer and author, and is Clinical Professor of Medical Psychology at the Cancer Research Center, S.F. He is also the founder of Shanti Project, a volunteer counseling program for patients and families facing life-threatening illnesses. Dr. Garfield is the editor of* Psychosocial Care of the Dying Patient *(McGraw-Hill, 1978) and* Rediscovery of the Body *(Dell, 1977) and co-author of* Consciousness East and West *(Harper and Row, 1976) and* Stress and Survival *(Mosby, 1979).*

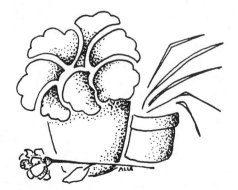

What We Can Learn from the Dying

Stephen and Ondrea Levine
in conversation with
Tom Ferguson, M.D.

MANY people think that if they came down with a fatal illness, they'd react by grabbing a giant bottle of whiskey and an attractive sexual partner and spending their remaining time at the nearest warm beach. But in working with thousands of dying people, we've found that virtually no one does that.

What people *do* is to begin looking into their own hearts and into the eyes of those with whom they share their lives. And all too often they find that these aren't places they've looked very deeply before.

Fred

We just spent some time with Fred, a 54-year-old bus driver for Greyhound. After Fred's diagnosis of terminal cancer, he and his family decided that he would prefer to die at home.

Because of his work, Fred had spent most of his married life away from home. He'd never had a very close relationship with his children. He and his wife had dealt with most major family difficulties—including some severe sexual problems—by totally ignoring them. Fred had always felt he needed to keep up a macho image, and his wife felt trapped in her role as wife and mother. His children only used the house as a place to eat and sleep.

But as his disease progressed, Fred reached the point where he could no longer play his accustomed roles. He couldn't be a tough guy any more. He had a lot of pain, and all the members of his family had to work like hell to take care of him. His teenage son—whom he formerly hardly spoke to—was now giving him baths and rubbing his back. His daughter would read to him when he had trouble sleeping.

Medical Self-Care, Fall 1983. P.O. Box 1000, Point Reyes, California 94956. Reprinted with permission.

As Fred's cancer progressed, he and his family broke through one barrier after another. It wasn't easy, but through it all the family members drew closer and closer. Everyone in the house learned to trust and confide in each other. Neighbors who came to visit would tell us, "I expected to find a house of death. Instead I find a house of life and love. This family has never been as close as they are now."

In observing the changes in Fred's family, we were reminded of the thousands of Brahma bulls that wander around India. They're considered sacred. If two men are trying to kill each other with knives, and a Brahma bull walks between them, they'll pull their knives away, because they mustn't scratch the bull.

Dying people are like Brahma bulls. In their presence, so many of our petty hassles are simply forgotten. We realize what's impermanent, and what's of permanent value.

For most of the people we've worked with, the diagnosis of a fatal disease comes as a frightening experience. One of their most frequent comments is: "I feel like I've wasted my life." So much of who they are has been held back. So much of their precious time was spent running away from their fears, waiting for the future, or remembering the past.

So little of their lives was spent actually *living*. Although they've been alive 40, 60, or 80 years, it suddenly feels to them as if they've hardly lived at all. They've been so busy striving for security and trying to live up to one ideal or another that they forgot to taste and savor the texture of their lives. They were so busy making a home, building their careers, becoming solid citizens, that they forgot to live.

Daren

We shared some time recently with Daren, a 38-year-old Los Angeles man dying from a degenerative nerve disease. Two years ago Daren was handsome, successful, and vibrantly healthy. He had reached the pinnacle of professional success. He was a singer, dancer, and virtuoso guitarist, and was greatly sought after by many of the major Hollywood studios. He had a wife and two children, a lovely home, and ran five miles a day.

Today Daren is strapped to a wheelchair, unable to support his own body's weight. His lungs are so weak that he must consciously draw in enough air to make his vocal cords work. He can no longer move his arms, legs, or body. He needs help to go to the bathroom. His flesh is slowly melting away from his bones.

At first Daren was in agony because he couldn't play, couldn't dance, couldn't earn money, couldn't drive his new Mercedes, couldn't make love—in short, he could no longer live up to his models of who he thought he should be. But after a time, he began to see that it was not his illness that was the problem.

"It was those damn models," he realized. "Those models were always a hassle for me. They're like balloons with holes in them—I've had to keep puffing and puffing all the time to keep them from collapsing. They're not really who I am." And gradually he's been able to let go of his identification with his models.

One day we were sitting and talking and he said to us, "You know, I've never felt so alive in my whole life. I can see now how all the things I used to do to 'be sombody' actually *separated* me from really being alive. For all my outward success, my life back then was just a sort of busy, numb dullness."

He laughed and shook his head. "We're such fools, aren't we? We spend so much time polishing our personalities, strengthening our bodies, keeping up our social positions, trying to achieve this and that. We make such serious business of it all. But now that I can no longer do the things I thought were so important, I have so much love for so many things. I'm discovering a place inside I'd never looked at, never knew. None of the praise I received in the world brought me half the satisfaction I experience right now from just being."

Few Well Prepared for Death

Very few of the people we see are well prepared for their deaths, and no wonder. We are taught to keep thoughts of death out of our consciousness, to ignore illness, to do our best to disguise the natural changes of aging. We grow up believing—and teaching our children—that we are not *supposed* to suffer. We are not *supposed* to grow old. We are not *supposed* to experience loss or pain.

We end up carrying a heavy load—a great deal of fear of illness and death. When Ondrea had cancer, people were afraid to visit her. They were afraid to touch her. And if they did come, they were terrified.

The Pepsi Generation

One of the things we can learn from the dying is simply that it's all right to die. It's all right to be ill. It's OK to be in pain. Sometimes we'll be working with a group of cancer patients, and we'll say, "You know, it's OK that you're suffering. It's OK to suffer." And there'll be a lot of shocked looks, like it has never occurred to them that it really *could* be OK.

It's the American way to be hale and hearty, and it's very difficult for us to accept the fact that illness and death

are a normal part of life. Everyone in the Pepsi generation must grow old and suffer and die just like all previous generations. But our conditioning makes it very hard to accept that.

It's hard for us to accept situations in which we are unable to live up to our models of what's OK. Elizabeth Kübler-Ross used to say that someday she would like to write a book titled *I'm Not OK and You're Not OK and That's OK*.

We learn to work hard to be OK—whatever that means for us. The dying can teach us a great deal about the ways we learn to distort ourselves, to diminish ourselves, to reshape ourselves in order to conform to that OK model, how we are raised to be constantly posturing, constantly inventing an acceptable reality.

A Mosaic of Awareness

The ebb and flow of our awareness is like a complex mosaic made up of many tiles. But because we learn that some of those tiles—parts of ourselves—are considered unacceptable, we begin, at a very early age, to pick out—or cover up—the offending tiles: "Oh, no, I'm not supposed to be angry," so we take that title away. "That part of my mind is too crazy for anybody to see." So we cover it up. "Oh, God, I don't want anybody to see my hatred. Or my jealousy. Or my confusion. Or my greed. Or my envy. That self-hatred, that guilt—that can't be who I really am. That's bad. That's unacceptable. That's crazy. That's neurotic." So out they go, until what is left is a pale caricature of who we really are.

But the dying tell us that *is* who we really are—that continually changing flow of thoughts, those conflicts in values, that continual confusion and not knowing. This is our life.

Accepting "Unacceptable" Feelings

The dying teach us that because of our efforts to drive those "unacceptable" feelings out of consciousness, we end up wondering if we have ever really lived. They teach that it is better to sit quietly with our unwanted states of mind, to accept the pain, accept the waves of unfashionable feelings, to accept our own confusion—rather than to let these painful events drive us out of awareness, into defenses that pull us away from life.

Perhaps the greatest gift the dying have to offer is the realization that we need not wait until we receive a terminal diagnosis to begin to relax our attachments to our images of who we think we should be. How much better, they tell us, to realize that we are *not* our fears, *not* our confusion, *not* our defenses. That it is possible to let those states of mind flow through us without identifying with them, without holding on to them, simply doing our best to stay open to awareness.

They teach us that it is possible to let whatever needs to happen, happen—without being driven into the life-denying reactions our fears would lead us to. It is possible to experience it all, to be threatened by nothing, to withdraw from nothing, not even death.

Learning to be Substantial

We are taught to make ourselves substantial, to take on certain roles and play them with utmost seriousness, to be responsible members of society. The dying teach us that

Dying at Home

In a recent survey, four out of five people said they would prefer to die at home; yet in practice, four out of five people die in institutions. To die at home is to die in the midst of life, in the midst of love. Many of the people we have taken home to die have found they needed less pain medication because of the support and relaxation available in the home environment.

Many have said in the last weeks of a loved one's dying in a hospital: "I wish I could do more." We always think to ourselves, "Take them home to die and don't worry, you will!"

Giving a loved one round-the-clock support may draw on energy reserves long unexplored, while feeding some place deeper than bodily fatigue. To bring loved ones home to die is like accompanying them on their last pilgrimage. There is no experience more intimate. To share that time with another, to encourage a loved one to let go gently while we ourselves practice what we preach, can bring beings together as no other situation can.

Here are a few things that can make the experience easier:

- A cassette recorder so the person can listen to a variety of music and guided meditations.
- A bedside bell so the person can feel in contact and summon help.
- Plastic bedpans, which aren't as cold as the metal ones.
- Daily baths, for human contact and protection against bedsores.
- Massage for decreasing tension and anxiety while deepening contact.
- Don't force someone to eat. You are sharing an openness and ease with what is. If the person wishes not to eat, so be it.
- A blender is useful when one does not wish to take in too much at a time.
- A hot plate or plug-in teapot in the person's room lets you have a cup of tea or light snack without having to leave the room.
- Water and juice should always be available.
- A hospital bed with side rails is convenient and comfortable, but many prefer to die in their own beds, and would rather use a foam wedge and a few extra pillows.

- Pain medications should be given as the person wishes. Don't push your own ideas of how they should work with pain.
- The best place for the bed may be in the living room, near the window. This lets the person maintain contact with the familiar.
- It is not uncommon for people who are dying to feel that their illness may be a punishment for past actions. Supportive measures that can help dissolve the guilt should be encouraged.
- You may wish to call the visiting nurses' association in your town for further information and support.

—Stephen Levine

Experiences That Will Give You Great Insight into Aging, Illness and Dying

1. Volunteer at a Nursing Home.
2. Volunteer at a Hospice.

People who've done either of the above—even if it's only for one week—invariably have a memorable experience. You'll see how your body is going to grow old some day, and all that entails—how difficult it can be just to sit up, just to lift your fork and eat, just to walk, just to sit in a chair. You'll see the way older people are treated. And you'll see how, for the elderly, the being inside has not changed a bit since they were 15. Highly recommended and unforgettable.

—Ondrea Levine

Choosing a Practice

We encourage the people we work with to adopt some kind of practice, one that suits their own life and preferences, but ideally a daily practice, one they can stay with, something to which they give first priority, something they do at a regular time, and do even if they don't feel like it on that particular day.

It might be meditation or yoga, tai chi, running, silent prayer, massage, playing an instrument, karate, judo, writing in a psychological diary, breathing exercises, or the practice of an art or craft—whatever is right for their temperament and their preferences. Something that will encourage them to pay attention. We find that this kind of a daily practice is perhaps the most powerful tool for building awareness.

—Stephen Levine

we must live more lightly, take ourselves less seriously, accept our own impermanence, our own not-knowing. Not to harden against life, but to soften into it. They teach us that real growth comes from coming to the edge of one's model, then letting that model go, and seeing what comes next. The dying can teach us that it's possible not to be "something" but just to be.

Thousands of years of meditation practice teach us that thinking in terms of "the mind" rather than "my mind" helps clarify what's really happening. When you look at

your flow of awareness as "my mind," there's confusion, because if it's *your* mind, then you must be responsible for what's in it. But when we look closely at our thought processes, we see that much of what arises in the mind is actually *uninvited*. We don't *invite* guilt. We don't *invite* anger. They come by themselves.

The Worst Possible Insult

Try this experiment: Think of the worst possible insult you can imagine, then suppose that you arrive home to

DEATH IN DREAMS

Jeremy Taylor

My experience is that death and the fear of death in dreams (and myth) are always associated at some level with the growth and transformation of personality and character. When we flee from death in dreams, we are most often fleeing from inner promptings that it is time to grow and change some more. This is also true of the images of death and dying in the world's

mythology. The Christian *mythos* offers a particularly clear and developed example of the archetypal drama of the Willing Sacrifice for whom death is consciously understood as the necessary prelude to rebirth and transformational reconnection with the energies of the Divine.

From Jeremy Taylor, *Dream Work: Techniques for Discovering the creative Power in Dreams*. Ramsey, N.J.: (Paulist Press, 1980.)

JEREMY TAYLOR *is a Unitarian Universalist Minister and dream worker residing in the San Francisco Bay Area.*

find your living space broken into and that message scrawled across your wall. You would experience—involuntarily—a state of mind that you did not invite, expect, or want. Whose mind did that?

The mind is constantly rating us on our behavior, constantly comparing things as they are to imagined models of things "as they should be." The mind finds everything wanting: us, others, and the world. It is never satisfied for long. Identification with the mind is the very definition of suffering.

To the extent that we identify with "my mind," our lives

will be in constant turmoil. We will be jerked up or down by any stray thought that drifts across our mind.

The dying teach us that to be able to accept ourselves in our true complexity, we must, without judgment, accept the craziness of the mind itself—accept it without mistaking it for who we really are.

Just Sleeping, Just Eating

For those of us who live in the mind, life is 99 percent an afterthought. It isn't tasting, touching, smelling, loving, being alive; it's mostly the mind thinking about what we

FORGIVENESS MEDITATION

Bring into your heart the image of someone for whom you feel much resentment. Take a moment to feel that person right there in the center of your chest.

And in your heart, say to that person, "For anything you may have done that caused me pain, anything you did either intentionally or unintentionally, through your thoughts, words, or actions, I forgive you."

Slowly allow that person to settle into your heart. No force, just opening to them at your own pace. Say to them, "I forgive you." Gently, gently open to them. If it hurts, let it hurt. Begin to relax the iron grip of your resentment, to let go of that incredible anger. Say to them "I forgive you." And allow them to be forgiven.

Now bring into your heart the image of someone you wish to ask for forgiveness. Say to them, "For anything I may have done that caused you pain, my thoughts, my actions, my words, I ask your forgiveness. For all those words that were said out of for-

getfulness or fear or confusion, I ask your forgiveness."

Don't allow any resentment you may hold for yourself to block your reception of that forgiveness. Let your heart soften to it. Allow yourself to be forgiven. Open to the possibility of forgiveness. Holding them in your heart, say to them, "For whatever I may have done that caused you pain, I ask your forgiveness."

Now bring an image of yourself into your heart, floating at the center of your chest. Bring yourself into your heart, and using your own first name, say to yourself, "For all that you have done in forgetfulness and fear and confusion, for all the words and thoughts and actions that may have caused pain to anyone, I forgive you."

Open to the possibility of self-forgiveness. Let go of all the bitterness, the hardness, the judgment of yourself.

Make room in your heart for yourself. Say "I forgive you" to you.

are doing. An action occurs, and a moment later we think of ourselves as acting. We see a bird, and a moment later we are no longer seeing the bird, but thinking of ourselves looking at a bird. At other times we live in fantasies of the future or the past. If we start to experience our flow of consciousness as just the mind "doing its thing," we find ourselves relating more directly to the world. It's as though the mind, the "I," disappears, and there is just smelling, just dancing, just seeing the sunset, just sleeping, just eating our food, just being with someone we love.

Letting Go

The dying teach us that happiness comes from learning to let go of the things that cause suffering. Though they've lost much that they desired, they've found much that is of even greater importance. Through their investigation of suffering, they have gotten in touch with something deeper.

The dying teach that it is possible to let go of wanting, that desire is only a cloud that obscures our real nature. We see that our true sources of satisfaction lie in what we already have, and have always had: simple awareness.

Before we began working with the dying, we used to think of those who had *not* suffered losses as the truly fortunate. No more. We feel sorry for them now.

These well-intentioned people who have, by luck or planning, isolated themselves so well from life may feel perfectly secure in their possessions and their loved ones. They may feel that the whole business of dying has nothing to do with them. They may feel that they have what they want in the world, that they are safe from the flow of change. But we can assure you that for them, the inevitable loss of possessions, the inevitable loss of loved ones, will be the most difficult.

The dying teach us that the real tragedy is not the loss of possessions, not even the loss of loved ones. The real tragedy is losing our connection with humanness, with compassion, with kindness, with forgiveness—for ourselves and those about us—closing off to life.

In their efforts to find a safe place, to avoid the inevitable suffering of life, these seemingly safe, secure people have merely saved up their suffering. They have put off their pain. They have carried it around without realizing it. And, in the meantime, they have piddled their lives away maintaining their defenses. We have come to feel deeply sorry for such people, because they will experience death with the greatest horror.

Who Dies?

Imagine that the time has now come when the energy in your body is no longer sufficient to allow you to participate in the world. You can no longer continue your former work, or earn the money you used to earn. You are lying in bed with your new car parked in the driveway outside your window. You realize that you will never drive that car again. You see your closet. You know that you will never wear your wardrobe again. Your children play in the next room. You are too weak to get up and join them.

In the kitchen, your mate cooks supper; you will have to be spoon-fed because you are too weak to feed yourself. You want to get up to help, but it is no longer possible. You sense that in the not too distant future, your mate will

be making love to someone else, that in a short time someone else will be raising your children.

You must let go of every model of yourself you have ever created—wife, husband, father, mother, lover, breadwinner, parent, teacher, doctor, nurse, businessperson. Those models are no longer available for you. Can you see how you might begin to wonder, "Who am I? Who is it lying here in this bed? Who is dying? Who is it that lived?"

For those who remain attached to how it *used* to be, to how they thought it would *always* be, dying can be hell. But dying doesn't *have* to be hell. It can be a remarkable opportunity for awakening.

Like Worn-out Clothing

We have seen people experiencing the same falling away of the body, the same inability to be the individual they thought they were, who are able to leave their old roles and duties behind like so much worn-out clothing. As their bodies grow weaker, their spirits and their participation in the moment grow stronger and stronger, until their old roles and old masks are seen as the bars of a cage, and they experience a joyful release from the part of their life that was made up of models and ideals of how they were *supposed* to be.

We have seen these remarkable people flow wholeheartedly into the vastness of what is, no longer kept captive by their models of the world. They see everything as present in each moment. It seems that all blocks to their perceptions are gone. They see how identifying with fantasies of the future and dreams of the past has kept them in prison for their whole lives. As one spiritual teacher said shortly before his death, "Today I am released from jail."

The Work of the Dying

It is from these remarkable people that we have learned that the work of the dying is to let go of self-protective control. To open, to live fully in the present moment, to accept the richness of each moment with an open heart, with a mind that does not cling to models.

These people are able to open up to an appreciation of all that is, beyond life, beyond death. They realize that they don't have to do or be anything to be who they really are. They have escaped from the tyranny of the mind, the tyranny of models and shoulds and musts.

We see them touch the real. We see them become part of what is. We see them let go of wanting things to be any other way.

Those who are able to open into the experience of dying are the most open-hearted, clear-minded people we know. If we might share a composite of what we hear them say, it would go something like this: "It's strange, but I've never been so happy in my life. I don't really know who I am, but it doesn't matter, because no matter who I think I am, I keep turning out to be something else.

"My knowing has always blocked my understanding, but now I am full of not-knowing, vulnerable, open. I had to lose it all to see how little of it was worth having. Somehow there is much more to me than I had ever imagined."

These people die in wholeness, without struggle. They seem to simply evaporate out of their bodies. Their death is like the rain falling gently back into the ocean.

Our best wish and hope for ourselves, our friends and family, and for you, is that we might, each in our own way, follow their example.

Resources

The Dying Project
Stephen and Ondrea Levine
P.O. Box 2228
Taos, New Mexico 87571
   The Levines welcome inquiries about workshops and lectures.

Who Dies? An Investigation of Conscious Living and Conscious Dying
Stephen Levine
1982/317 pages/$9.95 from:
Anchor Books
245 Park Avenue
New York, NY 10167
or Whole Earth
   A wise, insightful, readable book on conscious dying. It addresses many aspects of the dying process with both lightness and candor. There is much wisdom here—for people who are dying, for those close to them, and for readers interested in exploring their own attitudes and feelings toward death.

   Includes a number of useful meditations for those in pain, other guided meditations, a list of recommended music to help quiet the mind (from Chopin waltzes to birdsongs to Tibetan temple bells) and chapters on letting go of control, dying children, and working with the dying.

A Gradual Awakening
Stephen Levine
1979/173 pages/$5.95 from:
Anchor Books
245 Park Avenue
New York, NY 10167
   A readable, accessible book on the practice of mindfulness and meditation.

The Tape Library
P.O. Box 61498
Santa Cruz, CA 95061
   Write to this address to receive a catalog of audio tapes of lectures and workshops by the Levines, and to be placed on the Dying Project's mailing list.

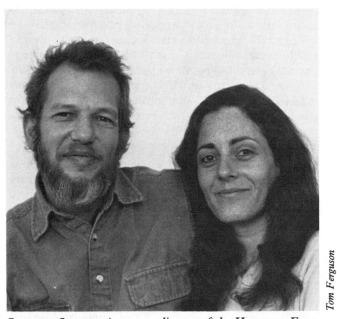

Tom Ferguson

ONDREA LEVINE *is past co-director of the Hanuman Foundation Dying Project. She began working with the elderly and convalescent in her mid-teens. While studying gerontology in college she continued working with the bedridden and dying. Counseling those in crisis on the East Coast for some years, she then moved to Taos, New Mexico, acting as a counselor to those with cancer (having worked with her own cancer for several years). Merging with Stephen Levine in 1979, she joined the work of the Dying Project and began teaching with her husband. Ondrea oversaw the creating of the free consultation phone and is a mainstay of its communication with those in crisis and growth. After three years of directing the "Dying Phone," Ondrea has deepened her focus on the teaching and sharing of healing techniques and the release of held suffering in the grieving process. She specializes in working with people in coma and sudden loss.*

For STEPHEN LEVINE, *the investigation of death becomes an investigation of life which uncovers "an exquisite opportunity for us to discover who we really are." Counseling the terminally ill, Stephen tells people to face their death fully aware of the process they are going through and to spend their remaining days living their dying in love and deep awareness.*

   Stephen's work with Ram Dass (a prominent American spiritual teacher and philosopher) was already quite well known, through their collaboration in writing Grist for the Mill, *when in 1977 Elisabeth Kübler-Ross invited him to teach meditation at her workshops on death and dying. He studied and taught with Kübler-Ross for two years before going on to develop techniques of adapting various meditative practices for the grieving and terminally ill.*

   In 1978 Ram Dass encouraged Stephen to undertake the organization and coordination of the Hanuman Foundation Dying Project. He has directed the Dying Project since that time, traveling three to four months a year offering workshops and intensive retreats for those confronting death and grief or working with others in crisis. He is a consultant to many hospices, hospitals, and service groups across the country. Stephen's book, Who Dies?, *is often used by hospices and universities as a main teaching text.*

   In the course of an evening or workshop with Stephen and Ondrea they investigate the process we all share in grief, dying, relationships, and a wide range of other topics. To any topic they bring a keen sense of humor and compassionate spaciousness that allows one to experience a deeper sense of being.

   "No longer (after 7 years) directing the Hanuman Foundation Dying Project allows us considerable expansion of our work with healing (we are working on a new book, Healing into Life), *relationship shops, nuclear workshops, and yet deeper levels of meeting the heart of the matter in those facing terminal illness and profound loss."*

Death Does Not Exist

Elisabeth Kübler-Ross, M.D.

In this powerful address, Dr. Ross relates some of the major experiences that have shaped her professional and personal life. She provides an overview of her world-renowned research into the nature of death and dying, but, more importantly, she spells out from her heart what the implications of her research and experiences are for our understanding of the spiritual nature of human beings.

I WAS thinking for a long time of what I'm going to talk about with you this morning. I'm going to share with you how a two-pound "nothing" found her way, her path in life. How I learned what I'm going to share with you, and how you too can be convinced that this life here, this time that you're in a physical body, is a very, very short span of your total existence. It's a very important time of your existence, because you're here for a very special purpose, which is yours and yours alone. If you live well, you will never have to worry about dying. You can do that even if you have only one day to live. The question of time is not terribly important; it is a man-made, artificial concept anyway.

To live well means basically to learn to love. I was very touched yesterday when the speaker mentioned, "Faith, hope, and love, but the biggest of the three is love." In Switzerland you have confirmation when you're 16, and you get a saying that is supposed to be a leading word throughout life. Since we were triplets, they had to find one for three of us; they picked love, faith, and hope, and I happened to be love.

I'm going to talk with you about love, which is life, and death; it is all the same thing.

I mentioned briefly that I was born an "unwanted" child. Not that my parents didn't want a child. They wanted a girl very badly, but a pretty, beautiful, ten-pound girl. They did not expect triplets, and when I came, I was only two pounds and very ugly, and no hair, and was a terrible, terrible, big disappointment. Then 15 minutes later the second child came, and after 20 minutes, a 6½-pound baby came, and they were very happy. But they would have liked to give two of them back.

I think that nothing in life is a coincidence. Not even that, because I had the feeling that I had to prove all my life that even a two-pound nothing...that I had to work really hard, like some blind people think that they have to work ten times as hard to keep a job. I had to prove very hard that I was worth living.

When I was a teenager, I needed and wanted to do something for this world, which was in a terrible mess at the end of the war. I had promised myself that if the war ever ended I would walk all the way to Poland and Russia and start first-aid stations and help stations. I kept my promise, and this is, I think where this whole work on death and dying started.

I personally saw the concentration camps. I personally saw trainloads of baby shoes, trainloads of human hair from the victims of the concentration camps taken to Germany to make pillows. When you smell the concentration camps with your own nose, when you see the crematoriums, when you're very young as I was, when you are really an adolescent in a way, you will never, ever be the same any more, after that. Because what you see is the inhumanity of man and that each one of us in this room is capable of becoming a Nazi monster. That part of you you have to acknowledge. But each one of you in this room also has the ability to become a Mother Teresa, if you know who she is. She's one of my saints—a woman in India who picks up dying children, starving, dying people, and believes very strongly that even if they're dying in her arms, if she has been able to love them for five minutes, it is worthwhile that they have lived. She is a very beautiful human being, if you ever have a chance of seeing her.

I had prepared my life to be a physician in India, like Schweitzer was in Africa. But two weeks before I was supposed to leave, I was notified that the whole project in India had fallen through. And instead of the jungles of India I ended up in the jungles of Brooklyn, New York, marrying an American, who took me to the one place in the world which was at the bottom of my list of where I ever wanted to live. And that too was not coincidence, because to go to a place that you love is easy, but to go to a place you hate every bit of, that is a test. That is given to you to see if you really mean it.

I ended up at Manhattan State Hospital, which is another dreadful place. Not really knowing any psychiatry, and being very lonely and miserable and unhappy, and not wanting to make my new husband unhappy, I opened up

This talk was originally given at a conference of the Association for Holistic Health in 1976, and first appeared in *Co-Evolution Quarterly* No. 14, Summer 1977. It is reprinted here by permission of Dr. Ross.

to the patients. I identified with their misery and their loneliness and their desperation, and suddenly my patients started to talk. People who didn't talk for twenty years started to verbalize, share their feeings, and I suddenly knew that I was not alone in my misery, though it wasn't half as miserable as living in a state hospital. For two years I did nothing else but live and work with these patients, sharing every Hanukkah, Christmas, Passover, and Easter with them, just to share their loneliness, not knowing much psychiatry, the theoretic psychiatry that one ought to know. I barely understood their English, but we loved each other. We really cared. After two years 94 percent of those patients were discharged, self-supporting, into New York City, many of them having their own jobs and able to function.

What I'm trying to say to you is that knowledge helps, but knowledge alone is not going to help anybody. If you do not use your head and your heart and your soul, you're not going to help a single human being. That is what so-called hopeless, schizophrenic patients taught me. In all my work with patients, I learned that whether they were chronic schizophrenics, or severely retarded children, or dying patients, each one has a purpose. Each one can not only learn and be helped by you, but can actually become your teacher. That is true of 6-month-old retarded babies who can't speak. That is true of hopeless schizophrenic patients, who behave like animals when you see them for the first time. But the best teachers in the world are dying patients.

Dying patients, when you take the time out and sit with them, teach you about the stages of dying. They teach you how they go through the denial and the anger, and the "Why me?" and question God and reject Him for a while. They bargain with Him, and then go through horrible depressions, and if they have another human being who cares, they may be able to reach a stage of acceptance. But that is not just typical of dying, really has nothing to do with dying. We only call it the "stages of dying" for lack of a better word. If you lose a boyfriend or a girlfriend, or if you lose your job, or if you are moved from your home where you have lived for 50 years and you have to go to a nursing home, if some people even lose a parakeet, or only their contact lenses, they go through the same stages of dying. This is, I think, the meaning of suffering.

All the hardships that you face in life, all the tests and tribulations, all the nightmares and all the losses, most people still view as curses, as punishment by God, as something negative. If you would only know that nothing that comes to you is negative. I mean *nothing*. All the trials and the tribulations, and the biggest losses that you ever experience, things that make you say, "If I had known about this, I would never have been able to make it through," are gifts to you. It's like somebody has to—what do you call that when you make the hot iron into a tool?—you have to temper the iron. It is an opportunity that you are given to grow. That is the sole purpose of existence on this planet Earth. You will not grow if you sit in a beautiful flower garden and somebody brings you gorgeous food on a silver platter. But you will grow if you are sick, if you are in pain, if you experience losses, and if you do not put your head in the sand, but take the pain and learn to accept

it, not as a curse or a punishment, but as a gift to you with a very, very specific purpose.

I will give you a clinical example of that. In one of my one-week workshops—they are one-week live-in retreats—there was a young woman. She did not have to face the death of a child, but she faced several of what we call "little deaths." Not very little in her eyes. When she gave birth to a second baby girl, which she was very much looking forward to, she was told in a not very human way that the child was severely retarded; in fact, that the child would never be able to even recognize her as her mother. When she became aware of this, her husband walked out on her, and she was suddenly faced with two young, very needy, very dependent children, no money, no income, and no help.

She went through a terrible denial. She couldn't even use the word retardation. She then went through fantastic anger at God, cursed Him out. First He didn't exist at all, and then He was a mean old you know what. Then she went through tremendous bargaining—if the child at least would be educable, or at least could recognize her as a mother. Then she found some genuine meaning in having this child, and I'll simply share with you how she finally resolved it. It began to dawn on her that nothing in life is coincidence. She tried to look at this child and tried to figure out what purpose a little vegetable-like human being has in this Earth. She found the solution, and I'm sharing this with you in the form of a poem that she wrote. She's not a poetess, but it's a moving poem. She identifies with her child and talks to her godmother. And she called the poem "To My Godmother."

What is a godmother?
I know you're very special,
You waited many months for my arrival.
You were there and saw me when only minutes old,
and changed my diapers when I had been there just
    a few days.
You had dreams of your first godchild.
She would be precocious like your sister.
You'd see her off to school, college, and marriage.
How would I turn out? A credit to those who have
    me?
God had other plans for me. I'm just me.
    No one ever used the word precocious about me.
Something hasn't hooked up right in my mind.
    I'll be a child of God for all time.
I'm happy. I love everyone, and they love me.
There aren't many words I can say,
But I can communicate and understand affection,
    warmth, softness and love.
There are special people in my life.
Sometimes I sit and smile and sometimes cry.
I wonder why?
I am happy and loved by special friends.
What more could I ask for?
Oh, sure, I'll never go to college, or marry.
But don't be sad. God made me very special.
I cannot hurt. Only love.
And maybe God sees some children who simply love.
Do you remember when I was baptized,

You held me, hoping I wouldn't cry and you wouldn't
    drop me?
Neither happened and it was a very happy day.
Is that why you are my godmother?
I know you are soft and warm, give me love, but there
    is something very special in your eyes.
I see that look and feel that love from others.
I must be special to have so many mothers.
No, I will never be a success in the eyes of the world,
But I promise you something very few people can,
Since all I know is love, goodness and innocence,
    Eternity will be ours to share, my godmother.

This is the same mother who, a few months before, was
willing to let this toddler crawl out near the swimming
pool and pretend to go to the kitchen, so the child would
fall into the swimming pool and drown. I hope that you
appreciate the change that had taken place in this mother.

This is what takes place in all of you if you are willing
to always look at anything that happens in your life from
both sides of the coin. There is never just one side to it.
You may be terminally ill, you may have a lot of pain, you
may not find somebody to talk to about it. You may feel
that it's unfair to take you away in the middle of your life,
that you haven't really started to live yet. Look at the other
side of the coin.

You're suddenly one of the few fortunate people who
can throw overboard all the "baloney" that you've carried
with you. You can go to somebody and say, "I love you,"
when he can still hear it, and then you can skip the schmaltzy
eulogies afterwards. Because you know that you are
here for a very short time, you can finally do the things
that you really want to do. How many of you in this room,
how many of you do not truly do the kind of work that
you really want to do from the bottom of your heart? You
should go home and change your work. Do you know what
I'm saying to you? Nobody should do something because
somebody tells him he ought to do that. This is like forcing
a child to learn a profession that is not its own. If you
listen to you own inner voice, to your own inner wisdom,
which is far greater than anybody else's as far as you're
concerned, you will not go wrong and you will know what
to do with your life. And then time is no longer relevant.

After working with dying patients for many years and
learning from them what life is all about, what regrets
people have at the end of their life when it seems to be too
late, I began to wonder what death is all about. Nobody
ever defines death except in physical language. First it was
no heartbeat, no blood pressure, no vital signs; then it
became more sophisticated and added EEG, and became
a several-page description. But that too is not sufficient,
because it only deals with the physical body.

One of my patients helped me to find out how to begin
research into what death really is, and with it, naturally,
the question of life after death. Mrs. S had been in and
out of the intensive-care unit 15 times, never was expected
to live, but always made a comeback. In one of her hospitalizations
she could not get to Chicago, and she was
hospitalized in a local hospital. She remembers being put
in a private room, very close to death, and could not make
up her mind whether she should call the nurse because

she suddenly sensed that she was moments away from
death. One part of her wanted very much to lean back on
the pillows and finally be at peace. But the other part of
her needed to make it through one more time because her
youngest son was not yet of age. Before she made the
decision to call the nurse and go through this whole rigamorole
once more, a nurse apparently walked into her
room, took one look at her, and dashed out.

At that moment, she saw herself floating out of her
physical body, floating a few feet above her body. She was
very surprised at seeing her corpse in that bed. She made
some funny remarks about how pale she looked, and then
to her utter amazement, described how the resuscitation
team dashed into her room. She described in minute details
how they worked on her, who was in the room first, who
was in last, what they wore, what they said—she even
repeated a joke of one of the residents, who apparently
was very apprehensive and started to joke. In the meantime,
while everybody worked very desperately to bring
her back to physical life, she floated a few feet above her
body and had only one need, one wish—to tell them down
there, "Cool it, relax, take it easy, it's OK."

Those are her own words. She could perceive absolutely
everything that was going on, but they could not perceive
her. And then she gave up on them. She was declared
dead, and three and a half hours later she made a comeback
and lived for another year and a half.

In my classroom this was our first account of a bed
patient who had this experience. This then led to a collection
of cases from all over the world. We have hundreds
of cases, from Australia to California. They all share the
same common denominator. They are all fully aware of
shedding their physical body. And death, as we understood
it in scientific language, does not really exist. Death is
simply a shedding of the physical body like the butterfly
coming out of a cocoon. It is a transition into a higher state
of consciousness, where you continue to perceive, to understand,
to laugh, to be able to grow, and the only thing
that you lose is something that you don't need anymore,
and that is your physical body. It's like putting away your
winter coat when spring comes, and you know that the
coat is too shabby and you don't want to wear it any more.
That's virtually what death is all about.

No one of the patients who had this experience was ever
again afraid to die. Not one of them, in all our cases. Many
of our patients also said that, besides the feeling of peace
and equanimity which all of them have, and the knowledge
that they can perceive but not be perceived, they also have
a sense of wholeness. That means that somebody who was
hit by a car and had a leg amputated sees his amputated
leg on the highway, and then he gets out of his physical
body and has both legs. One of our female patients was
blinded in a laboratory explosion, and the moment she was
out of her physical body she was able to see, was able to
describe the whole accident and describe people who dashed
into the laboratory. When she was brought back to life she
was totally blind again. Do you understand why many,
many of them resent our attempts to artificially bring them
back when they are in a far more gorgeous, more beautiful,
and more perfect place?

The most impressive part, perhaps, for me, has to do

WALT WHITMAN SPEAKS TO THE DYING

Shepherd Bliss

WHAT do you say to the dying, be it a lover, friend or patient? How do you comfort another human in the final throes of life, whether he or she is dying from a violent wound inflicted by war or by an auto accident or from the miserable slowness of cancer?

Whether a family member, friend, counselor, nurse or physician, where does one look for guidance for such an unexpected moment—when forced into the task of dealing with a dying person? Some psychologists can be helpful, as can some priests, rabbis or ministers. But many—even among the trained helping professions—are unable to adequately deal with the dying. They become confused and withdrawn and fear their own pending death.

Among those most helpful to us at such moments are poets, such as Walt Whitman. Known to us a century after his death mainly as a poet, Whitman was known to thousands of others by another work—serving as a nurse during the Civil War, that terrible time in our life of our country when brother fought brother.

The time was 1860—the year in which Lincoln was voted president. War followed. This was the year during which Whitman wrote the first of his "Whispers of Heavenly Death" poems. Most of these poems were written during the decade that followed. The Civil War began and ended in 1965—leaving behind many wounded men. Whitman tended these men, both during the height of battle and in the years to come. Whitman's contact with the dying and death was not abstract, but quite concrete. He worked from Washington, D.C., a few miles from where many were wounded. Some of Whitman's greatest poetry was written from these experiences, such as his tributes to Lincoln: "O Captain, My Captain" and "When Lilacs Last in the Dooryard Bloom'd."

From *Whole Life Times*, June 1982. 18 Shepard Street, Brighton, MA 02135. Reprinted by permission.

But a single short poem is especially helpful for the psychological insight it gives to working with the dying, though it is not among Whitman's best known or most anthologized. In this simple, direct poem one can get a sense of Whitman's longer poems and of his skill as a nurse ministering to the dying in practical ways:

To One Shortly to Die

*From all the rest I single you out, having
    a message for you,
You are to die—let others tell you what
    they please, I cannot prevaricate,
I am exact and merciless, but I love you—
    there is no escape for you.*

*Softly I lay my right hand upon you, you
    just feel it.
I do not argue, I bend my head close and
    half envelop it,
I sit quietly by, I remain faithful,
I am more than nurse, more than parent
    or neighbor,
I absolve you from all except yourself
    spiritual bodily, that is eternal, you
    yourself will surely escape,
The corpse you will leave will be but
    excrementitious.*

*The sun bursts through in unlooked-for
    directions,
Strong thoughts fill you and confidence,
    you smile,
You forget you are sick, as I forget you
    are sick.*

*You do not see the medicines, you do not
    mind the weeping friends, I am
    with you,*

with my recent work with dying children. Almost all my patients are children now. I take them home to die. I prepare the families and siblings in order to have my children die at home. The biggest fear of children is to be alone, to be lonely, not to be with someone. At that moment of transition, you're never, ever alone. You're never alone now, but you don't know it. But at the time of transition, your guides, your guardian angels, people whom you have loved and who have passed on before you, will be there to help you in this transition. We have verified this beyond

any shadow of a doubt, and I say this as a scientist. There will always be someone who helps you in this transition. Most of the time it is a mother or father, a grandparent, or a child if you have lost a child. It is sometimes people that you didn't even know were "on the other side" already.

I had the most moving experience, the gift of an Indian woman who was in her nineties, who came all the way to one of my lectures in Arizona and traveled an enormous distance from her reservation to share with me this incident. I have very few incidents of Indians. They do not

I exclude others from you, there is nothing
    to be commiserated,
I do not commiserate, I congratulate you.

Still intimate rather than distant after 120 years, these words remained relevant to those touched by the Vietnam War, and it could still guide those who might find themselves in combat or nursing victims of World War III.

This poem is as much a love poem as a death poem. It reveals tremendous intimacy and affection between the poet and the one soon to die—probably between one man and another. How does the poet approach the difficult assignment of lovingly telling someone he is to die? First, he does not hide behind the professionalism of those doctors who neglect to tell the patient he or she is to die soon. The poet realizes that this information must be communicated—clearly and yet compassionately. The victim probably intuitively knew that he was soon to die anyway. The poet subtly criticizes those doctors who would not tell—"let others tell you what they please, I cannot prevaricate." But in the same sentence, the poet adds the essential "I love you," sandwiching it between "I am exact and merciless" and "there is no escape for you." Some would communicate only the words of love, failing to share the essential medical information. Others would venture the medical information, but neglect the love. For the dying to hear, the two should come together. The poet does not participate in the 20th-century tendency to deny death.

Whereas too many doctors and nurses withdraw from their dying patients, this poet/nurse actually moves closer: "Softly I lay my right hand upon you, you just feel it." The healing touch facilitates the person's leaving this world. How essential it is to touch the dying, the aging and others in pain. Most of us like to be touched, in the right ways. Yet how often do family members out of fear withdraw their touch from the hospitalized. Dying and other pain is seldom contagious through touch.

The poet asks for nothing in return for his touch, a totally giving act, like mothers give their infants and like most of us still crave, whether we are dying or not. But of course, all of us are dying, only some are closer to that goal than others.

Notice the poet's posture. "I bend my head close and help envelop it. I sit quietly by. I remain faithful." What else would one ask from a lover or friend in those final minutes of life? "Come close; I want you close to me" is what the dying often seem to say. To some, staying close to a dying person is scary, but there is really nothing to fear.

So many people feel guilty as they die—for not having done something, or finished something, or said something. The poet is ready for this: "I absolve you from all...." Again, words relevant not only to the dying, but also to the living.

Eternally hopeful, the poet assures the dying man that "you will surely escape." Whitman's perspective here is spiritual, with the assurance of 19th-century transcendentalism. Once a person has died, he or she will leave only a corpse. But a person is not merely this physical reality and cannot be reduced to a body, but more, extending beyond the body, important though it is.

In these final minutes, the poet calls the dying man's attention to the "sun," which even now "bursts through in unlooked-for directions," filling the dying with "strong thoughts" and a "smile." He can even "forget you are sick," as can the dying man: "You forget you are sick."

But this kind of forgetting is not denial. It is a transcension and a turn of attention to the life-force even in these moments, as represented by the sun, over "the medicines" and "the weeping friends." They are there and important, but they are not all. The sun continues to rise above all else. Life continues, even in death.

The poet remains faithful: "I am with you." And his final attitude, his final posture, his final words: "I do not commiserate, I congratulate you."

The poet clearly feels this event as a commencement—an ending which brings a beginning, not something to be dreaded, but something which is an integral part of life, as the poet communicates in the immediately preceding poem in his famous *Leaves of Grass*, "O Living Always, Always Dying."

If you would speak to the dying, Whitman suggests, be unafraid, touch them, draw close to them, tell them the truth, share your love with them, remind them of the sun, let them know you are with them, be faithful.

talk about these things, and they are my most favorite people. This woman introduced me to her daughter; the woman was about 90, the daughter about 70. They came together to my workshop. The 70-year-old daughter told me that her sister was killed on the highway, hundreds of miles away from the reservation, by a hit-and-run driver. Another car stopped and the driver tried to help her. The dying woman told the stranger that he should make very, very sure to tell her mother that she was all right, because she was with her father, and she died after having shared

that. The patient's father had died one hour before on the reservation, hundreds of miles away from the accident scene and certainly unbeknownst to his traveling daughter.

Do you understand what I'm trying to say?

We've had one case of a child, a 12-year-old, who did not want to share with her mother that it was such a beautiful experience when she died, because no mommy likes to hear that her children found a place that's nicer than home; that's very understandable. But she had such a unique experience that she needed desperately to share it with somebody, and so one day she confided in her father. She told her father that it was such a beautiful experience when she died that she did not want to come back. What made it very special, besides the whole atmosphere and the fantastic love and light that most of them convey, was that her brother was there with her, and held her with great tenderness, love, and compassion. After sharing this she said to her father, "The only problem is that I don't have a brother."

Then the father started to cry, and confessed that she indeed did have a brother who died, I think three months before she was born, and they never told her.

Do you understand why I am bringing up examples like this? Because many people say, well, you know, they were not dead, and at the moment of their dying they naturally think of their loved ones, and so they naturally visualize them. Nobody could visualize that.

I ask all my terminally ill children whom they would love to see the most, whom they would love to have by their side always (meaning here and now, because many of them are nonbelieving people, and I could not talk about life after death. I do not impose that onto my patients). So I always ask my children, whom would you like to have with you always, if you could choose one person? About 99 percent of the children, except for black children, say mommy and daddy. (With black children, it is very often Aunties or Grandmas, because Aunty or Grandma are the ones who love them perhaps the most, or have the most time with them. But those are only cultural differences.) Most of the children say mommy and daddy, but not one of these children who nearly died has ever seen mommy and daddy, *unless* their parents had preceded them in death.

Many people say, well, this is a projection of wishful thinking. Somebody who dies is desperate, lonely, frightened, so they imagine somebody with all them whom they love. If this were true, 99 percent of all my dying children, many 5, 6, 7-year-olds, would see their mommies and their daddies. But not one of these children, in all these years that we've collected cases, when they died saw their mommies and daddies, because their mommies and daddies were still alive. The common denominator of who you are going to see is that they must have passed on before you, even if it's only one minute, and that you have genuinely loved them. That means many of my children see Jesus. A Jewish boy would not see Jesus, because a Jewish boy normally doesn't love Jesus. These are only religious differences. The common denominator is simply genuine love.

I have not finished telling you the story of Mrs. S and I'm going to run out of time, I'm sure. I want to add that she died two weeks after her son was of age. She was buried, and since she was one of many patients of mine, I'm sure I would have forgotten her if she had not visited me again.

Approximately ten months after she was dead and buried, I was in troubles. I'm always in troubles, but at that time I was in bigger troubles. My seminar on Death and Dying had started to deteriorate. The minister with whom I had worked and whom I love very dearly had left. The new minister was very conscious of publicity, and it became an accredited course. Every week we had to talk about the same stuff, and it was like the famous date show. It wasn't

worth it. It was like prolonging life when it's no longer worth living. It was something that was not me, and I decided that the only way that I could stop it was to physically leave the University of Chicago. Naturally my heart broke, because I really loved this work, but not that way. So I made the heroic decision that "I'm going to leave the University of Chicago, and today, immediately after my Death and Dying seminar, I'm going to give notice." The minister and I had a ritual. After the seminar we would go to the elevator, I would wait for his elevator to come, we would finish business talk, he would leave, and I would go back to my office, which was on the same floor at the end of a long hallway.

The minister's biggest problem was that he could not hear; that was just another of my grievances. And so, between the classroom and the elevator, I tried three times to tell him that it's all his, that I'm leaving. He didn't hear me. He kept talking about something else. I got very desperate, and when I'm desperate I become very active. Before the elevator arrived—he was a huge guy—I finally grabbed his collar, and I said, "You are gonna stay right here. I have made a horribly important decision, and I want you to know what it is."

I really felt like a hero to be able to do that. He didn't say anything.

At this moment a woman appeared in front of the elevator. I stared at her. I cannot tell you how this woman looked, but you can imagine what it's like when you see somebody that you know terribly well, but you suddenly block out who it is. I said to him, "God, who is this? I know this woman, and she's staring at me; she's just waiting until you go into the elevator, and then she'll come."

I was so preoccupied with who she was I forgot that I tried to grab him. She stopped that. She was very transparent, but not transparent enough that you could see very much behind her. I asked him once more, and he didn't tell me who it was, and I gave up on him. The last thing I said to him was kind of "Heck, I'm going over and tell her I just cannot remember her name." That was my last thought before he left.

The moment he entered the elevator, this woman walked straight toward me and said, "Dr. Ross, I had to come back. Do you mind if I walk you to your office? It will only take two minutes."

Something like this. And because she knew where my office was, and she knew my name, I was kind of safe, I didn't have to admit that I didn't know who she was. This was the longest path I ever had in my whole life. I am a psychiatrist. I work with schizophrenic patients all the time, and I love them. When they had visual hallucinations I told them a thousand times, "I know you see that Madonna on the wall, but I don't see it." I said to myself, "Elisabeth, I know you see this woman, but that can't be."

Do you understand what I'm doing? All the way from the elevator to my office I did reality testing on me. I said, "I'm tired, I need a vacation. I think I've seen too many schizophrenic patients. I'm beginning to see things. I have to touch her, if she's real."

I even touched her skin to see if it was cold or warm, or if the skin would disappear when I touched it. It was the most incredible walk I have ever taken, but not knowing all the way why I was doing what I was doing. I was both an observing psychiatrist and a patient. I was everything at one time. I didn't know why I did what I did, or who I thought she was. I even repressed the thought that this could actually be Mrs. S who had died and been buried months ago.

When we reached my door, she opened the door like I'm a guest in my own house. She opened the door with this incredible kindness and tenderness and love, and she said, "Dr. Ross, I had to come back for two reasons. One is to thank you and Reverend Gaines" (he was that beautiful black minister with whom I had this super-ideal symbiosis). "To thank you and him for what you did for me. But the real reason I had to come back is that you cannot stop this work on death and dying, not yet."

I looked at her, and I don't know if I thought by then that could be Mrs. S. I mean, this woman was buried for ten months and I didn't believe in all that stuff. I finally got to my desk. I touched my pen, my desk, and my chair, and it's real, you know, hoping that she would disappear. But she didn't disappear; she just stood there and stubbornly but lovingly said, "Dr. Ross, do you hear me? Your work is not finished. We will help you, and you will know when the time is right, but do not stop now, promise."

I thought, "My God, nobody would ever believe me if I told about this, even to my dearest friend." Little did I know I would say this to several hundred people. Then the scientist in me won, and I said to her something very shrewd, and a real big fat lie. I said to her, "You know Reverend Gaines is in Urbana now."

This was true; he had taken over a church there. I said, "He would just love to have a note from you. Would you mind?"

And I gave her a piece of paper and a pencil. You understand, I had no intention of sending this note to my friend, but I needed scientific proof. I mean, somebody who's buried can't write little love letters. And this woman, with the most human—no, not human—most loving smile, knowing every thought I had—and I knew, it was thought transference if I've ever experienced it—took this paper and wrote this note, which we naturally have framed in glass and treasure dearly. Then she said, but without words, she said, "Are you satisfied now?"

I looked at her and thought, I will never be able to share this with anybody, but I am going to really hold onto this. Then she got up, ready to leave, repeating: "Dr. Ross, you promise," implying not to give up this work yet. I said, "I promise." And the moment I said, "I promise," she left.

We still have her note.

My time is running out. I wanted to share with you many other things. I was told a year and a half ago that my work with dying patients is finished, that there are many people who can carry on now, that this was not my real job, why I'm on the Earth. The whole work with death and dying was simply a testing ground for me, to see if I can take hardship, abuse, resistance, and whatnot. And I passed that. The second test was to see if I can take fame. And that didn't affect me, so I passed that, too.

But my real job is, and that's why I need your help, to tell people that death does not exist. It is very important

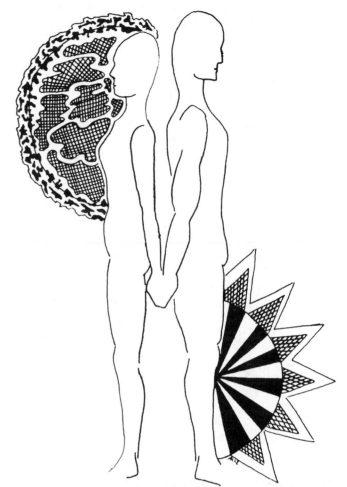

that mankind knows that, because we are at the beginning of a very difficult time. Not only for this country, but for the whole planet Earth. Because of our own destructiveness. Because of the nuclear weapons. Because of our greediness and materialism. Because we are piggish in terms of ecology. Because we have destroyed so many, many natural resources, and because we have lost all genuine spirituality. I'm exaggerating, but not too much. The only thing that will bring about the change into a new age is that the Earth is shaken, that we are shaken, and we're going to be shaken. We have already seen the beginning of it.

You have to know not to be afraid of that. Only if you keep a very, very open channel, an open mind, and no fear, will great insight and revelations come to you. They can happen to all of you in this room. You do not have to take a guru, you do not have to go to India, you don't even have to take a TM course. You don't have to do anything except learn to get in touch in silence within yourself, which doesn't cost one penny. Get in touch with your own inner self, and learn not to be afraid. And one way to not be afraid is to know that death does not exist, that everything in this life has a positive purpose. Get rid of all your negativity and begin to view life as a challenge, a testing ground of your own inner resources and strength.

There is no coincidence. God is not a punitive, nasty God. After you make the transition, then you come to what has been described as hell and heaven. That is not a right interpretation of the judgment, however.

What we hear from our friends who passed over, from people who came back to share with us, is that every human being, after this transition (which is peace and equanimity and wholeness and a loving someone who helps you in the transition), each one of you is going to have to face something that looks very much like a television screen, where you are given an opportunity, not to be judged by a judgmental God, but to judge yourself, by having to review every single action, every word, and every thought of your life. You make your own hell, or your own heaven, by the way you live.

Psychiatrist Elisabeth Kübler-Ross, world-renowned authority on death and dying, was born in Switzerland; she received her M.D. in 1957 from the University of Zurich. Her pioneer studies began with seminars on death and quickly expanded into interviews and therapeutic work with the terminally ill. Her books (On Death and Dying, Questions and Answers on Death and Dying, *and* Death—The Final Stage of Growth) *serve as guides to those investigating death as an integral part of human development.*

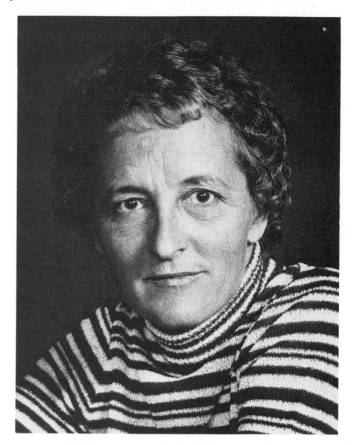

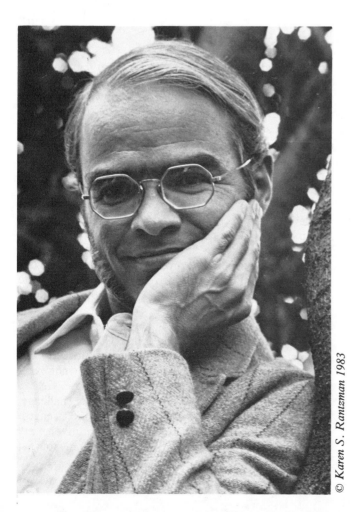

© *Karen S. Rantzman 1983*

DR. SHEPHERD BLISS *is a writer and Lecturer in Psychology at John F. Kennedy University in Orinda, CA, where he teaches Adult Development, Death Education, Men's Studies, and Aging.*

V

Bodywork and Movement

INTRODUCTION *by Naomi Steinfeld*

ALAS, OUR POOR bodies! We place them behind desks and hunch them over stacks of papers. Or we push and pull them through lunch-hour aerobics marathons. Or we treat them like convenient poles for propping up our heads.

We do everything for our bodies but listen to them.

Yet if only we would listen, what tales we would hear!

Tales of inspiration: a one- to two-year-old body valiantly making its first efforts to become vertical, as the elusive world outside the crib comes suddenly, exhilaratingly, within reach. To have the world at your fingertips, just because the legs will stay relatively steady and thus support the hips, the trunk, the neck, the head. "Here I come, world!" cries the toddler, lunging for it.

Tales of terror: a four-year-old falls from the jungle gym, and experiences in those few seconds a fear that is fully the equal of any felt by his cave-dwelling ancestors. He emerges with only minor bleeding and a wad of band-aids, but for the rest of his life he contracts his chest and hunches his shoulders in anticipation of "The Fall." It never recurs. However, he suffers shortness of breath, headaches, and chronic anxiety (breathing shallowly can be very anxiety-provoking). He is suffering not from "The Fall," but from his defense—his *body armoring*—against the possibility of falling.

Such tales of wonder sustain us, move us energetically through our lives; but such tales of terror hold us back, make us stiff, blocked, and tired. And the worst part is: We don't even know that we've told ourselves—*and are continuing to tell ourselves*—these terrible tales. We just think, "Well, that's how my body is." Or, "That's aging for you." Or, "That's life."

So this section, Bodywork and Movement, is intended to help you see what tales you have told yourself, and what tales you might tell yourself. Once you are released of your terrors on a physical level—whether through bodywork, massage, Reichian therapy, sports, chiropractic, laying on of hands, T'ai Chi Chuan, or sex—you can move toward your *real*, unarmored body—a body that knows *how* to move.

Think of the body as a kind of Rosetta stone, bearing encoded messages about your past, present, and future. You may think yourself as invisible as a turtle inside its shell, but the body is more like a crystal ball—or a neon sign—in which your physical, emotional, and spiritual history can be glimpsed by those who know how to look. Certainly, experienced bodyworkers can tell you astounding things about yourself just by looking at how you stand, breathe, walk—for example, "You were a first child, right?" "You had a neck injury between the ages of 8 and 12, right?" And so, incredibly, on.

An unterrorized body loves to move—it moves easily, naturally, with no extraneous motions; it moves with fluidity, wisdom, and grace. Because it expends no energy for the purpose of blocking energy, energy moves *through* it. And this has ramifications on nonphysical levels as well—emotional ("emotion," or "energy-in-motion"), sexual, and spiritual. According to the ancient texts, life *is* movement—ebb and flow, inhale and exhale, first this state of being and now that. And all are aspects of the one.

So the writings in this section tell their tales of wonder and of terror, and offer various ways of alleviating or transforming the embodied terrors. Most of the articles have to do with re-educating the body through bodywork or movement. Some disciplines—such as sports—are familiar. Others may be centuries old, but brand new to our western ways—T'ai Chi Chuan, for example, slows the body down enough so the mind can follow, then lead, then work together as a seamless unit. It is our hope that you will listen to these tales, measure them against what you already know about your body, and allow in something new.

In other words, it is our hope that you will let yourself be moved.

Sexuality and the Whole Person

Ken Dychtwald, Ph.D.

We are in a time when new ideas about sexuality are being explored. There is no model that is appropriate for every person. In this article we see two approaches to sexuality that are currently receiving a lot of attention, one from the East, one from the West. Their viewpoints differ greatly, but both support the premise that love, openness, and honesty are the basic ingredients for a rewarding intimate exchange.

WHAT ROLE does sexuality play in the quest for bodymind health and self-awareness? How are feelings and orgastic functioning related? Can sexuality be an aid to self-development? How do love and emotional openness relate to bodymind health and consciousness?

In the decades of the 1950s, 60s, and 70s, we have witnessed enormous upheavals in all areas of human experience. In particular, we have seen the strata of beliefs and practices that surround sexuality shift, quake, and separate. With the emergence of new images of human being, there has been a massive overturning of sexual styles, attitudes, and behaviors, as men and women of all ages strive to come to a more complete realization of their own bodies, minds, feelings, needs, and visions.

Although these years have provided us with many new tools with which to improve the quality of our lives, I don't feel that the development of more enlightened sexual attitudes and practices is complete. Instead, many of us have found that we are no longer satisfied with the beliefs and practices of yesterday, but have not as yet discovered the healthy and workable possibilities of tomorrow.

In this article I will be exploring several ways of viewing the relationships between sexuality and the body. My purpose is to present ways of understanding sexuality that lend themselves to fulfilling the needs, dreams, and passions in which many of us find ourselves immersed. I will not be dealing specifically with the social or political dynamics of sexuality in this article, even though they are of crucial concern to all who seek to understand and better the human condition. Rather, I prefer to deal with the

individual, personal, and energetic dimensions of sexual behavior, since this approach makes the most sense to me. As I see it, the various structures and mores of a culture are frequently projections from the internal psyches and somas of its people, and for this reason an effective way of understanding the picture can be to first examine the projector.

My Own Sexuality

Within my own bodymind, I experience a great deal of conflict about my sexuality. Although I am only 28 years old, I have had my share of sexual experiences and trials, which have been enhanced by ten years of deep immersion into the human potential movement. During these years I have experienced thousands of hours of encounter groups, yoga, meditation, massage, psychedelic drugs, Rolfing, Bioenergetics, and very much so on, both as a subject and as a practitioner/therapist. Yet, after all these adventures and self-explorational journeys, I still feel myself to be somewhat torn between two generations and between the opposing moralities that these generations represent.

On the one hand, I have grown up believing that sexuality is a private thing, something that you share with your wife. Sexuality is not something to be freely discussed and exchanged. Rather, it is a part of the special ritual of love and expression that is contained with the institution of marriage. Related to these beliefs are a whole series of statements and attitudes about relationships, family, sex roles, and emotional stability. Within the framework, man is most often the provider, the aggressor, the husband. Complimentarily, woman is the receiver, the nurturer, the mother, the wife. This was certainly the way of my grandparents, who before my grandfather's recent death had been happily married for 59 years. In a slightly modified form, it is also the way of my parents, who have been happily and monogamously married for 30 years.

I guess I have been lucky, for my parents are truly in love and share a deep respect for each other. The vows that they made long ago have been kept; commitments have been honored, responsibilities fulfilled. My parents seem to feel their relationship has worked, and that love, monogamy, respect, and sexual privacy have protected and reinforced the invisible tapestry of their human bond. For me, the monogamous love/life relationship offers beauty

Sections of this piece have been excerpted from *Bodymind* by Ken Dychtwald (Pantheon, 1977), and are reprinted here by permission of the author.

and stability. This kind of relationship seems to help develop trust, clarity, sensitivity, and commitment, qualities that are said to encourage the exchange of love between two people.

On the other hand, I have also grown up with a generation of men and women for whom sexuality is a changing, thrilling, playful thing. It is discussed openly, exchanged freely, experimented with, and often experienced casually. As more and more of us begin to travel, move to new regions, and enter into our own self-explorational adventures, we feel teasingly free to examine our mind, our bodies, our feelings, and, of course the dynamics of sexuality that had previously lived only on the edges of our fantasies. Along with these attitudes and practices, a new morality has been struggling to emerge, one that places a great deal of emphasis on personal freedom, inner awareness, independence, equality of the sexes, and the open experience/expression of feelings in the "here and now."

I feel that I have also been lucky on this side of sexuality and love, for throughout my life I have shared many warm and loving encounters with women whose bodies and souls seemed to be able to merge passionately with mine. These encounters have lasted at times for years, or on other occasions have been brief interludes of a few hours. I can honestly say that many of these interactions were enormously pleasurable and beautiful. Although long-term relationships often encourage a deeper connection than a short period of time allows, sometimes brief affairs can offer a closeness that no other relationship permits, since they are often free of the expectations, agendas, inhibitions, and history that enter into the marriage bed.

The unattached casual life of a lover in this new generation offers excitement, a variety of intimate exchanges, and freedom of movement. Long-term commitment and stability are sacrificed for short-term intensity and variety, as love and sexuality take on new shapes and meanings.

Surely there are many advantages as well as disadvantages to both of these generational preferences. I will not attempt to present the "correct" approach to sexuality, for I simply feel that there is none. Rather, with the enormous amount of sexual and lifestyle experimentation that is going on, as well as the rapid decrease in the number of successful long-term marriages, it seems there are many like myself who also seem to be stuck between two worlds and who apparently share my yearning and confusion.

I feel that a great deal of my uncertainty about sexuality is due to the unclear and sometimes irrelevant lessons I learned about sexuality as I was growing up. Hollywood movie screens, street corners, and pornographic novels offer images of sexuality that are at best amusing, but they certainly don't suggest viable and loving rituals of sexual interaction. As a result, I feel somewhat unsure about how to relate to my sexual activities. Do I join with another person for the energetic release? for emotional support? for the spiritual encounter? for the egotistical challenge? for the sheer sensory delight? for the opportunity for personal growth? for the psychic interchange? as a way of communicating my deep love? I know that at times my lovemaking experiences have taken on all these aspects, and I also know that each one of them is as much "me" as the next.

The existential conflicts that I feel about my own sexuality show up all over my bodymind and throughout my life. Sometimes I find myself wanting to open up and embrace the world; at other times I am closed, afraid of being rejected. Part of me wants to be free and independent; other parts desire security and relationship to one woman. Sometimes I feel as if I have internalized the unanswered questions of our times, and that while our culture is busy trying to find solutions to these problems, I too struggle for clarity.

In the last few years, however, with the increased interest in expanding awareness, improving health, and heightening the quality of life, several exciting myths of human sexuality have surfaced which have attracted a great deal of attention. Although individual sexual experience and behavior can never be isolated from the intricate tapestry of interpersonal relationships, these new myths are more directly related to the body, health, and self-development than they are to social and cultural behaviors. Underlying this perspective is the assumption that much of the sexual turmoil we are witnessing around us is a direct expression of the sexual conflict that exists within us as we try to move ourselves toward more joyful ways of being in this "new age." It is still far too early to tell if these seedlings of hope will grow to be healthy organisms, but I feel that it is indeed time for more conscious ways of understanding our own sexuality and the sexual energies that live within all of us.

While simultaneously exploring my own sexual feelings and beliefs and the different theories about sexuality that have developed, I have found myself attracted to two seemingly opposite approaches to sexuality and the bodymind: one comes from the West, the other from the East. Neither of them is actually new, but the enormous attention they have been receiving lately certainly indicates a new appreciation for the wisdom and relevance of these approaches.

The first of these perspectives is that developed by the late Wilhelm Reich; the other is the viewpoint that emerges from the theory and practice of tantric yoga. I will briefly explain the general principles and practices of these two systems, in order to identify and discuss ways that sexuality can be understood within a holistic appreciation of the bodymind.

My purpose in sharing specific pieces of information from these two fascinating approaches to bodymind development is not to present the "right" approach to sexual functioning and relating, for I feel that there is none. Rather, I believe that each of us must come to some functional understanding of how we relate to our own sexual attitudes, feelings, and activities, and that this understanding must fit without the overall scheme of our own unique self-developmental paths. My purpose in this discussion is therefore merely to present what I have found to be two of the most intriguing approaches to bodymind sexuality, with the hope that this information will be helpful or meaningful to you.

Reich and Sexuality

William Reich lived and practiced in the first half of the twentieth century. He received his medical and psychoanalytic training in Vienna in the early 1920s, and the major influence of his early development was Sigmund Freud. Much that Reich postulated in the 20s and 30s is just now being appreciated. In fact, I feel that the contributions Reich made to the understanding of bodymind sexuality in terms of character armor and psychosomatic tension have not been matched by any other contemporary Western thinker or healer.

For Reich, sexual energy was the most sublime of all energies, and sexual freedom the highest of all aspirations. This attitude is captured in an entry Reich made in his personal journal on March 1, 1919, the year in which he was to meet Freud: "Perhaps my own morality objects to it. However, from my own experience, and from observation of myself and others, I have become convinced that sexuality is the center around which revolves the whole of social life as well as the inner life of the individual."[1]

The healthy person, according to Reich, is one who regularly engages in lovingly uninhibited sexual exchange leading to a thoroughly satisfying orgasm. The unhealthy person, on the other hand, because of neurotic symptoms and rigid character traits, cannot give himself fully to the intensity of the sexual encounter, and, as a result, cannot experience a full orgasm and a full release of sexual energy. In fact, Reich postulated that all neurotic symptoms were in some way tied in to a dammed-up sexual energy.

In an attempt to understand more fully the relationship between the sexual experience and overall bodymind states, Reich questioned his patients explicitly about their sexual activity (an action that was considered extremely radical and improper by his fellow Viennese psychiatrists). He discovered that nearly all his female patients did not experience orgasms regularly, and that a similarly high percentage of his male patients also did not experience what Reich considered a true orgasm. He further discovered that different people were able to give in to the orgastic flow in different ways, and that there seemed to be qualitatively different degrees to which the orgasm was experienced, if it was experienced at all. He called the capacity for release of bodymind energy through the sexual experience "orgastic potency," and defined it as "the capacity for surrender to the flow of biological energy without inhibition; the capacity for complete discharge of all dammed-up sexual excitation through involuntary pleasurable contractions of the body."[2] In describing the ideal orgastic experience, which culminates in a total release of sexual energy, Reich identified four distinct and necessary stages of energetic processes. They are (1) tension, (2) charge, (3) discharge, and (4) relaxation. Together these stages make up what is called the "orgasm cycle."[3]

If this cycle is blocked or incomplete at any point in its progression, the person will not experience a full orgasm, and the energetic charge will continue to animate the bodymind, becoming stored in the neuromuscular system. Unreleased charge will continue to accumulate in this way, creating even more physical and emotional stress and conflict. The sexually potent individual, on the other hand, can move fluidly through the four stages of the orgasm cycle, and can therefore not only give in to the vegetative current of the sexual experience, but also benefit from the psychosomatic cleansing effects of the full orgastic release.

Reich put so much emphasis on sexuality and orgastic functioning because he felt that, of all the human bioenergetic mechanisms, the orgasm was the one process that was designed to release stress most effectively, through the sexual union and its accompanying release of tension. When this accumulated charge was not released successfully from the bodymind, it began to affect the character and behavior of the individual in unhealthy ways. Reich further postulated that not only were sexual dysfunction and neurotic behavior related, but that dammed sexual energy, in fact, encouraged neurotic behavior by rigidifying the unhealthy flow of feelings through the bodymind. When these feelings became frozen in this fashion, they were changed into what he called "character armor." Character armor was a "kind of illness in itself, a freezing of the once-spontaneous human personality into rigid patterns of behavior. Also [Reich] connected his theory of character to his theory of orgasm: character was something that developed out of blocked sexuality; the fully functioning 'genital' personality had Zen-like fluidity, scarcely a character at all."[4]

In his attempt to understand fully how character armor was formed and what effect it had on the individual's sexual functioning, Reich began to pay more and more attention to the various ways in which character armor seemed to be related to physical structure and vegetative functioning. He noticed that character armor and its related neurotic behavior seemed to correspond directly to specific bodily tensions and rigidities. His observation led him to the dramatic discovery that all psychoemotional conflicts and blockages took up residence in the muscular tissue of the body, forming what he called "body armor."

Body armor, the physical counterpart of character armor, encased the person in his own protective muscular shell. This shell not only kept out harmful or painful stimuli, but also limited the experience of fearful and painful emotions from within. The more armor there was, the less were the feelings able to flow through the bodymind; the important corollary was that healthy sexual functioning lessened also. Apparently, as the bodymind becomes more blocked, the orgasm becomes less vital, and simultaneously all feelings and interactions become somewhat limited and anesthetized. Since Reich viewed sexual functioning and orgastic potency as reflecting directly the degree to which his patients were truly alive and conscious, he proposed the armoring served to impede the flow of life through the organism.

His realization that psychoemotional energy (which Freud had called "libido") seemed to have actual physical substance to it (he called this bioenergy "orgone") caused a dramatic change in his therapeutic procedure. For if character armor, which contributed to bodymind unhappiness and disease, actually took up residence in the body, why not try to dissolve the armor, and therefore the neurosis, by working directly with the body, by means of physical manipulations, stretching postures, and breathing exercises?

As Reich proceeded to work with this new mode of therapy, he became convinced that the most effective way to relieve his patients of neurosis was first to therapeutically help them dissolve the character and body armor that encased them. When energetic blocks were released or removed, his patients became more able to experience full orgastic potency through full sexual exchange and release. Then the regular experience of a full bodymind orgasm helped maintain the individual's health and emotional stability. Reich not only considered sexual interaction to be necessary for an individual's bodymind development, but also considered healthy, loving, and regular sexual functioning to be the key to a healthy, well-adjusted life.

Reich's appreciation of orgastic functioning and its relation to bodymind awareness, health, and pleasure was the foundation out of which many of our contemporary bodymind therapies and practices (such as Reichian energetics, Bioenergetics, gestalt, encounter, Rolfing, sensory awareness, to name a few) as well as many of our current sexual/social mores have emerged. Certainly the growing interest in sensory awareness, body armoring and unarmoring, uninhibited sexuality, and the various "liberation" movements can be traced in part to Reich's pioneering efforts.

Tantric Yoga and Sexuality

Yoga is not a therapeutic methodology, but rather a vast and dynamic collection of existential principles and possibilities, whose various schools and practices emerge from a tradition that dates back to at least 1000 B.C. The word "yoga" derives from the word "yuj," and is roughly translated to mean "yoke" or "union." The implication of this name is that, by yogic self-exploration, an individual can achieve a state of union with himself and with the universe of which he is a part. Just as there is a wide range of personal styles and needs among individuals, there are a variety of yogic paths along which an individual might come to a more complete state of self-realization. Although here I will be focusing primarily on some aspects of tantric yoga, I will first share some of the general attitudes that underlie the yogic approach to body-mind development to give some background for my discussion.

The yoga perspective recognizes that each of us is made up of a great many forces, feelings, limits, possibilities, and passions. These aspects exist within my body and my mind, and collectively define the boundaries that I usually identify as "me." Therefore, at any one time, there is an infinity of limits and edges that await my explorations and growth. Physically, these limits are experienced as muscle tension, restricted movement, and pain. Psychologically, limits are experienced as dogma, ignorance, and fear. All limits can continually change and restructure themselves.

Now, if I sit on the floor and try to reach over to touch my toes, I notice that I can only stretch to about five inches away from my toes before I experience tension and slight pain. At this point, the muscles in my lower back and in the back of my legs are just too tight to allow me any further stretch; so here I am experiencing one of my boundaries. This point, this "edge," is a highly important place, for the yoga cosmology considers this edge to be my creative teacher, from whom I can learn about myself. If I approach this teacher/edge with love, sensitivity, and awareness, I will discover that my teacher/edge will move and allow me a greater range of motion. If I shy away from approaching my teacher/edge, I will learn nothing new; in time my own dogma/tightness will contract upon itself, and I will grow even tighter. If I try to blast past my edge, I might fool myself into thinking that I have learned and expanded, but in fact I am only impressing myself with a temporary surge of ambition, and this feeling may easily contract upon itself into insecurity, tension, and fear. Physically, when I approach my edge gently and consciously, my body responds by focusing energy and attention on this spot, encouraging the blood and energy to bathe the related muscles and organs with vitality, thus allowing me the experience of true growth and self-nourishment. But if I do not try to reach my edge, my body will have no point of focus, and will find it difficult to isolate the place and nourish it; so little growth and improvement will follow.[5]

Each of the yoga disciplines emphasizes a particular path to self-development, a path that comprises a certain set of beliefs, practices, and rituals. Common to many yoga paths is the belief that sexual involvement is a detriment to greater development of self and should, if possible, be avoided. In fact, a celibate approach to spiritual growth is quite common in many of the world's religious traditions. Within the vast and somewhat mysterious field of tantric yoga, however, it is believed that sexuality can be a powerful vehicle for increased self-awareness. Tantric yoga is thus unusual, in that it not only allows sexual feelings and contact, but in fact, uses the sexual experience as a means to enlightenment. According to William Irwin Thompson, "The Tantrics maintain that there is enormous energy locked into sexuality, which, if released from the lower end of the spine, can flow up the spinal column to bring divine illumination to the brain."[6] This concept is based on the belief that, within the interior of the spine, in a hollow region called the canalis centralis, there is an energy conduit that the Hindus call "Sushumna." Along this conduit, from the base of the perineum to the top of the head, flows the most powerful of all psychic energies, Kundalini energy. On either side of this canal are two additional energy channels, one called the "Ida," which originates on the right of the base of the spine, and the other the "Pingala," which begins on the left.

These two psychic currents, which correspond to the male (Ida) and the female (Pingala) life forces, are said to coil upward around the spine and the Sushumna like snakes, crossing at seven important locations. Each of these crossings creates a vortex called a "chakra," or "energy wheel," and each is viewed as a consciousness center. According to the ancient Hindu literature, each chakra is correlated with certain very specific aspects of human behavior and development. Since the psychosomatic nature of each chakra is related to a particular point along the spine as well as to a specific level of psychoemotional development, the Kundalini yogi's lifelong task is to evolve through the various chakra qualities and challenges, thereby bringing the focus of the Kundalini energy upward from the base of his spine to the top of his head.

Once the yogi has achieved mastery of self by relaxing body tension, silencing mental chatter, and releasing energy blocks, he is ready to join with a partner whose ener-

SEX IN DREAMS

Jeremy Taylor

MY experience is that explicitly sexual and erotic imagery and dream material is as multi-leveled and symbolic as any other dream experience. Most often, when overtly sexual dream images are explored beyond their more obvious references to waking sexual and emotional tensions, they reveal levels of significance associated with deep philosophical, religious, and spiritual concerns. Dreams with pleasant, enjoyable and rapturous sexual images are often associated with solving spiritual and moral problems, while dreams with frightening and repugnant sexuality are often associated with the repression of spiritual and ethical concerns and the inadequate resolution of religious and philosophical problems.

The conscious domination and control of sponta-

neous, "animal" sexual urges appears to be a primary metaphor of the development of human consciousness and individual self-awareness. The desire to foster this conscious domination is obviously at the root both of the prohibitions against spontaneous sexual expression imposed by so many of the world religions on the one hand, and of the complementary traditions which celebrate sexual encounter as a spiritual discipline on the other. These seeming contradictory approaches both affirm the deep association between sexuality and spirituality and the importance of gaining increasing consciousness amidst the flows of sexual energy. A more conscious and less repressed attitude toward ourselves as sexual beings is absolutely necessary for our collective survival.

From Jeremy Taylor, *Dream Work: Techniques for Discovering the Creative Power in Dreams.* (Ramsey, NJ: Paulist Press, 1983).

JEREMY TAYLOR *is a Unitarian Universalist Minister and dream worker residing in the San Francisco Bay Area.*

gies and spirit complement his own in such a way that together they form a "whole." This is the archetypal joining of Shiva and Shakti, of yang and yin, of masculine and feminine. Being ready to engage in tantric lovemaking demands much more than simple curiosity or a willingness to make love. Rather, the student of tantric yoga must first achieve a highly developed awareness within his own being, a process that might take lifetimes, before he is truly ready to engage in the tantric embrace.

In the tantric lovemaking experience, which is called "Maithuna," the lovers undergo a variety of meditations and rituals before they actually make physical contact. These preparations are designed to create a strong spiritual bond between the two lovers, and also to generate a mood of deep respect for the sexual joining which is to follow. Once the preparatory meditations have been completed, the two lovers proceed to make genital contact while maintaining the strong spiritual link that they have worked so devotedly to create.

By merging in this fashion, the "soul mates" together join bodies, hearts, and spirits. This full body-mind contact allows them to evaporate their own personal "edges" into the psychic space that they have created around and between themselves. When the lovers are united in this way, there is very little actual physical movement and no intellectual activity. Instead, the lovers attempt to "visualize the flow of pranic currents between them, the strongest being the point of contact between the sexual organs. Such concentration is not forced or tense, but performed in a detached, almost somnolent way. Gradually each partner will become aware of a rising tide of pleasureable sen-

sation, growing in intensity as psychic energy courses through the reproductive organs and the chakras."[7]

As the intensity of the experience builds toward orgasm, the psychic space between the lovers continues to expand, allowing each partner the feeling of openness and godliness. In tantric yoga, the lovers do not try to achieve orgasm. Actually, if they are trying anything at all, they are trying not to have orgasms. Instead, the tantric lovers are attempting to draw the forces of Kundalini energy upward through their bodyminds, thus releasing the power of the various chakras. According to Joseph Campbell, "This force transforms the yogi psychologically, changing his personality as the Kundalini rises to each succeeding chakra."[8]

As I have mentioned, we confront and transcend many edges as we explore our own limits. In hatha yoga, these edges are manifested as tension and strain, but there is another major edge against which both lovers are playing their bodymind: the *orgasm itself*. The lovers strive to come so close to its explosion that they experience its splendor without giving in to its consummation and termination.[9] By staying ever so close to the orgastic release and not allowing it to occur, the tantric lovers allow their energies to build and intensify, thus increasing the power available to them as the Kundalini energy continues to flow upward through their bodies, illuminating their beings. Although the trantric lovers are most definitely aware of and involved with their own bodies, and are also deeply connected to each other physically and spiritually, they are at the same time partly detached from the sexual aspects of the contact. For within the tantric embrace, the lovers are actually using their bodies and the joined magnitude of their complimentary forces as vehicles through which to achieve the rising of the Kundalini and the awakening of spiritual consciousness. In this eastern perspective the emphasis is not on sexual release as an end in and of itself, but rather on sex as a channel through which the evolution of self may proceed.

Although the classic tantric Maithuna seems to be a mysteriously rare experience, many contemporary students of yoga and bodymind development have modified the concept of tantric lovemaking to include all lovemaking in which the focus is on energetic and spiritual contact between two lovers, rather than on purely physical gratification and orgastic release. In this way, lovemaking that is shared by two sensitive, vital, self-aware individuals can be viewed as a form of tantric embrace. Here the achievement of orgasm by one or both of the lovers is not the primary goal of the experience; yet it is pleasantly accepted if it occurs during the fullness of the embrace.

I find this Eastern perspective fascinating because of both its similarities to and its differences from the liberated Western view of bodymind sexuality as epitomized in the work of Wilhelm Reich. In both perspectives, the body, mind, and spirit are viewed as aspects of the same whole. Both perspectives recognize that if an individual is blocked and self-unconscious, he will be unable to experience sexuality in its fullness. Both appreciate sexuality as an indication of the degree to which a person is alive, aware, and capable of honest loving and sharing with another individual, and both believe that, to change an individual's sexual practices and experience, the entire person must be prepared and open. The two systems also agree that the building of sexual energy and focus, rather than its continual dissipation and unfulfilled release, is something to be achieved and enjoyed. But here the similarities end.

Reich felt that the ultimate value of the sexual experience was in the emotional interaction between the lovers and orgastic release.

Tantra values the sexual experience more for its unique ability to allow two people to lovingly merge their bodyminds in such a way that they can playfully use the edge of the orgasm to guide the flow of Kundalini energy upward along the spine, and thus explore and develop higher centers and perspectives.

As I personally continue to search for some appropriate sexual path, I have discovered that techniques such as yoga, meditation, massage, Rolfing, and bioenergetics allow me to educate myself about the nature of my own bodymind, and put me in greater control of my own energy flow and expression. As a result, I have become more able to allow my whole being to feel alive and honest when I am engaged in lovemaking. It seems that the more conscious and sensitive I become, the more open my bodymind is, and the more beautiful are the sexual feelings I experience. And when I am honest, aware, and self-comfortable, I find that my interactions with my lover are more direct, more nourishing, and more loving.

At present I find the Reichian concepts especially meaningful, for they remind me that my thoughts, feelings, health, and dis-ease are all intimately connected, and that

my sexual experience is a direct expression of my state of being. The tantric approach supports this notion, and also suggests that sexual involvement with another person can be a starting point from which to climb to higher realms of self-development and interpersonal contact.

As these converging impressions of sexuality the most relevant and useful of all possible approaches to understanding the relationships between sexuality and the body? Will they give birth to healthy, viable, and loving relationships between people? I demur from offering pat answers. These suggestions offer only rough maps along which we might begin to plot our journeys. Nevertheless, I feel confident that their dynamic understandings of human experience contain at least the beginnings of solutions to many of our unanswered questions about sexuality.

Notes

[1] Wilhelm Reich, *The Function of the Orgasm*, p. 4.

[2] Wilhelm Reich, "Die Therapeutische Bedeutung der Genital Libido," *International Journal of Psychoanalysis*, No. 10 (1924), translated by Boadella, p. 16.

[3] For more detailed descriptions of the orgasm cycle, see Reich, *Function of the Orgasm*; Jack Rosenberg, *Total Orgasm*; and Ken Dychtwald, *Bodymind*.

[4] Walt Anderson, "Strange Prophet," *Human Behavior*, Jan. 1976, pp. 24–29.

[5] The implication of this yoga perspective is that health, disease, love, and personal growth are all aspects of the way in which you deal with yourself. So, rather than seeing the body and mind in terms of how they related to each other pathologically, with primary focus on therapeutic release from trauma and unconscious conflict, the yogic perspective approaches the opening and freeing of the body's energies as explorations and quests in search of self-awareness and higher understanding. Although the Reichian and yogic philosophies both recognize the importance of bodymind harmony, Reich, being heavily influenced by Freud and the Judaeo-Christian environment of Europe in the 1920s and 1930s, necessarily focused on sexual liberation and vegetative freedom; whereas the yogic viewpoint is deeply rooted in the Hindu concept of spiritual growth and a nonattached appreciation for the unity of mind, body, and spirit.

[6] William Thompson, *Passages About Earth*, p. 107.

[7] Omar Garrison, *Tantra, The Yoga of Sex*, p. 14.

[8] Joseph Campbell, "Seven Levels of Consciousness," *Psychology Today*, December 1975, p. 77.

[9] Actually, I have discovered some disagreement about whether the tantric lovers experience orgasm or not. Some sources say that both lovers simultaneously experience a spontaneous orgasm after a specific amount of time has elapsed. Other sources say that although the lovers do experience an energetic climax or zenith, it is not actually an orgasm that they are feeling.

Suggestions for Further Reading

Ellsworth Baker, *Man in the Trap*. Harper and Row, 1974.

Joseph Campbell, *Myths to Live By*. Bantam Books, 1973.

O. Hatch, *Sexual Energy and Yoga*. A.S.I. Publishers, 1972.

G. Krishna, *Kundalini, Evolutionary Energy in Man*. Shambhala, 1971.

H. Leadbeater, *The Chakras*. Theosophical Publishing House, 1972.

Swami Rama, Rudolph Ballentine, and Swami Ajaya, *Yoga and Psychotherapy*. Glenview, Ill.: Himalayan Institute, 1976.

C. Rendel, *Introduction to the Chakras*. Samuel Weiser, 1974.

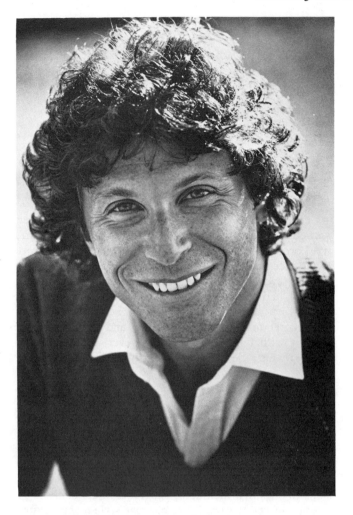

KEN DYCHTWALD, *Ph.D., is a psychologist, gerontologist, lecturer, author, and outspoken figure in the fields of human development, health promotion, and aging. He is President of a consulting firm, Dychtwald & Associates, with offices in Berkeley, California and Washington, D.C.; is the National Director of the "Institute on Aging, Health and Work" of the Washington Business Group on Health; is the Founding Director of the Bodymind Training Institute of Scandinavia; and serves on the national advisory panel for the "Technology and Aging" project of the Office of Technology Assessment, U.S. Congress.*

Dr. Dychtwald is also an adjunct instructor in psychology, gerontology and health related sciences at several colleges and universities, and frequently appears on television and radio shows throughout North America including Good Morning America, the Merv Griffin Show, CBS Morning, A.M. Los Angeles, and A.M. San Francisco.

His publications include: Bodymind *(translated into eight foreign languages),* Millennium: Glimpses into the 21st Century, Stress-Management: Take Charge of Your Life, The Aging of America, Wellness and Health Promotion for the Elderly, *and more than one hundred articles in professional journals and popular magazines.*

Bodywork

Neshama Franklin

I'M A PEOPLE watcher. As the crowds stream by in places like airports, I ask myself who looks good and why. My "winners" may or may not be "beautiful" in Hollywood terms. What attracts me is not how they look, but how they *move*: balanced, centered, and fully at home in their bodies.

Do you feel at home in yours? If you're often tired, tense, achy, or off-center, you might consider a body re-modelling project. We all have places where tension collects. For some, it's the shoulders, for others, the neck or back. As the years pass the tensions accumulate, they can lead to misalignments, but we're so adaptable, our maladaptations come to feel natural. We might not notice any specific medical problem, but we may experience fatigue, tension, or even chronic pain as a result. Self-care can help: Stress management can reduce tension, stretching can increase flexibility, and exercise can increase cardiovascular fitness. But it may take more to help us feel truly at home in our bodies. That's what bodywork is all about.

The term "bodywork" applies to a broad and sometimes bewildering range of massage-like therapies. Unlike massage, however, the effects tend to be more lasting. At its best, bodywork retrains the body's posture and movements for optimal functioning. Once you tune into the ways your body works best, you begin to recognize the early signs of imbalance and correct them before they develop into infirmities.

There are three basic schools of bodywork: movement re-education, deep-tissue manipulation, and meridian-based therapies. Other forms of bodywork combine the three basic approaches. Within each school there are many approaches, each with its own organization, training program, and therapeutic perspective (see Resources). (In this overview, I have omitted Bioenergetics and other similar therapies that basically focus on emotional well-being; and osteopathy and chiropractic because they concentrate primarily on illness problems. The approaches discussed here deal more with wellness.) All bodywork styles require a considerable investment of time and money. Sessions average $50 each, though individual practitioners may charge from $15 to $100 per session.

Each bodywork style has staunch supporters who insist that it is superior to all others. But from the consumer's perspective, how different are they? To find out, I sampled

From *Medical Self-Care* (Spring 1984), P.O. Box 1000, Point Reyes, CA 94956. Reprinted by permission.

six different styles in the San Francisco area, and interviewed colleagues who had experienced some styles I didn't try. I brought to the investigation some previous bodywork experience and a background in dance and t'ai chi.

After several months of being massaged, stretched, rolled, pressed, and realigned, I came away feeling that no single form of bodywork is intrinsically the best. What's "best" is a matter of personal preference, and one's feeling of rapport with the practitioner. However, the demonstrations gave me a clearer sense of the subtle differences among the styles in these four areas:

• Intensity of the touch: from light and gentle, to intense, even painful.

• Amount of client participation: from minimal—the practitioner does it to you, to extensive—you put your new kinesthetic insights into action by practicing the new movements.

• Amount of verbal interaction: from almost silent sessions to ones that include considerable discussion.

• Mix of "table work," i.e. massage-style manipulation, "floor work," i.e. exercises on a mat; and applications of new movements to everyday situations.

The various bodywork styles are difficult, if not impossible, to evaluate objectively, but the four elements above provide a good basis for comparison. Let me state my own personal preferences at the outset: (1) I enjoy various kinds of touch, from light to intense, but I prefer deeper, more intense manipulations. (2) I'd rather be active than passive. Practice gives me the change to experience bodywork more fully. (3) I'm a verbal person, so I prefer the approaches that emphasize discussion. (4) Finally, I like a thorough mix of table work, floor work, and applications.

Movement Re-Education

Alexander Technique. F.M. Alexander was a turn-of-the-century actor who lost his voice at crucial moments onstage. After painstaking observation, he discovered that an unconscious head motion and tensing of his neck muscles interfered with his voice. His experiments with counter-motions to stop the habit eliminated his problem, and launched the Alexander Technique. Through verbal instruction, demonstrations, and light touch, Alexander instructors show clients how to replace dysfunctional movements with more functional ones.

My Alexander session started on a massage table. The practitioner, a woman with exemplary posture and precise speech, lifted my head slightly to show me what Alexander called the "primary control," the area where the head and neck meet, an important key to releasing tension. She moved my head slightly forward and up, a small adjustment, but one that made a significant difference—I immediately felt relaxation spread along the length of my spine. Other minor adjustments led to a new feeling of ease across my hips and back. After each adjustment, I practiced replicating the movements that produced the new feelings of fluidity.

Off the table, the practitioner suggested that I make minor changes in several daily activities; under her guidance, the transition from sitting to rising changed from a sequence of hoists to an almost effortless float. I was struck by the difference a tiny, conscious movement could make.

Alexander teachers do not follow formal lesson plans. They tailor sessions to clients' individual needs. The technique uses no special exercises, but works with the movements of everyday life.

Touch: Very light.
Participation: Considerable, much practice of new movements.
Verbal Interaction: Moderate to high, depending on the practitioner.
Mix: Alternation of table work and applications.
Subjective: I found Alexander Technique relaxing and enjoyable, but a bit too subtle and cerebral for my taste.

Feldenkrais. An old soccer injury that caused chronic knee problems inspired Moshe Feldenkrais, now in his 80s, to apply his background in physics and engineering to the study of human movement. He cured his own affliction and made some intriguing discoveries about mind/body interactions in the process. The conventional wisdom is that the brain tells the body what to do. Feldenkrais discovered that the process is reversible. The body can also instruct the brain by demonstrating the easiest, most effective ways to move. This, in effect, reprograms the brain and incorporates the new pattern into everyday life. Feldenkrais bodywork comes in two forms: individual hands-on sessions called "Functional Integration" and movement re-education classes called "Awareness Through Movement" (ATM).

Functional Integration relies on a series of gentle manipulations that improve breathing and alignment, what Feldenkrais calls "showing the body how to move with functional intelligence." But it's more than physical manipulation. After a session I emerged with one shoulder perceptibly lower than the other. I expressed concern that I might have become permanently out of whack, but the practitioner, a small man with a soft voice and wry sense of humor, assured me that if my body liked how the lowered shoulder felt, the higher one would gradually drop to the same level. Within a few days, it happened, and my shoulders felt more relaxed than they had in years.

Touch: Light.
Participation: Minimal. It's mostly done to you.
Verbal Interaction: Minimal.
Mix: Almost all table work.

Subjective: I was impressed with the effect on my shoulders, but I prefer more participatory, more verbal styles.

Awareness Through Movement is noteworthy because it's the only form of bodywork I know of organized into formal classes, which makes it less expensive than individual sessions. ATM teaches a series of gentle nonaerobic motions designed to show participants how their bodies work. The key word is "awareness." Participants learn to scan their bodies for tension areas, often those that do not touch the floor when they lie on their backs. They also learn to compare their limbs; if right and left sides feel different, it's a clue to imbalance. Feldenkrais designed the lessons with many movement variations to minimize mechanical repetition. It may feel a little absurd to be in a room full of adults all rolling around on the floor (the process is quite similar to the one babies use to learn how their bodies work) but paying close attention to simple movements can be surprisingly demanding.

Touch: Does not apply.
Participation: Very high. You do it all.
Verbal Interaction: Minimal. You follow directions.
Mix: No table work. Mix of floor work and applications. ATM is the only bodywork style I sampled that used floor work.
Subjective: My attention tended to wander during the exercises. At times I got bored or found it hard to concentrate on discerning subtle differences.

Deep Tissue Manipulation

Rolfing. Ida Rolf, originally a biochemist, viewed the body as an architectural unit, ideally one that works as a balanced, aligned, graceful whole. Trauma and/or habits, however, distort ideal alignment. Rolfers re-align the body by manipulating the fascia, the connective tissue that envelopes the muscles. Rolf discovered that this tissue is amazingly plastic. It can be stretched and reshaped by careful manipulation. Rolfing is based on the premise that once fascial massage releases the body from old patterns, it can move toward greater balance and fluidity.

Rolfing is an intense process for both client and practitioner. It produces powerful, sometimes painful sensations, and many clients experience surprisingly strong emotions after long-accumulated tensions have been released. To provide access to the whole body, the client wears little clothing during the typical 10-session course.

Rolfing provided a friend of mine with a new sense of self. After 20 years of highly cerebral pursuits, he realized that he felt little connection with his body, and sought a therapy that would reintroduce him to it. His Rolfer, a quiet man who conveyed both firmness and sensitivity, continually asked him how he felt in response to the manipulations. At first, he had great difficulty verbalizing, but as he got more in touch with his body, the words flowed more easily. Rolfing also brought a flood of long-suppressed memories, particularly his fears during combat in World War II. Although some manipulations were painful, he was surprised to discover that the pain did not bother him.

MY FAVORITE BODYWORK

Neshama Franklin

AFTER sampling many forms of bodywork, Aston-Patterning emerged as my personal favorite. For me, it draws the best, most practical elements from all the other schools. The touch, which varies from light to intense depending on individual needs, felt right. There was lots of client participation; you practice your new movements a great deal. Practitioner and client converse extensively. And I found the mix of table work and applications especially valuable.

Judith Aston came to Ida Rolf for treatment after two auto accidents. Originally trained as a dancer, she went on to learn Rolfing, but was disturbed by her observation that Rolfed bodies tend to look alike. She also felt that Rolfing was unnecessarily painful, and that the same result could be achieved with less force. Aston uses the spiral as her logo because of her belief that all three-dimensional movement is asymmetrical. Rather than fastening on symmetry as the ultimate goal, Aston-Patterning encourages body parts to co-operate with one another however they move.

Aston-Patterning focuses on three areas: movement re-education with an emphasis on the individual; massage to relax chronic stress, restore flexibility, and expand movement range; and environmental redesign, which seeks to modify the objects in daily life to improve their "fit" with the user. The sequence and pace of Aston-Patterning sessions is determined by individual need. Some sessions concentrate on specific activities, for example, bicycling or housework.

My demonstration started with an evaluation of the way I walked. The practitioner, a quietly animated woman with a clear gaze, noted that my weight distribution was off balance—heavy on the heels, with my feet pointed at different angles. Then she explored my body with massage strokes. Whenever she located resistance or tension, she marked it on a chart. I liked the specific, graphic way the chart helped me see the patterns of tension in my body.

The practitioner then massaged me with firm yet gentle strokes, concentrating on my tension areas. Her spiral motions released much of the tension I was feeling. Aston-Patterning sessions include both massage and movement work so the client receives immediate feedback about how a release of tension in one part of the body produces a new way to move. The interplay of massage and movement work teaches the body to reconize the sensations of both the old and the new movements.

After the massage, we returned to walking. I explored ways to distribute my weight more evenly. The result was a new stride that felt springy and light. Six months later, I can still recapture that ease of movement when I focus on what I learned at the demonstration session.

The changes in my friend's body were striking. Rolfing improved his posture and made him look and feel healthier. He also reported an increase in energy and a better rapport with people. Three years later, many of these changes remain. "I once thought the mind and body were separate," he says, "but through Rolfing I experienced them as one."

Touch: Very intense, sometimes painful.
Participation: Minimal. It's mostly done to you.
Verbal Interaction: Depends on the Rolfer, but usually considerable.
Mix: Mostly table work, some applications.
Subjective: I did not try Rolfing because I had such a good first-hand report. But in general I find the method somewhat doctrinaire.

Meridian-Based Energy Therapies

These bodywork styles are derived from traditional Chinese medicine, which postulates that electromagnetic life energy ("ch'i" in chinese, "ki" in Japanese) flows along invisible body pathways, or meridians, and that illness occurs when energy becomes blocked at specific pressure points. Meridian-based healers practice a variety of approaches based on acupressure (acupuncture with finger pressure instead of needles) to unblock energy paths by manipulating the pressure points. This returns the body to proper balance and health.

Shiatsu. Literally "finger pressure," Shiatsu has been used widely in Japan for more than 1000 years, both for treatment of illness and for general health maintenance. the practitioner, a thin, tiny, incredibly strong woman, used her palms, thumbs, feet, even her knees to apply rhythmic, moderate pressure all over my body, sometimes gently stretching certain areas to bring the meridians closer to the surface. Shiatsu also includes deep breathing to help release tension and stimulate energy flow. Practitioner and recipient become linked by coordinated breathing and meditative focus. The result is a sense of communion, profound relaxation, and enhanced feelings of well-being that last long after sessions end.

Touch: Moderate.
Participation: Minimal. The practitioner does it to you.

EXPLORING REFLEXOLOGY

ASK the person to lie down. Sit on a low stool to provide easy access to the soles of the feet. Use your thumb as you work. Flex and extend the thumb as you work. (Make sure the thumbnail is cut short.) Press firmly, first over the entire sole, then up around the side of the heel to the anklebone. Check frequently for discomfort. If the person is willing, increase pressure somewhat on tender spots, but don't press anything tender for too long. Avoid areas that are cut or bruised. Keep sessions short. Even though tender areas may offer clues to problems in other parts of the body, do not use reflexology for diagnosis or treatment. Its purpose is overall relaxation—and it feels great!

Verbal interaction: Minimal.

Mix: All table work.

Subjective: Shiatsu feels good, but it's too passive for my taste. Also, the exclusive focus on table work is not for me.

Reflexology. A Western variation on pressure-point therapy, this style focuses exclusively on the feet. Reflexologists believe that points on the bottoms of the feet are linked to specific organs, and that massaging tender spots there promotes the health of the corresponding organs. How this linkage occurs is a matter of speculation. Some theorize that nerves or meridians serve as channels to the various organs. Reflexologists also believe that toxic deposits collect in the feet and that reflexology breaks them up and facilitates their elimination.

A skeptical MSC staff member reluctantly submitted to reflexology on a day when he had an upset stomach and tension in his neck, neither of which the reflexologist was aware of. The practitioner, a tall, curly-haired man with long fingers, asked him to speak up when he touched a tender area. As his feet were massaged, the staff member reported a tender spot. The reflexologist asked, "Do you have an upset stomach?" As he worked the spot, the indigestion disappeared. Later, another tender spot. "Do you feel tension in your neck?" Again, massaging the spot eliminated the problem. The staff member rose from his reflexology treatment a believer. Despite their often uncanny ability to detect physical problems, good reflexologists are careful not to diagnose illness. They concentrate on relieving tension.

Touch: Moderate to intense.

Participation: Minimal.

Verbal interaction: Minimal beyond identifying tender spots.

Mix: All table work.

Subjective: Foot massage feels wonderful. I prefer whole-body manipulation, but reflexology is simple, fun, and anyone can do it (see sidebar).

Combination Bodywork Styles

Aston Patterning. See sidebar: "My Favorite Bodywork," above.

Trager Psychophysical Integration. Milton Trager, M.D., now in his 70s, developed his style of bodywork over a 50-year period. It's based on a variety of gentle, rhythmic massage and stretching movements. At my demonstration session, I lay in briefs on a padded table as the practitioner, a gentle, plump young woman with warm brown eyes, led me on a kinesthetic journey that produced a degree of relaxation equivalent to an hour in a whirlpool bath.

She began by rolling my head gently in small figure-eight patterns. At first, I found it difficult to "let go" and simply allow the movement to happen without resisting or trying to help. She returned to this movement periodically throughout the session, and as my muscles relaxed and my trust increased, it became easier.

She then Tragered just about every part of me, swinging, stretching, pressing, bouncing, and rocking my limbs, torso, front, and back. It may sound like perpetual motion, but the effect was restful and meditative. I could feel motions as small as a foot-flex up and down my spine. I was surprised at how effortless Tragering felt, and how fluid my body became. My personal Achilles' heel is my lower back, which often feels stiff and fragile. But during Tragering, it moved without any strain.

By the end of the session, I felt so relaxed, it seemed by body had been poured onto the table. To my surprise, the experience also had humorous moments: At times, my limbs flapped with abandon and I found myself tickled both by a sense of the ridiculous and by a heady feeling of release and celebration. The practitioner also demonstrated a series of simple movements called "Mentastics," which Trager aficionados use at home to recapture the release achieved during Tragering sessions.

Touch: Moderate.

Participation: Minimal.

Verbal interaction: Depends on the practitioner, but usually minimal to moderate.

Mix: Mostly table work with some applications through Mentastics.

Subjective: Tragering feels great, and Mentastics is good self-help regimen, but I prefer more client participation.

Hellerwork. Joseph Heller was an aerospace engineer before Ida Rolf changed his life. He practiced Rolfing for seven

GIVE A FRIEND A MASSAGE

Lorin Piper

ONE of the premises of sensitive massage is that how the person giving the massage feels is just as important as how the person receiving it feels. The massage should be a relaxing and energizing experience for you both, a way to communicate caring without words. I don't deal here with the technical strokes. There is a good book on the subject: *The Massage Book*, by George Downing (Random House/Bookworks). Here I want to encourage you to try massage, with or without technical knowledge.

1. Arrange your massage area in a warm quiet room. Don't try to work on a couch or bed. Instead, spread out blankets or sleeping bags on the floor, enough for your friend to lie down on and for you to sit or kneel beside her. Cover this padding with an old sheet, one you won't mind getting oil on.

2. You can buy massage oil, or use a natural vegetable oil. If you use vegetable oil, you may want to scent it with a concentrated scented oil.

3. Tell your friend to close her eyes and take some deep relaxing breaths. You can take some too. During the massage, if either of you get tense, take some time out to breathe and relax.

4. Ask your friend not to talk unless she wants something special. This is a time for non-verbal communication.

5. Never pour cold oil directly onto the body. Squeeze the oil into your hands and rub them together until the oil feels warm. Then spread the oil over the area you are going to work on.

6. Always maintain contact with the body. When you need more oil, rest your left elbow or forearm lightly on your partner's body, and squeeze the oil into that hand with your right hand. When moving around the body, maintain contact by keeping your hands on the body.

7. The main stroke can be used on both sides of the arms, legs, and torso. I'll describe the stroke as done on the front of the leg. You can adapt the stroke on the arms in the same direction, and to the back and front torso, from the top of the head down.

Place your hands, left on top facing in, right facing out, across the ankle. Glide both hands from one end of the leg to the other, slowly and steadily, *lightly* over the knee (it's sensitive).

When you reach the top of the leg, the hands divide, the left going up over the hip, the right going slowly through the crease between thigh and pelvis. As the fingers circle and touch the floor, the hands move along, down the outsides of the leg, back to the foot.

When you do this stroke on the front and back torso, move your hands pointing down toward the feet, along the sides of the plumb line or the spine, turning out over the hips at the pelvis, and, bringing your hands along the outside, back up to the shoulders.

8. Another basic but different stroke is the alternating thumb circles. This is great for fleshy parts of the body; palms, soles, buttocks. Press directly with both thumbs, moving them in small alternating outward circles.

9. Use your hands to define the bone structure. Trace the hip tone, shoulder blade, spine. Get acquainted with the body. Remember to use all of your hand, molding it to fit the contours of the body. Keep your hands as relaxed and flexible as possible.

10. The feet and hands carry a lot of tension. Squeeze the fleshy parts of the palm and sole, and pull and squeeze the toes and fingers.

11. Experiment with different speeds and pressures, from slow and heavy to almost a light quick tickle. Ask your friend for feedback.

12. Keep a spare sheet or beach towel on hand. If your friend gets cold, you can cover the parts of her body you aren't working on.

13. When the massage is finished, maintain contact with your hands for a minute before you slowly move them away. You can both use this moment to take a deep breath and tune into how you feel.

14. If you don't know a stroke for a part of the body, experiment. Do something you think would feel good. Remember, you are massaging a person, not a machine made of skin, bone, and muscle. Love and care will go a lot farther than all the technique in the world.

years, then expanded Rolfing for seven years, then expanded it to include movement re-education. Hellerwork uses the same deep tissue manipulations as Rolfing, but includes verbal interactions that focus on the client's personality traits and attitudes toward life.

During my demonstration, I was introduced to deep tissue massage. The practitioner, a lean, smooth-talking young man, reminded me to use the magic word "stop" if I felt any discomfort. I never did. His long strokes were quite pleasurable. Periodically, he asked me to breathe deeply. When I did, I felt my tensions dissipate. Then I sampled Hellerwork's movement re-education component. Another Hellerwork practitioner, a stylishly dressed woman whose eyes glowed with new age-sincerity, had me sit at various angles until I found one that felt balanced and "right." A typical course of Hellerwork lasts 11 sessions. The final session is devoted to integrating the material into everyday life.

Touch: Moderate to intense.
Participation: Moderate.
Verbal interaction: Moderate to high.
Mix: Some alternation of table work and applications.
Subjective: I thought I'd enjoy Hellerwork more than I did. It contains many of the elements I like, but somehow it felt too "canned" for me. Also, the room was too cold, which interfered with the experience.

Other forms of bodywork, I did not sample include: *Touch for Health*, which combines massage, acupressure, and chiropractic; *Polarity Therapy*, which integrates massage and stretching postures with diet, nutrition, and spiritual concerns; *Naprapathy*, which focuses on stretching the muscles along the spine; and *Ortho-Bionomy*, which uses subtle physical manipulation to deal with chronic pain.

Which Bodywork For You?

The differences among the various schools can be subtle. If you're experienced with massage, shop for the bodywork style that appeals to you. If you've never had a good, professional massage, before you invest the money most bodywork requires, try a few sessions of Swedish- or Esalen-style massage. Both use light to moderate touch and emphasize relaxation, breathing, and the mind-body connection. It's a good way to become acquainted with your body's preferences.

The organizations in Resources can put you in touch with practitioners in your area, but as in all health-worker relationships, word-of-mouth recommendations are your best guide.

RESOURCES

The Alexander Technique, by Judith Stransky and Robert S. Stone, Ph.D. 1981, 308 pages, $14.95 from Beaufort Books, 9 East 40th Street, New York, NY 10016. A thorough introduction. Compares the Technique to other schools of bodywork and includes exercise for developing body awareness.

Awareness Through Movement, by Moshe Feldenkrais. 1972, 192 pages, $10.95 from Harper and Row, 10 East 53rd Street, New York, NY 10016. A series of health exercises for personal growth.

Your Body Works, Gerald Kogan, Ph.D., Ed., 1981, 177 pages, $9.95 from And/Or Press, P.O. Box 2246, Berkeley, CA 94702. A compendium of articles that provides a broad overview of several styles, including Rolfing and Feldenkrais.

Whole Body Healing, by Carl Lowe and James W. Nechas. 1983, 564 pages, $21.95 from Rodale Press, Emmaus, PA 18049. Vivid descriptions, with photos, of many body-involvement therapies, disciplines, and sports, from editors of *Prevention*.

The Complete Guide to Foot Reflexology, by Kevin and Barbara Kunz. 1980, 149 pages, $8.95 from Prentice-Hall, Englewood Cliffs, NJ 07632.

Bodymind, Ken Dychtwald, Ph.D. 1978, 298 pages, $3.50 from Jove Publications, 200 Madison Ave., New York, NY 10016. Reviewed in the *MSC* Book as "a useful and important effort to synthesize many seemingly different approaches."

Organizations

The American Center for the Alexander Technique, 142 West End Ave., New York, NY 10023; 9359 Olympic Blvd., Beverly Hills, CA 90211; c/o Joan and Alexander Murray, 508 W. Washington, Urbana, IL 61801, 931 Elizabeth St., San Francisco, CA 94114.

Rolf Institute, P.O. Box 1868, Boulder, CO 80302.

The Trager Institute, 10 Old Mill St., Mill Valley, CA 94941.

Aston-Patterning, P.O. Box 114, Tiburon, CA 92920.

Hellerwork, 147 Lomita Dr., Suite H, Mill Valley, CA 94941.

Feldenkrais Guild, P.O. Box 11145, San Francisco, CA 94101.

NESHAMA FRANKLIN, *associate editor of* Medical Self-Care *magazine in Point Reyes, California, has been involved with movement arts and related body practices for over 30 years.*

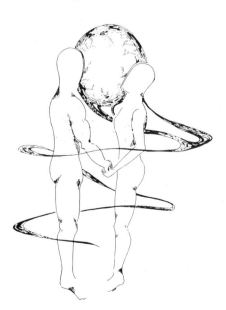

Overview of Reichian Therapy

Richard Hoff

Wilhelm Reich, an Austrian psychoanalyst, was born in 1897. After graduating from the University of Vienna, he spent six years (1922-1928) as clinical assistant to Sigmund Freud at the Vienna Psychoanalytic Polyclinic. By the late 1920s, Reich had broken with Freud, expounding controversial theories and doing pioneer work in relating neurosis to its physiological basis. It has become increasingly clear that Reich raised, sometimes decades in advance, many of the questions that concern us now.

In 1939 he settled in the U.S., where he began his work with orgone (life) energy. In 1954 he was arrested, ostensibly for selling orgone boxes, but more basically for the sexual tone of his work. He died in a Pennsylvania penitentiary in 1957, tired and bitter. A brilliant and emotional thinker, writer, and researcher, he is considered today the father of most body-oriented therapies. These include of course, Reichian therapy, which is presented here by Richard Hoff.

WILHELM REICH is the father of most present-day "body work," body-oriented therapies, and deep emotional therapies. His work, in turn, is really the natural and logical development of the work of his pioneering teacher, Sigmund Freud. However, Reich's penetrating genius and forthright courage led him into realms far beyond those explored by Freud, and brought him into sharp conflict with the psychoanalytic movement. I am referring here not to the later, more sensational "orgone" work, which lies beyond the scope of this article, but only to the therapeutic technique which Reich called "character-analytic vegetotherapy,"[1] which remains the core of all his later therapeutic work and is a complete and incredibly effective healing system in itself.

Whereas psychoanalysis is largely verbal and insight-oriented, Reich's system of therapy works directly with the body and the character structure, utilizing an ingenious array of powerful and original techniques to release repressed sexual-emotional energy through convulsive discharges. The ultimate aim of the therapy is to dissolve neurotic character structure and muscular armoring at the deepest biological levels, to restore free, natural energy flow, and, finally, to establish "full orgastic potency"—the ability to build up and release full energy at the moment of orgasm.

This concept of "full orgastic potency" lies at the very heart of Reichian Therapy. Like Freud, Reich was convinced that the root cause of neurosis is repressed sexual energy. Our society is obviously anxious and horrified about sex like nothing else. This anti-sexual attitude descends on us like a pall from earliest childhood, crushing down on our bubbling, spontaneous flow of erotic energy. Babies are denied the warm, sensual suckling and cuddling they crave.[2] The blissful release of excretion becomes tainted with anxiety and disgust. Our crotches become "dirty" and "nasty," too awful to be seen in public. Sex is enshrouded in secrecy and obscenity, shame and guilt. We learn to fear and resist our own deepest natural urges. The effort of resisting such a massive push of primal survival energy involves an equally massive contraction of the entire organism. The resulting pain and frustration arouse intense feelings of sadness and rage, which must also be suppressed. This entails yet more contraction. The contraction grows more and more entrenched and automatic; it becomes our habitual way of being. We lost much of the spontaneity and aliveness of childhood. We become stiffer, duller, more "armored." This armoring, and the underlying negative emotions surrounding sex, are incompatible with the surging currents and ecstatic convulsions of orgasm. The natural *orgasm reflex* has become disrupted by chronic *orgasm anxiety*.

Reich found that full orgasm is characterized by an enormous build-up of energy followed by a reflexive release, consisting of involuntary, wavelike convulsions of the entire body musculature, sensations of "melting" and "streaming," a loss of normal ego-awareness, and, finally, a profound feeling of peace, relaxation, fulfillment, and grateful tenderness toward the partner. When release is incomplete because of chronic armoring and orgasm anxiety, the surplus energy remains damned up inside. This reservoir of pent-up sexual energy, or "sexual stasis," is the immediate source of energy for the neuroses. The en-

---

[1] In German, "vegetative" refers to the primitive, involuntary, plasmatic level of biological functioning.

[2] Suckling is erotic for babies even to the point of "oral orgasm," and mothers may subconsciously fear this sensuality as well as the erotic stimulation they themselves naturally tend to feel through their nipples.

ergy simply has nowhere to go except into neurotic symptoms, such as anxiety, sadism, or compulsive behavior. Thus, neurotic defenses from the past block sexual release in the present, and the resulting sexual stasis supplies the driving power for the old neurotic patterns—which themselves originated from chronic sexual frustration—in an endless vicious circle.

Orgasm anxiety forms the basis of the general pleasure anxiety, fear of life, and particularly the fear of love, which is such an integral part of the prevailing human structure. Real love is more than a mental attitude of affection; it is a passionate emotion that involves powerful streamings of energy in the heart, the belly, the entire body. In an armored person such streamings arouse subconscious fears of passionate warmth, of sexual arousal, or "losing control." In other words, the block against the immense explosion of orgastic energy forms the *energetic basis* for a general block against all strong energy currents. In addition, the underlying rage and bitterness caused by the chronic sexual stasis poisons our natural feelings of love.

Reich believed that sexual stasis, because of its effect on the autonomic nervous system, is also the root cause of most disease. The autonomic nervous system is made up of two complementary systems, the *sympathetic* and the *parasympathetic*, which exert an opposing influence on every organ in the body. The sympathetic nervous system mobilizes the organism for emergency action—"fight or flight." It stimulates secretion of adrenalin and is involved in combating any kind of stress or infection. The parasympathetic, on the other hand, is involved in relaxation and pleasure, such as digestion or sexual arousal. Generally speaking, the sympathetic goes with *contraction*, the parasympathetic with *expansion*, of the total organism. A healthy organism would normally oscillate between these two poles in accordance with changing circumstances. But the armored, orgastically impotent organism is essentially in a chronic state of contraction. At the same time, the constant pressure of dammed-up energy acts as a continuous source of stress. Physiologically, this entails chronic activation of the sympathetic nervous system, or "chronic sympatheticotonia."

Perusal of Table 1, which lists the various functions of the autonomic nervous system, reveals a remarkable correlation between the type of disease that affects a specific organ and the effect of sympathetic activation of that organ. For example, *cardiovascular hypertension* corresponds to the effect of the sympathetic nervous system on the blood vessels, which is to contract them. Similar correlations can be found for constipation, ulcers, emphysema, rheumatism, arthritis, and many other common diseases—indirectly, even cancer. These observations seem to be well-substantiated by the experiments of Hans Selye, whose "stress syndrome" theory of disease has become widely accepted medical doctrine. Even where a pathogen is definitely involved, the susceptibility of the organism depends on the general state of the constitution. My own experiences have led me to a strong suspicion that flu and the common cold are largely sublimated or "disguised" releases of repressed emotions.

Orgasm anxiety and sexual stasis, according to Reich, are also the root cause of the mass social neurosis which now threatens our very survival as a species. War, racism, sexism, ruthless exploitation of one group by another, and fascism or dictatorship of all kinds—overt or covert—are all essentially based on *hatred*; and chronic sexual frustration is the primary source of hatred. This connection is particularly evident in the typically anti-sexual tone of racial bigotry, fascist torture techniques, and our common "cuss-words." Authoritarian, antilife political regimes are not merely imposed on the masses by a powerful few: they actually arise out of and are based on the authoritarian, antilife attitudes of the masses, which in turn emerge from the typical authoritarian, sexually repressive family upbringing. This type of upbringing tends to produce a resigned, impotent character structure, lacking in genuine self-confidence and submissive to authority, but with strong underlying sadistic and rebellious impulses. People with this structure may long for freedom and independence, but are actually deeply afraid of it. One is reminded here of the common practice of castrating a bull or a stallion to make it docile, "one of the herd." Such a character structure on a mass scale forms fertile soil for any sort of repressive, reactionary political movement, and constantly undermines the best efforts toward democracy and humanitarian reform.

Reich, then, saw neurosis not merely as isolated pockets of sickness in an otherwise healthy, "normal" society, but as a mass phenomenon, an "emotional plague" promulgated by the very structure of society. Neurosis *is* the norm. Similarly, a neurotic symptom is not an isolated defect in an otherwise healthy personality: the whole *character structure* is more or less neurotic. The symptom is only the most striking indication of the total underlying condition.

Increasingly Reich came to see the neurotic character structure as *a constellation of defenses against the free flow of sexual-emotional energy.* Accordingly, therapy meant identifying and dissolving these characterological resistances, step by step, so that the underlying emotions could emerge. Reich called this process "character analysis," contrasting it with the usual psychoanalytic practice of *symptom* analysis, in which the individual contents of the patient's unconscious were interpreted as soon as they arose, without due regard for the total characterological resistance. Symptom analysis usually had little emotional or therapeutic effect on the patient, but Reich found that careful and consistent character analysis led to powerful emotional release and more substantial cures.

By "character" Reich means the *how* of a person's behavior, as distinguished from the *what*. *How* a person talks, for example—the quality of his voice, his intonations, his expression—is more significant than the mere content of what he says. "Words may lie, but the character never lies." Similarly, such things as posture, carriage, gait, mannerisms, gestures, and facial expressions tend to have a set, habitual quality that makes a person uniquely recognizable to others, but of which he himself is largely unaware. The character analyst learns to feel the *expression* or emotional quality inherent in each of these traits and in the character as a whole. Based on his intuition, the analyst then proceeds to help the client become aware of his own character, primarily in a feeling or experimental way rather than merely intellectually. The analyst starts with the most

TABLE 1. ACTIONS OF THE AUTONOMIC NERVOUS SYSTEM.[a]

Organ	Sympathetic action	Parasympathetic action
Musculature of iris	Inhibition of m.sphincter pupillae: *Dilation of pupils*	Stimulation of m.sphincter pupillae: *Narrowing of pupils*
Lachrymal glands	Inhibition of lachrymal glands: *"Dry eyes"*	Stimulation of lachrymal glands: *"Bright eyes"*
Salivary glands	Inhibition of salivary glands: *"Dry mouth"*	Stimulation of salivary glands: *"Mouth waters"*
Sweat glands	Stimulation of sweat glands: *"Cold sweat"*	Inhibition of sweat glands: *Dry skin*
Arteries	Contraction of arteries: *"Cold sweat"; pallor*	Dilation of arteries: *Redness of skin, increased turgor*, without sweating
Arrectores pilorum	Stimulation of arrectores pilorum: *Hair is "raised". "Gooseflesh"*	Inhibition of arrectores pilorum: *Skin smooth*
Bronchial musculature	Inhibition of contracting musculature: *Relaxation of bronchi*	Stimulation of contracting musculature: *Bronchial spasm*
Heart	Stimulates heart action: *Palpitation, tachycardia*	Depresses heart action: *Heart quiet, pulse slow*
Gastrointestinal tract: liver, pancreas, kidneys; all digestive glands	*Inhibits peristalsis. Reduces secretion of digestive glands*	*Stimulates peristalsis and secretion of digestive glands*
Adrenals	*Stimulates secretion of adrenaline*	*Inhibits secretion of adrenaline*
Urinary bladder	Inhibits musculature which opens bladder, stimulates sphincter: *Inhibits micturition*	Stimulates musculature which opens bladder, inhibits sphincter: *Stimulates micturition*
Female sex organs	Stimulates smooth musculature, reduces secretion of all glands, decreases blood supply: *Decreased sexual sensation*	Relaxes smooth musculature, stimulates secretion of all glands, increases blood supply: *Increased sexual sensation*
Male sex organs	Stimulates smooth musculature of the scrotum, reduces glandular secretion, decreases blood supply: *Flaccid penis. Decreased sexual sensation*	Relaxes smooth musculature of the scrotum, stimulates glandular secretion, increases blood supply: *Erection. Increased sexual sensation*

[a]Adapted from W. Reich, *Function of the Orgasm* (Noonday Press, 1961), pp. 259-260.

obvious or superficial traits—those of which the client himself is most likely to have some awareness—and gradually proceeds to the deeper layers.

Suppose, for example, the client has a habitual smile. This smile might persist even when he is discussing the most painful emotions or experiences. Such a set expression, whether obvious or subtle, is clearly a block to the natural flow of feelings. The analyst would begin to point the smile out to the client, as it is happening, repeatedly, consistently. He would call attention to the incongruity between the smile and the painful content of what the client is saying. He might urge the client to wiggle his face around, or scowl, or make other expressions which contradict the smile, or he might have him exaggerate the smile. At the same time the analyst would be on the alert for signs of offense, resentment, anxiety, or any sort of resistance. He is well aware that in attacking the client's *character* he is attacking that which the client identifies most intimately with *himself*.

In fact the analyst's very position of "authority" inev-itably arouses latent negative emotions and attitudes which the client originally felt towards his parents and siblings. This is called the "negative transference." The analyst knows that it would be futile to try to push any therapeutic insights through this wall of negativity. Indeed, it is precisely these negative feelings that form the most important part of what lies concealed in the character armor and that the analysis needs to deal with. The analyst therefore tries to elicit these feeings and encourage the client to express them openly. As the negative feelings emerge, the defensive function of the smile will also become more apparent. This work with the latent negative reactions and transference is one of the most difficult, demanding, and subtle tasks of the therapy. Properly handled, the transference relationship is the royal road into the unconscious; bungled, it is the shipwreck of many a therapy.

If the character-analytic work proceeds correctly, the client will begin to become aware of his smile and his other traits as *symptoms* rather than inalienable parts of his true self. He will begin to feel the emotions immanent in the smile, as well as the underlying feelings which the smile is warding off. For example, the apparently polite or pleasant smile might harbor a concealed feeling of "Nothing touches me." Just beneath that might be a deeper feeling of "You can't get me, you bastard, I won't give you the satisfaction!" And beneath that, warded off by the defensive attitude, might be passionate feeings of pain, longing, sadness, and rage. There might be oral impulses to cry, scream, bite, or suck. If the transference has been properly dealt with, the client will become increasingly aware of the formerly covert feelings of mistrust, fear, anger, or longing which he feels toward the therapist, and of their roots in his earlier relationship with his parents. He will also begin to feel how his smile and other traits serve to disguise, contain, or ward off those feelings, and to sense the roots of these defensive patterns in his past. With the growth of awareness and deeper feeling, the defensive patterns will loosen their hold on the character, the underlying emotions will spontaneously emerge and find discharge, and the whole personality will become clearer, healthier, and more capable of seeking and enjoying real satisfaction in life and love.

Years of clinical experience with character analysis led Reich to his most original and extraordinary therapeutic discovery: the discovery of "muscular armoring" and the famous "Reichian body work." He found that neurotic character structure and repressed emotions are actually physiologically rooted in *chronic muscle spasms*. Emotions are not just feelings floating around in the brain—every emotion also involves an *impulse to action*. Sadness, for example, is a feeling—a psychic event—but it also involves an impulse to cry, which is a very physical event involving a certain kind of convulsive breathing, vocalizations, facial expressions, tearing, and even actions of the limbs. If the urge to cry has to be suppressed, all those convulsive muscular impulses have to be suppressed by means of a willful effort of holding or stiffening. Above all, one must hold the breath. This not only suppresses the sobs or screams, but lowers the energy level by decreasing the intake of oxygen. Also, the muscular tensions block the flow of energy which is an essential aspect of emotional excitation.

If the muscular holding has to become habitual, it turns into chronic spastic contractions of the musculature. These spasms become automatic, unconscious; they cannot be voluntarily relaxed; they persist even in sleep. *Suppression* has turned into *repression*. The forgotten memories and feelings lie dormant but intact in the form of *frozen impulses to action* in the muscles; and the totality of these chronic muscle spasms constitutes a system of *muscular armoring* which defends us against both stimuli from without and impulses from within.

Thus, muscular armoring is the physical aspect, and character armoring the psychical aspect, of our total defense system. One is truly inseparable from the other. For example, the neurotic smile we discussed earlier is not only an emotional defense or a psychic attitude—it is also a chronic spastic contraction of the musculature of the face. It can be effectively attacked by physical as well as by psychological means.

Reich developed a variety of ingenious techniques for dissolving the muscular armoring. These techniques have been further expanded and elaborated by his followers. Here is a list of some of the most typical:

WILHELM REICH ON EMOTIONS

Gerald Grow, Ph.D.

According to Reich, every human emotion can come in two forms. One form, which he called "primary," is an expression of the depth of the person. Expressing a "primary" emotion leads you back toward wholeness and balance. For example, under certain circumstances anger functions as a primary emotion; feeling and expressing anger is then the best, and perhaps only, way to become recentered.

In contrast, "secondary" emotions do *not* serve to rebalance you. Secondary impulses are part of a vicious circle in which an unsatisfying feeling keeps reinforcing itself.

Here's the important thing: secondary emotions only arise when primary emotions are suppressed. When a person's natural longings for love become blocked, secondary, perverse longings may appear: masochistic urges, sadistic impulses, compulsive sex that fails to satisfy, as well as feelings of emptiness, deadness, loss of direction, depression.

To Reich, people were basically good, and their deepest longings moved toward wholeness, community, and a profound, gentle, melting, loving passion. He explained everything that is "evil" or "destructive" in human nature as a "secondary" impulse, formed by suppressing the natural, primary, constructive impulses toward love and growth. In other words, destructiveness, masochism, perversion, neurosis, and the long list of human ills are life that is not lived deeply enough: emotions felt down only to the "secondary" layer, and not to the deep heart's core. Human problems come from frozen energy—energy that is held, dammed up, restrained from pulsing out its rhythms and transmitting its life wisdom into our actions.

1. *Deep breathing*, natural or in certain patterns suggested by the therapist. This in itself can produce energy streamings, prickling or tingling sensations, tremors, spasms, or even spontaneous emotional releases. The same is true for *repeated screaming*.

2. *Deep massage* of spastic areas, especially while having the client breathe deeply and express the pain with his voice, facial expression, and, when practical, his body. This is an extremely powerful route into the unconscious, either immediately or with time. Occasionally, pressure on a single muscle spasm will produce a spontaneous outburst of repressed emotion, with a specific memory of a forgotten traumatic event.

3. *Work with facial expressions*. This includes such actions as rolling the eyes around, wiggling the face and forehead, stretching the eyes and mouth wide open, and actually "making faces" which express various emotions, especially while maintaining eye contact with the therapist. These exercises are enhanced by deep breathing and making sounds. The face is a major organ of emotional expression, and the armoring there is a major block to feeling.

4. *Pushing down on the chest* while the client exhales or screams. The block to complete expiration is an important part of the breathing armoring. The work on this block also loosens up the block to complete inspiration.

5. *Work with the gag reflex*, the cough reflex, yawning, or any other convulsive reflex. Any convulsions tend to disrupt and break down the rigid armoring, and these three in particular reach deep internal armoring that would otherwise be inaccessible.

6. *Maintaining "stress positions,"* especially while breathing deeply and expressing the pain with voice and face. Stress positions loosen armoring by stretching it, tiring it, irritating it, and inducing tremors or clonisms." Clonisms, like any other convulsions, tend to break down armoring, and are also a sign that armoring is dissolving.

7. *Active "bioenergetic" movements*, such as pounding, stamping, kicking, tantrums, reaching out, and moving or shaking areas like the head, shoulders, arms, or pelvis. Needless to say, these should all be done with full breathing and appropriate sounds and facial expressions. Merely performing such actions as mechanical exercises is of limited benefit and usually indicates a latent resistance. On the other hand, even if the client doesn't seem to feel much at first, sincere work with these movements for a period of time tends to break down inhibitions and liberate genuine feeling.

There is a definite order to the application of these techniques and to the progression of the therapy. This order is never invariable or mechanical; it depends on the individual client, the vicissitudes of therapy, and the intuition of the therapist. Still, there are general laws that should never be overlooked.

The fundamental law of body work is the same as the fundamental law of character analysis: start with the most superficial defenses and work gradually into the deeper layers, at a rate that the client is able to handle. The client's fear and resistance—particularly the *latent* fear and resistance—should always be respected. It is there for good reason. The pain that we harbor within is monumental, and spectacular "breakthrough" now may be paid for later by increased resistance, severe anxiety, or in some cases even psychotic breakdown.

In body work this law has a very concrete application; and this brings us to yet another of Reich's incredible discoveries: *the segmental arrangement of the armoring*. It turns out that in general, the individual muscular blocks do not correspond to an individual muscle or nerve pathway; rather, they fall into a *segmental* arrangement. The segments function transversely, at right angles to the natural longitudinal flow of biological energy. They are like the rings of an earthworm: when the worm is pinched, its rings constrict, choking off and disrupting the natural sinuous flow of longitudinal energy streamings. Like the segmental arrangement of the spine, autonomic ganglia, and intestines, they represent the worm in man.

Reich identified seven major segments of armoring: the *ocular*; the *oral*; the *neck*; the *chest*; including the arms; the *diaphragmal*; the *abdominal*; and the *pelvic*, including the legs. Each segment is a ring of tension encircling the body, and also includes the underlying internal organs. The relative independence of these segments is shown by the fact that any emotional or bioenergetic activity in one part of a segment will tend to influence its other parts, while the adjacent segments will remain relatively unaffected. In fact, if bound-up energy is liberated in one segment, the adjacent segments will often show signs of *increased* armoring or resistance, as a defensive reaction to the pressure of the released energy, which is trying to push through.

Now, the torso and limbs are like a great reservoir of bound-up biological energy. Any energy which is liberated from this armoring will tend to collect in the chest and abdominal cavities, preparatory to being discharged through the head (as in screaming) or the genitals (as in orgasm). If these outlets are blocked, the pressure can build up to intolerable levels, causing acute anxiety or severe headaches. For this reason it is important to open up the head, throat, neck, and upper shoulder area before allowing too much dissolution of armoring in the lower body. It is the head, after all, that is the primary guardian of the repression in the first place; one might say that we must gain the head's "permission" before we can go very far in opening up the flow of repressed energy. Next the breathing can be gradually expanded, while the formidable energy of the pelvic segment is reserved for last. Thus we have the general rule that, in dissolving the armoring, *we should start with the topmost segments and gradually proceed downward*. Again, this rule should not be applied in a rigid, mechanical way. The organism is an intricately interrelated whole, and one can go only so far in dissolving the armoring in one area without working on the other areas as well.

Reichian body work is powerful. It cuts through the crap. It provides quicker, surer access to areas of the unconscious that used to be virtually inaccessible. Profound, convulsive, emotional releases, and even repressed memories from the earliest periods of life, emerge spontaneously, without special effort, simply as a by-product of the thoroughgoing softening of the resistances. The free-flowing energy that has been liberated pushes into the remaining blocks, further weakening them, and setting in motion a process of spontaneous dissolution of armoring that ultimately reaches down to the deepest levels of biological functioning, and paves the way for the full development of the orgasm reflex.

But, powerful as it is, the body work is only of limited effectiveness without character analysis. In the course of therapy, sometimes it is the body work that needs to be stressed, sometimes the character analysis. Both are indispensable, complementary parts of Reichian work. The body work gives teeth to the character work, but it is the character-analytic understanding that gives the whole process of therapy intelligence, meaning, and direction. Without this understanding, no matter how forcefully and diligently the body work is pursued, the therapy will bog down and founder at every turn.

Reichian therapy is no panacea. The process of dissolving the armoring requires courage, perseverance, and support. The further you go, the more your whole life has to become therapy. Your energy and life style have to become focused on opening up and getting into your feelings. Your occupation, living situation, and everyday habits all need to become supportive of that process. Above all, you need to cultivate supportive, intimate personal relationships dedicated to openness and growth. Only with loving support can we tolerate the fear and pain of our emerging inner depths. Also, love-related emotions that have been thwarted are at the core of our sickness, and only by means of love relationships can we really deal with those feelings. This means going behind the inevitable conflict syndromes that normally ruin our relationships, and openly getting into the underlying parental projections together. In other words, it is a matter of dealing with *transference*, making it conscious, getting into feelings or even fights together knowing that you're really screaming at your parents or siblings, and not primarily at each other. As you learn to let go more together and share your negative feelings, you build trust and open yourselves up to new possibilities of letting each other's love in. For although releasing your pain, fear, and rage is good for you, it is *letting the love in* that really cures. Loving surrender is also the basis of full orgastic potency.

Making your life therapy amounts to taking your therapy into your own hands. Once you get a feeling for it, it's amazing how much you can learn to do for yourself, especially with the help of friends who are involved in it with you. Approached in this way, Reichian Therapy can become the basis of a true yoga—a discipline or path of life designed to open one up to the highest energies. I call it *Primal Yoga*, using the word "primal" both in the ordinary sense and as it is used in Primal Therapy.[3] In its breathing, stretching, and convulsive energy-moving techniques Primal Yoga has much in common with established forms of yoga, such as Hatha and Kundalini. The seven segments of armoring even correspond rather closely with the seven chakras. But Primal Yoga differs above all in its specific emphasis on primal emotional release and systematic dissolution of armoring. To me this seems essential. How can we expect to face God when we can't face ourselves or each other; when we are tied up in knots of armoring and repressed emotions; when we are unable to tolerate high levels of energy, or bear the overwhelming ecstasy of full organic convulsions?

The path is hard, but the rewards are immense: reawakening of inner depths, release from crippling life-long burdens, and constant renewal of health, clarity, power, vitality, love, and the magic of existence.

Suggestions for Further Reading

Wilhelm Reich, *The Function of the Orgasm*, Noonday Press, 1971. The basic primer of Reichian therapy, tracing the evolution of Reich's work from psychoanalysis all the way through to orgone biophysics.

———, *Character Analysis*. Simon and Schuster, 1972. A more detailed exposition of character formation and character analysis, also tracing the development through vegetotherapy into orgone biophysics. Includes a fascinating case history of Reich's treatment of a schizophrenic.

Alexander Lowen, a pupil of Reich's and the founder of bioenergetics, has written many interesting and readable books, any of which are recommended.

RICHARD HOFF *is a self-taught Reichian practitioner and dedicated primal yogi. He loves nature, philosophy, science, classical music, art, dancing, gymnastics, and martial arts; he is also a craftsman and inventor. Richard's struggle to dissolve his own armoring led to his invention of the Knobble®, a small wooden self-massage tool that is effective on all parts of the body.*

A Sport for Everybody

Bob Kriegel

In ancient Greece, athletes were seen as heroic doers of great deeds, and their bodies as fit and shining temples for spirit. The great competitions, which actually originated as funeral games, were transpersonal events which could awaken the soul to higher and higher levels of transformation. Since then, many changes have come and gone, but sports are once again being seen as a medium for personal growth. As Bob Kriegel says, "America seems to have gone crazy discovering the joys of the body." In this article, he introduces and explains the new sports consciousness and its implications.

"Sports represent a key point in any society. How we play the game may turn out to be more important than we imagine, for it signifies nothing less than our way of being in the world."

George Leonard,
The Ultimate Athlete

VERYWHERE YOU look people are jogging, biking, hiking, swimming, playing tennis, skiing, doing yoga. It seems as if America has gone crazy rediscovering the joys of the body.

What happened to the America of not so long ago, when the big weekend activity was getting up for a can of beer during a commercial while watching a football game on TV? The new spirit of participation and body awareness seems to have its roots in the political and consciousness movements of the '60s, movements that shook us from the lethargy of the '50s to a realization of what was happening around us. Reflecting the political upheavals of the times, top-level athletes like Dave Meggyesy, Jim Bouton, Jack Scott, and Harry Edwards began to question the old structures. Politicians, the media, and parents began to raise voices against the inequities of organized sports from the majors on down to the little leagues. To the counterculture and the Left, the word "competition" took on unpleasant and devious connotations. In more than a few quarters, sports became passé.

At the same time, the first consciousness pioneers and environmental activists were being heard from. Attitudes about pollution, nutrition, sexuality, and sex roles changed—it became "OK" to share feelings, one's

"dharma" to seek transcendance, a "responsibility" and calling for all to seek political, social, and personal possibilities. Is it any wonder that the expression of our bodies would be the next frontier?

The New Sports

The athletic revolution gradually evolved from trying to break down the system to creating alternatives for achieving its goals. The revolution turned into an evolution: sport began to be looked at with vision rather than vengeance. This evolution was marked by the First New Games Tournament, organized by Stuart Brand (founder of the *Whole Earth Catalog*); the Symposium put on by the Esalen Sports Center, which brought together pioneers in this new movement; and the emergence of the martial arts (among them Aikido and T'ai Chi), which espoused values of blending, harmony, and centering.

Basically this evolutionary movement in sport took two general directions. One way was to change the principles and philosophy of traditional sports and games, as well as the manner in which they were taught (the inner approach). The other was to develop new alternative models for participation (the outer approach). The goal of these two approaches to sport and recreation is the same: to enhance the quality of participation.

Inner Games

Probably the best-known proponent of the inner approach is Tim Gallwey, the developer of the Inner Game, which is based on the thesis that we have the ability to perform at a much higher level than we normally do. Our most formidable opponent, Gallwey holds, is not across the net, but inside our own heads. What hinders our performance, ordinarily, is not poor equipment, bad conditions, or lack of technical knowledge or expertise, but our doubts, fears, and self-consciousness. To help overcome these innate obstacles and to maximize our capacities, the Inner Game approach focuses on developing nonjudgmental awareness, relaxed concentration, and the awareness of self—that part of us which learns naturally and performs effortlessly. The insights we can gain by means of the Inner Game approach can help us improve the quality of our lives—as well as develop a formidable backhand or a graceful parallel turn.

But Gallwey isn't alone. Many teachers are now combining elements of humanistic psychology, martial arts, yoga, and other movement and awareness disciplines. The sports thus approached range from rock climbing and kayaking to basketball and football. In their books on running and jogging, Mike Spino and Fred Rohe feature meditation, visualization, and Zen mind approaches. Dave Meggyesy and Robert Nideffer are only a few of those coaches using these inner approaches with college and pro athletes.

Outer Games

At the other end of the spectrum lies the outer approach—the attempt to develop alternatives to traditional sporting activities and to get more people to participate. The American Alliance for Health, Physical Education, and Recreation has been a major force in developing the "New Physical Education." The goal of the New P.E. is participation for all. Training starts in the lower grades, with body movement and success-oriented activities designed to help children develop a positive sense of their bodies—a key factor in their eventual self-images. The upper grades are introduced to "lifetime sports"—literally, sports they can participate in for the rest of their lives. The reaction to these sports has been overwhelming. Imagine taking sailing, skiing, tennis, or backpacking in high school—no wonder kids are "going out" for them in droves.

For the public at large, the New Games Foundation of San Francisco has been putting on play festivals in parks and recreation areas all over the country. A typical New Games event offers a variety of games, from ones invented on the spot to the rituals of ancient cultures, with every possible permutation in between. These happenings provide opportunities for whole families to play together and for people of disparate backgrounds, ages, and outlooks to come together in a joyous and fun-filled experience.

Utopian Games

One of the areas in which I have been working is to develop what I call "Utopian Games"—games espousing humanistic values. After outlining some parameters for this type of game, I realized that many examples already existed. They are the street and playground games we played as children, such as Hide and Seek, Kick the Can, Red Rover, Capture the Flag. The qualities they share are as follows.

No Time Limits. These games end only when interest wanes or parents call for dinner.

No Specific Play Space. These games can be played anywhere—in the street, playgrounds, fields, alleys. It's up to the players to be creative and adapt the game to the environment.

No Special Equipment. Players can wear whatever they want—no special uniforms or Adidas.

No Fixed Roles. Participants have the opportunity to play all different kinds of roles: to hide or to seek, to chase and to elude, to defend or to attack. In this way they are never restricted to one style of play (always being a guard, for instance, or a right fielder): instead, they learn to adapt to different situations and strategies.

No Spectators. The games are designed so that everyone can participate, regardless of age.

No Referees. All disputes are worked out by the players. This helps them learn how to come to agreements and to make concessions in order to achieve harmony: it also teaches them to stand up for themselves and something they believe is right. And, perhaps most important, it develops their sense of what's "fair." (In a way, referees actually foster cheating: often the attitude is "How much can I get away with without being caught?")

No Rewards. These games are designed to be autoletic; that is, the prize consists in the pleasure of playing. (Can you imagine a trophy for the best Hide and Seek player?) But the "nonrewards" can be considerable. A comment I keep hearing in the workshops I give is "I haven't had so much fun since I was a kid."

And that raises an interesting question: Is there any value in all this play, or are we just trying to relive our childhood? There *is* value in game-playing, and it takes many forms. One is the feeling that you get when the fun, the challenge, the excitement—the joy of the play itself—is the goal of the game. This alone is sufficient incentive for participation: in a culture that is so serious and goal-oriented, these activities provide us with needed lightness and teach us the value of the process as well as the goal.

But we get a great deal more from games. The health benefits of exercise are well-known (my own heartbeat has dropped from 76 to 55 since I started jogging). And since the body and mind are not separate, this sense of physical well-being transfers to our whole being. Feeling better about our bodies usually translates into feeling better about ourselves, having more confidence and self-assurance. Research has also shown that greater physical fitness leads to more imagination and creativity, more energy and vitality in every respect.

We can also learn valuable personal lessons from sports that can help us improve the quality of our lives. Those "breakthrough moments"—when, for no apparent reason, everything seems to click and we perform better than we thought possible—give us glimpses of the potentials that exist within us. From risk sports, such as skiing, rock climbing, and white-river rafting, we can learn how to deal with and overcome fear and anxiety, to develop courage. Running, swimming, or biking long distances can help us to develop endurance and will, and to learn how to deal with boredom. Through golf we can practice intense concentration and subtle control. Team sports can teach us the value of cooperation.

And, perhaps most importantly, all games—both traditional and revolutionary—make us realize we can't stand back and spectate while someone else establishes the rules and roles by which we live. When we start to take responsibility for being participants in the big game, actively involving ourselves in the choices that will affect our direction and destiny, that's called freedom. And that's what the new sports consciousness is all about.

BOB KRIEGEL, *a psychologist, was the co-founder and director of the Esalen Sports Center and the director of SAGAS, a training project for educators and therapists in the use of games and sports for self-development. He is the co-author, with Tim Gallwey, of* Inner Skiing (*Random House, 1977*).

LAYING ON OF HANDS

Chellis Glendinning, Ph.D.

IN my studies to become a holistic-health practitioner, I learned different healing systems which conceptualize energy flow in the body. I often found that different systems complemented each other, one adderssing itself to a type of imbalance which another took no notice of. I used breathing techniques, manipulations, and pressure points with the same person to great benefit. I also found that the various systems often contradicted each other. One described energy as flowing from head to toe, another from belly outward, another from right side to left side. I noticed that these contradictions usually arose from cultural or historical differences. In my work I wanted to go beyond cultural limitation and beyond system. To do this I began to pare down my use of techniques until I arrived at what is basic to all systems of healing: the life energy.

Laying on of hands is among the most direct approaches to healing. It is also one of the oldest and most widely used. Any mother who has held her child, any lover who has touched her mate, any friend who has comforted his friend has unwittingly practiced the laying on of hands. Touch is more than physical intimacy; it is a transmission of energy through one being to another.

Energy is that force which binds together all manifestations, visible and invisible, tangible and intangible, mental and physical. It is a phenomenon both physiological and mystical. Many people can see energy traveling through the body or emanating from its surface. We can all feel it if we take the time to notice.

Close your eyes and take note of how you feel. Where is your breathing? How are your feet connected to the Earth? Where are you relaxed? Where tense? What sensations do you find in your body? Allow yourself to explore.

Open your eyes and rub your hands together very quickly for a few seconds. Stop and hold them several inches apart at about belly level, palms facing each other. What do you feel between your hands? Allow

hands, arms, and shoulders to relax, so that the current can pass freely through them.

Now try experimenting with your hands. Bring them closer together. Draw them farther apart. At what point is the feeling between your hands strongest? At what point is it weakest? See if you can find out what shape this force is.

This exercise is a basic one for people who want to use their hands to channel energy. By doing it often, you may increase the flow and also your sensitivity to it. In order to channel energy through our hands, we need to have a good flow through our bodies. Some of us have this naturally. Others must develop and maintain it. Body work, martial arts, sport, dance, and meditation are all excellent ways to free up and strengthen the flow. Practicing laying on of hands on yourself is also a way to strengthen the current.

Lie down. Place a pillow under your knees if your back gets tired when you lie flat. Make sure you are comfortable. Now tune into what you are feeling. Allow yourself to breathe and relax.

Rub your hands together again, and hold them facing each other for a few moments. When you feel the energy between your hands, place them on your pelvic bones, right hand covering right pelvic bone and left over left. Focus your awareness on the exchange between hands and bone. After a while, feel yourself *being held* rather than doing the holding. You may close your eyes and lie in this position for as long as you like. I sometimes stay for half an hour. It is a self-healing meditation for me.

What are you feeling? Notice any body sensations, emotions, dream images, or memories which occur. When you feel finished, place your hands at your sides. How does your body feel different from when you started? As you emerge, give yourself time to assimilate the changes which have occurred. Rest. Stretch out. Come slowly up to sitting or standing.

Once you feel comfortable with the energy vibrating through your hands, you may want to try using it to strengthen another person's flow. Here is a simple method of diagnosis to help you decide where to place your hands. Hold your hands next to the person's body, about an inch or two from the skin. The energy emanating from the body is called the aura. Feel all around in some systematic way, from head to toes, for instance. Notice any changes: a place which feels stronger or weaker, congested or depleted. Look for heat, cold, irregular tingling (as opposed to clear vibration), numbness, pressure, electrical charges. Trust your hands; the place that needs contact is not always the place where a problem has been diagnosed.

Now both of you need to be comfortable, whether standing, sitting, or lying down. If either of you feel tense or uncomfortable in your position, the flow will be cut off. Don't be afraid to experiment with different positions or to change position at any time. When I work, I like to sit cross-legged on the floor with my client lying on a foam mat. Sometimes I rest my elbows on my knees.

Tell the person you are working with she may close her eyes so that she can focus inside. Tell her to be aware of her body, to notice the places which feel tense and the places which feel relaxed, to be aware of her breathing. Suggest to her that she stay aware of her self and any changes she may feel as you work together. You notice her too: her position, her breathing, her areas of tension, the parts of her body she holds, the expression on her face, etc.

Prepare to work by rubbing your hands together and feeling the energy between them. When you feel ready, place your hands directly on the place or places you have chosen for the laying on of hands. Allow your hands to be relaxed and to make full contact.

An important issue is closure. Practitioner Doris Breyer seldom stays in one place for more than a few minutes. Nurse-healer Dolores Krieger never uses her Therapeutic Touch technique for more than ten minutes. Spiritual healer Ambrose Worrall wrote that he sometimes practiced laying on of hands in one position for more than 45 minutes. I suggest that you maintain the contact for as long as you feel the connection. Perhaps the person lets go of a tense muscle or takes a deep breath. Perhaps what drew you to that place originally (heat, tingling, etc.) stops. Perhaps you intuitively feel that the connection has been made as deeply as is possible at this time. It is best to work too short a time than too long. You can always work again in a few days if more is needed, whereas staying too long can overstimulate a person's system and wreak energetic havoc! Have the person lie still for at least five to ten minutes after the treatment, so that she can assimilate the new pattern into her system rather than use her energy for some activity peripheral to healing.

Many people think of energy as "good" or "bad." They believe that when we work with an unbalanced person, we are in danger of "taking on" that person's "bad" energy. I think of energy as neutral. How we channel it through ourselves determines our vitality or imbalance. Don Boyles helped me understand the phenomenon of "taking on another's illness" in a new light. He explained we are like tuning forks, each of us vibrating like music within our own range of frequency. When we are open to another person, as we so often are during a therapy, health-counseling, or treatment session, we may begin to vibrate to that person's frequency! Many forms of protection and cleansing can help strenthen us, so that we are not affected when we don't want to be. Some are: meditation, imagining a white light surrounding yourself while you work, channeling energy through the feet into the floor while working, dipping the arms up to the elbows in water and epsom salts after working, taking a walk, airing out the room. I feel that the ultimate purpose of techniques is to help us understand how to channel the energy passing through us in ways which benefit our lives and growth.

Laying on of hands can be practiced for catalyzing a healing when imbalance has already manifested as a physical problem. It is also a "body therapy" for removing energy blockages, balancing, and improving one's healing journey through life. It can be an energizing experience for both the practitioner and the person worked on. We are all healers, and when we make ourselves open channels for the life energy, laying on of hands is available to us all.

CHELLIS GLENDINNING *is a published writer and feminist body therapist. She teaches and lectures all over the country. Her writings have appeared in many feminist publications, and she is co-author of* Chains Of Fires: A Rediscovery of Womanspirit.

Chiropractic

G.F. Riekeman, D.C.

One basic principle of chiropractic is that the human body, operating at its full potential, is capable of maintaining perfect health. Another is that the degree to which one's nervous system is operating efficiently is directly related to one's sense of well-being and totality. The spinal column is the life-line of the nervous system, and so deserves the best of care and maintenance. For this reason, chiropractic treatments can be greatly beneficial for treating any imbalance in the body. In this article, Dr. Riekeman introduces us to the modern system of chiropractice.

CHIROPRACTIC IS a New Age philosophy, science, and art which focuses on correcting interference with the nervous system, the coordinating mechanism of all body function. The goal of chiropractic is to enable people to manifest 100 per cent of their individual innate potentials, given their hereditary and environmental circumstances.

Chiropractic does not diagnose or treat diseases and infirmities; thus, it should not be classed with the so-called "healing arts."

In order to understand the ramifications of the art of chiropractic, it is important to recognize what health is. Health may be viewed as "A state of complete physical, mental, and social well-being, and not merely the absence of disease and infirmity" (Dorland's Medical Dictionary), and as "an integrated method of functioning which is oriented toward maximizing the potential of which an individual is capable within their hereditary and environmental framework" (Halpert Dunn, M.D.). In short, the word health should be understood as implying an ideal of coordination, evolution, and balance.

A second concept needed to understand chiropractic is the source from which health arises. Unfortunately, most people feel that health is obtained from outside the organism itself. During our first 18 years, we are conditioned by 330,000 television drug commercials to believe that if we have this ache or that pain, then we need medical product X or Y to solve the problem. Soon there is ingrained in our thoughts the belief that health is the absence of symptoms.

What chiropractic is suggesting is not a variation on what is already failing, but a completely new path: a path that looks for health within each person and which recognizes the orderly perfection of life and nature. For "nature needs no help, just no interference."

In one of his world travels, Dr. B. J. Palmer, the developer of chiropractic, visited an active volcanic pit that was one mile across and 1,000 feet deep. The volcano had erupted, filled, and overflowed into the surrounding terrain. That night, B. J. read an article which said, "Take Pill X in order to ASSIST NATURE." He thought, "If nature did what it did without Pill X, I wonder what would have happened if Pill X had been dropped into the crater."

It is life itself which heals, or, perhaps more accurately, the unfettered expression of life. Life and its unhampered expression (health) are conditions that come from within. The scientific law of homeostasis says that every organism in the universe has the innate ability to be whole and healthy and stable within itself and its environment. You have every potential that you'll ever need to live a balanced, coordinated existence: those potentials are not locked in cow pus, moondust, or any outside source, but rather flow from within. *In order to express more of your potential, you need only keep the channels for that expression open.*

This is where chiropractic enters. We recognize that the universe is perfectly organized and that, as extensions of that universal intelligence, we also have an unlimited potential for life and health.

In brief, health means being whole, having every part of your body functioning and adapting to its fullest potential. The question to be asked is not how do we treat disease, but *what controls* how efficiently my body is functioning.

All ancient and contemporary study of this question has led to an understanding of the nervous system as the link between innate potential and expression of that potential. Contemporary chiropractic studies have also discovered an increasing amount of evidence that vertebral (spinal) misplacement creates the most severe form of interference with the nervous system known today.

Let us then briefly discuss a few innate potentials, the role of the nervous system, and the contemporary practice of chiropractic.

The human organism has shown an ability to maintain homeostatic health in the face of almost any adversity. It has the potential, if functioning correctly, to protect itself from becoming cancerous. Dr. Robert Good, M.D., a noted researcher in the field of cancer, has found (*Time*, March 1973) that the body's immunological system is responsible

CHIROPRACTIC IN THEORY AND PRACTICE

T. A. Vondarhaar

IN human beings, the brain stem and spinal cord are protected by the vertebral column, which is the bony structure surrounding the nerve trunk from the upper neck to the lower back. If protection of the spinal cord were its only function, the spine could have become one long, solid, cylindrical bone, but, if it had, human beings would not be able to walk, sit, dance, run, or move at all. To allow motion, the backbone is segmented into 24 freely movable vertebrae.

Because of the various stresses to which the spine is subject, individual vertebrae can become misaligned. Such misalignments can create pressure on nerve tissue, and thus interfere with the conduction of nerve impulses to other parts of the body. Chiropractors call the condition a *subluxation*.

Nerves travel to various tissues and organs from each vertebra of the spine. A subluxation reduces the nerve signals to the affected tissue or organ, resulting in dysfunction and eventually disease. The subluxation of the spine, because it reduces nerve supply, is considered by doctors of chiropractic to be a main *cause* of disease. The point in the body at which disease becomes apparent is the *symptom*.

Physical trauma is one major cause of subluxations. One of the greatest burdens on the human spine is lack of motion, sitting, or lack of appropriate exercise. The designs of automobile seats and office furniture wreak havoc for the modern immobile man.

Mental stress is another cause of subluxation. Tightened muscles resulting from tension can pull the vertebrae out of alignment. Finally, chemical ingestion associated with faulty nutrition or consumption of drugs can cause misalignment of the vertebrae.

In 1895, Daniel David Palmer discovered the relationship between subluxations and dysfunction when the hearing of an employee was restored by Palmer's adjustment of the upper cervical spine. The employee had been deaf for seventeen years, D. D. Palmer remained in relative obscurity during his lifetime, but his son, Bartlett Joshua Palmer, directed the course of the chiropractic profession during the crucial early years of its growth and development.

Chiropractic has remained outside the mainstream of modern medicine because its major premise, that the body has inherent capacities for health, has simply been out of fashion in the United States and the Western world. The holistic view of health is regarded with suspicion by the medical establishment because it does not rely on technological intervention in the body. The internal mechanisms of the body, even in these modern times, are not completely understood, because they are not easily observed and are thus harder to research scientifically than is the impact of outside agents, such as chemicals, which can be measured and controlled.

Because no chemicals are used in chiropractic, there is no pharmaceutical industry, with its profits and resources, to support the profession. Drug manufacturers provide substantial support for biomedical research and political medicine. Their influence on the prescribing habits of physicians is well-documented. Drug-industry support of medical schools, hospitals, academic journals, and professional seminars creates symbiotic relationships that have shown themselves to be quite enduring.

Intraprofessional Differences

The chiropractic profession is divided into two basic groups. One group, called the "straights," adheres to a strict notion of chiropractic, that the vertebral subluxation is the fundamental cause of disease, and that the doctor of chiropractic should confine his work to adjusting the spine.

The primary function of the chiropractor, in the view of the straights, is to protect brain/nervous-system function by clearing the spine of vertebral subluxation, and allowing the intelligence within the body to function at its maximum.

(continued on next page)

(continued from previous page)

The *maxers*, on the other hand, are doctors of chiropractic who would broaden the scope of practice to include any modality of health care that is "natural." Some argue that chiropractic is whatever the law allows, or whatever is not drugs and surgery. Treatments often include clinical nutrition and physiotherapy. The mixers also generally argue for differential diagnosis and treatment of disease.

The differences between the straights and mixers are fundamental, representing opposing philosophical interpretations of chiropractic. Although members of both groups are usually rational and honest men and women, the debate is frequently ambiguous and occasionally intense.

When Should One See a Chiropractor?

Most patients of chiropractic are persons who have had specific complaints that have persisted despite medical treatment, and have often been made worse. Until recently, desperation was a chief motivation for seeking chiropractic care. Some patients see chiropractic as a type of medical specialty for low back pain or headaches. The concept of an appropriate amount of nerve energy is a valid one, however, and every person interested in holistic health should arrange for chiropractic analysis. The doctor of chiropractic will show the patient from his or her X-ray how the body is affected by vertebral misalignment, if the patient has any. X-rays before and after treatment, as well as the reduction or elimination of clinical manifestations, will make apparent the effectiveness of chiropractic care.

T. A. VONDARHAAR *was President of the Northern California College of Chiropractic.*

for keeping in check the cancerous cells that live inside each of us. In persons who develop cancer, there are definite signs that the immunological system is working at less than optimum. Recent studies have now raised the possible human life expectancy to close to 800 years of age. Dr. Ronald Pero, M.D., a leading geneticist, feels that a properly functioning body is necessary for the proper genetic unfoldment of our species. And various studies have shown that the human organism has a potential to interact with the universe in a more creative fashion on all levels of its existence. All this is possible only if the nervous system is free to perform its purpose, which, according to Gray's *Anatomy*, is "to control and coordinate every cell, organ, and structure in the body, and to adapt the organism to its enviornment."

Any interference with the nervous system will lessen its ability to function internally and to adapt to environmental and social stresses. As we mentioned previously, symptoms and disease have little to do with how well your body is functioning. Diarrhea, for example, is now considered a normal, *healthy* bodily function that is vital for eliminating cancerous growths from the intestinal tract. Conversely, some persons who have no "symptoms" are functioning so inefficiently that they may be dead tomorrow from a heart attack, with little or no prior warning.

Most interference to the nervous system that is caused by vertebral misalignment (subluxation) occurs before the age of two and goes unnoticed for years, or perhaps a lifetime. In fact, this first interference (subluxation) usually occurs during the birth process, not because of natural birthing, but, according to Dr. Joe Flesia, Chiropractor and Dean of Continuing Education at Sherman College of Straight Chiropractic, "this first subluxation is a result of the horrendous interference created by a sterile man-imposed technological birth process." Recent studies of Sudden Infant Deaths (crib deaths) at the University of Boston Medical Center have conclusively shown that the death was linked to cervical (neck) spinal-cord damage due to unnatural interference during the delivery process. As soon as this interference occurs, the child begins functioning at less than 100 percent. Studies at the University of Colorado by Dr. C. H. Suh, Director of Biomechanical Research, have shown that minimal pressure on a nerve root at the point where it leaves the spinal column will reduce the functioning of that nerve by some 60 percent.

The chiropractic philosophy is based on the deductive principle that the Universe is perfectly organized, and that we are extensions of this principle, designed to express life (health) and the universal laws. Since vertebral subluxations (spinal-nerve interference) are the grossest interference with the expression of life, the practice of chiropractic is designed to analyze and correct these subluxations, so that the organism will be free to evolve and express life to its fullest natural potential.

G. F. RIEKEMAN *was Dean of Philosophy at Sherman College of Chiropractic, South Carolina. He has co-founded Renaissance Chiropractic Organization, and is setting up an international headquarters and chiropractic college in the West Indies. Dr. Reikeman is an international lecturer on the subject of chiropractic.*

T'ai Chi Ch'uan as a Healing Art

Shandor Weiss

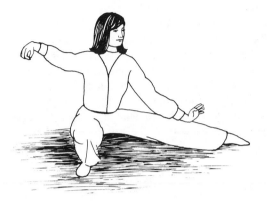

"The Tao is an empty vessel; it is used, but never filled.Oh, unfathomable source of the ten thousand things!"

Lao Tzu

IMAGINE RISING early, before the speed and noise of the day have begun, entering a quiet room or favorite outdoor place, and gathering yourself for practice. Nothing else in the world matters; there is nowhere to go, nothing else to do but the movements which await you. There is nothing to think about, for the body knows the sequence. As you flow into the movements, everything becomes suspended. Our descriptions of the world make it the way it is; thought creates patterns which are stored in the structure of body and mind.

T'ai Chi Ch'uan consists of a traditional series of movements that are intended to unite body and mind. However, to unite the body and mind, we must give up the desire to do so. As a therapy T'ai Chi is subversive, for if we *try* to improve ourselves it doesn't work. We never force anything. T'ai Chi works through nonexertion. Lao Tzu says,

"It is not wise to rush about.
Controlling the breath causes strain.
If too much energy is used, exhaustion follows.
This is not the way of Tao.
Whatever is contrary to Tao will not last long."

The usual reaction when an individual is directed to "push" is to respond with a physical/mental image of what it is to push, and begin by extending the arms as if to force something away. The body/mind is accustomed to dealing with the world by effort and struggle—until it learns another way. In T'ai Chi Ch'uan the movement called "push" really means something akin to "sink weight into ground, relax the arms and elbows, move the whole body as one unit." Hence, in pushing we actually relinquish the idea of pushing and let the elbows hang, the shoulders relax and the arms rest near the body, palms poised lightly to conform to one's partner.

In the next movement of the sequence, the hands remain in position as the body retreats over its firmly rooted feet. It is a movement of retreats, and the associated image of going back, yielding, and softness creates a different feeling. We allow ourselves to relax. The shoulders are gently pulled from the body as they round out the back. The elbows now open and extend without the effort associated with pushing. The wrists bend slowly as the fingers are allowed to open and spread. By moving very slowly, we trick the body's habitual movement responses. Although it seems as if little is happening, these flowing motions cause joints to open, chronic blocks to dissolve, and energy to circulate through the body once more.

It is probable that the basic principles of T'ai Chi—which is one of the few "internal" systems of martial arts—originated with early Taoists. The form itself, however, developed later. One story says that a thirteenth-century Taoist monk named Chang San-feng invented the movements one day while looking out a window. In the fields he saw a crane and snake fighting, and observed how softness and yielding combined so effectively in a combative situation. He devised a series of thirteen moves, which continued to be augmented until the 1800s, when the form emerged as we now know it. Once a secret art, T'ai Chi Ch'uan is now practiced for health, meditation, enjoyment, and self-defense by millions of people in China and around the world.

There are many other ways in which T'ai Chi promotes health and longevity. In China it is well-known for its healing powers, and is often prescribed by doctors in conjunction with other treatments or when other methods have failed. The gentle nature of T'ai Chi makes it suitable for the weak, old, infirm, or very young, as well as for those who enjoy excellent health. It strengthens without strain by the process of constant change from use to relaxation. Increased muscle tone improves circulation of the blood and lymph systems, which is vital to the maintenance of health. By opening the joints—especially the knees—T'ai Chi often alleviates and cures arthritis and rheumatism. It straightens the spine and strengthens the lower back. The slow, soft turning and bending massage the internal organs, and the gentle leg-raising movements strengthen the intestines and aid elimination. By calming the body/mind, it often relieves ulcers and nervous disorders. Deepened breathing supplies more oxygen to the blood and brain. The blood vessels become open and flexible, allowing the heart to function more smoothly.

By increasing the body's energy flow, the regular practice of T'ai Chi Ch'uan can ward off sickness and contagious disease. We know that disease germs are omnipresent, and only become a problem when our resistance is lowered. Similarly, chronic afflictions of the organs are often cured as blocks are removed, so that energy can flow through them once more. In Chinese medicine it is said that the kidneys supply energy to all the internal organs; when the kidneys are weak, the whole body feels drained of energy, and illness can result. In Western medicine this is called low blood sugar, or hypoglycemia, with symptoms of fatigue, dizziness, ringing ears, and blurred vision. In Chinese, it is simply called "low kidney energy," and an important part of the healing process for this condition is exercise. Although T'ai Chi appears soft, passive, and "yin" as an exercise, it actually has a very strengthening "yang" effect on the body/mind, partly because it stimulates one's kidney energy. Since this energy is not dissipated in the practice, T'ai Chi will leave one feeling energetic and eager to carry on the day's work.

Once the body becomes sensitive to this energy flow, the only health concern is losing that sensitivity. To truly practice, T'ai Chi Ch'uan is to be constantly aware of one's energy, and to cultivate it whenever one has the opportunity to do so. One well-known T'ai Chi master, T. T. Liang, took up the practice in midlife, after enduring prolonged illness and numerous surgical procedures. Doctors had given him only a short time to live. Now at age 77, Liang claims that T'ai Chi saved his life. In the preface of his book, *T'ai Chi Ch'uan for Health and Self-Defense*, he states, "At first I take up T'ai Chi as a hobby, gradually I become addicted to it, finally I can no longer get rid of it. I must keep on practicing for my whole life, for it is the only way to preserve health."

The movements in T'ai Chi are taken from nature, and they restore contact with the natural world. We learn how to be rooted like a tree, with our full weight resting on the ground. The breath becomes deep and natural, like the gentle swaying of a large tree in the breeze; the whole body becomes connected like a string of pearls. The waist is flexible, like clouds waving across the open sky; the mind is still and calm, like a large mountain; the spirit is allowed to soar, as though a graceful heron had just spread its wings. Our attention becomes like that of a hawk soaring effortlessly, waiting to seize a rabbit—or like a cat crouching, ready to pounce on its prey. We slide down like a snake and stand on one leg like a golden cock. In moving we flow like the current of a great river; in attitude we resemble the vast ocean, which is king of the waters because it lies lowest of all. By the practice of T'ai Chi Ch'uan we embody the essence of the natural world.

SHANDOR WEISS *studied T'ai Chi and other internal martial arts with Master T. T. Liang's senior student, Paul Gallagher, and others. He began teaching T'ai Chi Ch'uan in 1976 while working as an administrator for the Berkeley Holistic Health Center. Shandor has written several articles on T'ai Chi and natural healing, and co-authored a book on growing and using medicinal herbs, published by Rodale Press in 1984. Currently a student at the National College of Naturopathic Medicine, Shandor is also director of Arura Institute of Buddhist Medicine.*

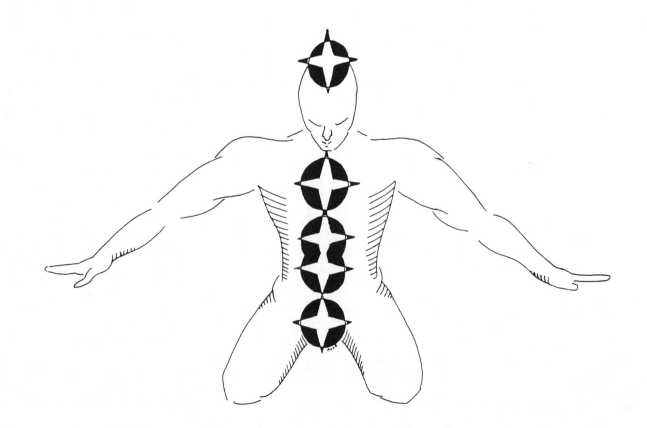

VI

The Growing Legitimacy of Holism

INTRODUCTION: *by Shepherd Bliss*

"To BE TRULY holistic, all parties must win: the business, the customer, the employees, the community, and the environment," says Carol Carpenter in the article which begins this section. She describes this holistic approach to business as "win-win." One of the major developments in holistic health in the 1980s has been its expansion into the business world—involving both major corporations and numerous smaller businesses. Corporate leaders are finding holistic health not only effective in terms of health, but also in terms of cost. As health-care costs have sky-rocketed, both individuals and businesses have had to explore creative alternatives. Linda Langan contributes an article on "Corporate Wellness: Wave of the Future." As director of Wellness Services at a major San Francisco Bay Area hospital, she has had ample hands-on experience of how such programs work. She reveals, "The areas typically included in a corporate program are exercise, smoking cessation, substance abuse, stress management, nutrition and safety practices."

Holistic Business:
How to Create Win-Win

Carol Carpenter

BECAUSE I am interested in holistic health, I had difficulty in coming to grips with the whole notion of doing business. To me, business dealings were the antithesis of holism. Business people seemed to be fueled by greed and self-serving interests, with little regard for the effect that their actions had on the other people involved or on the planet.

When I entered the holistic health field as a massage practitioner, and still later when I became the director of a holistic health training school, I had to come to grips with my feelings about business and learn how business and holism could interact. One day, after a distasteful negotiation for a possible new site for the school, I said to a friend of mine, "I am not going to do business this way. Where is consciousness in business?"

That question was the beginning of what has been a delightful journey of studying, practicing, and teaching a business methodology that I think is truly holistic. I call this methodology "win-win" because, to be truly holistic, all parties must win: the business, the customer, the employees, the community, and the environment.

Win-Win

The purpose of all business, including win-win business, is to make money. (For our purposes, barter is the equivalent of money, as long as the exchange is fair for all parties.) If we go into an activity without establishing its purpose as that of making money, then, by definition, it is not a business. It may be a hobby, a charity, or some other form of non-business, which we will not discuss here. What we are concerned with are those activities that are organized in such a way that the intended result is to make money.

However, a business can not be holistically sound unless it introduces the notion of "value added." The business must produce a product or service that is wanted and needed, and in the process the lives of everyone involved must be enhanced in some way.

Using this method to achieve the goal of making money

is what sets win-win business apart from win-lose, or lose-lose business. In win-win business everyone wins. And because value is added, money in the form of sales is the result.

A Model for Business

Once we understand that the underlying principle of win-win business is to be certain that everyone involved in the

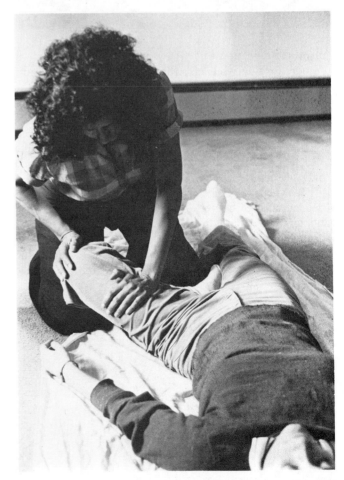

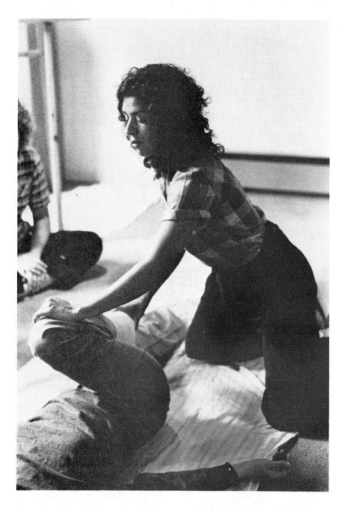

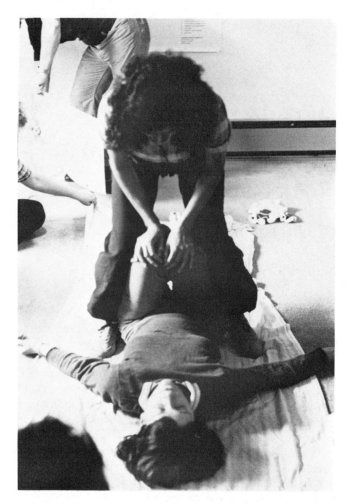

business transaction will have value added, we can look at a model for doing business that allows us to produce outstanding results for everyone. The model is based on the concept of synergy, which holds that the whole is greater than the sum of its parts. I know when my business is experiencing synergy because the results that are produced are beyond the ordinary. We're creating what looks like miracles to us. The results are greater than we imagined that they could be.

The synergy model can be thought of as a triangle with four levels. (See figure.) The niche is at the bottom level and this term stands for the business product or service through which the business adds value. In my own case, my niche was my massage service. Massage added value to my clients' lives, and I was rewarded for the service

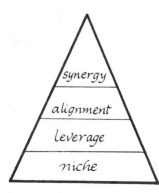

both financially and spiritually. When I became a school director, my niche became training others in massage.

When you define your own niche, I suggest that you choose something that you like so much that you would do it without pay. Before turning it into a business, practice until you are really good at it. In the meantime, keep your antennae out, researching whether your chosen niche is something that people want and need. Ask yourself, is there a market for it?

A number of people are satisfied at this level. In developing their niche, they have found something that they like to do, that adds value, and for which they are rewarded. They have a win-win one-person business. This was true for me both as a massage practitioner and as a beginning teacher of massage.

When I hired the school's first employee, however, I jumped to the second level of the business model, which this model calls leverage. You are leveraging yourself when you reproduce yourself or your activity in some way. In most cases, leveraging involves people. Each person in my school, from the head teacher to the person who cleans the school, is in some way a replication of me. I can, in effect, now be in more than one place at a time.

It is very important at this stage to be certain that everyone involved is united in the way they are doing business. Many businesses get into trouble at this point, when the group acts like a multi-headed monster, with all heads going off in different directions at once.

When we leverage with people, we move up to the third level, which is alignment. At this level, all of the people involved must be in complete agreement with regard to the business in order to avoid the multi-headed monster syndrome. Everyone must be clear and in agreement on how to do win-win business where value is added to everyone. They must understand and align on the purpose of the business, on what the product or service is that is adding value, and on the rules by which everyone is playing.

Alignment takes a lot of work. It is a very volatile state that organizations go in and out of easily. For me, it sometimes seemed that we were spending too much of our time trying to get everyone involved in alignment until I learned that some large companies like IBM spend approximately 25 percent of the company's time in planning and getting clarity. The Japanese businesses are masters at the alignment process by having the workers whose lives are affected by any decision or direction taken make the decisions in group meetings and set the direction. How many of us have worked in companies where decisions and policies are sent down from the top without having had any say or knowing any whys or wherefores?

When the group of people creating a business are in alignment, all is right with the world and miracles are happening. Work seems effortless, almost magical. Everyone involved thinks this place is the place to be, and to me it is worth all the time we spent hashing out ideas, goals, plans, and personalities.

How to Create Synergy Through Alignment

My organization has spent several years in working with this synergy model. We have learned something about what works. I would like to share with you some of the techniques that we use.

Three techniques that have made a big difference in the quality of our work lives are 1) clearly defining our purposes and goals, 2) learning how to make meetings work, and 3) establishing agreements by which we conduct ourselves at work.

Purpose and Goals

Any group should have an understanding of why it is coming together and what it expects to accomplish. This means that it needs to clearly state its purpose and short- and long-term goals.

The company's purpose is its guiding light. It is that which gets everyone up in the morning. The most inspiring kind of purpose is a lofty ideal that is not easily achievable. Our company's stated purpose is "personal and global transformation through professional training in holistic health practices, holistic education, and holistic business." We produce professional training in order to effect personal and global transformation. I am sure that you will agree that our purpose is lofty enough to keep us busy for years to come.

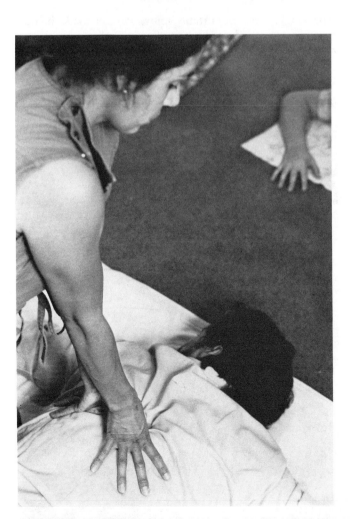

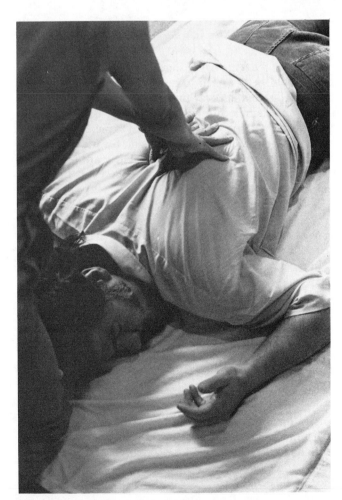

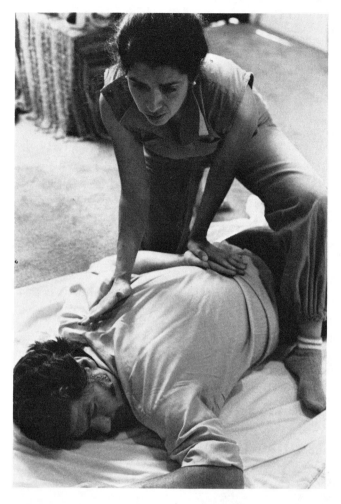

Goals, on the other hand, should be achievable, although they should be a stretch to meet. They should be measurable and stated in a way that allows us to tell if we reach them. An example of a measurable goal is "to increase enrollment by 30 percent," as opposed to merely, "increasing enrollment." Other goals that don't work as well are to "be happy," or "to enjoy work." These are nice ideas, but we have no way for everyone to see easily that the goal was indeed met.

Goals change as they are met, or as they are discarded or replaced with more appropriate goals. Purpose stays the same, unless the organization is willing to make a tremendous shift in its reason for existence.

In my organization both the purpose and the goals were established by the people in the group. We used meetings and the method outlined above to come to agreement on why we are together and what we want to accomplish by being here. Being involved in the creation of purpose is a powerful experience. That kind of involvement fuels people's participation and the energy generated contributes to the group achieving what it says it will do.

Making Meetings Work

Since most organizations spend upwards of 15 percent of their time in meetings, they should be effective. The best technique that I have found for conducting meetings is to use the interaction method. The interaction method, outlined in the book, *How to Make Meetings Work*, by Michael

Doyle and David Straus, suggests that you use a facilitator to conduct the meeting. The purpose of the facilitator is to be sure that everyone is heard, and not attacked or put down for his or her ideas. The facilitator also keeps the group on purpose so that people know that the meeting accomplished something worthwhile. The facilitator should be a person who has no vested interest in the issues of the meeting, so that he or she can orchestrate the meeting with no bias toward a particular outcome.

The interaction method makes use of "group memory," which is a record of the issues and possible solutions presented. The group memory is recorded on large paper pinned or taped to the wall in front of the group for all to see. This visible record of people's ideas allows everyone to participate freely with the certainty that their contribution was heard, recorded, and won't be forgotten. Our group uses colors, pictures, caricatures, and other fun and zany ways to have our group memory serve us and keep us awake and interested.

Meetings should create a safe space for people to really speak their minds with no fear of negative repercussions. The facilitator, and ultimately the boss, can insure this safety by reminding people that the meeting presents the opportunity to truly create miracles, but only by each person's full expression.

What Do You Feel Like Saying?

The single most important innovation we made in our meetings was the introduction of a process we call, "What do you feel like saying?" We start all of our gatherings this

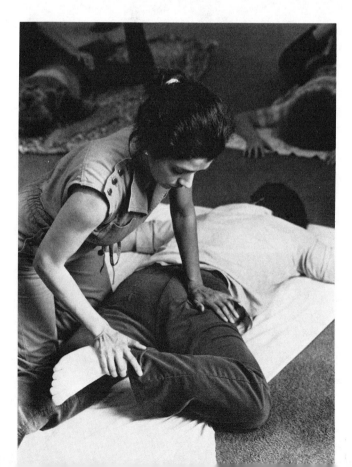

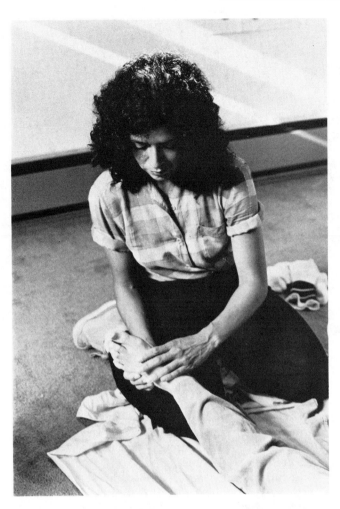

way, whether we are having a staff meeting or a two-person project work session.

The one rule in using this process is that everyone must agree to say nothing to the person speaking: no questions, comments, agreements. This rule insures that the person speaking says exactly what he or she wants to say without direction or inhibition from the group.

The purpose of "What do you feel like saying?" is three-fold. The first purpose is to allow everyone in the meeting to air anything that may be on his or her mind, whether or not it relates to the business or the meeting. The technique is especially useful if something is bothering the person whose turn it is to speak. For example, if the person was in a traffic jam on the way to the meeting, it is likely that his or her ability to contribute to the group will be impaired due to feelings of frustration or anxiety. By saying whatever he or she feels like saying, the participant can clear out feelings and get completion on that event, and be fully present for the job at hand.

This process also allows everyone in the group to perceive what state every other person is in. When each person speaks, and everyone else listens, an understanding and a rapport develop, so that the group can more easily get in sync with each other, which is a necessary condition of alignment. The group, then, has a better chance of accomplishing its goals for the meeting.

And thirdly, I have a notion that everyone likes to be heard, and to know that other people care about what they

have to say. Having an opportunity to say whatever I want to you creates a feeling in me that I am valuable to you and to the company.

Agreements, The Rules of the Game

It is important, I believe, to be clear about *how* we are going to work together. It would be very difficult to play any game without everyone knowing the rules and agreeing to play by them. In this game we call business we have some rules that we play by, which in our experience add to our ability to play well and to enjoy playing.

I believe that these agreements can work in any organization, and that they may even be useful in all relationships, work related or not.

Here are the agreements that we have established within our company.

1. Be willing to support our purpose, goals and agreements.
2. Speak supportively.

    We find that it is fairly easy to speak well of others. The more difficult challenge is to clean up how we refer to ourselves. For example, it is inappropriate to exclaim, "I am so stupid. Look at what I did!" because it is unsupportive to ourselves and others to call ourselves stupid. Also, we do not use profane language since, in our experience, profanity tends to muck up the atmosphere.

3. Acknowledge whatever is being communicated as true for the speaker at that moment.

    I may not like or agree with what you are saying, but acknowledging that it is true for you right now encourages me to listen to you, rather than to react to my beliefs about your statement. We can then speak to each other at a different level, and have a better chance of achieving true communication.

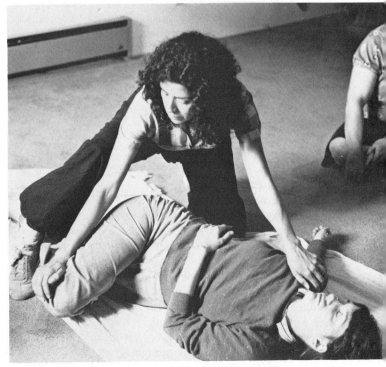

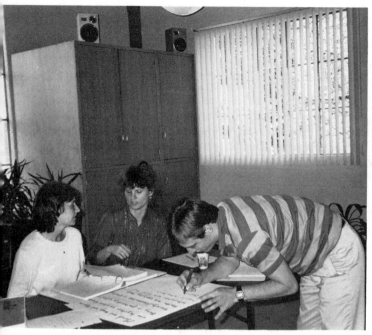

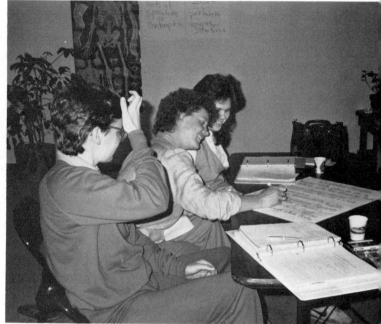

4. Tell the truth with compassion.

The truth is very powerful. When the truth is spoken, my entire being knows it. Share the truth with others, in a way that takes into account how it may be received by them at this time. It is important here not to sell out and refrain from saying what is true because you think that it will hurt someone's feelings. I know people are often grateful for having been told the truth. Almost everyone wants to learn about themselves and grow from their experiences.

5. Be accountable for your agreements.
   A. Make only agreements that you are willing and intend to keep.
   B. Communicate any potential broken agreement at the first appropriate time.
   C. Clear up any broken agreement at the first appropriate opportunity.

6. Be effective and efficient.

Effectiveness refers to doing the right thing. Efficiency is doing it the right way. So being effective and efficient will produce the best results while spending the least amount of time and energy.

7. If a problem arises, communicate it to the person who can do something about it.

This agreement is the best way to reduce griping and complaining about something that could be made to work.

8. Agree to agree.

Come to work with the mindset that we are going to agree, rather than having the work space be a place to express your negativity and resistance.

9. Have the willingness to win, and to allow others to win.

Have you known people who act as though there aren't enough good things out there for both of you to have some of them? They believe that if you have those good things, then they won't. A win-win attitude empowers all of us to do the very best we can, and to be rewarded for it. There is enough for everyone.

10. Focus on what works, and let go of what isn't working.

Pay attention to what gets results, and don't let old habits or tradition waste our valuable time and resources.

11. Be clear about your role in the organization, the contribution that you intend to make, and what you intend to create for yourself through your involvement.

12. Be present and on time.

It amazes me that we set up elaborate systems which actually reward people for not coming to work. A nurse who was a student at the Institute described how she actually made more money by taking sick leave since taxes were not deducted from sick pay.

In an organixation where all people are valued, and where their contribution is a real contribution to the whole, people cannot feel justified in not being there.

The same is true for time. Often people think 9 o'clock means 9:10. Those ten minutes lost could have made a difference in the integrity and the quality in our worklife. In our organization we do not hold a scheduled meeting if one person is absent. And, for the most part, people are on time. It makes a big difference.

Establishing your purpose and goals, using meeting time well, and having workable, supportive agreements create the condition for synergy, or outrageous results, to occur. Be prepared to hold onto your hat!

In *The Seven Laws of Money*, Michael Phillips states that if you are doing the right thing, money will come. By having found a niche that I would engage in without pay, leveraging it with people who are willing and able to play at a high level, and making a committment to staying in alignment with integrity has brought me much more than the money I set out to earn. It has added value to my life in ways that I did not foresee. Working in an organiztion that has such high ideals has contributed more to my personal growth, satisfaction, and self expression than anything I have ever done before. My own prosperity is only one indicator.

On the issue of prosperity, I would like to share something that was of great help to me. I had difficulty with the notion of taking money for my services. I wanted to be a good person with a strong spiritual influence, and it seemed to me that spiritual people should not have money. Then I read an article about Robert Schwartz and his Tarrytown, New York, group, in which the author asserted that spiritual people are precisely the people who deserve money. A spiritual person will earn money in a way that is in harmony with the universal principles and will spend it in the same way.

This view of the matter helped me resolve my ambivalent feeling about the seeming conflict between holism and business. I now believe that holism has much to offer a business in the process of becoming more effective, more efficient, and more nurturing.

Much success and prosperity to you!

Suggestions for Further Reading

Cole-Whitaker, Terry. *How To Have More In A Have-Not World.* N.Y., N.Y.: Rawson Associates, 1983.

Doyle, Michael and Straus, David. *How To Make Meetings Work.* Chicago, Illinois: Playboy Press, 1976.

Ferguson, Marilyn. *Aquarian Conspiracy.* Boston, Massachusetts: Houghton Mifflin Company, 1980.

Fuller, Buckminster. *Critical Path.* N.Y., N.Y.: St. Martins, 1982.

Kamoroff, Bernard, C.P.A. *Small-Time Operator.* Laytonville, California: Bell Springs Publishing, 1983.

Naisbitt, John. *Megatrends.* N.Y., N.Y.: Warner Books, 1982.

Ouchi, William. *Theory Z.* Reading, Massachusetts: Addison-Wesley Publishing Company, 1981.

Peters, Thomas. J. and Waterman, Robert H. Jr. *In Search of Excellence.* N.Y., N.Y. Harper and Row, Publishers, 1982.

Phillips, Michael. *The Seven Laws of Money.* Menlo Park, California: Word Wheel and Random House, 1974.

Phillips, Michael and Rasberry, Salli. *Honest Business.* N.Y., N.Y. Random House, 1981.

Tarrytown Newsletter. Tarrytown, New York: Published by the Tarrytown Group, 1983.

Toffler, Alvin. *The Third Wave.* N.Y., N.Y.: Bantam Books, 1980.

Seminars

Thurber, Marshal. Money and You. Burklyn Business School. La Jolla, California.

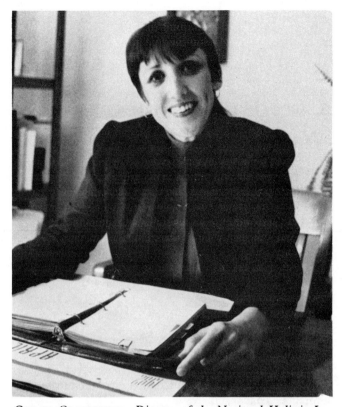

CAROL CARPENTER, *Director of the National Holistic Institute, received a B.A. in psychology from the University of North Carolina and is a graduate of Burklyn Business School. For many years she worked as a bodywork therapist on the East coast before coming to California to pursue the field more fully, and to dedicate her energies to educating others in the area of holistic health. She teaches seminars and workshops for small business people while also acting as a consultant for people who are setting up holistic practices. Ms. Carpenter is an acknowledged speaker and presenter of humanistic of "win-win" business practices.*

The National Holistic Institute, located in Oakland, California was founded in 1977. NHI trains people for careers in holistic health and wellness. The Institute conducts certification training in massage in 11-week or intensive 11-day formats. Advanced training as a certified Holistic Health Practitioner Educator is 1–2 years in length and includes state-of-the-art information in nutrition, stress management, fitness, business, and advanced bodywork. NHI's purpose is to transform life-style and health attitudes and to increase individual and community well-being.

Corporate Wellness: Wave of the Future

Linda Langan, M.P.H.

T O PREDICT that health care services in the next decade will be purchased and delivered in ways dramatically different than they are today is not just a forecast of the future, but a foregone conclusion.

A number of factors are creating more intense competition among health care providers and also leading to new kinds of provider-consumer relationships. These factors include rising costs, changing reimbursement patterns, an increased number of providers, and new or alternative settings for the delivery of health care services. Partnerships between hospitals and business for health care services will become commonplace.

Moving from the traditionally passive seller's market to the highly competitive buyer's market of the future will be difficult for many hospitals, since that transition requires the ability to manage and administer health services for large groups, rather than for individuals. In the evolving marketplace, the hospital of the future will need the ability to develop effective and comprehensive health risk management programs, and deliver cost effective medical care services to business and industry.

The realization that something has to be done to stem the rising tide of health care costs is not new. Medical care in the United States represents almost ten percent of the gross national product—an expenditure of some $325 billion each year. Business and industry pay half this staggering bill. In 1980, health insurance premiums alone consumed five percent of the total gross payroll, and represented an average yearly expenditure of $820 per employee. And this figure continues to climb.

Corporate medical care expenditures include both direct medical care costs and indirect costs, such as those related to absenteeism, substandard performance, employee replacement, training and non-productive time.

Understandably, corporations are alarmed and are looking for solutions to their health care bills. A one percent savings to a large corporation translates into a substantial sum of money. As "informed consumers," corporations have the ability to interject free market economics into the health care system. Corporations are already involved in some innovative insurance plans which promote more appropriate individual utilization of health services. Hospital utilization review boards, regional health planning, negotiated rate setting, employee assistance programs and business coalitions are additional examples of corporate involvement.

Despite these measures, corporations are having to face the grim fact that their astronomical expenditures are not resulting in a healthier, more productive employee. Nor do they help address the critical issues of turnover, absenteeism or recruitment costs.

An employee wellness program is a viable cost-containment strategy. It is now generally acknowledged that the worksite has a major impact on the health of employees, and in turn, on the health care costs of the corporation. A comprehensive health promotion program can make an impact on employee health, and subsequently, corporate health care expenditures. By the same token, wellness programs offer a new perspective for the health care provider. Historically, the major focus of medical care has been on the *individual*, the patient who needs to be cured of a disease. It has not been on the prevention of disease or the promotion of a healthy lifestyle.

In fact, less than two percent of current health expenditures are devoted to disease prevention, yet one-half of all current diseases are related to individual lifestyles and thus, are potentially preventable. Consider this: an employee works eight hours a day, often in a sedentary job. During the course of the day, he or she tends to drink too much coffee, eat too much junk food, smoke too many cigarettes, and ineffectively handle the stress created by work-related problems and relationships. Today, many cor-

Linda Langan, M.P.H., "Corporate Wellness: Wave Of The Future." *Bay City Business Journal*, April, 1984, Vol. 2, No. 9, p. 25.

porate executives are concerned about employee's lifestyles and health. The costs related to poor employee health is motivating that concern.

A study conducted by the Center for Disease Control revealed that lifestyle-related diseases result in the highest percentage of deaths for those under age 65. Experts now agree that chronic lifestyle-related diseases are best addressed through preventative medicine and health promotion. For example, smoking is related to cardiac, vascular, and respiratory disease, and twenty percent of all cancers. It is estimated that the average pack-a-day smoker costs industry a minimum of $625 per employee each year. These costs are related to increased medical expenses, and to an absenteeism rate some forty to fifty percent greater than non-smokers. The goal of corporate wellness programs is to have a positive impact on employee lifestyle habits.

The areas typically included in a corporate program are exercise, smoking cessation, substance abuse, stress management, nutrition and safety practices.

Many organizations are under the impression that a properly motivated individual can make a permanent, positive behavior change without outside help. However, it is becoming increasingly clear that permanent behavior changes require the motivational impetus of the employee *and* the organization. The organization's environment directly affects employee health.

Let's consider the individual who is initially successful with his decision to quit smoking. He returns to the working setting where he is surrounded by smokers who may not be helpful or supportive. The organization supports the negative behavior of smoking with cigarette vending machines and smoking lounges. The organization's norm then appears to be at odds with the individual's efforts to quit smoking. The individual finds himself trying to "buck the system," and the organization in effect undermines its very efforts to contain costs.

Other effective aspects of an employee wellness program include an employee assistance program and a risk-screening component. Statistically ten percent of all employees have serious personal problems; the most common of these are alcohol-related. An alcohol abuser's use of health insurance is three times higher than that of a non-alcoholic employee. Industry's cost for alcoholism is estimated at $51 billion a year. Employee assistance programs can first identify the employees in need, and then aid them in dealing with the problem while saving substantial health care dollars.

A screening component to identify prevalent risk factors in the employee population can also have a positive impact on the "bottom line." Heart disease, cancer and accidents are the leading causes of employment-age death today. These conditions account for nearly 75% of the total deaths and, are logical targets for wellness or health promotion efforts.

The development of these conditions has been linked to the presence of several "risk facors." Most of these risks are lifestyle-related: smoking, high cholesterol levels, obes-

ity. High risk individuals account for forty to sixty percent of all corporate spending. Intervention programs can help individuals change negative habits to reduce risk factors, and significantly lower corporate medical spending. It is estimated that if only twenty-five out of every one-hundred high risk individuals significantly reduce these factors, the cost of corporate medical care could be reduced by ten to fifteen percent.

Also important to a corporation considering a wellness program is that it grows out of the company's specific needs. Since each company is different, each has unique employee health needs and interests. It would not be cost-effective for a corporation to develop a wellness program that failed to meet their unique needs or contained unnecessary components. A comprehensive analysis done prior to program development can prevent these failings.

A number of corporations across the country have developed wellness programs for their employees and are claiming substantial savings. However, the corporation seriously considering such a program should realize that a quick return on the investment is probably unrealistic. A wellness program should be viewed as a *long-term* investment whose eventual financial return could be substantial.

When contemplating the implementation of a wellness program, it should be remembered that the employees represent the corporation's greatest asset. A real contributing factor to a corporation's profit/loss statement, the health of employees directly impacts the value of their contributions to corporate activity, productivity, and profit margin.

Suggestions for Further Reading

Berry, Charles A., M.D., "Health Cost Saving: An Approach to Good Health For Employees and Reduced Health Care Costs for Industry," *Health Insurance Association of America*.

"Cashing In On Wellness," *Business Insurance*, September 21, 1981.

Laughlin, Judith A., R.N., Ph.D., "Wellness at Work: A Seven-Step 'Dollars and Sense' Approach," *Occupational Health Nursing*, November, 1982, pg. 9–13.

Levine, Art, "American Business is Bullish on 'Wellness'," *Medical World News*, March 29, 1982.

"Make Cancer Control Your Business," N.Y.: *American Cancer Society*, 1981.

LINDA LANGAN, *M.S., M.P.H., has 14 years of experience in health, first in clinical research and later in community health. Her areas of expertise include senior health care services, community and corporate health education and hospital and corporate employee health promotion programming. Linda is currently Director of Wellness Services for John Muir Memorial Hospital in Walnut Creek, California, where she is responsible for the planning, development, marketing and implementation of corporate health care cost-containment strategies and programming and for individual and community wellness programs.*

The Health Care Contract:
A Model for Sharing Responsibility

Jerry A. Green, J.D.

This article summarizes the scientific assumptions of medicine and holistic practice as a basis for clarifying the professional responsibilities of health practitioners. The basic elements of contracting are then applied to the dynamics of clinical relationships, creating a mutually defined plan as framework for allocating responsibility among doctors, patients, holistic practitioners and clients. The legal aspects of health contracts are discussed and it is suggested how contract principles may be tools for sharing responsibility.

- *How does one define one's roles and responsibilities in health care?*
- *What can health professionals and individuals do to share responsibility for making their relationship work?*
- *How can health care relationships be created which satisfy both practitioners' and clients' interests and needs?*
- *How does one sort out the many different services being offered by health practitioners?*

MY RESEARCH of medical malpractice cases began in 1972 with the curiosity to explore a suspicion that the holistic perspective may have something to do with the solution to our crisis in medicine. I learned that many malpractice cases were generated by unfulfilled expectations about the role of the doctor. I postulate that by clarifying the responsibilities of both the doctor and the patient, a framework can be developed in which each party can discover the dynamics of a successful working relationship. This is the process of contracting.

The problems generated by not making clear agreements in medicine start when practitioners assume more professional responsibility than what medical science is designed to deal with. It is unnecessary for doctors and hospitals to assume more responsibility than diagnosing and treating pathology. Their failure to define their roles in a manner

limited to their scientific purpose makes the identification of patient responsibility difficult. Health professionals should assist individuals to go beyond the banner of "self-responsibility" as a simple admonition by helping them construct a plan for their action.

Contracting in health care relationships should not be approached as a legal issue. The process of developing contracts is primarily an educational tool. The terms and conditions of a contract create a framework within which practitioners and clients work together. Contracting enables us to define individual goals, purposes, preferences and expectations, and choices as well as explicitly allocate responsibility for decision making to the appropriate person.

Nobody Can Give Us Freedom of Choice

Many people involved in today's health renaissance seem to be clamoring over the issue of freedom of choice in health care. They feel that the prime strategy for creating a more responsive health care system is through legislative modifications amending current civil and criminal codes that govern the practice of medicine. Their premise is that the medical professions and the law deny the individual's freedom of choice. They fail to realize, however, that our freedom of choice is one of those inalienable rights that courts have difficulty recognizing precisely because the source of this freedom is fundamental to our social nature. Freedom of choice in the marketplace is one of these inalienable rights. The law does not prohibit people from choosing any health practice. It only defines what certain services can be provided by licensed practitioners.

However, the legislative process can encourage freer choice among health care systems by requiring full and fair disclosure by medical and health practitioners and requiring ethical standards for all kinds of practitioners. More importantly, the legislature can encourage and support broad health education programs.

The only risk to our freedom of choice in health care is our failure to exercise that right. It is through the exercise of our fundamental rights that we recognize their nature and protect them from abuse. Making an agreement is the way we recognize our rights regarding any matter and assume the obligations necessary to enjoy them. This is how responsibility as a concept is transformed into action. Agreements are thought-out opportunities for taking responsibility.

A Process, Not a Product

The first task is to clarify needs for pathological services and distinguish them from desire for health promotion and holistic health service. Many problems are generated by classifying holistic perspectives as diagnosis or treatment of pathology. Physicians risk professional censure and civil liability for violating standards or practice when holistic services are thought of as alternative treatments.

Consider whether holistic practices are really alternative treatments. Clarifying their nature will enable individuals to make more meaningful contracts utilizing them. History provides a good place to start exploring the assumptions in which our health care relationships are rooted.

Holistic Practices are Schools of Thought, Not Just Alternative Treatments

What is commonly understood as "alternative treatments," "techniques," "practices," or "systems," I would call *schools of thought*. These schools are simply names that are given to the process of study by which people associate with certain teachers. The holistic perspective provides a *point of view* from which to evaluate all of the elements of the personal health plan and the plans made with health professionals.

Two Traditions of Scientific Inquiry

Schools of thought are fundamentally historical phenomena. In three volumes entitled *Divided Legacy*, medical historian Harris Coulter (1975) has documented the history of conflicts between the two predominant traditions of thought.

Coulter guides us in examining a fundamental vocabulary of scientific assumptions that will help clarify roles and responsibilities in health care. These assumptions have been visible in medical thought and practice for 2000 years and are more apparent than ever today.

Coulter observed that the most significant contributions to medicine were made by the purest thinkers of either school. Practicing physicians have drawn upon both viewpoints, taking information which most suited their interests, skills, and abilities. By understanding the scope of this spectrum, the nature of skills or services can be determined that suit one's needs and desires at any particular point in time. This dipolar conceptual framework also offers a basis for clarifying the relationships between medicine and holistic practice. It will also reduce the kinds of misunderstandings which lead to malpractice litigation. Granted, some malpractice cases are clearly actual physician errors (sponges remaining inside surgical patients, or patients with ruptured appendices being treated for gas pains, for example). Other cases may arise from the failure of a physician to disclose vital information about risks to the patient and subsequently leading to the patient's suffering consequences from a treatment which had risks the patient did not expect or consent to. However, most medical malpractice cases suggest that a fundamental misunderstanding of the allocation of responsibility between doctor and patient could be clarified by making contracts which identify medical responsibility in terms of diagnosis and treatment of pathology, (Green, 1976). This framework will also encourage new professional roles to emerged in a meaningful way.

Assumptions of Empirical and Rational Traditions

Coulter (1975) notes that the Empirical tradition considered observation and experience to be the only source of knowledge, while the Rational tradition placed a premium on logical analysis. The Rationalists relied upon hypotheses to give structure to experimentation and research in order to focus on cause and effect. Empirics were not interested in causation. They sought to stimulate the growth or balance of the "life force," which they confessed inability to explain and even questioned whether its dynamics were

SCIENTIFIC ASSUMPTIONS OF THE EMPIRICAL AND RATIONAL SCHOOLS OF HEALTH AND HEALING

Empirical School		Rational School
Observation and experience are source of knowledge	**Premise**	Logical analysis is the source of knowledge
Studies growth or balance of "life force" or vital energy	**Object**	Studies disease entities
Workings of life force unknowable	**Hypothesis**	Established hypothesis of causation
Studies peculiar symptoms to determine uniqueness of individual	**Subject**	Classified common symptoms into disease entities
Subjective sources of data	**Source**	Objective sources of data
Individual is energetic and has a spiritual dimension	**Nature**	Individual is material or mechanistic, chemical
Treatment by similars sometimes creating healing crisis	**Treatment** (or treatment approach)	Treatment by contraries sought removal of symptoms
Health is internal and environmental balance	**Context**	Health is absence of disease
Holistic Methodology	**Methodology**	Atomistic or reductionistic methodology
Client	**Authority**	Doctor

knowable by man. The Rational tradition evolved the concept of the disease entity (pathological condition), which was arrived at by identifying "common symptoms" in a class of patients. The Empirics said that the "peculiar symptoms" were the most important ones because they indicated the uniqueness of the individual. These peculiar symptoms suggested the basis for selecting a remedy or therapy which acted on the whole person rather than just on the disease. Rationalists sought to eliminate the disease and its symptoms usually by treating with *contraries*, attempting to stop the symptoms. Empirics saw symptoms as manifestations of the healing process. They offered treatments *similar* to the symptoms, often generating an aggravation of symptoms perceived as a healing crisis. From the Empiric viewpoint, cure lay in the pattern of change in the symptoms, not just their palliation or amelioration.

The Rational physicians took an atomistic or reductionistic view, focusing upon progressively smaller components. They evolved a rather mechanical concern for the efficient workings of the various body parts. Empirics emphasized the relatedness of mind, body and emotions and could be described as being more concerned with energetics than mechanics. For example, homeopathy and Chinese medicine are Empirical sciences. The use of antibiotics for infections is based in Rational Science.

Examining the assumptions of the two traditions in medical philosophy leads to the following comparisons. (Figure 1).

Pathology and Holistic Practice

In the past century, medical thinking has been so dominated by the Rational tradition that its practice is legally defined in terms of the diagnosis and treatment of pathological conditions (Note 1).

Standards of practice have almost completely forced Empirical practices out of the profession by labeling them as unscientific. Rational medicine's success is marked by a current Webster's definition of Empiricism as "unscientific" and "quackery," while Coulter's work indicated that Empirical science simply proceeds on the basis of different assumptions. He suggests that a "science" is fundamentally a methodology for collecting information.

If today's holistic practices are viewed in Empirical terms as a means of nourishing the life force (which is not prohibited by §2052) a framework can be constructed for understanding the relationship between responsibilities of holistic practitioners and physicians.

Since the early 1900's when the Flexner Report determined teaching Empirical practices to be unscientific, medical education in the United States has focused on and

Note 1: The California Medical Practices Act, Section 2052 of the Business and Professions Code, states: "Any person who practices or attempts to practice, or who advertises or holds himself out as practicing, any system or mode of treating the sick or afflicted in this state, or who diagnoses, treats, operates for, or prescribes for any ailment, blemish, deformity, disease, disfigurement, disorder, injury, or other mental or physical condition of any person, without having at the time of so doing a valid, unrevoked certificate as provided in this chapter, or without being authorized to perform such act pursuant to a certificate obtained in accordance with other provision of law, is guilty of a misdemeanor."

is dominated by the diagnosis and treatment of pathological conditions. Health is viewed in this pathology model as the absence of disease, and not (as "holistic" practitioners would say) entire in its own right and incorporating the human environment. Thus the tools at the physician's disposal are diagnosis and treatment tools, not "growth and prevention" tools. The physician, in our society, sees the sick in the professional setting, and rarely the healthy.

Today's physicians are practitioners of the Rational tradition. Their science has evolved to a degree of specialization and clarity worthy of respect and admiration, but should not be confused with attempts to stimulate and nourish the growth balance of the life force. The Rational posture of medical education makes it difficult for the best physicians to practice Empirical perspectives, as their training is dominated by the pathology model. Physicians who have approached the mastery of any holistic practice tend to go through a long and painful struggle attempting to fit new information into familiar analysis and thought forms.

Dissecting Medical Responsibility

Physicians often play the role of sympathetic ear, father figure, information source or confidant. If the client's purpose in talking to a doctor is any of the above, have them state it at the outset. However, if they want to hire a doctor for what he is trained to do, it is helpful to think about the specific skills for which they are well trained.

Why People Seek Health Professionals

Professional responsibilities in health care realtionships may include:

1) Diagnosis of a pathological condition.
2) Treatment of a pathological condition.
3) Monitor changes in a pathological condition.
4) Watch for the development of a latent or potential pathological condition.
5) Advise regarding likely outcome or prognosis.
6) Nourish or balance the life force/vital energy.

Only the first five are exclusively reserved to licensed doctors.

Other responsibilities, frequently assumed by health professionals, though not always necessary to the performance of their professional responsibility, include:

1) Being someone to talk to.
2) Providing sympathy.
3) Being an authority figure.
4) Providing moral or emotional support.
5) Making decisions for clients.
6) Providing information to clients concerning health and/or pathology.

The first skill is diagnosis. Does the client manifest any set of symptoms which puts him in a recognized class of patients associated with a recognized disease? What does medicine know about this disease, its course and consequence? Another skill is providing information about or performing the accepted treatment for this disease. A third skill is the ability to monitor a disease during self-healing. This skill is particularly valuable in holistic health, because vital energies may be restored to a point where a regular prescription for medical treatment becomes an overdose in cases where holistic practitioners are working in conjunction with medical practitioners.

If physicians are offering holistic practices, understand that the medical training did not prepare them for this work. Learn about their training and ability to provide this service. Recognize that many "holistic doctors" apply holistic practice as alternative treatments for pathology. Competency may be sacrificed by trying to get both kinds of services from the same person.

One should consider making separate plans that address both concerns about pathology and the stimulation of the body's self-healing abilities/mechanisms. This will help demystify medicine and give some perspective on clarifying expectations with physicians. Treat the issues separately, especially when both kinds of services are sought from a "holistic physician."

A plan to satisfy *concern* about pathology may not require seeing a physician. It may be appropriate, though, to plan to see a doctor when the client's concern about pathology reaches a certain level. Diagnostic services may be retained without contracting for treatment.

How Do We Recognize Expressions of Vital Energy

The purpose of a plan to obtain holistic health services in the Empiric tradition should relate to changes of the following kind: (Not an all-inclusive list.)

Pain	Creativity
Physical balance	Self esteem
Behavior patterns	Energy level
Tension patterns	Mental clarity
Breathing patterns	Spontaneity
Patterns of emotional expression	Centeredness
Ability to become calm	Spirit

Government programs to nourish the vital energy should be developed that are distinct from current programs aimed at treatment of diseases (National Cancer Institute, Center for Disease Prevention and Control, etc.).

Defining Professional Responsibility in Holistic Practice

Methodical thinking about the roles of holistic practitioners has not yet begun in earnest. If holistic work is to be appreciated as distinct from and complementary to medical practice, discovering the differences between the two is necessary to structuring relationships with holistic practitioners more precisely. This delineation will also moderate the possessiveness over perceived professional territory. What kinds of agreements are appropriate to nourishing vital energy (Note 2.) The purpose of making

plans with holistic practitioners should relate to how these practitioners perceive and work with vital energy. Satisfaction in the relationship will depend on how well a practitioner's skill lines up with a client's interests. Suggest to the client that they examine how they experience their own vital energy when they are defining their objectives.

Each person is unique; individual interests will lead to the right practitioner for any given moment. Each individual has his or her own sequence for exploring different paths of growth. Learning to perceive and follow this inner sense of timing is an important part of understanding what healing really is about.

Remember that holistic perspectives may promote an aggravation of experiences which are seen as symptoms of pathology by the Rational medical tradition. These experiences can sometimes be expressions of healing.

Plans with holistic practitioners should include discussions about healing crises. Anticipate that working from this perspective may entail feeling worse before getting better. Also, consider that Empirical means of healing tend to work more slowly than the remedies of Rational medicine.

Examples of Means by Which We Can Nourish, Stimulate or Balance Vital Energy

Love	Homeopathic remedies
Touch	Colors
Suggestion	Fasting
Meditation	Harmonic sounds
Awareness training	Herbal cleansing
Nutritional changes	Colonic irrigation
Emotional expression	The essence of flowers
Spiritual fulfillment	Acupuncture
(Not an all-inclusive list).	

The Use of Written Instruments

Contracts with health professionals need not be in writing. They could be written down, but they must be negotiated verbally. They need not be written up as "contract." Written notes of either party are legal evidence of the agreement. Professional records and correspondence between the parties can also evidence the agreement. Written instruments should contain as much information as is deemed necessary by both practitioner and client and should acknowledge risks, if any, of procedures which are experimental. Attractive brochures given to the client may describe the practice and the practitioners' experience. Written instruments can and should outline the patient's rights and responsibilities. At the bottom line, however, the best evidence is always the conduct of the parties.

Elements of a Contract

A contract is an agreement between two people about the essential elements of a plan to do a job. The best contracts are the simplest plans. Three basic elements of a contract are: (a) purpose, (b) complementary responsibilities, and (c) term. The first element explains what the job is. The second says what each person may be expected to do. The

Note 2: Hereafter, "vital energy" is used to suggest the current thinking about what has been referred to historically as the "life force."

third defines the time frame in which the job is planned. Defining a term provides an opportunity to modify or renew the agreement.

Access to and Ownership of Medical/Health Records

Client/patient access to medical/health records is an unsettled question, legally. The client/patient has a right to the information, but the practitioner or facility owns the document. Access to records is a negotiable issue. Make an agreement about the availability of records at the outset. All parties can then rely on the agreement in the future. Making these agreements will create the right which courts are now only beginning to examine. Arbitration agreements are becoming widespread in the medical profession. Typically, they are not explained to the patients in any way, but are handed with a bundle of other papers to the patients who are told to sign them before the doctor will see them. Patients do not realize they are waiving substantial legal rights, such as the right to a jury trial.

Self-Awareness Journal

Personal journal entries are valuable not only as evidence of the agreement between the client and the practitioner, but as tools for focusing awareness, an essential element of Empirical health practices. Change in self awareness is a manifestation of the growth of the life force. Self awareness journal keeping is an aid in working with all Empirical practitioners. For example, homeopathic case-taking records impressions in the patient's exact words, relying totally on the subjective experience.

Arbitration

Written agreements may be used to substitute arbitration for litigation as the process for settling disputes. Arbitration agreements are the first expression of contract thinking in health relations. Unfortunately, they deal with only one issue; the choice of forum for resolving disputes. They do nothing to suggest how to make the relationship work. They focus attention upon both party's anticipation of failure. If arbitration is the desired choice of the parties, agreement upon this issue should be seen in the context of agreement on the responsibilities that are necessary to making the relationship succeed.

Beware of Disclaimers

Watch out for written statements purporting to be disclaimers or waivers of liability. They are usually unnecessary and may be used to argue knowledge of unlawful intent. They are likely to be disregarded by courts as being against public policy unless they appear in the larger context of a well defined relationship. When the relationship is called into question, it will be judged by what the parties do, not by what they say they are doing.

On the other hand, written answers to questions concerning elements of progress in the relationship are statements about the nature of the work being done. A questionnaire about body awareness would read quite differently than a history of symptoms, though both provide a valuable clinical focus for their respective practitioners.

The Legal Authority for Contract in Health Relationships

The idea of contracting individual responsibilities in health care relationships is relatively new, historically speaking. University of Chicago Law Professor Richard Epstein (1977) has laid the foundation for legislative and judicial acceptance of medical contracts in two articles which describe the natural evolution toward contract-thinking in other fields. He shows how other fields of law have progressed to where principles of contract govern risks which have previously been decided by principles of common law negligence.

Court-made law on health contracts will not appear until courts examine controversies in which the parties have made contracts. The courts will evolve doctrines of contract as they decide these cases. The Dana Ullman Case (1977) was the first judicial recognition of health contracts. There, the district attorney and the trial court recognized "a regular practice of contracting with clients in order to clarify the role of non-medical health practitioner" as a basis for dismissing criminal charges for practicing medicine without a license. However, other courts are not bound by this settlement because the case was dismissed without trial. Consequently, there was no issue for the appellate courts and appellate courts possess the exclusive power to bind other courts.

The judicial recognition of contracts defining professional responsibility will require a test case. Eventually, there will be many cases in which the issue will be recognized because the court will not be so interested in the question of contract as in deciding which party should prevail in a dispute over the contract. However, both the test case and those that follow will be those in which the parties failed to make *clear* agreements and consequently generated a dispute. Most legal problems start this way.

Since provider-client agreements are an evolutionary step in health care relations, courts will assess the validity of such contracts on an individual basis. The principle factor in deciding to uphold such agreements will be their reasonableness, given the likely disparity in apparent bargaining power created by professional comprehension and client need. Disclosure of information which is known or should be known to the practitioner will be a crucial element in evaluating the reasonableness of the circumstances. All contracts are vulnerable to attack on the grounds that the parties failed to achieve a meeting of the minds about issues fundamental to their agreement. If the making of agreements is undertaken as clarification of the planning process and its purpose is to further the working relationship, then it will increase the likelihood of achieving expectations. The making of agreements will minimize the risk of misunderstandings which can lead to failure in the relationship and disputes over responsibility. The thoughtfulness with which agreements are made will be the bottom line in determining whether the agreement will withstand a challenge to its validity.

Since health care relationships are fundamentally contractual in nature (their terms are *implied* when they are not expressly defined), there is really no avoiding the issue. Either good agreements are made or some kind of trouble and dispute ensues.

Financial Responsibility

The means of payment is an essential element of agreements. Questions about payment for holistic services by MediCal and other third-party sources (Medi-care, private insurance companies) are only beginning to surface. Perhaps it is only American to focus on financial responsibility before exploring working responsibilities very thoroughly. Requesting payment for holistic services through our current MediCal (California) system requires describing the work as diagnosis or treatment for some specific pathology. If the State is told this, is the patient's view of themselves set into pathological terms as well? And what model is the doctor working in?

The incidence of disease and the cost of medical treatment form an actuarial basis for insurance companies to determine their income (your premiums), expenditures and reimbursement schedules. In the end, less money may be spent on treating disease if more is spent on promoting health. However, the functional relationships between medicine and holistic practice should be examined more fully before compensation schemes or government regulation are further developed. Meaningful policy changes will then become apparent.

Planning for Health

Before establishing a relationship with a health care practitioner, clients should decide their purpose and time frame on their own, understanding that they may change as needs change and as more is learned. In order to make this first plan, and before seeking professional advice, clients should answer the following questions:

1. How do you experience your self now?
2. What changes do you feel might be considered?
3. What might you ask a health educator or counselor to help you clarify your needs?
4. How can these changes be brought about without the assistance of a health practitioner?
5. What do you want from a physician or other health practitioner?
6. How and when might you evaluate your progress and consider redefining your purpose?
7. How much time and money do you wish to commit to this job?

Having a plan with oneself assists in shopping for services that help implement the plan. This will involve making new plans with others who are the resources for the fulfillment of the plan. Clients should be prepared for negotiation, collaboration and further clarification of their goals.

Make Any Simple Plan

When it comes to making an agreement, discuss any plan which increases the likelihood of achieving your client's purpose. Make it simple at first. The plan can always be changed. Whatever the plan, it will acquaint everyone with the process of clarifying implied expectations by making expressed agreements. Where achieving a working agreement fails, expectations will have been uncovered which would likely have led to disappointment later had they remained implicit.

Misunderstandings About Holistic Health Practices

Currently, there is widespread misunderstanding about the fundamental nature of holistic practice. Does each practice constitute a separate technique or system of healing? Is it the client's job to find out which technique will work or which practitioner knows the most techniques? These questions represent only the tip of the iceberg.

There are many reasons why one might seek the services of a physician or health practitioner. In addition, every health professional has his or her own unique skills and abilities. Individual responsibility for health includes being responsible for obtaining quality health care. Making clear agreements is necessary for getting this or any job done.

Clients Should Have a Purpose in Mind When Choosing a Health Practitioner

By interviewing health practitioners concerning a specific purpose before engaging their services, clients can learn about the practitioner's willingness and ability to satisfy that purpose. The objective in the interview should be to reach an agreement on the basic elements of a plan that will define complementary responsibilities and assist in fulfilling the client's purpose. For example, if a client's primary purpose is to recover from a back injury, their plan may include seeking the services of a doctor to diagnose any tissue damage and offer advice about available medical treatments. The client may also want to learn to reverse patterns of accumulating tension from a holistic practitioner.

The initial interview with a health professional should be approached as if an agent were to be hired to help implement a plan. The client's job in the interview is to learn what unique skills the practitioner has that can help fulfill the client's purpose, what the practitioner can be relied on for, and what is necessary to work with that person. These complementary responsibilities must be negotiated because they are interdependent. Also, making an agreement with a health professional is distinct from the process of looking for someone to work with. Shopping around, seeing at least two people, will help develop clarity on the client's basic plan.

Where is the Power to Make Change?

Until now, most of my work with contract principles has been solving legal problems generated by the failure to make clear agreements. The greatest value of thinking contractually about health is that it helps identify responsibility. This enables the responsibilities of evolving nonmedical roles to be examined and defined more clearly.

The Rational model of pathology has been the only context within which we have thought about health in the past century. We are unaccustomed to thinking about nourishing the "life force," let alone taking seriously those who attempt to address this challenge scientifically. Coulter demonstrates that while there has been little public recognition of Empirical concepts in the Western world, some doctors have explored Empirical premises for years, attesting to their value while fighting a losing battle for recognition within their profession. Understanding the distinctions between the Rational and Empirical assumptions will permit appreciation of both perspectives and their practices.

The holistic health movement is today's expression of the Empiric tradition. Its strength is among practitioners who are not medically trained. As it appears that most "holistic doctors" work in a Rational model and employ holistic practices as alternative treatments for disease, medical training may even be an obstacle to study and applying Empirical practices. Today, the Rational influence is not just the strongest tradition in the medical profession; it is the only operative model. If medical thinking governs our development about holistic health practices, we will forfeit whatever benefit there may be in having a health industry which offers us a balance of Rational and Empirical services.

Rational standards of practice in medicine have already judged Empirical perspectives to be unscientific. The influence of Rational standards within the profession has determined the direction of research (Note 3) and will control professional responsibilities in the field unless the professional community and an educated public recognize the need for a different kind of service.

Complaints that our current system of health care takes advantage of people are growing louder. Most people think that someone—the state, the American Medical Association, Uncle Sam—should do something about it. Enough, already! Every gardener has the power to determine how his garden grows. Contracts are tools. Use them to create changes that are important to you personally, and we will all work together to incorporate these needs at institutional levels.

The holistic practitioners of the 19th century were homeopaths, herbalists and osteopaths. The Empiric practitioners of the 21st century are the holistic practitioners of today. If preservation of the integrity of both Rational and Empirical traditions of thought about health is desired, independent professional recognition of holistic practitioners is necessary. The groundwork for this is initiated by recognizing individual needs for health services in the Empiric tradition and by making agreements with all health professionals which provide for both forms of service.

References

Coulter, H. *Divided Legacy: A History of the Schism in Medical Thought*. Washington, D.C.: Wehawken Books, 1975. Three Voumes.

Epstein, R. Medical malpractice: The case for contract. *American Bar Foundation Resources Journal*, 1976, *1*, 87.

Epstein, R. Contracting out of the medical malpractice crisis. *Perspectives in Biology and Medicine*, Winter 1977, 228.

Green, J. Responsibility for health. *Journal of Holistic Health*, 1976, *1*, 76.

The People of the State of California vs. Dana Ullman, March 9, 1977. Municipal Court Oakland-Piedmont Judicial District. County of Alameda, No. 98158.

Suggestions for Further Reading

"Holistic Practitioners Unite—It's time to learn to fly" Somatics, V. 3 N. 4, Spring 1982, which may be obtained, together with a membership packet describing the structure of a model practitioners association, from California Health Practitioners Association, P.O. Box 8467, La Jolla, CA 92038.

"Patients Who Refuse Medical Treatment" Applebaum & Roth, M.D.s JAMA V. 250, No. 10, Sept. 9, 1983.

"Adding Insult to Injury: Usurping Patient's Prerogatives" J. P. Kassirer, M.D., New England Journal of Medicine, 4/14/83.

"Allocating Responsibility by Contract" J. Green, Medicolegal News, V. 8 N. 5, 10/80 Amer. Soc. of Law & Medicine.

"Contracting Out of the Medical Malpractice Crisis" R. Epstein, JD Perspectives in Biology and Medicine, Winter 1977.

"The Health Care Contract: Key to Minimizing Malpractice" Prof. Liab. Newsl., March '82 Insurance Corp. of America.

"Contracts With Your Doctor?" J. Green, New Realities, V. 2, N. 1, 1978

These published and several unpublished works comprise the reading for a Professional Responsibility Training designed and conducted by the author for health practitioners, continuing education programs, and private practices. For information about the availability of these readings, and the programs, lectures, and related consulting services, write the author in care of P.O. Box 5094, Mill Valley CA 94942.

JERRY A. GREEN, *J. D., graduated from U. C. Berkeley in 1964 and from Boalt Law School in 1967. He practices in Mill Valley, California and specializes in medicine and health care. He is a member of the American Society of Law and Medicine, a Medical Arbitrator for the American Arbitration Association, and an Advisor to the Health Advocates Coalition. He lectures on the health care contract, and conducts professional education programs for health practitioners. He is the author of "Seven Keys to Creating Successful Health Care Relaitonships—A Consumer's Guide."*

Note 3: Most scientific research concerning stress has been conducted in the context of stress-related pathology. An example of holistic research into stress may be seen in Peter Levine's work which evaluates stress as a function of the dynamic capacity of an organism to interact with its environment. It is measured in terms of homeostatic resiliance on motoric, automatic, and metabolic levels.

Levine, P. Accumulated stress, reserve capacity and disease (Doctoral dissertation, University of California, 1976).

Microfilms International, 1976, 77–15, 760, 265.

Unorthodox Healing and the Law

Leonard Worthington, LL.B., J.D.

There is no social merit to the suppression and rejection of the right of qualified healers to exercise their talents. As we begin to recognize these gifted individuals, the scope of our health-delivery system will broaden substantially. Leonard Worthington, one of California's most distinguished attorneys, suggests guidelines for replacing the old laws with sensible legislation.

THE EXISTENCE of restrictive laws concerning the healing arts is understandable to a degree, since such laws are plausible as a way to protect the public from charlatans and others who would profit from the sick and ailing without providing any form of relief. But what happens when these restrictions actually contribute to human suffering and death?

What of the great "no man's land" between laboratory-induced cures and defeats, and that vast field known as paranormal healing—which for the most part has been officially forgotten, ignored, or declared illegal?

Any honest and impartial research into the histories of spiritual, psychic, and energy healing will convince all but the preconditioned skeptic that there exist in the universe strange and unusual powers whose use has resulted in substantial benefits for humanity.

Should those who possess such powers be denied their use? I think not.

Is there some way in which we can allow these honest healers to practice their art and can still protect the public from charlatans? I believe so, and will show specifically how we can and should do it through legislation. First, though, I think we should put medicine itself into proper historical perspective.

From the time God first looked upon his original creation and "found it to be good," we have consistently devoted great efforts toward harming or destroying this perfectly created vehicle—the human body.

The causes of some disease were known to early peoples; others have been discovered only in recent times. However, at all times in our history, including today, there have existed many unknown factors which, singly or in combination, induce various disabling or fatal ailments.

In our early history, we depended solely on priests and priestesses for both our spiritual and our physical needs, the former because of their religious studies, the latter because of their study of plants and herbs. *They recognized that the only real healer was nature.*

The role of such "medicine men" was to study every possible factor which might produce beneficial results for the members of their tribes. They would carefully assemble herbs and plants, experiment with them, and analyze the results for future use. Through this open-minded approach to medicine, miraculous cures were effected, many of which have been lost to succeeding generations because ignorant observers elected to classify these practices as "witchcraft" and therefore as unacceptable to a "civilized" society.

When the priesthood lost exclusive jurisdiction over the field of healing practices, a chasm was created which has widened so greatly over the centuries that the breach may never be healed. The now-separate medical profession focused its attention on strictly empirical approaches to specific problems, totally excluding the fact, known and accepted by the medicine man, that nature is the only real healer.

There have been some practitioners of medicine who recognized that the laboratory did not contain all the secrets of the universe and that results defying human explanation could be secured. They reached greatness, while their colleagues remained mired in their laboratory mediocrity.

Today's doctor, whatever his/her specialty, actually does no more than recognize the signs of an unfavorable condition, attempt to diagnose some of its causative factors, and, within the limits of his/her knowledge, remove these factors so that nature may take over and supply the healing energies necessary to bring about a cure.

Now, I do not intend these statements to be a wholesale criticism of the modern medical profession as such: many of its members are dedicated individuals, serving humanity with honor and distinction. What I am criticizing is the law which insists that these doctors are the *sole* possessors of healing abilities, a law which denies the existence of other forces and which, indeed, forbids their existence.

I practice law in the state of California and, although its statutes are not unlike those of other states, I shall confine my comments and criticism to my home ground.

As the California statute (Section 2141 of the Business and Professional Code) is worded, the law actually denies the Creator the right to maintain His creation as "good"—unless, of course, He makes use of the small segment of the population that possesses a medical degree, a degree earned from professors whose own knowledge is necessarily limited by the qualifications of their predecessors, by their own restricted experience, and by the available literature on the subject.

Under a strict interpretation of the code, a member of the public is denied even the right to suggest to another person that he use specific remedies for the alleviation of pain or the cure of disease—be it only a banana, a glass of water, or even a Band-Aid! (Prosecution has actually resulted from such innocent suggestions.) I see this not only as a denial of a person's right of free speech, but as a limitation of the free use of his talents.

Let us talk about unequal enforcement of the law for a moment. Not a day goes by without television viewers being bombarded by annoying ads prescribing in no uncertain terms specific remedies for ailments. On listening wearily to these repetitious suggestions, I have wondered how a person on TV can get away with things for which another member of the public would surely be prosecuted for practicing medicine without a license. Whereas the one violation of the act on TV reaches hundreds of thousands in a few seconds, a member of the public who is sincerely attempting to help his fellow man, usually gratuitously or for a nominal fee, is transmitting his message of hope only from person to person, one at a time. Why the favoritism?

Is it because the pharmaceutical firms so greatly influence the Medical Boards, the Federal Food and Drug Administration, or the enforcement agencies that they can escape prosecution where a private citizen cannot? I have wondered what would happen if the law-enforcement agencies issued warrants for the arrest of every firm which prescribed remedies for a disease or for the relief of pain, if every advertisement prescribing a remedy for any physical condition were declared unlawful and the media prohibited from accepting them? I wager that the Medical Practice Act would soon be amended to exempt advertising from its provisions—but individuals would still be prohibited from doing precisely the same thing.

The principle of law that says every person is innocent until proven guilty loses its value if you are accused of violating the Medical Practice Act. Merely to suggest that a person take a specific medicine automatically assures that you will be convicted of some misdemeanor and that you may be fined or jailed, even if you produce 100 witnesses in court to testify that your methods are effective and beneficial, and that you have never harmed a human being in any of your treatments. Operators of health-food stores, for instance, have been prosecuted for suggesting harmless herbs; nutritional consultants for recommending safe foods or vitamin/mineral supplements.

Here is how the California law is worded:

"Any person who practices or attempts to practice, or who advertises or holds himself out as practicing, any system or mode of treating the sick or afflicted in this State, or who diagnoses, treats, operates for, or prescribes for any ailment, blemish, deformity, disease, disfigurement, disorder, injury, or other mental or physical condition of any person, without having at the time of so doing a valid unrevoked certificate as provided in this chapter, or without being authorized to perform such act pursuant to a certificate obtained in accordance with some other provision of law, is guilty of a misdemeanor."

Now, there are laws concerning acts which in themselves are admittedly dangerous to society and likely to lead to injury, such as driving while drunk or carrying a concealed weapon. The mere commission of such an act "in and of itself" is sufficient to warrant a prosecution and a conviction. But where the act complained of has proven to be beneficial to mankind and is not "in and of itself" clearly injurious to the public welfare, it is a poor law which makes that act automatically a crime.

The law should be changed so that only in cases where the evidence shows that persons have been harmed by the treatment (or by the prescribing of a remedy) will the person be subject to criminal prosecution, and then only where fraud or misrepresentation has been used.

There are adequate civil and criminal laws on the statute books to protect the public from persons who would trick or deceive them. We do not need a statute which is so broad that it traps the unwary person who seeks nothing more than to help his fellow man.

As it now reads, this act, along with other similarly worded statutes in various states, allows the Department of Consumer Affairs (or any other enforcement agencies) to select at random the persons whom they elect to prosecute, regardless of their value to society. A single complaint by a disgruntled or selfishly motivated person or group is sufficient to begin legal harassment of any innocent, well-meaning individual whose only statutory (but not moral) wrong has been to use his or her valuable talents for the good of ailing individuals, often ones who have not obtained relief through the regularly recognized channels.

The public is taxed to meet the payrolls of such enforcement agencies, yet is not represented in their composition. If such broad power is to be delegated, it should be done only with the greatest of care, lest those vested with authority abuse their positions of public trust and thwart the very purpose of the legislation.

One rigid rule should be firmly established by all appointing powers, to the effect that no board, agency, or commission shall ever consist of a majority of members whose personal or financial interests can be benefitted by the functions of that agency or board. For example, a medical board should consist of a majority of qualified "outsiders," with the minority of members being from the medical profession; the latter could thus act as advisors, but their vote alone could not control or establish policy. And so it should be with every appointed board in each industry and profession. Only then will the public have unbiased representation for the highest good of all its citizens.

Since a Board of Medical Examiners consisting solely of doctors would be oriented toward self-preservation, its recommendations to the Legislature would naturally tend to favor statutes that preserve its status quo, solidify its entrenched position, and provide personal benefits to its members. However, this very human trait is certainly not restricted to members of the medical profession. It is as American as apple pie or motherhood, and is to be found in practically every other profession, business, union, or industry, wherever the elements of money, power, prestige, or control rear their heads.

When members are appointed to a board or commission, it should be policy that no person be appointed who has a conflict of interest in the matters upon which that board would pass a decision, except to the extent that professional advice is required to guide and assist the Board on subjects where expert advice is integral to the field; even then, such members should remain in the minority.

As amendments to the Medical Practice Act, I would propose that additional exceptions be inserted in the act itself to allow certain forms of healing to be practiced by qualified persons; to set up standards for others, under which their abilities could be explored, tested, and determined; and, if their abilities are found beneficial to mankind, to provide for the qualification and licensing of such persons, as we approved by the California Legislature for acupuncturists during the 1974 session.

Whereas Section 2146 of the Medical Practice Act now states that "*Nothing in this Chapter shall be construed so as to discriminate against any particular school of medicine or surgery, school of podiatry, or any other treatment, nor shall it regulate, prohibit, or apply to any kind of treatment by prayer, nor interfere in any way with the practice of religion,*" this exception has not always been understood or noted by enforcement agencies or the courts. It requires explanatory assistance in order that it not continue to be improperly enforced.

I would suggest, along these lines, that an amendment be introduced in the legislative bodies in order to provide for the general licensing of natural healers who have somewhat the following qualifications.

1. "Persons who possess or claim to possess special healing powers, or who are able to direct healing energies which have proven effective in the alleviation of pain, relief, or cure of illnesses in the past, shall, upon establishing satisfactory proof of their abilities, be licensed under this Act and shall be permitted to continue such practices, provided that they publicly display in their place of treatment a notice, of which they shall give a copy in writing, stating in clear and plain language that they do not have medical educational training or certificates, and that the patient should also seek medical advice about the nature of his illness and about the possible effect of this type of treatment on his condition."

2. "Such licenses shall be renewable annually and shall require the licensee to report the name and address of each patient treated by him during the preceding year, the nature of each patient's complaint, the type and cost of treatment afforded, and the results of the same."

3. "Persons unable to substantiate past case histories as required above will, under certain conditions, be granted probationary licenses which will allow them to accept only cases referred by a physician and will require them to file monthly reports of the kind described above, until such time as the effectiveness of such treatment has been established, whereupon an annual license will be granted."

4. "In any case of alleged violation of the Medical Prac-

tice Act the burden of proof shall be upon the prosecuting authorities to establish their case as in all other criminal matters."

Such amendments would open the door for a physician who recognizes that his services are no longer effective to refer a patient to a natural healer, something which is being done now, but only under cover and with fear of detection. It would permit qualified healers to appear and practice publicly instead of clandestinely, and would enable the medical profession and the authorities to learn from the reports and treatment methods of such persons about matters which are not covered in the average medical schools. It would provide a field of knowledge from which both the public and the medical profession could well benefit.

Only by a complete exposure of this important field of healing and an objective and unbiased investigation of it can the general public reap the benefits which the Creator intended when He endowed upon selected persons knowledge, divine powers, and energies which are as yet not accepted or understood.

Had the healing professions adequately met the challenge of the centuries, the restrictive and punitive provisions of the California Medical Practice Act would have been justified. Such, however, is not the case. Thousands of patients have failed to obtain relief or cures for their conditions. Often discouraged by the inability of the medical profession to help them, or despondent at the admonition to "live with it" or a prognosis of death staring them in the face, patients have turned in desperation to quacks and charlatans, as well as to qualified natural healers who employ unorthodox methods of treatment. It is often after hospitalization and medical treatments have exhausted their funds that these persons are forced to seek relief from spiritual or natural healers, and confirmed reports record surprising relief and even permanent cures from many of these so-called unorthodox sources.

This poses the very tantalizing question whether society has the right to deprive its ailing citizens of such services solely on the grounds that not all the practitioners might be qualified to render beneficial aid in certain cases.

If this argument justifies the absolute rejection of the right of qualified healers to exercise their talents, then the sale of liquor or automobiles could also be banned, on the theory that, if the product sold is misused, such sales can result in injury or loss of life to members of the general public.

The right to drive a motor vehicle is both a benefit and a threat to public welfare. An ambulance or a police car, if properly operated, can alleviate suffering and misery as well as save lives, but if carelessly driven can also maim and kill.

A member of the medical profession, regardless of university training, can be guilty of malpractice or manslaughter, yet it would be wrong to condemn the entire profession for the incompetence of the few. The benefits from this profession so greatly outweigh the detriments that to repeal the Medical Practice Act and prohibit anyone from aiding the sick, regardless of his qualifications, would be a grievous mistake.

The services and talents of the unique persons we have discussed should be universally recognized, legalized, and utilized either by State statutes or by the United States government under the auspices of the Department of Health, Education, and Welfare for the benefit of all of our citizens.

If justice is to be dispensed, it must be done without discrimination, whether it be racial or religious, or the favoring of a corporation against the ordinary citizen. The only remedy is for the voters to rise up in protest against this unjust discrimination which now exists concerning the healing arts and to force their elected representatives to change the law.

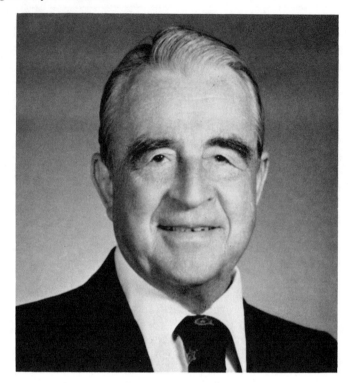

LEONARD A. WORTHINGTON *Attorney, A.B., LL.B, J.D.*
Past Pres. *S.F. Lawyer's Club, A.U.M. Foundation, S.F. Democratic Club, Native Sons, Great Western University.*

Board of Directors *Psychic Research, Hasting's College of Law, Aletheia, A.U.M. Foundation, St. Francis Hospital, St. Francis Pavilion, American Academy of Asian Studies, S.F. Bar Association.*

He is a lecturer, writer on Metaphysical & Healing subjects, and an attorney for hundreds of Foundations, Holistic & Metaphysical Groups, churches, and individuals all over the world.

Tone Up at the Terminals

AN EXERCISE GUIDE FOR COMPUTER AND WORD PROCESSING OPERATORS

Denise Austin

Numerous studies have shown conclusively that appropriate exercise improves the ability to relax, both immediately and over a sustained period. Findings indicate that a relaxed person works and thinks more efficiently. It has been noted that physical activity increases circulation through the body and exercising helps all the brain cells receive the nutrients they need. Increased circulation through exercise can reduce or eliminate "nervous fatigue," as well as improve memory and cognition.

During a hectic day, your muscles store up tension. This tension can lead to back pain, stiff neck or tension headaches. If muscles are not given relief from tension by relaxation, exercises or change of activity, the muscle fibers physiologically "adapt" to the states of increased tension. The tension can be released by purposeful exercises and you can select the exercises that fit your individual needs.

The exercises illustrated here can be done at your work station in a matter of minutes. No special skills or athletic abilities are required. You can even try them at home or on the train, plane or bus. Better still, do the exercises while you're watching TV.

For best results, supplement them with a balanced program of regular cardiovascular conditioning, muscular flexibility, strength training and sound nutrition.

Eyestrain Tips*

- Take visual breaks every two to three minutes, more frequent if your work is intense. Relax your eyes by changing focus and look away into the distance.
- If you have other tasks that don't require work at your video display terminal, vary the tasks to eliminate long periods at your terminal.
- Make a point to consciously blink and take deep

*Information courtesy of Vision Care Clinic, San Jose, CA.

Tone Up At the Terminals by Denise Austin (Sunnyvale, California): The Verbatim Corporation.

breaths. Sometimes intense work can prevent you from proper breathing and regular blinking.
- If you wear glasses and have a sensitivity to glare or flicker, a tint in your lenses can be helpful.
- Consider using a terminal screen with a light background and dark characters or a polarizing filter that mounts on your screen and deflects glare.

Warm Up Exercises

Shake: Loosen up by moving your neck, shoulders, arms, thighs, legs and feet. Promotes blood circulation through the body.

Reach: Slowly raise your arms and draw the stomach fully in. Then let your arms drop. Repeat twice. A good stretch for the rib cage and can help posture.

Deep Breathing: Close your eyes and direct your attention to the breathing process. Think of nothing but your breathing. Inhale deeply through the nose and exhale forcefully out the mouth. Repeat six times. Benefit—Aids in relaxing and reducing tension.

Tensing the Muscles: Most people generally have very little awareness of the sensation of relaxation. Therefore, you must first produce tension sensations, then slowly release them. This will allow you to feel the difference internally between tension and relaxation.

Shoulder Roll

Slowly roll your shoulders forward five times in a circular motion using your full range of movement. Then roll your shoulders backward with the same circular motion. Benefit—Releases nervous tension buildup in neck and shoulders.

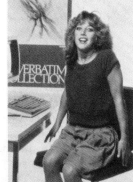

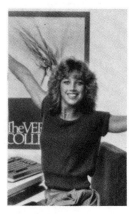

Arm Circles

Raise your arms out to the side with your elbows straight. Slowly rotate your arms in small circles forward and then backward. Benefit—To increase joint mobility in the shoulders.

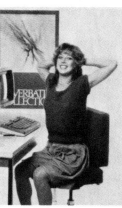

Pectoral Stretch

Grasp your hands behind your neck and press your elbows back as far as you can. Return to starting position, then drop arms and relax. Repeat. Benefit—Good stretch to do when you find yourself slouching. Stretches the front of your chest.

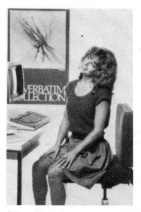

Neck

Let your head drop slowly to the left, then to the right. Slowly drop your chin to your chest and then raise your chin as high as you can. Turn your head all the way to the left, return it to the normal position and then turn your head all the way to the right. Return to normal position.

Benefit—Stimulates the neck muscles to alleviate a stiff neck.

Upper Back Stretch

Sit on a chair with your hands on your shoulders. Try to cross your elbows in front of you until you feel the stretch across your upper back. Return to starting position, drop your hands, relax. Repeat. Benefit—Reduce muscle stiffness of the upper back.

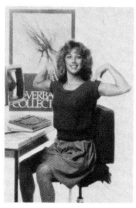

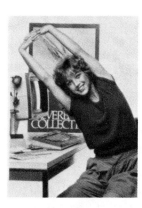

Side Stretch

Interlace your fingers. Lift your arms up over your head keeping your elbows straight. Press your arms backwards as far as you can. Then slowly lean first to the left and then to the right until you can feel the stretch along the sides of your body. Benefit—Will stretch the muscles along side of your body from your arm to your hips.

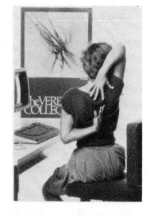

Shoulder Stretch

Bring your right hand to your upper back from above. Bring your left hand to your upper back from below and hook fingers of your two hands. Repeat to the other side. Benefit—It reduces tension and increases flexibility.

Wrist Flex

Put your elbow on a table with your hand raised. With your other hand, hyperextend your wrist to bend your hand so that the back of your hand is aiming to the top of your forearm. Repeat with opposite hand. Benefit—This releases tension in your hand and wrist.

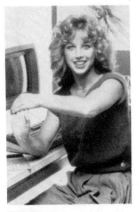

Fingers

With palms down, spread your thumb and fingers as far apart as you can. Hold it for the count of five. Relax. Repeat. Benefit—To relase the tension build-up in your hands and fingers.

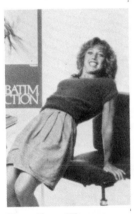

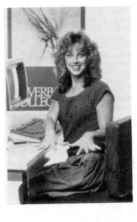

Derrière Firmer

Place hands on chair, feet flat on the floor, and lift your hips and buttocks up. Tighten your buttocks. Hold for five seconds, then sit back and relax. Repeat twice. Benefit—To firm and tone your legs and buttocks.

Strengthen the Quadriceps

Bring legs straight out in front of body to hold an L-shape position. Hold for five seconds and make sure you are sitting up straight with good posture. Relax. Repeat. Benefit—Strengthens the quadriceps and abdominal muscles.

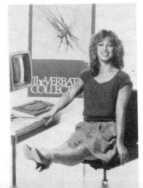

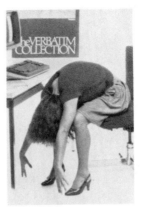

Back Relaxer

Sit on chair. Drop your neck, your shoulders and your arms, then bend down between your knees, as far as you can. Return to upright position, straighten out and relax. Benefit—This will take pressure off your lower back.

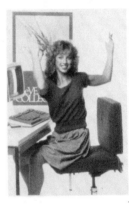

Trunk Twists

Turn at your trunk. Turn your head in the direction of your trunk. Twist 3 times in each direction. Benefit—Excellent for trimming the waistline and improving flexibility.

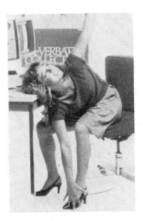

Windmill

Sit in a chair. Place your feet apart on the floor. Bend over and touch your right hand to your left foot with your left arm extended up. Alternate sides repeatedly. Benefit—To trim your hips and waistline.

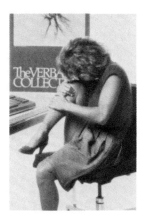

Knee Kiss

Sit in a chair. Pull one leg to your chest, grasp with both hands and hold for the count of five. Repeat with opposite leg. Benefit—Excellent stretch for the hamstrings.

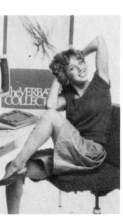

Trimming the Waist

Interlace fingers behind your neck. Lift right knee, and touch the left elbow to the right knee. Alternate sides repeatedly 5 times. Benefit—Trim and tone the waistline.

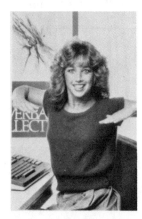

For Your Arms

Bend your elbows, parallel to the floor, fingers in front of chest. Then push arms way out to the sides with arms straight. (Try to push arms as far as possible.) Repeat 5 times. Keep firm. Benefit—Tones the muscles of the arms.

Middle-Upper Back Stretch

Hold your right arm just above the elbow with your left hand. Now gently pull your elbow toward your left shoulder as you feel the stretch. Hold stretch for 5 seconds. Do both sides. Benefit—To stretch and increase flexibility of the middle-upper back.

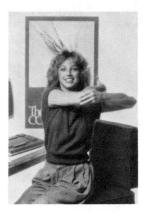

Hug Yourself

Cross arms in front of chest and reach fingertips towards your shoulder blades. Benefit—Relieves tension from shoulders and upper back.

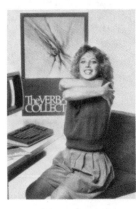

Exercise physiology specialist DENISE AUSTIN *(formerly Katnich) has offices in Los Angeles and Washington, D.C. and serves as a clinician with the President's Council on Physical Fitness and Sports. Her field of expertise is employee fitness, stress management and aerobics.*

A former nationally prominent gymnast, Denise attended the University of Arizona on a gymnastics scholarship. She received her degree in physical education from California State University, Long Beach.

Denise has hosted her own television exercise show in Los Angeles, called "Daybreak." In addition, she has appeared on a number of major TV programs such as Hour Magazine, Merv Griffin Show, AM Los Angeles and Alive & Well (U.S.A. Cable Network). Denise has also been featured in national magazines including Glamour, Cosmopolitan and Shape.

VII

Out Into the Wider World— Beyond the Individual

INTRODUCTION *by Shepherd Bliss*

"BEYOND THE INDIVIDUAL" is the key phrase here. Looking at health certainly begins with the individual, but it must include consideration of the wider world—the ecological, cultural, social, and political environments within which we live.

We begin by offering an acupuncturist's historical and political perspective on social responsibility. We then move to a homeopath's provocative consideration of holistic health as "friend and foe." The prominent physicist Fritjof Capra—author of *The Tao of Physics*—then relates holistic health to what he calls "holistic peace."

Though we are tempted to deny the possibility of nuclear annihilation, which confronts us daily during the 1980s, Joanna Macy and Chellis Glendinning provide us theoretical and practical tools for living during this Nuclear Age—not through denial, but by dealing with feelings such as grief and despair. They are two of a growing number of citizens concerned with the effects of the ongoing threat of nuclear war.

We end the book with two projections into the future by interesting sources—the American Council of Life Insurance and a top United Nations official. The Council's report is optimistic. The U.N.'s Robert Muller concludes that we should "consult the wise old people who are transmitters of world wisdom from generation to generation," and hold open the vision that, "humanity is on a further evolutionary ascent and we have magnificent frontiers in front of us."

Holistic Health and Social Responsibility: An Historical and Political Perspective

Michael W. Hussin

LIKE AN individual, particular event, or society, holistic medicine cannot be fully understood outside of particular social contexts. With an historical approach, we can begin to discern our direction by understanding where we have been; by examining the past we may find that our predecessors have struggled with similar questions and we can learn from their triumphs and failures.

Consequently, I will present a brief history of the Popular Health movement, which took place in the early 19th century, and reached its peak just before the Civil War. It was born at a time when people were questioning the very foundations upon which the country stood: it was a time of upheaval when members of the abolitionist movement, women's rights organizations, workingmen's unions, and the popular health movement were working together. The movement offered a holistic and political understanding of health.

The popular health movement was created to defend the medical practices used by the overwhelming majority of the people against an attack by an elite class seeking to monopolize medicine and eliminate the popular systems. These popular medical practices were based on a combination of European, African, and native American folk medicines that gave birth to a rich new North American healing tradition.[1] At the time of the American Revolution, medical practice was open to anyone who could demonstrate healing skills regardless of training, race, or sex.[2] Practiced mainly by females, healing was a neighborly service in stable communities where skills could be passed on for generations, where practitioners knew what roots and herbs were available in their environment; healers knew their patients and the families of their patients. Whereas the experience of lay healers had accumulated over the ages and healers were rooted in their communities, those who attempted to usurp their positions had no theoretical or experiential knowledge.[3] Thomas Jefferson called them "an inexperienced and presumptuous band of medical tyros at loose upon the world." The usurpers were inspired by their British counterparts who had made medicine a gentlemanly profession, fit only for those who studied the classics. They believed medicine should not be the province of illiterate rural women and farmers.

Many of those self-styled "regular" doctors, however, were not men of wealth and status. E. Richard Brown notes that, "The inexpensive and widely dispersed medical colleges encouraged large numbers of young men and some women to attempt careers in medicine. Graduates, many of them from yeoman farming and working-class families, filled the cities, towns, and countryside of America."[4] Their survival depended on convincing large numbers of people that healing was a *commodity*, something to be paid for, determined by the healing involved.[5] Healing would no longer take the form of neighborly advice but would be a commodity entirely detached from personal relations. When it became a profession and a source of wealth, women healers were cast aside as unfit for such pursuits, and it became nearly the sole province of men.

Between 1800 and 1820, the organized forces of regular medicine succeeded in restricting the practice of medicine in 17 states. It was a premature move because there was no mass support for medical professionalism, much less for the healers who claimed that professionalism.[6] Lay healers were spread throughout the countryside, making enforcement of restrictions impossible. Ironically, it was the development of this "professionalism" within medical practice that inspired a radical health movement, seeking to reclaim healing from the marketplace and prevent the domination of medicine by an elite class.

This reaction developed into a mass movement by the 1830s, after thousands of people were dissatisfied with the profession and practice of regular medicine. The constituency of this movement was small farmers, shopkeepers, artisans, and housewives.[7] Their resistance was not only due to the rise of regular medicine but also to the social and economic disruption caused by the rise of industrial capitalism. At this time the factory system swept up skilled craftsmen; stable communities were threatened as people relocated to find work. People no longer produced for themselves what they and their communities needed but instead had to sell themselves as wage laborers. Medicine became a reflection of the values inherent in industrial capitalism. Healing became just another product, a consumer good bought and sold in the marketplace. It reflected a very basic competitive tenet: "May the best man win."

Many Americans were outraged by the failure of the Revolution to free the slaves and guarantee the rights of women. Out of this dissatisfaction, many popular movements appeared, such as abolitionist, women's rights, unions, and the popular health movement, whose advocates often actively supported each others' causes. Leading abolitionists often followed one of the natural life-style disciplines. Leading members of women's rights groups often joined women's "physiological societies," organized to explore the female reproductive anatomy and give advice and instructions in self-examination and birth control.

Many abolitionists and members of women's organizations followed Samuel Thompson or Sylvester Graham. Samuel Thompson compiled lists of herbal remedies from Mrs. Benton, a lay healer in Vermont. Between 1822 and 1839, his *New Guide to Health* sold 100,000 copies. At this same time he started a movement to keep healing from the marketplace. He wanted to democratize medicine and advocated that every person should be his or her own healer. Thompsonian magazines sprang up with controversial ideas about popular health, including attacks on male doctors' medical abuse of women. Thompson himself disapproved of male regular obstetrical practice and said such practitioners had no experience compared to that of midwives.[8]

Sylvester Graham joined Thompson as a forerunner of the Wholistic Health movement. His followers advocated a diet of whole breads, fresh fruit and vegetables, and encouraged the use of natural remedies. Both Grahamists and Thompsonians were political activists working with abolitionists and women's rights activists and were supported by them in return. In 1835, Thompsonians joined forces with a slave insurrection in Mississippi. Grahamists were just as radical, equating natural living habits with liberty and classlessness.[9] Sarah and Angelina Grimke, Elizabeth Cady Stanton, William Lloyd Garrison, and Henry David Thoreau were but a few of the leaders of this period, for whom there was no difference between individual well-being and social well-being, between personal responsibility and social responsibility.

This unity of radical politics and health was not to last. By the middle of the 19th century, many Thompsonians began to hanker for respectability and something very much like professionalism. These aspiring professionals decided it was time to take healing out of the hands of the masses and grant diplomas to certain approved healers. They began to set up their own schools, grant degrees, distinguish lay from professional healers, and push for strict licensing laws. By 1900 nonregular doctors participated in medical licensing in 33 of the 45 states. By co-operating in licensure, the nonregular profession won inclusion among the "respectable" and wealthy.[10] Any radical movements connected with popular health were now seen as a hindrance to the desire for upward mobility and respectability.[11] Samuel Thompson protested, saying healing was being "taken

from the people generally, and like all other crafts monopolized by a few learned individuals."[12]

The popular health movement had always ridden along with the social unrest of the time, whence it derived its mass constituency. When the coalitions gave way to individual self-interest, the strength of a mass movement declined. E. Richard Brown has noted that "competition between the sects and the lack of decisive public support for any one of them, left none of the sects in a position to establish control...." This division within the movement left it easy prey for the "regular" practitioners who—in 1847—created the American Medical Association. Thus, the regulars consolidated power and money to use against the divided "irregular" practitioners.

The women's movement turned away from "body" issues and focussed on the vote; many women were lured into the Jacksonian Democratic Party. With the rise of a new industrial working class, the health movement lost its connections and base. The desire for professionalism turned it into another elite group and it lost its identification with the people it served. Without this mass energy and direction from below, the Thompsonians easily succumbed to the very forces they had set out to challenge. Where they had once denounced the transformation of healing into a commodity, they now sought to package their own alternative into a new kind of commodity.[13] Eventually, regular medicine became dominant, even adopting principles from the popular movement such as fresh air, fresh fruit and vegetables, and less meat in the diet. Regular medicine was credited with the decline in the death rate, which was, in fact, largely a result of better hygiene, something instituted by a parallel movement then starting in Europe. People were led to believe that this new "scientific" medicine, which promoted the germ theory, was solely responsible for increased longevity and better health. Brown notes, however, "In the great majority of cases the toll of the major killing diseases of the 19th century declined dramatically *before* the discovery of medical cures and immunization.... Improvements in general living and working conditions as well as sanitation, all brought about by labor struggles and social reform movements, are most responsible for improved health status.... Nineteenth-century reformers brought dramatic declines in mortality without the benefit of even the germ theory."[14]

The popular health movement, then, had grown from a radical movement intent on societal change, to one which became indistinguishable from regular medicine in its politcs. Its ideas were assimilated as reforms and its roots soon forgotten. Self-help, hygiene, and egalitarian socialistic-economic structures were not ideologically or economically viable in a society turning its people into consumers and health into a commodity.

The rise and development of capitalism and industrialism in the United States paralleled the growth of professional medicine. The American dream in the 19th century held the hope that capitalism would bring peace and prosperity. One hundred and fifty years later, we are seeing the results of this system. Our country is now being poisoned by chemical and radioactive wastes in our air, food, and water. It is turning into a military state whose chief export and cash crop is weapons.[15] The U.S. government fights against people struggling for self-determination in the Third World, while supporting brutal regimes in El Salvador, Guatemala, Honduras, Chile, and South Africa. Money is reallocated from human service agncies to weapons of mass destruction. Each day, the United States adds three new nuclear warheads to its stockpile of over 9200 strategic nuclear warheads.[16]

Just as many of our predecessors were dissatisfied with the "status quo," many of us have built mass movements to change present conditions. In the last 20 years, movements such as Civil Rights, Peace, Women's Liberation, and Environmental Protection have grown in strength and numbers. Out of this soil, the natural health movement was reborn and became a new popular health movement. Many of the political activists of the '60s became the developers of the holistic health movement as the criticism of the social system was extended to the health care system.

Ten years ago many people doing yoga, meditation, massage, etc., were part of these movements and espoused sweeping social change. But by the mid-1980s the social and political concerns of alternative healers are being neglected. The conferences, workshops, publications, and journals of the wholistic health movement are, except in rare cases, involved with the personal fulfillment of individuals, making one's practice cost-effective, and the hyping of new-age consumer products. We find our politics often limited to obtaining third-party payments, licensing laws, and acceptance by "regular" medicine.

Ironically, the focus of treatment and prevention in holistic health care is not all that different from the orthodox ideal. Both systems concentrate solely on the treatment of the individual and downplay the significance of the social genesis of disease. The approach to cancer is a good example of this convergence of thought. Orthodox medicine has focused most of its energy and resources on finding the "magic bullet" that will cure cancer in an individual, and a multibillion dollar industry has developed from this approach. However, it is generally acknowledged that about 80 percent of cancers are environmentally caused,[17] 30 to 40 percent through industrial pollution, and 20 to 40 percent through occupational hazards.[18] Comparatively little research, time, and effort is given to eradicating these causes. Holistic practitioners can fall into the same trap as Western medicine.

It is incumbent upon proponents of holistic health care to treat not just the whole *individual* but the whole society. Our society is generating disease at an incredible rate through occupational hazards, environmental cancers, stressful work conditions, and the ever-increasing threat of war. Much of the sickness of the individuals coming into our practices is but the result, the symptom, of these deteriorating social conditions. It is unrealistic to think we can treat enough individuals to turn things around; there are too many sick individuals, and conditions are deteriorating too quickly. Treating individuals, getting them balanced, and sending them back into an environment that overhelms the healthiest can be a cruel hoax. We must simultaneously treat individuals *and* address the social conditions that cause disease.

If we are to avoid repeating the mistakes of the past, we must understand and struggle to change the social and political causes of the diseases we aim to cure. The holistic health movement must once again join forces with other movements to change this country, and we must hoist the banner of social activism so proudly carried by health movements of former days.

MICHAEL W. HUSSIN *lives in Cambridge, Massachusetts, and has been practicing Chinese acupuncture for seven years. A faculty member of the Traditional Acupuncture Institute in Columbia, Maryland, and Vice-President of the Massachusetts Acupuncture Society, he currently works in a group practice in Boston. He has been an activist since the Vietnam War era and continues to work on peace, justice, social, and environmental issues. He draws inspiration from the past and present women's movement, the struggles of Black-Americans, Native-Americans, the artists, singers, poets, revolutionaries from around the world, and above all from his friends and lovers who enable him to cry more deeply, laugh more easily, and think a bit more wisely.*

Notes

1. Barbara Ehrenreich and Deirdre English, *For Her Own Good: 150 Years of Experts' Advice to Women* (Garden City, New York: Anchor Press/Doubleday, 1979), p. 40.
2. *Ibid.*, p. 39.
3. In their work cited above, Ehrenreich and English state: ". . . at the heart of professional medicine there still lay a frightful theoretical void. Air and water were blamed as bringers of disease." (p. 43) and "In the first half of the 18th century, male, regular obstetrical practitioners tried to replace midwives but most regular physicians received their degrees without having witnessed a delivery." (p. 53)
4. E. Richard Brown, *Rockefeller Medicine Men: Medicine and Capitalism in America* (Berkeley and Los Angeles: University of California Press, 1979), p. 64–65.
5. Ehrenreich and English, *Experts' Advice to Women*, p. 44.
6. *Ibid.*, p. 47–48.
7. *Ibid.*, p. 48.
8. *Ibid.*, p. 52.
9. *Ibid.*, p. 52.
10. Brown, *Medicine and Capitalism in America*, p. 89–90.
11. Ehrenreich and English, *Experts' Advice to Women*, p. 55–56.
12. *Ibid.*, p. 56.
13. *Ibid.*, p. 56.
13. *Ibid.*, p. 57.
14. Brown, *Medicine and Capitalism in America*, p. 219–21.
15. American Friends Service Committee, *Questions and Answers on the Soviet Threat and National Security*, p. 3.
16. AFSC, *Soviet Threat and National Security*, p. 3.
17. David Driebel, "Cancer: Some Notes for Activists," *Science for the People Magazine* (May-June, 1980), p. 6.
18. Bob Ginsburg, Book Review: The Politics of Cancer, in *Science for the People Magazine* (May-June, 1980), p. 17.

Holistic Health:
Friend and Foe of
Progressive Health Care

Dana Ullman, M.P.H.

T HE WORD "holistic," like the words "revolutionary," "love," and "health," means so much and yet so little. Its overuse by individuals who seem to have little interest in its usage has devalued its meaning and has created much confusion in its application. Still, like other overly used words that begin to mean so little, their various meanings indicate the need in our language to describe new and/or particularly valuable perceptions, experiences, and understandings. Although I too cringe when I hear people use the word "holistic," I feel it is too good a word to let others less interested in its precise meaning define it for us.

Before defining "holistic health," however, it is first important to clarify what I mean by "progressive health care." Basically, I define progressive health care as health care which is predominantly of, by and for the people it serves. Specifically, it is health care that significantly involves the individual and the community in its own care and, as appropriate, in the decisions how, where, when and by whom it should be delivered. Progressive health care should also significantly involve the community it serves in the development, implementation and evaluation of public policies that have considerable effects upon community health. In this definition, progressive health care still makes use of clinical and policy expertise of professionals, however the consumers of health care are considered the most important members of the health care team.

Holistic health has been defined as a set of modalities, as a movement, and as a systems approach to health and disease (Carlson, 1979). Probably more than any other definition, most people initially assume that holistic health is an alternative set of therapeutic modalities or health educational processes that somehow treat "the whole person." Becoming aware of and working with the physical, emotional, mental and spiritual characteristics of the per-

son is often considered treatment of the whole person; however, the degree of attention to each different level of the person varies from practitioners to practitioner. Another major problem with this definition is its tendency toward ignoring physical and social environmental effects upon the whole person, which then certainly questions the degree of holism that advocates utilize.

Holistic health is also understood as a movement of any "unorthodox" (to Western standards) healing or health educational practice. There is however nothing that is inherently holistic in any health practice or educational approach since any person can utilize these methods in a reductionistic manner. In fact, our Western upbringing encourages reductionistic orientations, and as such, significant numbers of practitioners and their clients still look for specific treatments for specific diseases, tending to neglect individualized health care for the patient's unique condition.

Understanding holistic health as a systems approach to health and disease is, in my mind, the most appropriate way of utilizing the holistic health concept. This definition primarily emphasizes that holistic health is an approach to understanding and working with health and disease and is not necessarily a specific modality. Also, with this definition every unorthodox healing method would not automatically be considered "holistic" since more emphasis is placed on the way one practices or teaches and less on what method one specifically uses. Lalonde's (1974) health field concept and Brody and Sobel's (1979) systems hierarchy have created a skeletal structure by which the systems approach can be applied to health care.

Holistic health did not emerge from nowhere. In fact, an almost predictable set of historical developments set the stage for its growth. Harris Coulter (1973, 1975, 1977) has documented in a three-volume treatise on the Western medical history how a school of thought pre-dating Hippocrates (350 B.C.) emphasized a holstic approach to health. This Empirical school of thought was countered

Published in the *International Journal of Holistic Health & Medicine.* Winter, 1984, and reprinted by permission.

by the Rational school. The Rational school analytically developed their system of health practice. A physiochemical diagnosis is made, a disease entity and the physiochemical cause is hypothesized, and a reductionistic treatment to the disease is offered. In comparison, the Empirical school developed their practice from their own time-honored experience, rarely seeking rational basis for explaining why their methods worked. A diagnosis of an imbalance in their energy system is made, a body-mind disease process is assessed, and a treatment to raise the person's defense system is offered. Whereas orthodox medicine evolved from the Rationalist's school, holistic health has sprung from Empiricist's roots.

Although the word "holism" wasn't formally coined until 1926 (Smuts), the deep roots of the holistic approach to health only needed to be tapped for this school of thought to grow. Various social movements during the past 20 years have begun to tap these roots. Specifically, the human potential movement, the Eastern philosophy/spiritualism movement, the self-care movement, the women's movement, and the environmental movement have each contributed important concepts and perspectives that have helped form the holistic health movement today.

The way I'd like to present how holistic health is both a friend and foe to progressive health care is to discuss some of the major contributions of the above mentioned movements and then evaluate the degree to which the holistic health movement has incorporated the progressive characteristics for change from them.

The Human Potential Movement and Holistic Health

Recognition that health is more than the absence of disease is one of the important contributions of the human potential movement to holistic health. Health then is understood as a high level of wellness that fosters the freedom and the power to think, feel and act in ways conducive to individual and collective growth.

Another contribution from the human potential movement is the recognition of and respect for symptoms as positive phenomena. Symptoms are understood as efforts of the organism to heal itself and are learning experiences from which to understand the individual's imbalances with his/her environment. Having respect, rather than contempt, for symptoms has not yet been realized for its truly radical potential. If one understands symptoms as efforts of the organism to call attention to a problem, to obtain homeostasis between one's internal and external environment and to begin to heal itself, one's attitude toward symptoms and toward their treatment must change significantly. Viewing symptoms in this beneficial context also changes our views toward protests, strikes, and boycotts of various sorts. If one understands protests as attempts to call attention to a problem and to re-establish some type of fair balance, it becomes clear that they, like symptoms, should not be ignored or suppressed. This viewpoint does *not* mean that all protests or all symptoms are good or are always successful. Indeed, sometimes protests and symptoms create further problems. However, it is still true that protests and symptoms are efforts to call attention to a problem and neither should be ignored or suppressed.

The Eastern Philosophy/Spiritualism Movement and Holistic Health

The Eastern philosophy/spiritualism movement has contributed to holistic health in many similar ways as the human potential movement, but its unique contributions have helped holistic health advocates become aware of and accept some of the mysteries of nature and human nature. The "let it be" Eastern approach, rather than the "let's help it" Western approach, has helped holistic health advocates appreciate the inherent wisdom of natural systems to seek their own homeostasis and has cautioned us against too often or too rapid "therapeutic" intervention. Although Eastern philosophers will generally recognize the value of both "let it be" and "let's help it" approaches, the "let it be" approach tends to be sorely missing in the Westerner's ways of dealing with problems.

The Eastern philosophy/spiritualism movement has also contributed to holistic health by its appreciation of a unifying invisible dynamic force within and around the human body that is called "chi" by the Chinese, "ki" by the Japanese, "prana" by the yogis and numerous other names by various cultures throughout the world. Unlike the word "spirit" in the West, the words for this energetic force in the East generally have a very practical meaning and have direct and specific influences upon health. It is my personal feeling that our efforts to understand and work with the energetic processes within the human body will provide extremely valuable diagnostic and therapeutic tools for medicine in the future (Ullman, 1981).

This conceptualization of energetic processes within and around the organism is a part of progressive health care because it helps us understand the direct, though subtle, connection between body, mind and nature. Also, since it is now clearly understood from physics that energy and matter are a part of the same dynamic continuum, understanding energetic processes in the body will help us predict and prevent diseased physiological processes.

The Self-Care Movement and Holistic Health

The self-care movement also provides important concepts to holistic health. The basic premise of self-care is that the individual is an essential and valuable member of the health care team. The cooperative, rather than paternalistic, practitioner-client relationship is a significant contribution to progressive health care. Participation in one's own health care not only reduces the individual's medical care costs, more important it tends to empower individuals to take responsibility for their own health and life. Such empowerment is therapeutically and socially valuable both in times of sickness and in varying degrees of health. Such empowerment is particularly socially valuable when self-care becomes mutual aid with another person or with a group of people. Although self-care has sometimes been inaccurately construed as a selfish, narcissistic act, more and more of the self-care literature is encouraging mutual aid, various types of group action and acknowledgement of stresses outside of the individual's control (Ferguson, 1981; *Medical Self-Care*, 1976–1981).

Before leaving this topic, it should also be mentioned that certain degrees of selfishness and narcissism can be valuable therapeutically when a person is sick. Extra attention to one's self and learning to love oneself certainly should not always be understood as bad. Such attention is sometimes invaluable in developing one's own center so that the individual can be more effective working with and for others. Although these statements certainly can be considered statements of the obvious, it seems that many leftist politicos directly or indirectly tend to condemn anything but "the struggle over the tools of production."

The Women's Movement and Holistic Health

The women's movement has added innumerable concepts and understandings to the holistic health movement. Perhaps its most significant contribution is the ongoing use of feminine principles in understanding ourselves and the universe and in learning to act within and change our environment. Utilizing our intuition, expressing our emotions, understanding the symbols, myths, and dreams of our past and present, and sensitizing ourselves to our environment are all basic attributes of a traditionally feminine principle that the women's movement has reaffirmed and that are integral parts of a holistic approach to health.

The Environmental Movement and Holistic Health

The environmental movement has made some significant contributions to the development of the holistic health movement, even though many holistic health advocates sometimes forget their real importance or don't understand their deep significance. The environmental movement contributes to holistic health more than just awareness of the effects that air, water, food, modern living and the economy have on us. The environmental movement has also contributed its orientation towards perceiving whole systems and towards assessing direct and indirect effects from interventions in the short and long term. Differentiating short- and long-term solutions is particularly important in health care since many therapeutic measures may be effective in getting rid of symptoms . . . temporarily. But if the disease is not actually cured, the symptoms may persist, or worse, they could be suppressed to a deeper level which then threatens a person's health even more seriously. An important evaluative measure used by some involved in holistic health is one that differentiates between cure, palliation and suppression of disease (Vithoulkas, 1979).

Despite the contributions that each of these movements have made to holistic health to help it form a progressive health care movement, there are also elements from each of these movements that holistic health has either not assimilated or has done so in a distorted form.

The most obvious way in which the holistic health movement has become a foe of progressive health care has been in its tendency to assume that individuals are not only responsible for their health but also to blame for their disease. The human potential movement, the Eastern philosophy/spiritualism movement and the self-care movement, in particular, have elements in them that reinforce

this victim blaming. The distinction between being responsible for one's health and for one's disease is rarely clearly made, and reactionary tendencies result from this foggy conceptualization. Jesse Jackson, reverend and civil rights leader, inadvertently clarified this distinction in an address to a black high school student body, saying, "You may not be responsible for being down, but you are responsible for getting up." In relation to health and disease, it then can be recognized that the individual may or may not be responsible for her/his disease, but she/he *is* responsible for doing something about it.

Before moving on to describing other reactionary tendencies in the holistic health movement, it is important to place victim blaming in a broader perspective. Commonly, leftists tend to encourage individuals to see various social and economic stresses over which individuals have little or no control, thereby absolving individual responsibility for one's state of health. Ultimately, this type of logic also has victim blaming tendencies since it victimizes individuals by emphasizing that they are the unfortunate prey of systems and forces over which they have little or no control.

A healthy avoidance of victim blaming is difficult and carries no simple answers. Various degrees of individual and/or collective action are needed at different times to deal with different personal and social stresses.

The influences of the Eastern philosophy/spiritualism movement has given birth to the notion that individuals choose their disease, including genetic and environmentally related diseases. Although more and more of us are having metaphysical experiences that are teaching us that we tend to know more than our conscious mind makes us think, the synergistic effects of the innumerable stresses in our current lives today makes it uncertain at best if even the totally conscious being can understand the health implications of day-to-day behavior.

The perspective that we choose our own disease further reinforces a victim blaming ideology. It tends to encourage individuals to learn to accept their condition and to adapt to their world rather than work to change it. The "let's take responsibility" attitude of holistic health proponents primarily refers to taking responsibility to change oneself and rarely refers to changing the system one is in. Even symptoms, which are recognized as the organism's efforts to heal itself, tend to be understood as something the individual isn't doing correctly, rather than something that may be amiss from external sources.

Oddly enough, even though spiritually minded individuals will be the first to tell you that "we are all one," they often assume that the only way they can help the world is by helping themselves reach enlightenment. If, in fact, we are one, then it seems that one can equally help oneself by helping others. The twisted, self-serving logic that maintains a social amnesia certainly diminishes collective good.

The women's movement contributions to holistic health haven't been fully adopted and occasionally have been inappropriately manipulated. Holistic health proponents have sometimes disguised their sexism by cloaking it in yin-yang terminology that encourages widespread stereotyping. Also, the women's movement respect for one's intuition and one's emotions has sometimes been interpreted by holistic health proponents as reasons to neglect intellectual analysis. A pomposity and lack of humility is an occasional further outgrowth from an overconfidence in one's feelings.

The environmental movement's contribution to holistic health has forced some people in holistic health to see the contradictions in their health philosophy. Also, since the environmental movement is a naturalistic oriented movement that maintains a political posture, this movement has created a bridge by which personal growth oriented people are becoming politically active. The environmental movement has reminded holistic health proponents that there are some issues, like nuclear power and toxic substance exposure, that are more critical than many lifestyle issues. Since many holistic health proponents are "health chauvinists" who assume that one's lifestyle and one's consciousness creates one's entire universe, the critical environmental issues are waking up holistic health people to harsh realities of the present world. The environmental movement is beginning to make it obvious that those who primarily baste themselves in personal growth activities are not just exhibiting bourgeois behavior, but are indulging in reactionary behavior due to their neglect of critical problems.

One movement which holistic health has only just begun to learn from is the community health movement. Although the holistic health movement has a grassroots orientation to the provision of health care, the movement still seriously lacks organizational development (both regionally and nationally), direct ties to community organizations, and commitment to providing health care to all those who need it.

I have tried to show how holistic health is both a friend and foe of progressive health care. Since the holistic health field is presently so vaguely defined, my analysis can only at best apply to the general characteristics of the movement

as it is at present. Its rapidly changing nature makes predictions of its future development uncertain. I am hopeful that your involvement in this field will further help make it become an important contribution to progressive health care.

References

Brody, Howard and David Sobel, "A Systems View of Health and Disease," *Ways of Health: Holistic Approaches to Ancient and Contemporary Medicine.* New York: Harcourt Brace Jovanovich, 1979, pp. 87–105.

Carlson, Rick, "Holistic Health: Will the Promise be Realized?" *Holistic Health Review.* Fall 1979.

Coulter, Harris, *Divided Legacy: A History of the Schism in Medical Thought.* Washington, D.C.: Wehawken, 1973, 1975, 1977. (For a summary and review of these volumes, see Dana Ullman, "The Philosophical and Historical Roots of Holism in Health," *Holistic Health Review,* Winter, 1979).

Ferguson, Tom, *Medical Self-Care: Access to Health Tools.* New York: Simon and Schuster, 1980.

Lalone, Marc, *A New Perspective on the Health of Canadians.* Ottawa: Government of Canada, 1974.

Medical Self-Care, 1976–1981.

Smuts, Jan Christiaan, *Holism and Evolution.* New York: Viking. 1926.

Ullman, Dana, "Conceptualizing Energetic Medicine: An Emerging Model for Healing." *American Journal of Acupuncture.* Sept., 1981.

Vithoulkas, George, *The Science of Homeopathy.* New York: Grove, 1979.

DANA ULLMAN, *M.P.H., authored* Everybody's Guide to Homeopathic Medicines *(Tarcher, 1984) and is also known for his work on legal issues of alternative health care.*

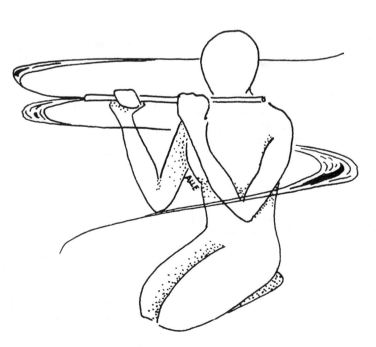

Holistic Health—Holistic Peace

Fritjof Capra

The Paradigm Shift

THE THREAT of nuclear war is the most dramatic symptom of a multifaceted, global crisis that touches every aspect of our lives: our health and livelihood, the quality of our environment and our social relationships, our economy, technology, our politics—our very survival on this planet. Conventional politicians no longer know where to turn to minimize the damage. They argue about priorities and about the relative merits of short-term technological and economic "fixes" without realizing that the major problems of our time are simply different facets of a single systemic crisis. They are closely interconnected and interdependent and cannot be understood through the fragmented approaches pursued by our academic disciplines and government agencies. Rather than solving any of the difficulties, such approaches merely shift them around in the complex web of social and ecological relations. A resolution can be found only if the structure of the web itself is changed, and this will involve profound transformations of our social and political institutions, values, and ideas.

The first step in overcoming the crisis, in my view, is to recognize that the required profound cultural transformation is, in fact, already beginning to take place. This transformation has many aspects. At its core is a dramatic shift of paradigms, or world views— a shift from a mechanistic to a holistic and ecological vision of reality. The paradigm now beginning to recede has dominated our culture for several hundred years, during which it has significantly influenced the rest of the world. This world view consists of a number of ideas and values, among them the belief that the universe is a mechanical system composed of elementary material building blocks, the view of the human body as a machine, the view of life in society as a competitive struggle for existence, the belief in unlimited material progress to be achieved through economic and technological growth, and—last, not least—the belief that a society in which the female is everywhere subsumed

under the male is one that follows a basic law of nature. During recent decades all of these assumptions have been found severely limited and in need of radical revision.

The mechanistic world view was formulated most succinctly in 17th-century science by Galileo, Descartes, Newton, Bacon, and several others. During the subsequent 300 years it was extremely successful and dominated all scientific thought. Today, however, its limitations have become clearly visible, and scientists and nonscientists alike will have to change their underlying philosophies in profound ways in order to participate in the current cultural transformation.

Mechanistic Views of Health and Peace

I would like to illustrate the limitations of Cartesian-Newtonian thinking with two examples—health and peace; these two examples turn out to show some striking parallels. The mechanistic view of health still dominates our medical institutions and the mechanistic view of peace dominates the thinking of our politicians and the military. In both cases we have to realize, of course, that the mechanistic view and the "engineering approach," are of great value. But they are limited and must be integrated into a larger holistic framework.

Descartes compared the human organism to a clockwork. "I consider the human body as a machine," he wrote. "My thought compares a sick man and an ill-made clock with my idea of a healthy man and a well-made clock." Many characteristics of current medical theory and practice can be traced back to this Cartesian imagery. Health is often defined as the absence of disease, and disease is seen as a malfunctioning of biological mechanisms which are studied from the point of view of cellular and molecular biology. The doctor's role is to intervene, using medical technology, to correct the malfunctioning of a specific mechanism, different parts of the body being treated by different specialists.

As medical scientists define health as the absence of disease, so military strategists define peace as the absence of war, and the engineering approach to health has its

---

Keynote Address to the Fourth Medical Congress for the Prevention of Nuclear War, Tubingen, West Germany, 30 March, 1984.

counterpart in the engineering approach to peace. Politicians and military men tend to perceive all problems of defense simply as problems of technology. The idea that social and psychological considerations—let alone philosophy or poetry—could also be relevant is not entertained. Moreover, questions of security and defense are analyzed predominantly in Newtonian terms—"power blocks," "action and reaction," the "political vacuum," and so on.

In contemporary health care the human organism is generally dissociated from the natural and social environment in which it is embedded, and the large network of phenomena that influence health is reduced to its physiological and biochemical aspects. In very similar ways, the conventional approach to defense reduces the large network of phenomena that influence peace to its strategic and technological aspects. And even those aspects are further reduced as politicians and the military continue to talk about national security without recognizing the dangerous fallacy of this simplistic and fragmented notion. Most of our politicians, led by the American president, still seem to think that we can increase our own security by making others feel insecure. Since the threats made with today's nuclear weapons threaten to extinguish life on the entire planet, the new thinking about peace must necessarily be global thinking. In the nuclear age, the entire concept of national security has become outdated; there can only be global security.

In conventional medical thinking, the therapy involves technological intervention. The self-organizing and self-healing potential of the patient is not taken into account. Similarly, conventional military thinking holds that conflicts are best resolved by technological intervention and does not take into account the self-organizing potential of people, communities, and nations—see Afghanistan, Grenada, Poland, Nicaragua, and many other examples.

The conceptual problem at the center of contemporary health care is the confusion between disease processes and disease origins. Instead of asking why an illness occurs and trying to remove the conditions that lead to it, medical researchers try to understand the mechanisms through which the disease operates, so that they can then interfere with them. Very often their research is guided by the idea of a single mechanism that dominates all the others and can be corrected by technological intervention. Similarly, politicians tend to be blind to the origins of conflicts and concentrate instead on the external processes; for example, on the visible acts of individual violence rather than the hidden structural and institutional violence. An extreme example of reductionist thinking is President Reagan, who believes that he has found the key mechanism of all conflicts around the world—Communist infiltration by the Soviet Union—and that he can correct it by intervening with massive military technology.

Patriarchal Values

The mechanistic world view has been complemented by a value system that is much older than Cartesian-Newtonian science. The values, attitudes, and behavior patterns which dominate our culture and are embodied in our social institutions are typical traits of patriarchal culture. Like all patriarchal societies, our society tends to favor self-assertion over integration, analysis over synthesis, rational knowledge over intuitive wisdom, competition over cooperation, expansion over conservation.

None of these values and attitudes is intrinsically good or bad, but the imbalance characteristic of our society today is unhealthy and dangerous. The most severe consequence of this imbalance is the ever-increasing threat of nuclear war, brought about by an over-emphasis on self-assertion, control and power, excessive competition, and a pathological obsession with "winning" in a situation where the whole concept of winning has lost its meaning, because there can be no winners in a nuclear war.

There is now a rich feminist literature on the roots of militarism and war in patriarchal values and patriarchal thinking. Patriarchy, these authors point out, operates within the context of dominance/submission. Thus parity of nuclear weapons is not enough for American generals; they want superiority. This "macho" competition in the arms race extends even to the size of missiles. During the Carter Administration, military lobbyists persuaded politicians to spend more money on defense by showing them upright models of Soviet and American missiles, in which the Soviet missiles were larger, although it was known that the larger missiles were technically inferior. The phallic shape of these missiles makes the sexual connotation of this competition in missile size obvious.

Patriarchy equates aggression and dominance with masculinity, and warfare is held to be the ultimate initiation into true manhood. In prepatriarchal cultures, the menstrual blood of women was the source of sacred mysteries, a blood associated with giving life and nurturing. Patriarchy transformed this association. The sacred blood became the blood of death. Honor became associated with the blood shed in the warrior's glorious death on the battlefield. When I went to school in Austria, I learned that the colors of the Austrian flag, red-white-red, were inspired by the white uniform of a hero soaked in red blood after a battle. But in a nuclear war, there are no white uniforms and no battlefields. The patriarchal codes of honor have become outdated.

To conclude my illustrations of the parallels between concepts of health and concepts of peace within the old paradigm, I should mention that in both areas the mechanistic views are perpetuated not only by scientists, politicians, and generals, but also—and perhaps even more forcefully—by the pharmaceutical and military industries, which have invested heavily in the old paradigm. The scientific establishment and the corporate community match each other perfectly, since the outdated Cartesian world view underlies both the theoretical framework of the former and the technologies and economic motives of the latter. To change this situation is now absolutely vital for our well-being and survival, and change will only be possible if we are able, as a society, to shift to the new holistic and ecological paradigm.

The Systems View

Indeed, such a shift is now occurring. Researchers on the leading edge of science, various social movements, and numerous alternative networks are now developing a new vision of reality that will form the basis of our future technologies, economic systems, and social institutions. The new world view emphasizes the interconnectedness and interdependence of all phenomena, as well as the embeddedness of individuals and societies in the cyclical processes of nature. It is profoundly ecological in a sense that goes far beyond the immediate concerns with environmental protection. It is supported by modern science but is rooted in a perception of reality that goes beyond the scientific framework to an intuitive awareness of the oneness of all life, the interdependence of its multiple manifestations and its cycles of change and transformation. Ultimately, such deep ecological awareness is spiritual, or religious, awareness. In fact, the root of the word "religion"—from *religare* ("to bind strongly")—points to that awareness of being connected to the cosmos as a whole. Ecological awareness, then, is truly spiritual at its deepest level.

In science, the most coherent formulation of the ecological paradigm is found in the new systems theory of life that was developed in the 1970s by a number of researchers from various disciplines—Prigogine, Jantsch, Bateson, Maturana, Eigen, etc. The systems view looks at the world in terms of relationships and integration. Systems are integrated wholes whose properties cannot be reduced to those of smaller units. Instead of concentrating on basic building blocks, the systems approach emphasizes basic principles of organization. Examples of systems abound in nature. Every organism—from the smallest bacterium through the wide range of plants and animals to humans—is an integrated whole and thus a living system. Cells are living systems, and so are the various tissues and organs of the body. But living systems are not confined to individual organisms and their parts. The same aspects of wholeness are exhibited by social systems—such as a family or a community—and by ecosystems that consist of a variety of organisms and inanimate matter in mutual interaction.

All these natural systems are wholes whose specific structures arise from the interactions and interdependence of their parts. Systemic properties are destroyed when a system is dissected, either physically or theoretically, into isolated elements. Although we can discern individual parts in any sytem, the nature of the whole is always different from the mere sum of its parts. Another important aspect of systems is their intrinsically dynamic nature. Their forms are not rigid structures, but flexible manifestations of underlying processes. Systems thinking is process thinking; form becomes associated with process, interrelation with interaction, and opposites are unified through oscillation.

An important aspect of living systems is their tendency to form multilevel structures of systems within systems. For example, the human body contains organ systems composed of several organs, each organ being made of tissues and each tissue made up of cells. All these are living systems that consist of smaller parts and, at the same time, act as parts of larger wholes. The entire organism, furthermore, is embedded in larger social and ecological systems. Each living system, then, is a part and a whole at the same time, and accordingly it has two opposite tendencies: an integrative tendency to function as part of the larger whole, and a self-assertive tendency to preserve its individual autonomy. In a healthy system, there is a balance between self-assertion and integration. This balance is not static but consists of a dynamic interplay between the two opposite but complementary tendencies, which makes the whole system flexible and open to change.

Systems Views of Health and Peace

The systems view of living organisms seems to provide an ideal basis for a holistic approach to health, an approach that is profoundly ecological and thus in harmony with the Hippocratic tradition, which lies at the roots of Western medicine. At the same time, the parallels between health and peace can be carried further: corresponding to the systems view of health there is also a systems view of peace.

At the core of the systems view of health lies the notion of dynamic balance. Health is an experience of well-being resulting from a dynamic balance that involves the physical and psychological aspects of the organism, as well as its interactions with its natural and social environment. The natural balance of living organisms includes, in particular, the balance between their self-assertive and integrative tendencies. To be healthy an organism has to preserve its individual autonomy, but at the same time it has to be able to integrate itself harmoniously into larger systems. Imbalance manifests itself as stress, and excessive stress is harmful and will often lead to illness.

The health and dynamic balance of social systems is a necessary condition for true peace. To be in such a healthy and peaceful state, a social group, or nation, has to preserve its automony and, at the same time, has to be able to integrate itself harmoniously into the larger national, or global, community. As in the case of individual health, imbalances manifest themselves as stress, or conflict, and excessive conflict is harmful and likely to lead to violence and war.

From the systems point of view, effective health care consists largely in finding healthy ways of managing stress. This means restoring and maintaining the dynamic balance of individuals and social groups by recognizing the web of interrelated patterns which leads to ill health and changing it in such a way that the stress is minimized. Such a holistic approach to health will involve a whole range of therapies—from psychological and social counseling to "bodywork," various techniques of relaxation, nutritonal therapy, herbal medicine, etc. It will, of course, also include standard medical therapies.

Similarly, a holistic approach to peace will consist largely in finding healthy, nonviolent ways of conflict resolution. This will mean, first of all, developing a holistic view of the network of economic, social, and political patterns out of which conflicts arise. Once these patterns have been understood, a wide range of methods may be used to resolve the conflicts. Humanistic psychologists, family therapists, and social workers have spent the last two decades studying group dynamics and have developed a whole spectrum of techniques of stress management and conflict resolution. It is now time to apply these techniques at the political level—nationally, between nations, and globally.

DREAMS AND PLANETARY CONSCIOUSNESS

Jeremy Taylor

For centuries, great world religions, mystics, and artists of all cultures and periods have proclaimed that all humanity and all the world is one. But they have essentially been ignored by the vast majority of humankind, who persist in making ultimate distinctions between "us" and "them," and acting as though local ecosystems were hermetically sealed and separated from the rest of the world. Now the collective unconscious, acting through the agency of human consciousness, has generated the "nightmare" possibilities of nuclear war, accident, and planning failure. Horrible though the nightmare of nuclear menace is, it has—like all nightmares—made its positive point more memorably and effectively than have the gentler admonitions of the world's spiritual teachers over the past 4000 years or so: WE ARE ONE! (And the terrible shadow of nuclear disaster falls alike on *everyone*.)

Our collective perils are real and pressing. We have manufactured them for ourselves, and we must look at them consciously and clearly in order to find ways of disarming ourselves, reforming our institutions, and reconciling ourselves with our planetary neighbors and with the ultimate ecological and spiritual interconnectedness of all beings. Dream work can enhance and energize these efforts by breaking down our prematurely closed prejudices, opinions, ideologies, and world views. Paying attention to our dreams opens us regularly to the creative impulse, and offers new ways of understanding our as-yet-unrealized developmental and evolutionary potential. Group dream work can also create a community of support and understanding that can sustain us in the efforts to remake global society in a wiser, more humane, and more just form, as well as offering specific insights and ideas to accomplish this vitally important task.

The search for wholistic health and healing always extends beyond the individual into the environment, and ultimately involves the health of the entire human species, of all species, and of the planet as a whole. The health of each depends upon the health of all. Dream work offers a unique avenue of both individual and collective healing and reconciliation, because the symbolic language and grammar of dreams and dreaming is universal—all people dream in essentially the same way, and the dreams bring their messages of healing and growth alike to us all.

JEREMY TAYLOR *is a Unitarian Universalist Minister and dream worker living in the San Francisco Bay Area.*

The Rising Culture

All this is not going to be easy, because the majority of politicians, military strategists, and corporate leaders are more interested in maintaining the status quo than in our health, peace, and survival. They will do everything they can to oppose any changes that might curtail their power and profit expectations. However, they will not be able to prevent the paradigm shift and cultural transformation that has already begun. The '60s and '70s have generated a whole series of social movements which all seem to go in the same direction; they all emphasize different aspects of the same new vision of reality.

There is a rising concern with ecology, expressed by citizens' movements that are forming around environmental issues—first and foremost the death of the forests—pointing out the limits to growth, advocating a new ecological ethic, and developing appropriate "soft" technologies. They are also the sources of emerging counter-economies (self-help networks, etc.) based on decentralized, cooperative, and ecologically harmonious life-styles. In the political arena, the peace movement is opposing the nuclear missiles—the most extreme outgrowth of an overly self-assertive, "macho" technology—calling on both Moscow and Washington to de-escalate the arms race and proposing phases of demilitarization.

The peace and ecology movements are active in Europe as well as in America, and there are now many contacts and initiatives of collaboration between individuals and organizations on both sides of the Atlantic; between people who feel that solidarity with the human family and with all of living nature is more meaningful than any allegiance to a nation-state. In fact, these contacts are beginning to include the Soviet Union. There are several American initiatives to meet Russians, bypassing all government channels, in order to communicate their common interests in health and peace.

At the same time, there is the beginning of a significant shift in values, from the admiration of large-scale enterprises and institutions to the notion of "small is beautiful," from material consumption to voluntary simplicity, from economic and technological growth to inner growth and development. These new values are being promoted by the human-potential movement, the holistic health movement, and by spiritual movements that re-emphasize the quest for meaning and the spiritual dimension of life. Lastly, but perhaps most importantly, the old value system is being challenged and profoundly changed by the rise of feminist awareness, originating in the women's movement.

During the 1970s, most of these movements operated separately and did not recognize how their purposes interrelate. In the last few years, however, several important coalitions have been formed, mainly between the ecology, peace, and women's movements. Thus people now speak of "Oko-Pax," "ecofeminism," or the "Frauenfriedensbewegung" (women's peace movement). Finally, this merging of ideas, concerns, and movements has been translated into political practice by the Greens, who have begun to change the political culture of West Germany in ways that are inspiring alternative movements around the world.

In this coalescence of movements, which I have called "the rising culture," the collaboration between physicians, health professionals, and the peace movement is extremely important. Many have already been very successful in raising the public consciousness through discussions and testimonies about the medical consequences of nuclear war.

I am suggesting that you could go even further. By applying experience in holistic health care to conflict resolution and stress management within social groups, nations, and the global community, corresponding holistic approaches can be developed to peace. This would be a further step in the coalescence of movements subscribing to the new vision of reality; a further step in the evolution of our cultural transformation. Many social and political forces will oppose such a step, but the realization that evolutionary changes of this kind cannot be prevented by short-term political activities provides great hope for the future.

FRITJOF CAPRA *received his Ph.D. from the University of Vienna and has done research in high-energy physics at several European and American universities. In addition to his many technical research papers, Dr. Capra has written and lectured extensively about the philosophical implications of modern science. He is the author of* The Tao of Physics, *an international bestseller that has sold a half a million copies and has been translated into a dozen languages.*

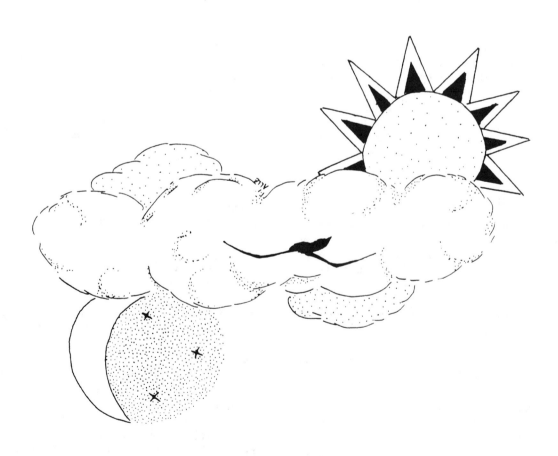

How to Deal with Despair

Joanna Rogers Macy, Ph.D.

I do not wish to seem overdramatic but I can only conclude from the information that is available to me as Secretary-General, that the Members of the United Nations have perhaps ten years left in which to subordinate their ancient quarrels and launch a global partnership to curb the arms race, to improve the human environment, to defuse the population explosion, and to supply the required momentum to development efforts. If such a global partnership is not forged within the next decade, then I very much fear that the problems I have mentioned will have reached such staggering proportions that they will be beyond our capacity to control.

—U. Thant (1969)

OUR TIME bombards us with signals of distress—of ecological destruction, waning resources, social breakdown, and uncontrolled nuclear proliferation. Not surprisingly, people are feeling despair—a despair well merited by the hair-trigger machinery of mass death that we have created and continue to serve. What is surprising is the extent to which we hide this despair from ourselves and one another. If we are, as Arthur Koestler suggested, undergoing an age of anxiety, we are also growing adept at sweeping this anxiety under the rug. As a society, we are caught between a sense of impending apocalypse and an inability to acknowledge it.

Political activists, who would arouse us to the fact that our very survival is at stake, decry public apathy. The cause of this apathy, however, is not mere indifference; it derives also from dread. It stems from a fear of confronting the despair that lurks subliminally beneath the tenor of life-as-usual. If anything, the alarms raised by protestors have an anesthetic effect, numbing us to our despair. Our dread of what is happening to our future is banished to the fringes of awareness, too deep for most of us to name, too fearsome to face. Sometimes it manifests in dreams of mass destruction—and is exorcised in the morning jog and shower, or in the public fantasies of disaster entertainment. But it is rarely acknowledged or expressed directly. Because of social taboos against despair and because of fear of pain, it is kept at bay.

The suppression of despair, like that of any deep recurrent response, produces a partial numbing of the psyche: expressions of anger or terror are muted, deadened as if a nerve had been cut. This refusal of feeling takes a heavy toll: not only an impoverishment of emotional and sensory life (the flowers dimmer and less fragrant, loves less ecstatic), but a lessened capacity to process and respond to information. The energy expended in pushing down despair is diverted from more creative uses, depleting resilience and imagination needed for fresh visions and strategies. Furthermore, the *fear* of despair can erect an invisible screen, selectively filtering out anxiety-provoking data. Since organisms require feedback in order to adapt and survive, such evasion is suicidal. Now, just when we most urgently need to measure the effects of our acts, attention and curiosity slacken—as if we were already preparing for the Big Sleep. Many of us, doggedly attending to business-as-usual, deny both our despair and our ability to cope with it.

Despair cannot be banished by sermons on "positive thinking" or injections of optimism. Like grief, it must be worked through. It must be named, and validated as a healthy, normal, human response to the planetary situation. Faced and experienced, despair can be *used*: as the psyche's defenses drop away, new energies are released.

I am convinced that we can come to terms with apocalyptic anxieties in ways that are integrative and liberating, opening awareness not only to planetary distress, but also to the hope inherent in our own capacity to change. To do so, a process analogous to grief work is in order. "Despair work" is distinct in that its aim is not acceptance of loss (indeed, the "loss" has not yet occurred and is hardly to be "accepted"), but similar in the dynamics unleashed by the willingness to acknowledge, feel, and express inner pain.

Reprinted by permission from *New Age Magazine*, June 1979 issue
Copyright© New Age Communication Inc.

Ingredients of Despair

Regardless of whether we choose to accord them serious attention, we are daily barraged by data that render questionable, for the first time in recorded history, the survival of our culture and our species, and even of our planet as a viable home for conscious life. These warning signals prefigure, to those who do take them seriously, probabilities of apocalypse that are mind-boggling in scope. While varied, each scenario presents its own relentless logic. Poisoned by oil spills, sludge, and plutonium, the seas are dying; when the plankton disappear (in 30 years at present pollution rates, says Jean-Jacques Cousteau), we will suffocate from lack of oxygen. *Or* carbon dioxide from industrial and automotive combustion will saturate the atmosphere, creating a greenhouse effect that will melt the polar icecaps. *Or* radioactive poisoning from nuclear reactors and their wastes will not only induce plagues of cancer that will decimate populations, but cause fearful mutations in the survivors. *Or* deforestation and desertification of the planet, now rapidly advancing, will produce giant dustbowls, unimaginable famines. The probability of each of these perils is amply and soberly documented by scientific studies (many of which are summarized in Lester Brown's *The 29th Day*). The list of such scenarios could continue; the most immediate and likely stem from the use of nuclear bombs, by terrorists or superpowers. That eventually presents vistas of such horror that, as is said, "The survivors will envy the dead."

Despair, in this context, is not a macabre certainty of doom, nor a pathological condition of depression and futility. It is not a nihilism denying meaning or efficacy to human effort. Rather, as it is being experienced by increasing numbers across a broad spectrum of society, despair is the loss of the assumption that the species will inevitably pull through. It represents a genuine accession to the possibility that this planetary "experiment" may fail.

Symptoms and Suppressions

Years ago, at a leprosarium in India, I met a young woman, a mother of four. Her case was advanced, the doctor pointed out, because for so long she had hidden its signs. Fearing ostracism and banishment, she had covered her sores with her sari, pulled the shoulder drape around so that no one would see. In a similar fashion did I once hide despair for our world, cloaking it like a shameful disease—and so, I have learned, do others.

When the sensations aroused by the serious contemplation of a likely, but avoidable end to human existence break through the censorship we tend to impose on them, they can be intense and physical. A friend, who left her career to work as a full-time antinuclear organizer, tells me her onslaughts of grief came as a cold, heavy weight on the chest and a sense of her body breaking. Mine, which began two years ago, after an all-day symposium on threats to our biosphere, were sudden and wrenching: I would be alone in my study, working, and the next moment would find me on the floor, curled like a fetus and shaking. In company I was more controlled, but even then in those

early months, unused to despair, occasionally I would be caught off guard: a line from Shakespeare or a Bach phrase would pierce me with pain, as I found myself wondering how much longer it would be heard, before fading out forever in the galactic silences.

At the prospect of the extinction of our civilization, feelings of grief and horror are natural. We tend to hide them, though, from ourselves and each other. Why? The reasons are both social and psychological.

Despair is resisted so tenaciously because it represents a loss of control, an admission of powerlessness. Our culture dodges it by demanding instant solutions. "Don't come to me with a problem unless you have a solution": that tacit injunction, operative even in public policy-making, rings like my mother's words to me as a child, "If you can't say something nice, don't say anything at all."

In a culture committed to the American dream, it is hard to own up to despair. This is still the land of Dale Carnegie and Norman Vincent Peale, where an unflagging optimism is taken as means and measure of success. As commercials for products and campaigns of politicians attest, the healthy, admirable person smiles a lot. Feelings of depression, loneliness, and anxiety—to which this thinking animal has always been heir—carry here an added burden: One feels bad about feeling bad. The failure to hope, in a country built and nurtured on utopian expectations, can seem downright un-American, a betrayal.

In a religious context, despair can appear as a lapse of faith. Speaking at a vigil held in a church before a demonstration against nuclear weapons at the Pentagon last fall, Daniel Berrigan spoke of the necessity of hope to carry us through. Others chimed in, affirming their belief in the vision of a "New Jerusalem," and their gratitude for having that hope. After a pause, a young man who planned to participate in the week's civil disobedience actions spoke up falteringly: he questioned whether hope was really prerequisite, because—and he admitted this with difficulty—he was not feeling it. Even among friends committed to the same goal, it was clearly hard for him (and brave of him, I thought) to admit despair. Evidently, he feared he would be misunderstood, taken as cowardly or cynical—a fear validated by the response of some present.

"There is nothing more feared and less faced," writes Jesuit essayist William Lynch, "than the possibility of despair." This is one reason, he notes, why the mentally ill are so thoroughly isolated from the well—or why, one might add, expressions of anguish for the future are considered a breach of etiquette. Our culture discourages the acknowledgement of despair: this inhibition amounts to a social taboo. Those who break this taboo—to express their concern about nuclear holocaust, for example—are generally considered "crazy," or at least "depressed and depressing." No one wants a Cassandra around or welcomes a Banquo at the feast. Nor, indeed, are such roles enjoyable to play.

When the prospect of collective suicide first hit me as a serious possibility—and I remember the day and hour my defenses against this despair suddenly collapsed—I felt there were no one to whom I could turn in my grief. If there were—and indeed there was, for I have loving, intelligent friends and family—what is there to say? Do I want them to feel this horror, too? What can be said without casting a pall, or without seeming to ask for unacceptable word of comfort and cheer?

To feel despair in such a cultural setting brings on a sense of isolation. The psychic dissonance can be so acute as to seem to border on madness. The distance between our inklings of apocalypse and the tenor of business-as-usual is so great that, though we may respect our own cognitive reading of the signs, our affective response is frequently the conclusion that it is we, not society, who are insane.

Psychotherapy, by and large, offers little help for coping with these feelings, and indeed compounds the problem by reducing social despair to private pathology. Practitioners have trouble crediting the notion that concerns for the general welfare might be genuine, and acute enough to cause distress. Assuming that all our drives are ego-centered, they tend to treat expressions of this distress reductionistically, as manifestations of private neurosis. (In my own case, which is far from unique, deep dismay over destruction of the wilderness was diagnosed as fear of my own libido—symbolized by bulldozers!—and my painful preoccupation with U.S. bombings of Vietnam was interpreted as an unwholesome hangover of Puritan guilt.) Such "therapy," of course, only intensifies the sense of isolation and craziness that despair can bring, while inhibiting its recognition and expression.

Our culture makes it hard to get in touch with the genuine dimensions of our despair, and until we do, our power of creative response to planetary crisis will be crippled. Until we can grieve for our planet and its future inhabitants, we cannot fully feel or enact our love for them. Such grief is frequently suppressed, not only because it is socially awkward, but also because it is both hard to credit and very painful. At the root of both these inhibitions lies a dysfunctional notion of the self, as an isolated and fragile entity. Such a self has no reason to weep for the unseen and the unborn, and such a self, if it did, might shatter with pain and futility.

So long as we see ourselves as essentially separate, competitive, and ego-identified beings, it is difficult to respect the validity of our social despair, deriving as it does from interconnectedness. As open systems, we are sustained by flows of energy and information that extend beyond the reach of conscious ego. Both our capacity to grieve for others and our power to cope with this grief spring from the great matrix of relationships in which we take our being. Just as our pain is more than private, so is our resilience.

Validation

You can hold yourself back from the suffering world: this is something you are free to do . . . , but perhaps precisely this holding back is the only suffering you might be able to avoid.

—Elie Wiesel

The first step in despair work is to disabuse oneself of the notion that grief for our world is morbid. To experience anguish and anxiety in face of the perils threatening humanity is a healthy reaction. This pain, far from being crazy, is rather a testimony to the unity of life, to the deep interconnections that relate us to all beings.

Such pain for the world becomes masochistic only when one assumes personal guilt for its plight or personal responsibility for the solution. No individual is that powerful. True, by participating in society, each shares in a collective accountability, but acknowledging despair, like faith, means letting go of the manipulative assumption that conscious ego can or should control all events. Each of us is but one little nexus in a vast web. As the recognition of that interdependence breaches our sense of isolation, so also does it free our despair of self-recrimination.

Most world religions corroborate the goals of despair work, offering constructs and symbols attesting to the creative role of this kind of distress. In the Mahayana Buddhist tradition, for example, *bodhisattvas* vow to forswear Nirvana until all beings are enlightened. Their compassion is said to endow them with supranormal senses: they can hear not only the music of the spheres, but also all cries of distress. All griefs are registered and owned in the bodhisattva's deep knowledge that we are not separate from one another.

Positive Disintegration

The process of internalizing the possibility of planetary demise is bound to cause deep psychic disarray. How to confront what we scarcely dare think? How to think about it without going to pieces?

It is helpful in despair work to realize that going to pieces or falling apart is not such a bad thing. Indeed, it is as essential to evolutionary and psychic transformations as the cracking of outgrown shells. What Kazimierz Dabrowski calls "positive disintegration" has been operative in every global development of humankind, especially during periods of accelerated change; it permits, he argues, the emergence of "higher psychic structures and awareness." Occurring when individuals internalize painful contradictions in human experience, positive disintegration can appear as a dark night of the soul, a time of spiritual void and turbulence. But the anxieites and doubts are, Dabrowski maintains, "essentially healthy and creative"—not only for the person but for society, because they permit new and original approaches to reality.

What "disintegrates" in periods of rapid transformation is not the self, of course, but its defenses and ideas. We are not objects that can break. As open systems, we are, as Norbert Wiener writes in *The Human Use of Human Beings* (Doubleday, 1954), "but whirlpools in a river of everflowing water. We are not stuff that abides, but patterns that perpetuate themselves." We do not need to protect ourselves from change, for our very nature is change. Defensive self-protection, restricting vision and movement like a suit of armor, makes it harder to adapt; it not only reduces flexibility, but blocks the flow of information we need to survive. Our "going to pieces," however uncomfortable a process, can open us up to new perceptions, new data, new responses.

Feeling

No matter how safe and comfortable our personal lives or engrossing our private concerns may be, grief for those who suffer now, and may suffer in the future, is present in us all on some level. Given the flows of information circling our globe, our psyches, however inattentive or callous they may appear, have registered the signals of distress. We do not need to be exhorted or scolded into feelings of concern and compassion, for they inhere in us already, by virtue of our nature as open systems, interdependent with the rest of life. We need only to be encouraged and empowered to open our consciousness to the griefs and apprehensions that are within us.

We cannot experience these feelings without pain, but it is a healthy pain, like the kind felt as circulation is restored to a limb that has gone "to sleep": it gives evidence that the tissue is still alive. In dealing with these feelings, as with a cramped limb, exercises can help. I have found meditational exercises useful, particularly ones from the Buddhist tradition. Practices such as the *Brahmaviharas*, or "Abodes of the Buddha," designed to increase the capacity to experience such feelings as loving-kindness and compassion, can get us in touch with those concerns in us that extend beyond ego—and, in so doing, with our social despair.

In one workshop I led, entitled "Being Bodhisattvas," we did a meditation on compassion which involved giving oneself permission to experience the sufferings of others (imaginatively, but in as concrete a fashion as possible), and then taking these sufferings in with the breath, visualizing them as a dark stream drawn in with each inhalation, into and through the heart.

Afterwards, one participant, Marianna, described her experience in this meditation. She had been resistant, and her resistance had localized as a pain in her back. In encouraging the participants to open themselves to their inner awareness of the sufferings of others, I had primed the pump with some brief verbal cues, mentioning our fellow beings in hospitals and prisons, a mother with dried breasts holding a hungry infant . . . That image awoke in Marianna an episode she had buried. Three years earlier she had listened to a record by Harry Chapin with a song about a starving child; she had, as she put it, "trouble" with it. She put away the record, never to play it again, and the "trouble" remained undigested. With her recollection of her experience with the song, the pain in her back moved into her chest. It intensified and hardened, piercing her heart. It seemed for a moment excruciating, but as she continued the exercise, accepting and breathing in the pain, it suddenly, inexplicably, felt right, felt even good. It turned into a golden cone or funnel, aimed point downward into the depths of her heart. Through it poured the despair she had refused, griefs reconnecting her with the rest of humanity.

Marianna emerged from this experience with a sense of release and empowerment. She felt empowered, she said, not to *do* so much as to *be*—open, ready to act. She also believed that she had allowed herself to open up because I had not asked her to "do" something about the griefs of others, or to come up with any answers, but only to experience them.

Sometimes the blocked emotions of despair become accessible through dreams. A very vivid dream came to me one night after I had spent hours perusing statistics on nuclear pollution; before going to bed I had leafed through baby pictures of our three children to find a snapshot for my daughter's high-school yearbook.

In my dream I behold the three of them as they appeared in the old photos, and I am struck most by the sweet wholesomeness of their flesh. My husband and I are journeying with them across an unfamiliar landscape. The land is becoming dreary, treeless and strewn with rocks; Peggy, the youngest, can barely clamber over the boulders in the path. Just as the going is getting very difficult, even frightening, I suddenly realize that, by some thoughtless but unalterable prearrangement, their father and I must leave them. I can see the grimness of the way that lies ahead of them, bleak and craggy as a moonscape and with a flesh-burning, sickly tinge to the air. I am maddened with sorrow that my children must face this ordeal without me. I kiss them each and tell them we will meet again, but I know no place to name where we will meet. Perhaps another planet, I say. Innocent of terror, they try to reassure me, ready to be off. Removed, from a height in the sky, I watch them go—three small solitary figures trudging across that angry wasteland, holding one another by the hand and not stopping to look back. In spite of the widening distance, I see with a surrealist's precision the ulcerating of their flesh. I see how the skin bubbles and curls back to expose raw tissue, as they doggedly go forward, the boys helping the little sister across the rocks.

I woke up, brushed my teeth, showered, had an early breakfast meeting, took notes for a research proposal. Still the dream would not let me go. As I woke Peggy for school, I sank beside her bed. "Hold me," I said, "I had a bad dream." With my face in her warm nightie, inhaling her fragrance, I found myself sobbing. I sobbed against her body, against her 17-year old womb, as the knowledge of all that assails it surfaced in me. Statistical studies of the effects of ionizing radiation, columns of figures on cancers and genetic damage, their inutterable import turned into tears—speechless, wracking.

What good does it do to let go and allow ourselves to *feel* the possibilities we dread? For all the discomfort, there is healing in such openness, for ourselves and perhaps for our world. To drop our defenses and let grief surface brings not only release but connection. Opening to our despair opens us also to the love that is within us, for it is in deep caring that our anguish is rooted. The caring and connection are real, but we cut ourselves off from their power when we hide from the grief they bring.

Imagining

To acknowledge and express our despair, we need images and symbols. Images, more than arguments, tap the springs of consciousness, the creative powers by which we make meaning of experience. In the challenge to survival that we now face, exercise of the imagination is especially necessary, because existing verbal constructs seem inadequate to what many of us are sensing.

Recognizing the creative powers of imagery, many call upon us today to come up with visions of a benign future—visions that can beckon and inspire. Images of hope *are* potent, necessary: they can shape our goals and give us impetus for reaching them. Often they are invoked too soon, however, diverting us from painful, but fruitful confrontation with the causes of our crisis and our own deep feelings. Sometimes it takes a while, in the slow alchemy of the soul, for hope to signal, and longer still for it to take form in concrete plans and projects. Genuine visioning happens from the roots up, and right now, for many of us, those roots are shriveled by unacknowledged despair. This is an in-between time: we are groping in the dark, with shattered beliefs and faltering hopes, and we need images for this phase if we are to work through it.

Working together in groups is a good way to evoke powerful images to express—and thereby own—our despair. Quaker-style meetings, especially, in which a group sits and shares out of open silence, are an excellent way of letting images appear and interact.

In a workshop I once gave on planetary survival, I explored means by which we could share our apprehensions on an affective as well as cognitive level. I asked the participants to offer, as they introduced themselves, a personal experience or image of how, in the past year, the global crisis had impinged on their consciousness. Those brief introductions were potent. Some offered a vignette from work on world hunger or arms. A young physicist simply said, very quietly, "My child was born." A social worker recalled a day her small daughter talked about growing up and having babies; with dull shock she encountered her own doubt that the world would last that long. Some offered images: fishkill washed up at a summer cottage, strip mines leaching like open wounds. Most encompassing in its simplicity was John's image: the view from space of planet Earth, so small that it could be covered by the astronaut's raised thumb. That vision of our home, so finite that it can be blotted out by a single human gesture, functioned as a symbol in our week's work. It touched a raw nerve in us all—desperate concern.

In the sharing of despair that our imagery permitted, energy was released which vitalized our work. As pent-up feelings were expressed and compared, there came laughter, solidarity, and a resurgence of commitment to our common human project.

In that same workshop, John showed slides of a trek he took up Mount Katahdin with some of his students at Yale. Between two high peaks was a narrow, knife-edge trail that they had to cross: it was scary and dangerous because fog had rolled up, blanketing their destination and everything but the path itself. The picture of that trail, cutting through the clouds into the unknown, became a strong symbol for us, expressing the existential situation in which we find ourselves, and helping us to proceed patiently, even though we can see no more than a step at a time.

Waiting

> *I said to my soul, be still, and wait without hope,*
> *For hope would be hope of the wrong thing.*
> —T.S. Eliot

And so we wait; even as we work, we wait. Only out of that open expectancy can images and visions arise that strike deep enough to summon our faith in them. "The ability to wait," writes William Lynch, "is central to hope."

Waiting does not mean inaction, but staying in touch with our pain and confusion *as* we act, not banishing them to grab for sedatives, ideologies, or final solutions. Jacob Needleman suggests that part of the great danger in this time of crisis is that we may, in impatience and fear, short-circuit despair—and thereby lose the revelations that may open to us:

> ... For there is nothing to guarantee that we will be able to remain long enough or deeply enough in front of the unknown, a psychological state which the traditional paths have always recognized as sacred. In that fleeting state between dreams, which is called "despair" in some Western teachings and "self-questioning" in Eastern traditions, a man is said to be able to receive the truth, both about nature and his own possible role in the universal order.

In my own feelings of despair, I was haunted by the question, What do you substitute for hope? I had always assumed that a sanguine confidence in the future was as essential as oxygen. Without it, I had thought, one would collapse into apathy and nihilism. It puzzled me that in owning my despair, I found the hours I spent working for peace, environmental, and antinuclear causes did not lessen, but rather increased.

One day I was talking with Jim Douglass, the theologian and writer who left his university post to devote all his efforts to resisting nuclear weapons; jailed repeatedly for civil disobedience, he is now involved in the citizens' campaign against the Trident submarine. He said, in passing, that he believed we had five years left before it was too late—too late to avert the use of our nuclear arsenal in a first-strike strategy. I reflected on the implications of that remark and watched his face as he squinted in the sun, with an air of presence and serenity I could not fathom. "What do you substitute for hope?," I asked. He looked at me and smiled. "Possibilities," he said. "Possibilities. You can't predict—just make space for them. There are so many." That, too, is a form of waiting, active waiting—moving out along the fog-bound trail, even though we cannot see the way ahead.

Community

When we face the darkness of our time, openly and together, we tap deep reserves of strength within us. Many of us fear that confrontation with despair will bring loneliness and isolation, but—on the contrary—in the letting go of old defenses, truer community is found. In the synergy of sharing comes power.

Suggestions for Further Reading

Brown, Lester. *The 29th Day*. W. W. Norton, 1978.
Dabrowski, Kazimierz. *Positive Disintegration*. Little, Brown, 1964.

Douglass, James. *Resistance and Contemplation*. Doubleday, 1972.

Lifton, Robert. *Boundaries*. Simon & Schuster, 1967.

Lynch, William. *Images of Hope: Imagination as Healer of the Hopeless*. University of Notre Dame Press, 1974.

Needleman, Jacob. *A Sense of the Cosmos: The Encounter of Modern Science and Ancient Truth*. Dutton, 1977.

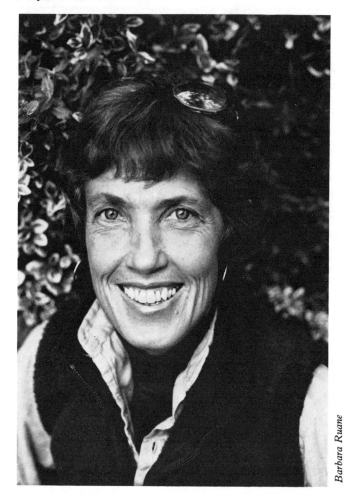

JOANNA ROGERS MACY, *Ph.D., is the originator of Despair and Empowerment work, a process for overcoming political apathy and powerlessness in the nuclear age. Her ground breaking article,* Despairwork *(1979) has been reprinted and excerpted in over 30 publications around the world. Some 50,000 people in the U.S. and Europe have participated in the workshops, whose theory and methods are described in her recent book* Despair and Personal Power in the Nuclear Age *(1983).*

Dr. Macy is cofounder of Interhelp, an organization of people engaged in this work, which is active in the U.S., Canada, U.K., Germany, and now Australia. Macy also works with the Sarvodaya Movement, a Buddhist-inspired village self-help organization in Sri Lanka, and is the author of Dharma and Development *(1983).*

Barbara Ruane

Workshop Exercise:
Ground/Earth/Speak

Chellis Glendinning, Ph.D.

THIS EXERCISE serves to introduce members of the workshop to each other in an intimate but non-threatening way—one that binds people together in its acknowledgment and support of our common concerns. It introduces us to our own feelings about nuclear war and the deterioration of the biosphere as it grounds us to one of our greatest resources, our connection to the Earth. It can be used in a group of varying size (from 12 to 500), in a room or outdoor space that is large and comfortable enough for everyone to lie down. If there are people present who cannot lie down or cannot walk, they may participate even so. They may sit or stand during the entire exercise and not miss any part of it. Estimated time for this exercise is 45–60 minutes.

To begin, the facilitator says:

Lie down on your back with your legs outstretched and your arms at your sides. Make sure you are comfortable. With your eyes closed begin to breathe with your mouth open. As you inhale through your mouth, let the breath come into your belly first, then into your chest. Long and deep. Then exhale...

(Estimated time is 2–3 minutes)

Now when you exhale, let there be a pause at the end of the exhale. Let there be a pause, and let your body decide when it wants to inhale again... then inhale. Deep into your belly and chest... exhale... let there be a pause... inhale...

(Estimated time is 2–3 minutes. If the belly is the place of breathing which activates the unconscious mind, as in deep sleep, the chest is the location of breath that best uses the conscious mind. In this breathing pattern, we dip into the unconscious by sending the breath to the belly. Then we make any messages, symbols or deep feelings accessible to the conscious mind by sending the breath to the chest. It is a pattern used and popularized by San Francisco therapist Magda Proskauer.)

Now as you inhale, visualize a light growing in your belly, expanding as you let in more air. If you are lifting your right leg let the light grow. If you are resting your leg let the light grow. As you exhale, let that light travel down your right leg and out the bottom of your right foot. If you are letting your leg drop, let it move through your leg and foot. If you are resting your leg, let it travel down and out the bottom of your foot. Continue the breath-leg lift pattern and continue to visualize the light.

(Estimated time is 2–3 minutes. This visualization establishes a conscious energy connection from the pelvis down the leg to the foot.)

Relax your right leg. Relax your breathing. Tune into how your body is feeling. Do you notice any differences between the right side of your body and your left? Notice any thoughts or images that come to mind.

(Estimated time is one minute)

Now begin the long deep breath again. Let your belly, then your chest expand as you inhale. Exhale. Allow a pause until your body wants to breath in again.

(Estimated time is one minute)

As you inhale, lift your left leg two or three inches off the floor...

(See instructions for right leg. Estimated time is 3–4 minutes)

Now let a light shine in your belly as you inhale. Let that light travel down your left leg as you exhale and out the bottom of your left foot...

(See instructions for right leg. Estimated time is 2–3 minutes)

Relax your breathing. Relax your leg. Notice how your body is feeling. Notice any images or thoughts you may be having.

(Estimated time is one minute)

With your eyes still closed, begin the long deep breath again. Inhale. Let your belly and chest expand. Exhale. Let yourself pause. Now as you exhale, make a movement towards coming to a sitting position...as you inhale, let yourself be still in the new position...take your time...exhale and let yourself be propelled by the breath to bring you to another position closer to sitting...inhale and rest...now as you exhale, let the breath move you towards a standing position...take your time...when you inhale be still, gaining energy for the next movement...

(Estimated time is 2–3 minutes. This is a way to get up without losing the sense of deep connection with one's self, the calm, the centeredness.)

Now you are standing. With eyes still closed, continue the long, deep breath. As you inhale, let your belly fill up with light. As you exhale, let the light travel down your legs, out the bottom of your feet into the floor and now, all the way down into the core of the earth.

(Estimated time is one minute. While the breathing pattern enhances our utilization of both unconscious and conscious mind, this visualization enhances our experience of being grounded, solidly placed on the Earth, and therefore strong.)

Now open your eyes. Allow the light, space, objects and people in this room to fill your vision. At the same time, keep breathing. Stay aware of the light in your belly and the light that connects you to the core of the earth...if you need to close your eyes to regain that connection, do so...begin to walk around the room. Explore and at the same time breathe. Let the light into your belly as you inhale. Exhale and send it down to the earth. Stay connected.

(Estimated time is two minutes. We learn to maintain contact with our deepest selves and the earth as we include seeing and walking.)

When you feel ready, come together with another person. (If the group contains an odd number of people, one "pair" can be made up of three people.) Stand before this person, make eye contact. At the same time stay aware of the light...if you feel distracted, close your eyes for a moment, breathe, visualize the light. Then try to open your eyes and face your partner ...be aware you are connected to the earth. Be aware your partner is connected to the earth.

Now I am going to say a sentence, an unfinished sentence. After I say it, one of you repeat the sentence and finish it with just one sentence. As you do, stay connected to the light.... Then the other partner repeat the sentence and finish it too.

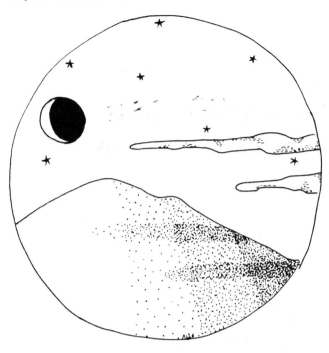

I came to this workshop because....

When you feel ready, return your attention inside to your breathing and the light.

(Estimated time is 1–2 minutes.)

Begin walking around the room...Take time to ground yourself...when you feel ready, come together with another person. Make eye contact.

I shall say another sentence. One of you repeat it and finish it. Then the other repeat it and finish it.

My worst fear for the future is...

Remember your breath. Remember the light. Make contact with your partner however you like with your eyes, with a touch, with a hug...

When you feel ready, begin to walk again...when you need to, stop and close your eyes, tune into the light...

(Follow similar instructions for the following unfinished sentences. As people understand the procedure, you can explain less of it. Occasionally remind them to be aware of the light. Estimated time for each change of partners and unfinished sentence is 1–2 minutes. If people become highly emotional, allow for more time.)

My picture of a nuclear plant accident is...
My picture of a slow death of the planet is...
My picture of a nuclear war is...
My feeling about children growing up right now is...
The way I numb myself from feeling these things is...
The way I cope when I am not numb is...
The way I find hope and strength is...
My best hope for the future is...

Slowly now, stay aware of your breathing and walk to the center of the room to form a large circle with everyone...

Let us breathe together...
Let us send our light down to the core of the Earth together...
Let us image our own lights and everyone else's lights...
Let us know the power of this circle, or us together, and let us remember it wherever we go...

(Estimated time is 3–5 minutes. Reconnection with the group as a whole, affirmation of our individual and collective power and beauty. At this point allow for any spontaneous prayers, singing, chanting, testimony or movement initiated by the group that further affirms the power and beauty of our being.)

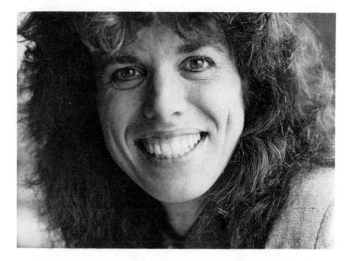

CHELLIS GLENDINNING, *Ph.D., is a Fellow at Peace and Common Security Institute (PACS) in San Francisco and a pioneer in psychological approaches to dealing with living with the nuclear menace. She co-founded the national network Interhelp and the Bay Area's Psychotherapists for Social Re-sponsibility, and her writing appears in* The Politics of Women's Spirituality *(Doubleday),* The Present Nuclear War *(New Society Publishers),* Mother Jones *and* Not Man Apart. *She is the author of the forthcoming* Changing Our Mode of Thinking: A Psychology for the Nuclear Age.

Comprehensive Report of the Cooperative Commission on Wellness 2030

BY THE end of the 20th Century, most people believed that physical disease was a symptom of some underlying emotional, mental, social-psychological or spiritual pathology. It was also widely accepted that a society's assumptions about the world and the way people were expected to behave had a great deal to do with the health status of its population.

For example, it is now realized that the 20th century emphasis on the individual, or on ego separateness, was a primary cause of many diseases. The stress associated with maximizing profit, survival of the fittest and other forms of competition were seen as triggers that broke down the body's ability to maintain equilibrium. And the end results of this emphasis on the individual, such as unequal distribution of food, were responsible for most of the health problems associated with both affluence and poverty.

A cultural transformation has touched every aspect of Western industrial civilization, and as we all know, a change in the conceptual model of the world has an all-pervading influence on the forms of human life and its institutions. Perhaps the intensity of the recent cultural transformation is best illustrated by a look at developments in health and health care—the subject of this comprehensive report issued by the Cooperative Commission on Wellness.

This transformation was pioneered back in the 1970s, but it used ideas as old as the most ancient cultures. Before the turn of the century, the transformational approach was called holistic. The assumption was that health care involved a focus on all dimensions of an individual related to health improvement: physical, psychological and spiritual.

Upon this basic concept rested two other premises: that medicine had little or nothing to do with health and that there were few limits to an individual's responsibility for his health. These building blocks of a wellness system were consistent with other new values.

This concept of health meant that every component of society—the workplace, educational institutions, transportation networks and urban environment in general—was considered part of the health-care system.

For example, the relationship between stress and illness had at last been comprehended by the 1990s. Employers were expected to take responsibility for eliminating stressful or "dis-ease" producing environments. Early programs in stress management became commonplace. Efforts were made to reduce stress between family and work roles by legislating flexibility in work and non-work schedules. Even so, parents of young children frequently chose unpaid leave as a benefit, until knowledge industry workers (about 75 percent of service workers) routinely had the option of using computers to work away from the office—typically at home.

Working at home strengthened the ties of "newfamily" groups, whose members had markedly increased when energy costs made single person households untenable. Newfamily groups were the target of quite a few wellness education programs, since members of a group could care for each other's needs in ways that were impossible for one or two persons living alone. For example, collective meetings to heal mentally or physically ill members were very successful. Multi-family dwellings also seemed more appropriate to the simple life-style many people felt was conducive to wellness.

Other health problems—including morbidity and mortality resulting from traffic accidents and crime—that used to be regarded as primarily an individual's problem were redefined as symptoms of a diseased community.

"Comprehensive Report of the Cooperative Commission on Wellness 2030." Trend Analysis Program Report TAP #19, American Council of Life Insurance, Spring 1980, pp. 8–13, reprinted by permission.

As governments were forced to connect health with everything else, funding for non-medical interventions (such as providing human-powered vehicles to encourage exercise) was generally increased in so-called health and welfare budgets.

Most readers of this report will recall the high price paid for this shift away from a disease-oriented medical system. The traditional health care delivery system had been one of the nation's largest employers and it could not be altered without higher unemployment and legislative battles.

When the dust settled in the early 21st century, it became clear that several things had happened: there were more entrepreneurs, more cottage industries and more diversified enterprises. Much to the federal government's chagrin there was continued growth in the already swollen invisible economy, when health care providers relied more heavily on barters and other unrecorded transactions than on fees for service. Comprehensive National Health Insurance bills failed to pass since the public had grown to recognize the ineffectiveness of such programs and place such great emphasis on individual responsibility. Membership in the American Association for the Advancement of Medical Technology had dwindled to a handful.

But other anticipated changes did take place. For example, women began to play much more important roles in health-care delivery. The roots of this trend reached back to the middle of the 20th century, when it became clear that women were assuming a larger role in alternative health care (such as free clinics) than they ever had in traditional medicine. Trends in health care indicate that androgyny, or the realization of both masculine and feminine attributes in every individual, has become a cultural goal.

By 2010, most of the old hospitals were gone; a few remained as regional repair centers, for the limited amount of crisis intervention that was still necessary. The grand old medical institutions, including the Mayo Clinic, were typically converted into health education and fitness centers. Now that many Americans have substituted retreats for vacations, these centers are well-frequented.

One of the reasons for the demise of the hospital was that other structures were devised to do what hospitals used to do—only better. Indeed, as early as the 1980s, an individual with any life transition or psychosocial problem (pregnancy, mid-life crisis, alcohol addiction, terminal disease) could find a care unit or group specifically designed to support him or her through that experience.

Traditional care providers faced unexpected competition, then obsolescence. Professionals, particularly MDs, had an especially difficult time adjusting to the decreased reliance on professionals and more egalitarian relationships between professionals and consumers. The proposed 1994 integration of the county medical societies into the American Holistic Health Association was sabotaged.

However, by the 21st century, the traditional health care providers who remained primarily defined their role as evaluating their clients' level of wellness. The newly established Cooperative Commission on Wellness placed substantial rewiance on community-based healers as educators. Osteopaths, acupuncturists, massage therapists, ethnic healers and allopathically trained diagnosticians had equal status—and roughly equal earnings. Earnings were much lower than physicians' fees had been when they enjoyed elevated status. There was some feeling that fee for service arrangements were inappropriate and should be scrapped entirely since spiritual/healing traditions do not fit easily into a payment structure.

Methods of care emphasized the client's need to gain a better understanding of his or her individual health status. A typical late 20th-century client entering into a wellness contract with a healer or self-help group was usually asked what threats, losses and gains their sickness represented to them. Did their chronic pain give them time off from a boring job? Did their obesity provide a certain comfort? Clients were reminded that they often had physical restrictions because, ultimately, they chose to have them.

The majority of chronic cases were treated by helping the client alter his or her lifestyle. In any wellness contract or evaluation, nutritional guidance was of paramount importance. Often, body chemistry was analyzed automatically with very accurate instruments from samples of urine, saliva, blood, hair, etc. This iris and sclera of the eye were photographed and analyzed to determine conditions throughout the body. These techniques (which provided sophisticated readings of an individual's mineral and vitamin needs) and others were routinely used to provide individualized diet plans. Many Americans turned to vegetarianism or a reliance on fish protein not only out of necessity, but choice. Today most diets include an emphasis on fruits and vegetables grown for higher vitamin C content. Since sugar is now used for energy, it is no longer heavily present in the average diet. As nutritional patterns have changed, public health has improved markedly.

Wellness evaluations are expected to become more sophisticated in the future since most clients now have been educated in wellness-enhancing behaviors since they were children. Pioneer efforts in the early 1980s—such as wellness camps—opened the door to a redefinition of education as a system of developing all human potentials. By the early 1990s most people accepted the fact that the body was its own finest laboratory and children were taught techniques which allowed the body to follow its best adaptive course when they were ill.

As the first generation of children educated in this manner reach adulthood, it seems clear that a significant percentage of them have gained control over their bodies equivalent to that exercised by Eastern mystics. Abilities which had been thought involuntary by Western medicine (raising one's body temperature, stopping the flow of blood when there is a wound, having organs cleanse themselves of pollutants) currently are well within the self-regulatory capacity of those individuals. It seems human beings may have an innate biological awareness of their physical state down to the level of the single cell and that the human mind can intervene in and direct any physiologic function.

While there has been some change in the mortality rates as the population becomes wellness-oriented, many believe that future cohorts will show major improvement in mortality rates. It remains to be seen, of course, but there are further expectations that these cohorts have dramatically improved life expectancies, and that they will live well beyond what has been thought of as the human life span.

This possibility has heightened attention to the needs of the aged. Publicly funded support programs for mid-life transitions and retraining are only a first step in this direction. Since health promotion has worked so well, the population has already begun to increase rapidly in older age brackets. In the third decade of the 21st century our greatest challenge is to find healthful and meaningful work opportunities for our very large senior population. Remembering that advances in wellness were accomplished at the expense of disease-care medical systems, a few of the "old-old" still long for the high-technology that used to keep terminal patients alive long after they would have achieved natural death. But most are much more accepting of death than their grandparents and increasingly view the process of dying as an opportunity for spiritual growth.

Thus objective indicators of improvement in morbidity and mortality have been achieved at the same time that belief in objective, or "value-free" medical care waned. For example, it is now clear that one value of the old medical system was that it assumed all illnesses were undesirable and should be eliminated at any cost.

Values—the client's and the provider's—are now an explicit part of any discussion of wellness strategy. Weak signals of this change appeared before the turn of the century and culminated in increased participation of consumers in health care policy development, the bill of rights that gave institutionalized patients the right to refuse "chemical straightjackets" (tranquilizers), and the recognition that clients needed to find healers whose value system was compatible with theirs.

It was within this climate of increased options that some technologies actually have gained in acceptance. During the major rejection of high technologies in the last two decades of the 20th century, holistic health advocates argued that humans could develop non-invasive techniques for diagnosis using as-yet-undeveloped powers of the brain and mind. Third World and religious experiences were offered as models of these technologies, many of which were introduced by immigrants. However, we now recognize that some appropriate technologies are necessary, particularly for older people who believe in their efficacy and who are unwilling to look beyond symptoms for a cure.

Harbingers of doom warned that rejection of objective medical care would spell the end of scientific research. And it is true that research efforts were redirected because of the feeling that biomedical research could no longer rest on reductionist assumptions (e.g., separation of body/mind/spirit) which directed 20th century medicine. Throughout the closing years of the 20th century, researchers devoted themselves to finding techniques for motivating wellness-enhancing behavior in populations that were not so inclined.

There was also a great deal of research on the healthy. At first, it was directed toward finding out what wellness was for various groups, by determining normative values for different subsets of the healthy population. But recognizing that organisms are biochemically unique, research moved to a concentration on determining wellness for given individuals and finding out why some people were super-healthy, even in seemingly stressful situations.

The brain/mind also held great fascination for wellness researchers. In fact, some people argued that the value shift that has taken place resulted from breakthroughs in science. Physicists and biologists, as far back as Pribram in the 1970s, presented evidence that our lack of understanding of the brain had limited our understanding of the world. Breakthroughs in brain/mind research showed that while the world of appearances was a real world, it was not the only order of reality. Different explanations of the brain yielded different realities, which explained paranormal phenomena including remote viewing and visualizing reality on either side of the infra-red to ultra-violet range. This made it easier to heal the body/mind schism that had dominated medicine for so long and to explain how thoughts and emotions were related to illness. One of the immediate changes resulting from a new understanding of the brain was the realization that it was foolish to maintain separate systems to treat mental and physical illness.

When reviewing the advances in wellness in the last 50 years, it is important to place them in context. New attitudes toward health went hand-in-hand with a greater sense of respect for the environment. The goals of growth and development have been balanced against a greater awareness of biohazards. Freedom and dignity are related to the resource consequences of individual decisions. In other words, we now understand that individual health and social health cannot be separated.

Since 2000, more than 80 percent of the population in the developed world has lived in urban areas. We have daily reminders of global interdependence. The developed northern hemisphere and the developing southern hemisphere have had to learn new ways of sharing resources.

In this context, energy wasting behavior, chemical pollution and dehumanizing work (or out-of-work) conditions are as much disease states as the cholera, typhus and malnutrition of the 19th century.

On the other hand, individual health offers the opportunity for societal growth. Our hope for the future is that new directions in wellness are a vehicle for greater human happiness, health and consciousness. The need for a disease care system and the concept of patient have faded. The ideal future is one where the wellness system empowers people to transform themselves.

Healing Ourselves and Healing Our Planet

Dr. Robert Muller

I T IS with much humility that I speak to doctors, health workers, social workers, and people who are experts in the art of healing, while I am an economist, a lawyer, and a political man. The only wisdom I can share with you is to draw certain conclusions from my 34 years in the first global organization of this planet. My daily work is to deal with most of the world's and humanity's problems and to hear the complaints, the dreams and the wishes of human communities from all around the globe. Nevertheless, I can derive from my many years of observation a number of hopeful conclusions for our future. I have learned enormously from the United Nations, much more than from any university on earth. I am grateful for these years spent in a global observation post. To begin with, let me tell you what my basic beliefs are today, after a life of war and peace.

My first belief is that we are part of a cosmic process or evolution; that there is a reason for our being on this planet; that something of momentous importance in the universe is happening on this particular planet; and that progressively our fate is being revealed to us as making sense and as having an objective. In a job like mine where you have to deal on a daily basis with problems reaching from astrophysics and outer space to atomic science, from the total humanity to individual human rights, from development to ecology, from preserving the past to planning for the future, I could drown—and I did so for many years—if I did not assume that there is a sense and an objective in the multi-billion-year evolution of this planet. There must be a logic and an ultimate purpose in all that. From the moment I assumed that there was a cosmic pattern, much became clear to me and I will try to explain to you what this consciousness is. I believe that the human race is undergoing a very fundamental transformation and transcendence, of which we have completed only the first part.

Having received at one point of evolution eyes to see, ears to hear, minds to understand, hands to handle and legs to walk, we have accomplished a series of kirst miracles: we have extended our eyesight into the infinitely large and infinitely small. Through astronomical observatories, telescopes, microscopes and atomic bubble chambers, we have multiplied the scope of our vision millions of times. We have extended our hands with tools, machines and factories. We have analyzed matter of the moon, of Mars and of other planets. We have multiplied our mind's capacity through books and computers, storing information and calculating to an extent out of reach to us. We can hear across the continents and seas via telephones. We can teleeview things that happen on the other side of the earth. We have extended the scope and speed of our legs through boats, trains, cars, aircraft and satellites. This has been a tremendous page of success in the story of the human species. All along the line, every invention has had its good and its bad sides. The fundamental problem of good and evil is still with us at every progress we make. This first page being turned, there are further transcendences to take place.

My second fundamental belief is that life is sacred. Human life is a prodigy, something truly mind-boggling, incredible and unique. As I grew through my observation of life, I came more and more to the conclusion that a human being is a miracle in the universe which will never be repeated again in exactly the same form or in the same circumstances in the entire eternity. My respect for life has grown for all forms of life, from the handicapped to the greatest genius. We are all sacred units in the universe. From this I have drawn the conclusion that no one should ever be asked to kill or to be killed, not even in the name of a nation. It is no longer a question of conscientious objection. It is a fundamental human right, inseverable from our nature, a right derived from the uniqueness and preciousness of life. In front of tribunals I would not say what my moral objections are; I would ask governments to prove what right they have to ask me to kill other human beings in the name of nations which have existed only for

This article is a statement presented by Robert Muller, Assistant Secretary-General, UN, to the San Diego Holistic Health Conference, 28 August, 1982.

the last few hundred years and which run counter to the oneness of our planet and of the human family.

My third fundamental belief is that I am the ruler, the guide, the manager, the caretaker of my own cosmos or cosmic unit. I am a very complicated system of cells, mechanisms and senses, and I have the basic responsibility to guide this little satellite through his environment. I cannot turn to others for doing that. My trillions of cells have to receive guidance from me. I have to give them hope and spur them toward the fulfilment of the consciousness I have received in the universe. A doctor, another person or society cannot do that for me. It is *my* sacred responsibility to manage my cosmos well, to validate it to the fullest among the four and a half billion other cosmoses, in the human society, in nature and in the universe. My love, kindness, cooperation, and understanding are simply the reflection of my graitutude for having received in the mysterious universe a tremendous few years of consciousness of that universe.

There are my three basic beliefs derived over the years. Now, with such beliefs, how can I guide myself in the present world?

In the first place, it is not a world where everyone can see a clear cosmic evolution. It is a world which is utterly confused, a world of noise, of competing claims, a world where not a single philosopher can give you an answer or a clear view of the future. Perhaps the only person who came close to giving me a hopeful view of the future was Teilhard de Chardin and his philosophy of the transcendent evolution of humanity into a spiritual dimension. In his view and also in mine, this particular planet and humanity are a tremendous case of a planet and of a species becoming conscious of the universe or in which the universe is becoming conscious of itself. This, in my opinion is the ultimate destination of the great adventure which the human race is living in the cosmos. But as yet it is a confused world. The law of sacredness of life is not yet shared by all: we still kill in the name of nations, religions or ideologies and receive medals for it. The individual is not given responsibility over his life. Close to two-thirds of the governments of this planet are dictatorships. And where there are no dictatorships, you are exposed from morning to evening to sounds, images, words, and advertisements which try to impose on you certain values. As a result, in a democracy, too, you may be a prisoner of values, desires, objectives which are not really your own. You are offered ladders to climb and once you are on the top you wonder whether they were really worth wasting your life.

How do I react to that? Should I protest and proclaim that this is not the type of world in which my beliefs and life can unfold in happiness? No. I would say that the state of the world today has its good dose of justification. Let us not forget that the world of today is the result of a very complicated past. We have entered the global age with over 5000 languages and 5000 religions, with more than 150 nations which usually do not make much sense, with cultures, beliefs, social systems, and ideologies which obscure the fact that we are one human race on one planet with one future. All these past ingredients were brought together over a very years after World War II. When I was a young man after that war, I had no hope for humanity.

I was convinced that we would blow each other up. How could communists and capitalists, black and white, rich and poor, the Chinese, the Americans, the Russians, the old and the new nations ever survive their differences and confrontations? To my utter astonishment, this planet has not been blown up and we are still alive! I saw during my young years two civilized nations, France and Germany, on tiny Europe, slaughter each other like savages. My grandfather had five nationalities and saw three wars. My father had three nationalities and saw two wars. I saw one war and half of my family in French uniforms and the other in German uniforms. After living through and observing all of that, how could I believe that the world would make it? The miracle is that despite all the enormous nonsense that is going on, we are still here. I derive great hope from the mere fact that the four-and-a-half billion people of this planet have not done worse than they did. Please remember that today's confrontations are the result of the long and checkered history of our species. How to outgrow, how to transcend this conflictual situation, that is our new great evolutionary challenge to which we should give all our attention.

There are hosts of areas and fields of turbulence and of potential conflicts on this planet. We have seen a couple of them since the beginning of this year. When you work in an organization like the United Nations you feel almost like being in a clinic. And as a doctor you must have faith, you must believe that you can save patients even if you do not always succeed. Often the patient is brought in too late. For the world as a whole we must develop a preventive medicine. We ought to try to prevent conflicts rather than to let them occur. We have prevented many conflicts in the UN, but nobody speaks about it. A conflict which has not broken out is not a conflict. And yet it is a thousand times preferable to one that has broken out.

As world doctors or clinicians we can take two approaches. In the first place there are what you call emergency measures or the emergency clinic. Secondly, there are the numerous measures aimed at improving the overall health. While dealing with emergency situations, you must also try to improve, by every possible means, the total health, peace, and happiness of humanity. As a matter of fact, while we often compare world expenditures on armaments with the trickles we spend on peace development, we seldom compare world expenditures on the health of its 4.5 billion individuals with those for the peace, i.e., the health of the world. I will briefly review what is being done and what should be further done under the two above categories.

Under the category of emergency measures, the most immediate priority is, of course, nuclear disarmament. We have held two special disarmament sessions at the United Nations. They have led to no results but this is not a reason for despair. On the contrary, we must continue and never give up, because humans have a fundamental right to a disarmed planet. We have the right to be born, to live, and to die on a disarmed planet. There can be no compromise on this basic cosmos issue. There can be no excuse for arms whatsoever in a global world, on a miraculous planet such as ours in the universe. This fight must continue even if it takes years as it did in the past against slavery which was also considered to be hopeless. It might be a wearisome fight, but it has at long last started and it will be irreversible, as is human evolution. At the UN we have been waiting many years for the public's support. It is only now, at this last session that hundreds of thousands of people did wake up and march. But they should not wake up only against armaments, they should go on the streets and protest against any conflict on this planet. Leaders move into other territories because the public does not react. Every government, when it joins the United Nations, makes the solemn pledge not to have recourse to arms and conflict before having exhausted all the peaceful means spelled out in the Charter. But when it comes to their interests, they often invade another country and they are applauded by their national public. The world's public should never accept this and fall into the trap. We need demonstrations and protests against any military intervention and conflict, so that governments will learn to behave according to the principles of the Charter and to the supreme interests of the human race. This is very fundamental.

There are many other emergency measures I could mention. There is a whole encyclopedia of them. There are hunger situations on this planet which are intolerable and which must be alleviated. The UN is shipping millions of tons of food from surplus countries to needy ones. The UN World Food Program today is one of the biggest programs of international aid on this planet. When there is a disaster anywhere, an immediate coordinated relief operation is set up. We have a world warning system against epidemics, the first ever on this planet. I receive on my desk every day telegrams on hunger situations, emergencies or natural disasters, and the international machinery enters forthwith into action. Nations in these cases are working together in a novel effort of solidarity which I would not have dared to dream of 30 years ago. There are twelve million refugees on this planet due to political nonsense. The UN High Commissioner for Refugees has thousands of workers who protect, receive and take care of these people in provisional camps and arrange for their settlement in willing countries around the world. Twelve million refugees represent a lot of emergency situations! I would advise every journalist on earth to visit at least once a refugee camp of the UN. A good part of the UN system is busy round the clock dealing with emergencies. I often pity our Secretary General who has to spend so much time on emergency situations: flare-ups in the Middle East or elsewhere, highjackings, human rights violations, etc. Sometimes he says to me: "Robert, I came to this house with the hope that I could help build a better world and here I am every day dealing with the innumerable wounds of the planet, with practically no time left to work on the fundamentals." This is how he talked to me just a few days ago before leaving for Beijing. His time is eaten up by the daily emergencies of this planet while there is so much need for the long-term construction of the planet. But governments in their narrowness do not take this into account. They consider that their problem or interest should occupy the front scene of the world, as if they were the magnetic pole of it.

Be it war, drugs, alcoholism, traffic accidents or the environment, all comes up in one of the 32 United Nations specialized agencies or world programs which I have the privilege and task to coordinate. I could write volumes about them but let me now turn to even more fundmental and perhaps more promising issues of the human condition. Basically they deal with the healing and the creation of one human family on this planet. It is a challenge of unprecedented, beautiful magnitude.

In my view, the agenda of the human race in the years to come will turn around five fundamental harmonies. The Hopi people whom I visited recently spoke about the same subject but they used the word "balance" which is practically the same.

The first harmony is *the harmony between the human species and our planetary home*. This has never been put to us in such terms in our entire previous human history. But today we are confronted with the problem of finding our right relationships with our planetary home. It is only recently that we have explored that home in its entirety. Now the question is: how can we live optimally within this planet's given conditions which we can change only up to certain limits? We know now every segment of it from the seas and oceans to the atmosphere, the biosphere, the deserts, our energy resources, our living resources, our minerals, our plants, etc. Grosso modo the inventory of our planet is complete. Great problems have arisen in this category: the population explosion, the environmental crisis, the energy crisis, the food problem, the habitat question. These are all great warnings that we need to find a harmony with our planet in order not to let our home deteriorate and the quality of life diminish. This is the first great agenda on which humanity has to work. You know it from your own personal lives as we know it on a global level in the United Nations.

The second great harmony we have to achieve is *the harmony of the human family itself*. As I noted earlier, we have so many religions, nations, cultures, beliefs and entities on this planet, including new ones like the multinational corporations. The great problem is to determine how these groups and entities can contribute to the maximum fulfillment of the human family and not battle each other at enormous cost. This, too, is an unprecedented problem for humanity on a planetary scale. It does not only concern nations. Many other entities on this planet are playing the game, "My nation, right or wrong," "My religion, right or wrong," "My race, right or wrong," "My ideology, right or wrong." We must build bridges, tear down walls, open doors and get people to cooperate because cooperation and prevention are the only ways to avoid conflicts. There can be conflicts between sexes, races, generations, levels of wealth, the valids and the invalids, etc. To foster cooperation, we convene one world conference after the other: on women, on races, on aging. We proclaim international years: for the child, for youth, for the disabled, for the homeless. It is an enormous problem to get four and a half billion people (and in the year 2000 six billion people) grouped in multiple entities to live in harmony and peace with each other and to transform the diversity of the human species from something negative into something positive. Then we will have achieved a major evolutionary objective: unity in diversity.

The third harmony we have to achieve is *our harmony with time*. This planet will be around for another six to eight billion years. We have to think about the future and we have to preserve our past. This is a problem with which humanity has never been confronted on such a scale. If you raise a good child, you will have made a contribution to a good future of humanity. If you raise a bad child, if you are an alcoholic or a drug addict you will prepare a generation of abnormal children. Hence, the problem concerns not only our environment and natural resources, but also the human species itself.

There is fourth harmony which the religions know very well: *our harmony with the heavens*. As I have advanced in my work in the United Nations, I have come to the conclusion that this planet will not be in peace and will not find its fulfillment as long as we do not recognize and lay down the cosmic or divine laws which must regulate our lives on this planet. We cannot do it by human means alone. We must elevate ourselves into the totality of the universe in order to understand our place in it and what rules we must obey. The great religions knew this well. They all proclaimed: "Thou shall not kill," which should be the first world commandment. We need to agree on the universal commandments for the behavior of the human species on this planet. I recommend ceaselessly that the religions get together and draft the great commandments of human behavior. We can call them divine commandments or cosmic commandments. We are part of the universe. We are not separate from it. The universe is in us and we are in the universe. It is therefore, high time that we find our harmony with the heavens. Confucius said it already 600 years before Christ, the Greeks said it. Kepler said it, and we must say it again. It is the only way out.

Finally and last but not least, there is *our personal harmony*. We have to find our personal peace, health, and harmony so that we can contribute to the total harmony. We must understand the world in which we live and contribute to it our personal health, happiness, kindness, and love. We cannot expect others to do it, and not do it ourselves. This is one of the greatest requirements today in a world of four and a half billion people. It is the ultimate key, the alpha and omega of the success of humanity. It rests in each single individual. Multiplied by 4.5 billion each of us is the key to the world's future. When we become heads of family, of an institution, of a government, of a corporation or of a class, we are still individuals and we can radiate the qualities which are needed to bring about a fulfilled, peaceful society on our beautiful planet.

So, as you see, there remains an immense amount of work to do and each of us must find a suitable task and do our share. When asked to write this article, I reviewed in my mind the work of the World Health Organization which, as part of the UN system, deals with the world's health. It is a beautiful organization of which humanity can truly be proud. The Ministers of Health from every nation meet in it every year to review the health of the world. Six thousand people work for it. And yet, sadly enough, there is no University on earth that would teach its students about the existence, endeavors and works of that global organization. The world possesses in it a marvelous institution which has been able to eradicate prac-

tically every major epidemic on this planet. The eradication of smallpox alone saves the world 2 billion dollars a year, not to speak of the human suffering spared. From it, I get every year a clear picture of the total health of this planet. And yet, it scratches only the surface, because it is dealing only with the physical health of humanity (major diseases, accidents, environmental hazards, viral diseases, hunger, disabilities, etc.). The World Health Organization does not deal with the emotional health of humanity. It does not deal with the spiritual well-being of humanity.

Take the emotional health of humanity: there is a famous exchange of letters between Einstein and Freud in 1932. Einstein had come to the conclusion that as a scientist and as a political activist he had no answer to the armaments race. So he turned to Freud and asked him: Perhaps you, the psychologist, have the answer. Freud answered that the problem was as much in Einstein's field as in his: humanity is divided between tendencies of aggression and of love which correspond to the laws of attraction and repulsion in the physical field. If we want to win the battle for peace we must do everything we can to multiply the ties of sentiment among the peoples of the world. We have been able to develop the love for nation. We must now develop the love for all humanity. This is why he considered the League of Nations to be an experiment without precedent to develop ties of sentiments among all humans on a political basis. We have done it before for religions, for nations, for every conceivable group, but it has never been attempted for the entire humanity.

Politicians today seldom dare to use the word "love" which is probably the key to our success in the universe. Love for life, love for light, love for the greatness of Creation, a positive attitude from the moment we have received life. Love that holds the heavens together, as Dante said. With a few exceptions such as Dag Hammarskjold and U Thant in the United Nations, you find little love among political leaders. Recently, we had a marvelous experience with the Hopi people. We listened to their elders in their sacred kivas. They gave me their prophecy for the future, which was very simple: perhaps humanity will continue on its present path, separated from the Great Spirit, and humanity will perish. Gourds filled with ashes (atomic bombs) will fall from the sky and destroy us. The only salvation—and they did not speak about arms or politics—is the return of humanity to the fold and the rules of the Great Spirit. In its simplicity it was for me an answer to a fundamental question, because we are extremely diversified individuals. We have many ideals, dreams and wishes but there is only one element which binds us together: the original source of energy which is still being diffused in the universe in an endless variety of forms. God or a Creator. In the end it is only by unifying ourselves in our lives, in our minds, in our hearts and in our souls with this cosmic spirit that we can find the answers to our problems. The Hopis or Peaceful People continue to believe that peace depends entirely on our remaining within the will of the Creator and being part at every moment of our lives of the great impulses of nature and creation. It was a most moving experience to listen to the great simple truths expressed by the elders of a very wise people. As a matter of fact, we do not consult enough anymore the wise old people who are transmittors of world wisdom from generation to generation.

So there is a lot to do. Some of you are doctors. You are experts in micromedicine, namely the healing of individuals. Where is macromedicine, or the healing of the whole human race? We have courses and entire libraries on individual psychology, but where is the psychology of the entire human species, of our collective anxieties, hopes, dreams, and feelings? Where are the great philosophers developing a philosophy for the entire human family? Where are the global political scientists working on the way this planet should be managed and be taken care of? Where are the global psychiatrists who would be looking into the psychiatry of the whole human species? Where are all the globalists the world so desperately needs at this juncture of its evolution?

The macrosciences in the social field are almost nonexistent. They are not supposed to exist. They stop at the national level, which seems to be the supreme level and mental block. We need a completely new education, a world, a global education. Some of you are educators, I wish that I could show you copies of my World Core Curriculum which I would like to see refined and adopted in every school on earth. Education speaks first about the nation, but first comes the planet, the human family, the heavens and myself. When I was young, I was told that France was the greatest and then that Germany was the greatest, and each time I was given a gun to shoot in opposite directions on my human brethren. I could not understand it. We are all programmed by national education, but when there is someone like me who has been programmed twice, you become suspicious, you deprogram yourself and you program yourself into the only right environments: the planet, humanity and the heavens.

So, at this stage of my life, despite many idiosyncrasies, follies, contradictions and confusions, I have gained great hope in the United Nations. I have gained it, because I am convinced that humanity is on a further evolutionary ascent and that we have magnificent frontiers in front of us. After having succeeded in the material and scientific fields, we will now discover the incredible potentials of the heart and of the spirit. This is the next stage in civilization, in our cosmic journey, in our transcendence and consciousness, our identification with the universe. The holistic health movement is only the beginning of it. Your belief in the whole human being—physical, mental, emotional, and spiritual—is no less true for the entire humanity.

The global, cosmic agenda in front of us is tremendous. You might say: "Well, what is my role in this?" It is fundamental, because your personal health, your whole health—physical, mental, moral, and spiritual—is part of the world's physical, mental, moral, and spiritual health. Whatever you and I do for a better world will bring about a better world. I find it arrogant for governments to ask that people should be peaceful when they themselves are armed, quarrelling and violent. How can they expect the individual to be peaceful when they give such insane examples of large scale violence?

Our agenda will reach from the total to the individual, from the global to the local. I have great hope in humanity. Every day I am more respectful for what humans can do. It is a tremendous species. We have a special purpose, an incredible destiny in the universe. I would throw in my gauntlet for the human species at any time. I will never give up. It is a magnificent adventure, probably one of the greatest in the universe, and we must succeed. Our comprehension goes from the infinitely large to the infinitely small, from the beginnings to the apocalypse, from the total humanity to the individual. Instead of being frightened by this magnitude, we must rejoice in it. Our minds are broad enough to take it in and to love it. I would therefore, beg you to feel proud to be human and to do everything in your power in thousands of ways and through thousands of people you meet in your life, through your letters, through what you say, to contribute your personal health, consciousness, peace and happiness to the health, peace and spiritual transcendence of the proud human race.

As Darwin said at the end of The Origin of Species: ". . . whilst this planet has gone cycling on according to the fixed law of gravity, from so simple a beginning endless forms most beautiful and most wonderful have been and are being evolved."

DR. ROBERT MULLER *has been serving the United Nations in various capacities since 1948. He is also an author and essayist:* Most of All, They Taught Me Happiness, *(Doubleday, 1978),* New Genesis, Shaping of Global Spirituality *(Doubleday, 1982),* Dialogues of Hope *(Crossroads, 1983),* The Desire to be Human *(a compendium on Teilhard de Chardin, co-edited with Leo Zonneveld, Mirananda, Holland, 1983),* Sima, mon amour *(a French novel, Pierron, France, 1983).*

The World Core Curriculum can be obtained by writing to the author at the United Nations, New York, N.Y. 10017.

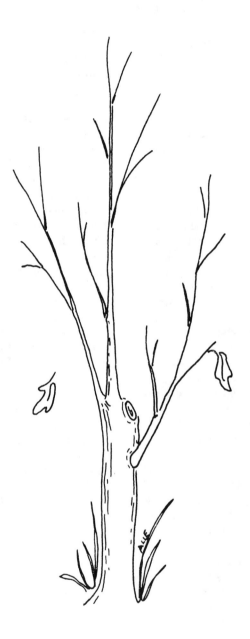

Bibliography

I. HOLISTIC HEALTH IN THE 1980s

Bland, Jeffrey. *Your Health Under Siege.* Lexington, MA: The Stephen Greene Press, 1982.

Capra, Fritjof. *The Turning Point: Science, Society, and the Rising Culture.* New York: Simon and Schuster, 1982.

Ferguson, Tom, ed. *Medical Self Care.* Summit Books, 1980.

Stanway, Andrew. *Alternative Medicine.* Pelican Books, 1979.

II. HEALING SYSTEMS FROM AROUND THE WORLD

Coulter, Harris, Ph.D. *Divided Legacy: The Conflict Between Homeopathy and the American Medical Association.* Berkeley, CA: North Atlantic, 1973.

Coulter, Harris, Ph.D. *Homeopathic Science and Modern Medicine: The Physics of Healing with Microdoses.* Berkeley, CA: North Atlantic, 1981.

Cummings, Stephen, F.N.P., and Ullman, Dana, M.P.H. *Everybody's Guide to Homeopathic Medicines.* Los Angeles: J. P. Tarcher, 1984.

Eliade, Mircea. *Yoga: Immortality and Freedom.* Translated by W. R. Trask. New Jersey: Princeton University Press, 1958.

Feuerstein, George. *The Essence of Yoga.* New York: Grove Press, 1974.

Iyengar, B. K. S. *Light on Yoga.* Schocken Books, 1970.

Kent, James, M.D. *Lectures on the Homeopathic Philosophy.*

Rama, Swami; Ballentine, Rudolph, M.D.; Ajaya, Swami, Ph.D. *Yoga and Psychotherapy: The Evolution of Consciousness.* Glenview, Illinois: Himalayan Institute, 1976.

Sharma, C. H. *A Manual of Homeopathy and Natural Medicine.*

Shepherd, Dorothy, M.D. *Homeopathy for the First Aider.*

Vithoulkas, George, and Gray, Bill, M.D. *The Science of Homeopathy: A Modern Textbook.* New York: Grove, 1979.

Whitmont, Edward C., M.D. *Psyche and Substance: Essays on Homeopathy in Light of Jungian Psychology.* Berkeley, CA: North Atlantic, 1980.

Woods, Ernest E. *Yoga.* Penguin Books, 1968.

III. TOOLS FOR KEEPING HEALTHY

Amanta, Charles A. Jr., D.D.S., and Brachett, Robert C., D.D.S., M.S. *Dialogue on Preventive Dentistry.* March Publishing, 1971.

Assagioli, Roberto. *Psychosynthesis.* Hobbs & Dunn, 1965.

Assagioli, Roberto. *Psychosynthesis: A Manual of Principles and Techniques.* New York: Psychosynthesis Foundation, 1965.

Ballantyne, Sheila. *Imaginary Crimes.* New York: Viking, 1982.

Ballentine, R. *Diet and Nutrition.* Honesdale, PA: Himalayan International Institute, 1978.

Bennett, John G. *Understanding Subud.* University Books, 1959.

Benson, H. *The Relaxation Response.* William Morrow, 1975.

Bentove, I. *Stalking the Wild Pendulum.* New York: E. P. Dutton, 1977.

Berkson, Devaki. *The Foot Book: Healing with the Integrated Treatment of Foot Reflexology.* Funk and Wagnalls, 1977.

Brown, B. *New Mind, New Body.* New York: Harper and Row, 1975.

Campbell, Don. *Introduction to the Musical Brain.* Magnamusic-Baton Inc., 1983.

Capra, Fritjof. *The Tao of Physics.* New York: Bantam, 1975.

Capra, Fritjof. *The Turning Point.* New York: Simon and Schuster, 1982.

Carrington, P. "Using Modern Forms of Meditation in Psychotherapy," Boorstein, S., and Speeth, K., eds. *Explorations in Transpersonal Therapy.* Aronson, 1978.

Carter, Mildred. *Helping Yourself with Foot Reflexology.* Parker Publishing, 1969.

Castleton, Virginia. *The Calendar Book of Natural Beauty.* New York: Harper & Row, 1973.

Christopher, John R., N.D. *School of Natural Healing.* Provo, UT: Bi-World Publishers, 1976.

Cooley, M. *Architect or Bee.* Boston: South End Press, 1980.

Cooper, C. *Current Concerns in Occupational Stress.* New York: John Wiley & Sons, 1980.

Corbett, Margaret. *Help Yourself to Better Sight.* Wilshire Books, 1949.

Crile, George. *Surgery: Your Choices, Your Alternatives.* New York: Dell Publishing Co., Inc., 1978.

Davidson, Roy W. *Documents on Contemporary Dervish Communities.* London: Hoopoe, 1966.

Desoille, R. *Theorie et Pratique du Reve Eveille Dirige.* Geneva: Editions du Mont Blanc, 1961.

The Dream Network Bulletin. 487 Fourth Street, Brooklyn, NY 11215.

Dreissens, Georges, ed. *The Preliminary Practices of Tibetan Buddhism.* Burton, WA: Tusum Ling Publications, 1974.

Dreyfus, H. *What Computers Can't Do.* New York: Harper & Row, 1972.

Edelwich, Herry. *Burnout: Stages of Disillusionment in the Helping Professions.* Human Sciences Press.

Faraday, Ann. *The Dream Game.* New York: Harper & Row, 1974.

Faraday, Ann. *Dream Power.* New York: Berkeley, 1972.

Freudenberger, H. J. *Burnout: The High Cost of Achievement.* Anchor/Doubleday.

Friedman, M. and Rosenman, R. H. *Type A Behavior and Your Heart.* New York: Alfred A. Knopf, 1974.

Fromm, E. *The Revolution of Hope: Toward a Humanized Technology.* New York: Harper & Row, 1968.

Gardner, H. *Art, Mind, and Brain: A Cognitive Approach to Creativity.* New York: Basic Books, 1982.

Garfield, Patricia. *Creative Dreaming.* New York: Simon & Schuster, 1974.

Glasser, R. *The Body is the Hero.* New York: Random House, 1976.

Green, Elmer, and Green, Alice. *Beyond Biofeedback.* New York: Delacorte, 1977.

Hales, Dianne. *The Complete Book of Sleep.* Belmont, CA: Addison Wesley, 1981.

Hall, R. H. *Food for Nought: The Decline in Nutrition.* New York: Harper & Row, 1974.

Hamel, Peter Michael. *Through Music to the Self.* Shambala, 1976.

Harmonic Choir. *Hearing the Solar Winds.* A recording: LP 106, Cassette CS 106 (import).

Hogan, M. *Histology of the Human Eye.* Sanders, 1971.

Hutschnecker, A. A. *The Will to Live.* Cornerstone Library, 1977.

Huxley, Aldous. *The Art of Seeing.* Montana Books, 1975.

Ingham, Eunice D. *Stories the Feet Have Told.* Rochester, NY: Ingham Publishing.

Isenberg, Seymore, and Elting, L. M. *The Consumer's Guide to Successful Surgery.* New York: St. Martins Press, 1976.

Jaffe, Dennis. *Healing from Within.* New York: Bantam, 1982.

Jensen, Bernard, D. C. *The Science and Practice of Iridology.* Escondido, CA: Jensen, 1952.

Johari, Harish. *Dhanwantari.* San Francisco, CA: Rams Head, 1974.

Jung, Carl G. *Man and His Symbols.* New York: Dell, 1968.

Keyes, Laurel Elizabeth. *Toning: The Creative Power of the Voice.* DeVorss, 1973.

Khan, Hazrat Inayat. *The Soul: Whence and Whither.* New Lebanon, NY: Sufi Order Publications, 1977.

Kriege, Theodore. *Fundamental Basis of Irisdiagnosis.* London: Fowler, 1969.

LeShan, Lawrence. *You Can Fight for Your Life.* Evans, 1977.

Lindermann, Hannes. *How to Overcome Stress the Autogenic Way.* Germany: Berpelsmann, 1973.

Lindlahr, Henry, M.D. *Iridiagnosis and Other Diagnostic Methods.* Chicago: Lindlahr, 1922.

Lings, Martin. *What is Sufism?* University of California Press, 1977.

Lust, John. *The Herb Book.* Sun Valley, CA: Lust Publications, 1974.

Luthe, Wolfgang. *Creativity Mobilization Technique.* Grune and Stratton, 1976.

Luthe, Wolfgang, and Schultz, Johannes. *Autogenic Therapy.* Grune and Stratton, 6 vols., 1959–1973.

Marcus; Shakti; and Noj. *Reunion: Tools for Transformation.* Mill Valley, CA: Whatever Publishing, 1978.

McGuire, Thomas, D.D.S. *The Tooth Trip: An Oral Experience.* Random House/Bookworks, 1972.

McKeown, Joe, D.D.S. *Everybody's Tooth Book.* Santa Cruz, CA: Happy Valley Apple Press, 1973.

Miller, Alice. *The Drama of the Gifted Child: How Narcissistic Parents Form and Deform the Emotional Lives of Their Talented Children.* New York: Basic Books, 1981.

Naboru, Muramoto. *Healing Ourselves.* Swan House and Avon Books, 1973.

Nebelkopf, Ethan. *The Herbal Connection.* Orem, UT: Bi-World Press, 1981.

Nebelkopf, Ethan. "Herbs and Drug Addiction." *Well-Being,* #28, 1978.

Nebelkopf, Ethan. "Holistic Programs for the Drug Addict & Alcoholic." *Journal of Psychoactive Drugs,* Volume 13(4), 1981.

Nebelkopf, Ethan. *The New Herbalism.* Orem, UT: Bi-World Press, 1980.

Nebelkopf, Ethan. *White Bird Flies to Phoenix: Confessions of a Free Clinic Burn-out.* Eugene, OR: Jackrabbitt Press, 1974.

Ouspensky, P. *In Search of the Miraculous.* Harcourt, Brace, and World, 1949.

Patanjali. *The Yoga Aphorisms of Patanjal: How to Know God.* Translated by Swami Parbhavananda and Christopher Isherwood. Signet Books, 1969.

Peale, Norman Vincent. *Positive Imaging.* New York: Ballantine Books, 1982.

Peck, M. Scott. *The Road Less Traveled: A New Psychology of Love, Traditional Values and Spiritual Growth.* New York: Simon and Schuster/Touchstone, 1978.

Peller, S. *Cancer in Man.* New York International University Press, 1952.

Pelletier, Kenneth. *Healthy People in Unhealthy Places.* New York: Delacorte Press/Seymour Lawrence.

Pelletier, Kenneth. *Holistic Medicine: From Stress to Optimum Health.* New York: Delacorte Press, 1979.

Pelletier, Kenneth. *Mind as Healer, Mind as Slayer.* Delta, 1977.

Rajneesh, Bhavagau. *Meditation: The Art of Ecstasy.* Harper Colophon, 1976.

Reed, Henry. *Dream Realizations Workbook.* Virginia Beach, VA: Henry Reed.

Regardie, Israel. *The Art of True Healing.* Weiser.

Remen, Naomi. *The Human Patient.* New York: Anchor Pess, 1980.

Revici, E. *A New Concept of the Pathophysiology of Cancer with Implications for Therapy.* Yale University Press.

Roberts, Jane. *The Nature of Personal Reality.* Englewood Cliffs, NJ: Prentice-Hall, 1975.

Rosa, Karl. *You and A.T.: Autogenic Training.* New York: E. P. Dutton, 1976.

Rose, Jeanne. *The Herbal Body Book.* Grosset & Dunlap, 1976.

Rose, Jeanne. *Herbs and Things.* Grosset & Dunlap, 1974.

Rudhyar, Dane. *The Magic of Tone and the Art of Music.* Shambala, 1982.

Samuels, Michael, and Samuels, Nancy. *Seeing with the Mind's Eye.* New York: Random House, 1975.

Sannella, Lee. *Kundalini: Psychosis or Transcendence?* San Francisco, CA: Sanella, 1976.

Sayadaw, M. *Practical Insight Meditation.* Santa Cruz, CA: Unity Press, 1972.

Schneck, J. M. *Hypnosis in Modern Medicine.* Charles Thomas, 1959.

Seligman, M. E. P. *Helplessness.* W. H. Freeman, 1975.

Selye, Hans. *The Stress of Life.* McGraw-Hill, 1956.

Shah, I. *Islamic Sufism.* Weiser, 1971.

Shakti, Gawain. *Creative Visualization.* Mill Valley, CA: Whatever Publishing, 1979.

Shealy, Norman. *Ninety Days to Self-Health.* New York: Ballantine Books, 1982.

Shook, Edward E., N.D., D.C. *Advanced Treatise on Herbology.* Mokelumne Hill, CA: Health Research, 1976.

Silva, Jose. *The Silva Mind-Control Method.* New York: Simon and Schuster, 1977.

Simonton, Carl. O., and Simonton, Stephanie Matthews. *Getting Well Again.* New York: Bantam, 1980.

Spaniol, Leroy. *Managing Professional Stress and Burnout: A Workbook.* Belmont, MA: Human Services Association.

Speeth, K. *The Gurdjieff Work.* Berkeley, CA: And/Or Press, 1976.

Spiegelberg, F. *Spiritual Practices of India.* Citadel Press, 1962.

The Sufi Message, Vol. IV. Published for the International Headquarters of the Sufi Movement, Geneva. London: Barrie Books, 1962.

Suzuki, Roshi. *Zen Mind, Beginner's Mind.* Weatherhill, 1970.

Taylor, Jeremy. *Dream Work: Techniques for Discovering the Creative Power in Dreams.* Ramsey, NJ: Paulist Press, 1983.

Tuktu, Tarthang. *Gesture of Balance.* Dharma Press, 1976.

Ullman, Montague, and Zimmerman, Nan. *Working with Dreams.* New York: Delacorte, 1979.

Vargiu, J., et al. *Synthesis.* Vol. 1, no. 1 (1974) and no. 2 (1975). Redwood City, CA: Psychosynthesis Press.

Weitzenhoffer, A. M. *Hypnotism: An Objective Study in Suggestibility.* Wiley, 1953.

Wolf, Harri. *Applied Iridology.* San Diego, CA: Wolf, 1979.

Zukav, Gray. *The Dancing Wu Li Masters.* New York: Bantam, 1979.

IV. LIFE CYCLES

Adams, Richard N. "An Inquiry into the Nature of the Family," from Dole, G. E., and Carneiro, R. L., eds. *Essays in the Science of Culture in Honor of Leslie A. White,* pp. 30–49. Crowel, 1960.

Airola, Paavo. *Sex and Nutrition.* Health Plus, 1974.

Ardell, Donald B. *High Level Wellness: An Alternative to Doctors, Drugs, and Disease.* Emmaus, PA: Rodale Press, 1977.

Bell, Norman W., and Vogel, Ezra F., eds. *The Family: A Modern Introduction.* New York: The Free Press, 1968.

Bieler, H. G. *Food is Your Best Medicine.* Neville Spearman, 1968.

Bieler, H. G. *Natural Way to Sexual Health.* Charles, 1972.

Billings, John. *Natural Family Planning: The Ovulation Method.* Collegeville, MN: Liturgical Press, 1972.

Butler, Robert N. *Why Survive? Being Old in America.* New York: Harper & Row, 1975.

Dextreit, Raymond. *Our Earth, Our Cure.* Swan House, 1974.

Ehret, Arnold. *Mucusless Diet Healing System.* Ehret Literature, 1972.

Engels, Friedrich. *The Origins of the Family, Private Property, and the State.* Translated by Untermann, E. Chicago: Chas. H. Kerr, 1902.

Finch, Caleb E., and Hayflick, Leonard. *Handbook of the Biology of Aging.* New York: Van Nostrand Reinhold Company, 1977.

Fries, James F., and Crapo, Lawrence M. *Vitality and Aging.* San Francisco: W. H. Freeman and Company, 1981.

Kluckholm, Florence R. "Variations on the Basic Values of the Family System," *Social Casework,* Feb./Mar. 1958, pp. 63–72.

Kulvinkas, Victoras. *Love Your Body.* Omangod Press, 1975.

Kulvinkas, Victoras. *Survival in the Twenty-First Century.* Omangod Press, 1975.

Lacey, Louise. *Lunaception.* New York: Warner Books, 1976.

Leaf, Alexander. *Youth in Old Age.* New York: McGraw Hill, 1975.

Lidz, Theodore. *The Person: His Development Throughout the Life Cycle.* Basic Books, 1968.

Luce, Gay Gear. *Body Time.* Pantheon, 1971.

Malstrom, Stan. *Herbal Remedies II.* Family Press, 1975.

Mofziger, Margaret. *A Cooperative Method of Natural Birth Control.* Summertown, TN: Book Publishing Company, 1976.

Osherson, S. *Holding On or Letting Go: Men and Career Change at Midlife.* New York: The Free Press, 1980.

Osherson, S. *The Silent Wound: Why Men Don't Talk.* New York: The Free Press, due 1985.

Osherson, S., and AmaraSingham, L. "The Machine Metaphor in Medicine," from Mishler, Osherson, et al, *Social Contexts of Health, Illness and Patient Care.* Cambridge University Press, 1983.

Osherson, S. and Dill, D. "Varying Work and Family Choices: Their Impact on Men's Work Satisfaction," *Journal of Marriage and the Family,* pp. 339–346, May 1983.

Parsons, Talcott, and Fox, Renee. "Illness, Therapy, and the Modern Urban American Family," *Journal of Social Issues,* XIII, no. 4, pp. 31–44. 1952.

Parvati, Jeannine. *Hygieia: A Woman's Herbal.* Freestone Publishing Collective, 1978.

Pelletier, Kenneth R. *Holistic Medicine: From Stress to Optimum Health.* New York: Delacorte and Delta, 1979.

Pelletier, Kenneth R. *Longevity: Fulfilling Our Biological Potential.* New York: Delacorte and Delta, 1981.

Rosenblum, Art. *The Natural Birth Control Book.* Philadelphia, PA: Aquaraian Research Foundation, 1976.

V. BODYWORK AND MOVEMENT

Baker, Ellsworth. *Man in the Trap.* New York: Harper and Row, 1974.

Campbell, Joseph. *Myths to Live By.* New York: Bantam Books, 1973.

Dychtwald, Ken. *Bodymind.* New York: Jove Publications, 1978.

Feldenkrais, Moshe. *Awareness Through Movement.* New York: Harper and Row, 1972.

Hatch, O. *Sexual Energy and Yoga.* A.S.I. Publishers, 1972.

Kogan, Gerald. *Your Body Works.* Berkeley, CA: And/Or Press, 1981.

Krishna, G. *Kundalini, Evolutionary Energy in Man.* Shambala, 1971.

Kunz, Kevin, and Kunz, Barbara. *The Complete Guide to Foot Reflexology.* Englewood Cliffs, NJ: Prentice-Hall, 1980.

Leadbeater, H. *The Chakras.* Theosophical Publishing House, 1972.

Lowe, Carl, and Nechas, James W. *Whole Body Healing.* Emmaus, PA: Rodale Press, 1983.

Rama, Swami; Ballentine, Rudolph; and Ajaya, Swami. *Yoga and Psychotherapy.* Glenview, IL: Himalayan Institute, 1976.

Reich, Wilhelm. *Character Analysis.* New York: Simon and Schuster, 1972.

Reich, Wilhelm. *The Function of the Orgasm.* Noonday Press, 1971.

Rendel, C. *Introduction to the Chakras.* Samuel Weiser, 1974.

Stransky, Judith, and Stone, Robert S. *The Alexander Technique.* New York: Beaufort Books, 1981.

VI. THE GROWING LEGITIMACY OF HOLISM

American Cancer Society. *Make Cancer Control Your Business.* New York, 1981.

Applebaum and Roth. "Patients Who Refuse Medical Treatment," *JAMA,* Vol. 250, no. 10, September 9, 1983.

Berry, Charles A. "Health Cost Saving: An Approach to Good Health For Employees and Reduced Health Care Costs for Industry," *Health Insurance Association of America.*

California Health Practitioners Association. "Holistic Practitioners Unite—It's Time to Learn to Fly," *Somatics,* Vol. 3, no. 4, Spring 1982.

"Cashing in on Wellness," *Business Insurance,* September 21, 1981.

Cole-Whitaker, Terry. *How to Have More in a Have-Not World.* New York: Rawson Associates, 1983.

Doyle, Michael, and Straus, David. *How to Make Meetings Work.* Chicago: Playboy Press, 1976.

Epstein, R. "Contracting Out of the Medical Malpractice Crisis," *JD Perspectives in Biology and Medicine,* Winter 1977.

Ferguson, Marilyn. *Aquarian Conspiracy.* Boston: Houghton Mifflin Company, 1980.

Fuller, Buckminster. *Critical Path.* New York: St. Martins Press, 1982.

Green J. "Allocating Responsibility by Contract," *Medicolegal News,* Vol. 8, no. 5, October 1980. American Society of Law and Medicine.

Green, J. "Contracts with Your Doctor?" *New Realities,* Vol. 2, no. 1, 1978.

Insurance Corporation of America. "The Health Care Contract: Key to Minimizing Malpractice," *Professional Liab. Newsletter,* March 1982.

Kamoroff, Bernard, C.P.A. *Small-Time Operator.* Laytonville, CA: Bell Springs Publishing, 1983.

Kassirer, J. P. "Adding Insult to Injury: Usurping Patient's Prerogatives," *New England Journal of Medicine,* April 14, 1983.

Laughlin, Judith A. "Wellness at Work: A Seven-Step 'Dollars and Sense' Approach," *Occupational Health Nursing,* pp. 9–13, November, 1982.

Levine, Art. "American Business is Bullish on 'Wellness'," *Medical World News*, March 29, 1982.

Naisbitt, John. *Megatrends*. New York: Warner Books, 1982.

Ouchi, William. *Theory Z*. Reading, MA: Addison-Wesley Publishing Company, 1981.

Peters, Thomas J., and Waterman, Robert H. Jr. *In Search of Excellence*. New York: Harper & Row, 1982.

Phillips, Michael. *The Seven Laws of Money*. Menlo Park, CA: Word Wheel and Random House, 1974.

Phillips, Michael, and Rasberry, Salli. *Honest Business*. New York: Random House, 1981.

Tarrytown Newsletter. Tarrytown, NY: Tarrytown Group, 1983.

Toffler, Alvin. *The Third Wave*. New York: Bantam Books, 1980.

VII. OUT INTO THE WIDER WORLD—BEYOND THE INDIVIDUAL

Brody, Howard, and Sobel, David. "A Systems View of Health and Disease," *Ways of Health: Holistic Approaches to Ancient and Contemporary Medicine*, pp. 87–105. New York: Harcourt, Brace, Jovanovich, 1979.

Brown, Lester. *The 29th Day*. W. W. Norton, 1978.

Carlson, Rick. "Holistic Health: Will the Promise be Realized?" *Holistic Health Review*. Fall 1979.

Coulter, Harris. *Divided Legacy: A History of the Schism in Medical Thought*. Washington D.C.: Wehawken, 1973, 1975, 1977.

Dabrowski, Kazimierz. *Positive Disintegration*. Boston: Little, Brown, 1964.

Douglass, James. *Resistance and Contemplation*. Doubleday, 1972.

Ferguson, Thomas. *Medical Self-Care: Access to Health Tools*. New York: Simon and Schuster, 1980.

Lalone, Marc. *A New Perspective on the Health of Canadians*. Ottawa: Govt. of Canada, 1974.

Lifton, Robert. *Boundaries*. New York: Simon and Schuster, 1967.

Lynch, William. *Images of Hope: Imagination as Healer of the Hopeless*. University of Notre Dame Press, 1974.

Medical Self-Care, 1976–1981.

Needleman, Jacob. *A Sense of the Cosmos: The Encounter of Modern Science and Ancient Truth*. New York: E. P. Dutton, 1977.

Smuts, Jan Christiaan. *Holism and Evolution*. New York: Viking, 1926.

Ullman, Dana. "Conceptualizing Energetic Medicine: An Emerging Model for Healing," *American Journal of Acupuncture*. September 1981.

Vithoulkas, George. *The Science of Homeopathy*. New York: Grove, 1979.

Recommended Magazines

Among the growing number of magazines on holistic health, the following were the most helpful in compiling this book:

Medical Self-Care, P.O. Box 1000, Point Reyes, CA 94956. $15 per year for 4 issues. Tom Ferguson, M.D., editor, and Michael Castleman, managing editor. Excellently researched and popularly written articles. Also see *Medical Self Care*, 1980, a book which brings together the best of the first eight issues of the magazine plus other articles.

Whole Life Times, 18 Shepard Street, Brighton, MA. 02135, $11.95 per year for 10 issues. This "journal for personal and planetary health" is distinguished by its blend of holistic health and current events. The magazine also sponsors the Whole Life Expos, health fairs which occur in cities such as San Francisco, Los Angeles, New York, and Boston. Some regional editions; the New England edition, edited by Randy Showstack, is particularly good.

Yoga Journal, 2054 University Ave., Berkeley, CA. 94704, $12 a year for 6 issues. Based on the practice of yoga, which means "unity," this "magazine for conscious living" features special issues on such subjects as "Relationships" and "Men in Changing Times" and excellent articles on aerobics, message, meditation, longevity, shamanism, childbirth, peace, and "healing touch."

In addition to these three magazines which aided us greatly, we would also like to draw attention to two other fine publications: 1) *New Age*, 342 Western Ave., Brighton, MA. 02135. A general publication with some health articles; Rick Ingrasci, M.D., is health editor. 2) *East West Journal*, 17 Station St., Brookline, MA. 02147. A monthly published by the macrobiotic Kushi Foundation.

Holistic Health Centers

PLEASE NOTE: DISCLAIMER

The definition of what constitutes a "Holistic Health Center" was left very broad for the purposes of compilation of this directory. These facilities do not all offer alternative treatments nor do all follow proscribed "usual and customary" medical practices.

The inclusion of any listing is not an endorsement of the services offered. Centers did not pay to be listed in this directory. We intend to provide access to these groups; it is up to the consumer to make the determination of quality, safety and effectiveness. These organizations were included on the basis of unsolicited promotional materials sent to our office. *Please be very careful in your considerations and thorough in your investigations before engaging any services or payment of any fees. THERE ARE NO STANDARDS OF PRACTICE FOR THESE FACILITIES.*

Additional copies of this directory and of a National Directory of *Schools: Healing and Alternative* are also available. Please remit $5.00 for each and a large self-addressed stamped envelope to the Holistic Health Organizing Committee at the address in the footnote below.

ALASKA

Radiant Health Center   907-349-5916
209 West Diamond
Anchorage, AK 99502

ARKANSAS

Ozark Life Center   501-361-2155
Rt. 4, Box 540
Grandview Road
Springdale, AR 72764

ARIZONA

A.R.E. Clinic   602-955-0551
4018 North 40th Street
Phoenix, AZ 85018

International Holistic Center   602-957-2181
P.O. Box 15103
Phoenix, AZ 85060

Lukats Prevention & Regeneration   602-428-2881
  Resort
Route 1, Box 955
Safford, AZ 85546

CALIFORNIA

Actualism Wholistic Health Center   714-741-7827
739 E. Pennsylvania, Suite D
Escondido, CA 92026

Alive Fellowship of Harmonious   707-942-0997
  Living
1880 Lincoln Avenue
Calistoga, CA 95415

Alternative Therapies Unit   415-821-5139
San Francisco General Hospital
2550 23rd Street, Bldg. 9, Room 130
San Francisco, CA 94110

Aquarian Institute   415-534-1856
2939 Galindo Street
Oakland, CA 94601

Astara   714-981-4941
800 West Arrow Highway
Upland, CA 91786

Balance and Wholesome Seminar   714-236-1409
P.O. Box 1705
San Diego, CA 92102

Berkeley Holistic Health Center   415-845-4430
3099 Telegraph Avenue
Berkeley, CA 94705

Berkeley Massage Studio   415-845-5998
1962 University Avenue
Berkeley, CA 94707

Berkeley Women's Health Collective   415-843-6194
2908 Ellsworth
Berkeley, CA 94705

Biofeedback & Family Therapy   415-841-7227
  Institute
2236 Derby Street
Berkeley, CA 94705

Brahma Kumari's Raja Yoga Center   213-635-4846
11600 Atlantic Avenue
Los Angeles, CA 90262

Steven Markell and Wendy Worsley © 1982
Sponsored by: Holistic Health Organizing Committee
4169 Park Blvd
Oakland, CA 94601

Bresler Center for Allied Therapeutics
12401 Wilshire Blvd.
Los Angeles, CA 90025
213-826-5669

Buena Vista Women's Health Center
2000 Van Ness Avenue
San Francisco, CA 94109
415-771-5000

Center for Attitudinal Healing
19 Main Street
Tiburon, CA 94920
415-435-5022

Center for Chinese Medicine
230 South Garfield Avenue
Monterey Park, CA 91754
213-573-4141
572-0424

Center for Creative Health
3501 4th Avenue
San Diego, CA 92103
714-296-2178

Center for Counseling &
Psychotherapy
3017 Santa Monica Blvd.
Santa Monica, CA 90404
213-829-7407

Center for the Healing Arts
11081 Missouri Avenue
Los Angeles, CA 90025
213-477-3981

Center for Health and Healing
8631 West Third Street, Suite 1140E
Los Angeles, CA 90048
213-652-2101

Center for the Form
1453-B 14th Street
Santa Monica, CA 90404
213-395-0063

Center for Metabolic Research
Pacific Center for Advanced Studies
1312 North Stanley Avenue
Los Angeles, CA 90046
213-876-0474

Center for Release and Integration
1057 Steiner Street
San Francisco, CA 94115
415-929-0119

Cooperative Healing Center
1201 Parducci Road
Ukiah, CA 95482
707-462-9473

Cotati Holistic Health Center
65 W. Cotati Avenue
Cotati, CA 94928
707-795-8584

Dolphin Holistic Center
3641 Diamond
Oakland, CA 94611
415-531-5509

Dovetail Institute
160 Bret Harte Road
San Rafael, CA 94901
415-461-9521

Duzhan Center
15445 Ventura Blvd., #10–150
Sherman Oaks, CA 91403
213-788-6424

East West Health Center
61 Camino Alto, No. 103
Mill Valley, CA 94941
415-388-0646
383-1585

Farallones Institute Rural Center
15290 Coleman Valley Road
Occidental, CA 95465
707-874-3060

Flower Essence Society
P.O. Box 459
Nevada City, CA 95959
916-265-9163

Fort Help Counseling Center
169 Eleventh Street
San Francisco, CA 94103
415-864-4357

Gerson Institute
P.O. Box 430
Bonita, CA 92002
714-267-1150

Habitat Center
P.O. Box 2363
Berkeley, CA 94702
415-526-0869

Haight Ashbury Free Clinic
1696 Haight Street
San Francisco, CA 94117
415-864-6090

Healing Center of San Francisco
465 Brussels
San Francisco, CA 94134
415-468-4680

Healing Light Center
138 N. Maryland Avenue
Glendale, CA 91206
213-244-8607

Health Enhancement Center
930 Mission Street #3
Santa Cruz, CA 95060
408-429-8161

Health Evaluations
P.O. Box 187
Hayward, CA 94543
415-582-0286

Health Analysis Institute
1001 Bridgeway, Suite 305
Sausalito, CA 94965
415-331-3462

Health Integration Center
1625 Olympic Blvd.
Santa Monica, CA 90404
213-450-9998

Health Training Center
420 Walnut Street
San Diego, CA 92103
714-296-2178

High Point Foundation
5337 North Millbrook
Fresno, CA 93710
209-222-5695

Holistic Health Center
2872 Folsom Street
San Francisco, CA 94110
415-285-2909

Holistic Health Center
8907 Wilshire Blvd., Suite 200
Beverly Hills, CA 90211
213-851-7044

Holistic Family Service Health Clinic
16260 Ventura Blvd., #630
Encino, CA 91436
213-990-1190

Holistic Healing Arts Clinic
312 South Cedros
Solano Beach, CA 92075
714-755-6681

Holistic Healing Center
1050 Chestnut Street, Suite 202
Menlo Park, CA 94025
415-321-8020

Holistic Medical Group
3031 Tisch Way, Drawer 106
San Jose, CA 95128
408-249-1991

Holmes Center
600 South New Hampshire
Los Angeles, CA 90075
213-380-6176

Homecoming Clinic
3829 22nd Street
San Francisco, CA 94114
415-821-9134

Homelight Birthing
458 9th Avenue
San Francisco, CA 94112
415-387-6445

Human Relations Center
5200 Hollister Avenue
Santa Barbara, CA 93111
805-967-4557

Humboldt Open Door Clinic
P.O. Box 367
Arcata, CA 95521
707-822-2957

Hypnosis Clearing House
1504 Franklin Street
Oakland, CA 94612
415-451-6440

Institute of Colon Hygiene
807-A Fourth Street
San Rafael, CA 94901
415-459-3253

Institute for the Study of Conscious
Evolution
2418 Clement Street
San Francisco, CA 94121
415-221-9222

Integral Health Center
905 Sir Francis Drake Blvd.
Kentfield, CA 94904
415-454-9690

Julian Preventive Medical Clinic
1654 Cahuenga
Hollywood, CA 90028
213-466-0126

Kairos
P.O. Box 111
Encinitas, CA 92024
714-753-9018

La Jolla Clinic of Preventive Medicine
8950 Villa La Jolla Drive, #2161
La Jolla, CA 92037
714-457-2360

Learning for Health
1314 Westwood Blvd., #107
Los Angeles, CA 90024
213-474-6929

Meadowlark Friendly Hills Fellowship
12626 Fairview Avenue
Hemet, CA 92343
714-927-1343

Mid-Peninsula Health Service
704 Webster
Palo Alto, CA 94301
415-324-1940

Min An Health Center
1144 Pacific Avenue
San Francisco, CA 94133
415-771-4040

National Androgeny Center
P.O. Box 7429
San Diego, CA 92107
714-270-4900

National Center for the Exploration of
Human Potential
P.O. Box 1233
Del Mar, CA 92014
714-481-7751

Natural Environmental Health Center
P.O. Box 11
Brookdale, CA 95007
408-338-2363

New Ways of Consciousness
3118 Washington Street
San Francisco, CA 94115
415-346-5671

Nyingma Institute
1815 Highland Place
Berkeley, CA 94709
415-843-6812

Pacific Heights Healing Arts Center
3198 Ninth Street, Suite A
Del Mar, CA 92014
714-481-2541

Pain Rehabilitation Center
Bay General Community Hospital
435 H Street
Chula Vista, CA 92010
714-420-8182

Pierre Pannetier Polarity Center
410 North Glassell Street
Orange, CA 92666
714-532-3035

Preventative Medicine & Health
Center
3330 Third Avenue, Suite 400
San Diego, CA 92103
714-291-0261

Price Pottenger Nutrition Foundation
P.O. Box 2614
La Mesa, CA 92041
714-582-4168

Proteus Institute
330 Ellis Street, Suite 206
San Francisco, CA 94102
415-771-9997

Radiant Life Center
824 5th Street
San Rafael, CA 94901
415-459-6798

Radiant Life Medical Center
Highway 53 @ 40th Avenue
Clearlake, CA
707-994-9486

Religious School of Natural Hygiene
6344 Pacheco Pass Highway
Hollister, CA 95023
408-637-1920

Riverwinds
1545 Franklin Street
San Francisco, CA 94109
415-673-3462

Rockridge Health Care Services
430 40th Street
Oakland, CA 94609
415-658-8517

Round Valley Indian Health Center
P.O. Box 247
Covelo, CA 95428
707-983-2981

Sacramento Holistic Health Institute
1822 21st Street
Sacramento, CA 95814
916-454-4470

SAGE Project
491 65th Street
Oakland, CA 94609
415-763-0965

San Diego Sport Psychology Center
6505 Alvarado Road #207
San Diego, CA 92120
714-286-5156

San Andreas Health Council
531 Cowper Street
Palo Alto, CA 94301
415-324-9350

Self Realization Fellowship
3880 San Rafael Avenue
Los Angeles, CA 90065
213-225-2471

Shanti Nilaya
P.O. Box 2396
Escondido, CA 92025
714-749-2008

Shanti Project
1314 Addison Street
Berkeley, CA 94702
415-849-4980

Shaw Health Center
5336 Fountain Avenue
Los Angeles, CA 90029
213-467-5200

Shaw Health Center
Torrance, CA

South Bay Institute
819 Harbor Drive
Redondo Beach, CA 90277
213-376-4440

St. George Homes
1515 Arch Street
Berkeley, CA 94708
415-848-2393

Sufi Islamia Ruhaniat Society &
Center
410 Precita Avenue
San Francisco, CA 94110
415-285-5208

S.Y.D.A. Foundation & Meditation
Center
1107 Stanford Avenue
Oakland, CA 94611
415-655-8677

Teen Reach/Center for Living with
Dying
1542 Los Padres Blvd.
Santa Clara, CA 95050
408-243-0700

Theta Seminars
301 Lyon Street
San Francisco, CA 94117
415-929-1743

Trager Institute
300 Poplar Avenue #5
Mill Valley, CA 94941
415-388-2688

Ultra Nutrition Institute
780 Charcot Avenue
San Jose, CA 95131
408-263-5540

Village Oz
P.O. Box 147
Point Arena, CA 95468
707-882-2449

Watercourse Way
165 Channing Avenue
Palo Alto, CA 94301
415-329-8827

Well Being Community Center
788 Ferguson Road
Sebastopol, CA 95472
707-823-1489

Willow Women's Center
6517 Dry Creek Road
Napa, CA 94558
707-944-8173

Whole Life Center
3437 Alma Street, #28
Palo Alto, CA 94306
415-493-0561

Wholistic Health & Nutrition
Institute
150 Shoreline Highway
Mill Valley, CA 94941
415-332-2933

Wholistic Medicine & Counseling
Center
1703 Wilshire Blvd.
Santa Monica, CA 90403
213-451-9997

Womankind Health Clinic
1003 40th Street
Sacramento, CA 95819
916-452-KIND

Women's Community Clinic
696 East Santa Clara Street
San Jose, CA 95112

Wellness Counseling Center
173 Seminary Avenue
Ukiah, CA 95482

World Synergy Institute
P.O. Box 24242
Los Angeles, CA 90024

Yoga Society of San Francisco
2872 Folsom Street
San Francisco, CA 94110

Vital Health Center
17200 Ventura Blvd., Suite 305
Encino, CA 91316

Lela Center for Creative Service to
Humanity
320 2nd Street #2H
Eureka, CA 95501

National Arthritis Medical Clinic
13–630 Mountain View Road
Desert Hot Springs, CA 92240
714-32

COLORADO

Colorado Health Center
1640 Welton
Denver, CO 80202
303-623-3166

Denver Pain & Health Rehabilitation
Center
3005 E. 16th Avenue
Denver, CO 80201
303-377-9619

Whole Life Learning Center
1912 W. Colorado Avenue
Colorado Springs, CO 80904
303-475-7322

Womanwise Health Care
1829 High Street
Denver, CO 80218
303-320-1020

CONNECTICUT

Integral Health Services
245 School Street
Putnam, CT 06260
203-928-7729

FLORIDA

Shangri-La Natural Hygiene Institute
Bonita Springs, FL 33923
813-992-3811

Ultra Nutrition Institute
1825 N.E. 149th Street
Miami, FL 33181
305-945-2020

GEORGIA

Chrysalis at Kingswood
P.O. Box 725
Claytin, GA 30525
404-782-4278

ILLINOIS

Center for Appropriate Nutrition
P.O. Box 10696
Chicago, IL 60610
312-764-5470

'7

408-287-4322

707-462-0609

419

213-821-1302

415-285-5537

213-986-0886

07-442-6641

-0532

_6422

504-568-1201

207-655-7624

...s
.. 279
..d, ME 04071

MARYLAND

Center for Studies of Human Systems
8604 Jones Mill Road
Chevy Chase, MD 20015 — 301-657-8299

Center for Traditional Acupuncture
Suite 108
American Cities Building
Columbia, MD 21044 — 301-752-5425

Koinonia
1400 Greenspring Valley Road
Stevenson, MD 21153 — 301-486-6262

New Life Clinic
1301 Asbury Road
Baltimore, MD 21209 — 301-435-9736

Rockville Health Association
4808 Macon Road
Rockville, MD 20852 — 301-881-2406

Wellness Center
1015 Wisconsin Avenue, N.W.
Georgetown, MD 21930 — 301-338-7171

MASSACHUSETTS

Acupuncture Center of Cambridge
380 Green Street
Cambridge, MA 02139 — 617-864-4600

Beacon Hill Health Associates
14 Beacon Street, Suite 620
Boston, MA 02108 — 617-523-8017

Biofeedback Institute of Boston
110 Francis Street, Suite 7E
Boston, MA 02215 — 617-734-7181

Center of the Light
P.O. Box 540
Great Barrington, MA 01230 — 413-229-2396

East-West Medical Center
51 Brattle Street, Suite 1A
Cambridge, MA 02138 — 617-661-0700

.artspring Health Center
'empstead Road
a Plain, MA 02130 — 617-738-4366

.erface
230 Central Street
Newton, MA 02116 — 617-964-0500

New England Health Foundations
2 Nutting Road
Cambridge, MA 02138 — 617-661-6225

Soma Center
595 Massachusetts Avenue
Cambridge, MA 02139 — 617-491-8694

Synthesis Center
P.O. Box 575
Amherst, MA 01004 — 413-256-0772

MINNESOTA

Center for Health Promotion
2810 57th Avenue, Suite 601
Brookdale Towers
Minneapolis, MN 55430 — 612-574-7800

Center for Holistic Healing
569 Selby Avenue
St. Paul, MN 55102 — 612-291-7637

MISSOURI

Natural Health Institute
7624 S. Broadway
St. Louis, MO 63111 — 314-631-4514
-4839

NEW HAMPSHIRE

Another Place
Route 123
Greenville, NH 03048 — 603-878-1510

NEW JERSEY

Better Health & Nutrition Center
1 Woodbridge Center
Woodbridge, NJ 07095 — 201-636-6228

Jamie Schuman Center
600 Blue Hill Road
River Vale, NJ 07675 — 201-291-4473

Yoga and Growth Center of Bergen
County
84 East Ridgewood Avenue
Ridgewood, NJ 07450 — 201-447-2474

NEW MEXICO

Healing Arts of Santa Fe
P.O. Box 1445
Santa Fe, NM 87501 — 505-988-4122

NEW YORK

Creative Aging 212-864-1523
700 West End Avenue, #11B
New York, NY 10025

Dialogue House 212-673-5880
80 East 11th Street
New York, NY 10003

Fryer Research Center 212-265-5805
200 West 57th Street
New York, NY 10019

Health Associates 212-298-1295
13 East 71st Street, #2A
New York, NY 10021

Heights Holistic Health Association 212-625-4802
100 Remsen Street
Brooklyn Heights, NY 11201

Himalayan Institute 212-243-5995
78 Fifth Avenue
New York, NY 10011

Institute for Self Development/ 516-627-0309
Wholistic Health Center
50 Maple Place
Manhasset, NY 11030

Institute for the New Age 212-737-8808
45 East 78th Street
New York, NY 10021

Institute of Behavioral Kinesiology 914-268-5144
P.O. Drawer 37
Valley Cottage, NY 10989

Matagiri Sri Aurobindo Center 914-679-8322
Mt. Tremper, NY 12547

New York Zendo 212-861-3333
223 East 67th Street
New York, NY 11021

Omega Institute for Holistic Studies 518-794-8850
P.O. Box 396
New Lebanon, NY 12125

Rochester Center for the Healing Arts 716-461-3130
8 Prince Street
Rochester, NY 14607

Serenity 212-472-3104
310 East 72nd Street
New York, NY 10021

Wholistic Health Education Center 716-442-5480
715 Monroe Avenue
Rochester, NY 14607

Pawling Health Manor 914-889-4141
P.O. Box 401
Hyde Park, NY 12538

OREGON

Academy of Predictive Cell Health 503-636-8167
8 State Street, Lakeside Plaza
Lake Oswego, OR 97034

Aletheia Foundation 503-479-4855
515 N.E. 8th Street
Grants Pass, OR 97526

Atlantis Rising Health Education 503-253-4031
Center
7915 S.E. Stark Street
Portland, OR 97215

Eugene Center for the Healing Arts 503-895-4967
82644 N. Howe Lane
Creswell, OR 97426

Healthworks 503-231-0090
2917 N.E. Everett
Portland, OR 97232

Institute of Preventive Medicine 503-246-7616
6171 S.W. Capitol Highway
Portland, OR 97201

Naturopathic Clinic at the National 503-226-3717
College of Naturopathic Medicine
510 S.W. Third Avenue
Portland, OR 97204

White Bird Sociomedical Aid Station 503-342-8255
341 E. 12th Street
Eugene, OR 97401

PENNSYLVANIA

Himalaya International Institute 717-253-5551
P.O. Box 88
Honesdale, PA 18431

Kripalu Center for Holistic Health 717-754-3051
P.O. Box 120
Summit Station, PA 17979

Performance Training Systems 215-535-3413
5931 Tackawanna Street
Philadelphia, PA 19135

Center for Well Being 215-923-6600
716 South Street
Philadelphia, PA 19147

TEXAS

Austin Wellness Center 512-451-6519
1801 W. Koening Lane
Austin, TX 78756

Cancer Counseling & Research Center 214-373-7444
6060 N. Central Expressway
Dallas, TX 75206

Institute for the Study of Stress & the 817-776-0400
Family
4901 Bosque Blvd., Suite 223
Waco, TX 76710

VIRGINIA

American Center for Homeopathy 703-534-2600
7297 H Lee Highway
Falls Church, VA 22042

Association for Research & 804-428-3588
Enlightenment
P.O. Box 595
Virginia Beach, VA 23451

Nutritional Analysis & Health Design 703-836-7636
3104 Old Dominion Blvd.
Alexandria, VA 22305

National Center for Homeopathy   703-698-5783
7810 Helena Drive
Falls Church, VA 22043

Simonton Cancer Self-Help Education   703-524-1639
    Center
1327 N. Lynbrook Drive
Arlington, VA 22201

Spiritual Science Healing Institute   703-361-9877
8718 Yorkshire Lane
Manassa, VA 22110

WASHINGTON

Balance and Wholesome Seminar   206-671-3194
    Center
1111 High Street
Bellingham, WA 98225

Polarity Health Institute   206-376-2291
P.O. Box 68   -4755
Olga, WA 98279

Psychosynthesis Center   206-282-1171
311 West McGraw
Seattle, WA 98119

WASHINGTON, D.C.

Columbia Road Wholistic Health   202-462-1337
    Center
2700 Ontario Road, N.W.
Washington, D.C. 20009

Healing Arts Center   202-232-3040
1449 Rhode Island Avenue, N.W.
Washington, D.C. 20005

Holistic Medical Clinic   202-723-4510
5605 16th Street, N.W.
Washington, D.C. 20011

Naturopathic Health Clinic   202-667-5162
1455 Harvard Street, N.W.
Washington, D.C. 20009

Potomac Massage Therapy Institute   202-829-4201
421 Butternut Street, N.W.
Washington, D.C. 20012

3HO Center for Holistic Living   202-435-5599
1704 Q Street, N.W.   -4411
Washington, D.C. 20009

CANADIAN HOLISTIC HEALTH CENTERS

ONTARIO

Voie Suchness Way   613-256-2665
RR #3
Almont, Ontario K0A 1A0

Positive Alternatives Wellness   416-454-2688
    Education Centre
123 Queen Street West
Brampton, Ontario L6Y 1M3

Chestnut Hill   416-888-1231
Box 454
RR #1
Gormley, Ontario L0H 1G0

Santosa Yoga and Health Centre   519-837-3022
16A Wyndham
Guelph, Ontario

Total Health Gateway   519-837-3022
P.O. Box 1386   416-598-3117
Guelph, Ontario N1H 4E5   (Toronto
    telephone)

Life Space Centre for Holistic   416-533-1903
    Psychotherapy and Counselor
    Training
1527 Davenport Road
Toronto, Ontario M6H 2H9

Toronto Healing Arts   416-535-8777
715 Bloor Street West
Toronto, Ontario M6G 1L5

Toronto Health Education Centre   416-926-1782
258 Dupont Street
Toronto, Ontario M5R 1V7

West End Holistic Health Centre   416-763-3211
12 Heintzman Street
Toronto, Ontario M6P 2J6

BRITISH COLUMBIA

Atlin Holistic Health Centre   604-651-7655
Box 284
Atlin, British Columbia V0W 1A0

Hollyhock Farm   604-935-6465
127 Mansons Landing
Cortes Island, British Columbia V0P
    1K0

The Salt Spring Island Health Clinic   604-653-4216
Box 4
Fulford Harbour, British Columbia
    V0S 1C0

Bright Farm   604-537-2378
c/o Coleman
RR #1
Tripp Road
Ganges, British Columbia V0S 1E0

The Salt Spring Centre   604-537-2326
Box 1133
Ganges, British Columbia V0S 1E0

The Hailos Society for Wholistic   604-547-9680
    Living
P.O. Box 8
Lumby, British Columbia V0E 2G0

Health Enhancement Centre   604-876-5955
2021 Columbia Street
Vancouver, British Columbia V5Y 3C9

Inner Garden Activity Centre   604-875-8828
535 West 10th Avenue
Vancouver, British Columbia

Integrated Health Centre   604-879-2319
4676 Main Street
Vancouver, British Columbia V5V
    3R7

Preventive Medicine Centre   604-224-1515
3743 West 10th Avenue
Vancouver, British Columbia

Well-Quest Holistic Health Centre   604-567-9959
c/o Bobby J. Ford
RR #2
Birch Road
Site 6, Box 6
Vanderhoof, British Columbia V0J
    3A0

Dispensable Healing Centre   604-384-5560
403A Kingston Street
Victoria, British Columbia V8V 1V8

Islands Association of Holistic Health   604-389-1290
   Professionals
1126A Dallas Road
Victoria, British Columbia V8V 1V9

Victoria Attunement Centre   604-383-1243
Suite #1
2727 Quadra Street
Victoria, British Columbia V8T 4E5

Victoria Stress and Pain Centre   604-247-9211
5575 West Saanich Road
Victoria, British Columbia V8X 4M6

Self Health Herbal Centre   604-383-1913
   Practitioners
1221 Wharf Street
Victoria, British Columbia V8W 1T8

HOLISTIC HEALTH CENTERS—INTERNATIONAL

Centro Medico del Mar   908-387-1850
Paseo de Tijuana 1-A
Apdo. Postal 179
Playas de Tijuana, B.C. MEXICO
or: P.O. Box 3793
      San Ysidro, CA 92073

Clinica Cydel S.A.   706-687-1502
Apartado 3437
Tijuana, B.C. MEXICO

Dr. Edward Bach Centre
Mt. Vernon, Sotwell
Wallingford, Oxon. 0X10 OPZ
   ENGLAND

Fairfield Medical Center   305-462-0206
Montego Bay, Jamaica, WI
or: P.O. Box 13042
         Fort Lauderdale, FL 33316

Immunology Research Center   809-352-7455
P.O. Box F 2689
Freeport, Grand Bahamas Island

Institut Holistique De La Sante   022-28 08-81
36 bis, rue de Carouge
CH 1205 Geneva SWITZERLAND

Institute of Regeneration   706-688-1972
P.O. Box 1822
Ensenada, B.C. MEXICO

Radient Health Clinic   092-71-2372
17 Iverness Cres.
Menora 6050 WEST AUSTRALIA

Ringberg Klinik   0-80-22/2-20-37
Postfach 149
8182 Bad Wiesse, GERMANY

Lemington Spa
10A Beauchamp Avenue
Warwickshire, ENGLAND

Renaissance Revitalization Spa   809-327-8441
Cable Beach, P.O. Box N4854
Nassau, BAHAMAS

Rio Caliente, CA
APDO 1-1187
Guadalajara, Jalisco MEXICO

For additional listings, write: Cancer Control Society
                              2043 North Berendo Street
                              Los Angeles, CA 90027
                              213-663-7801

Index

About the Editors

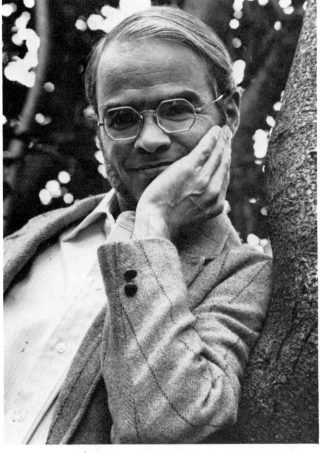

© Karen S. Rantzman 1983

DR. SHEPHERD BLISS, D.MN., divides his time between Berkeley, California, and Cambridge, Massachusetts. Professor of Psychology at John F. Kennedy University in Orinda, CA., since 1981, he spent most of the 1970's associated with Harvard University and Radcliffe College as an administrator, counselor, teacher, and post-doctoral student. He has also taught at the California School of Professional Psychology (CSPP), Starr King School of Ministry (part of the Graduate Theological Union), Suffolk University, and Goddard College. Graduated from Benson High in Omaha and the University of Kansas, he went to seminary at Drew University and received the Doctor of Ministry degree from the University of Chicago. Commissioned an officer in the U.S. Army and ordained a Methodist minister, Dr. Bliss is now active in Psychotherapists for Social Responsibility, Interhelp, and the Association for Humanistic Psychology. A member of the National Writers Union, he is a contributing editor to *Yoga Journal* and *Awakening in the Nuclear Age* and a staff writer for *Whole Life Times*, and was a foreign correspondent in Latin America. A popular lecturer and workshop leader on Holistic Health and Men's Studies at colleges, health fairs and churches around the country, he is interviewed frequently in newspapers and on radio and television.

EDWARD BAUMAN is a nutrition mentor and pioneer in holistic health. He received a Master of Education degree from the University of Massachusetts in 1971 and a Master of Arts degree from Heartwood College in Natural Health Education in 1985. Edward's seven year participation with the Berkeley Holistic Health Center produced an exciting educational and clinical prototype of holistic services. He authored *Nutrition and Your Health* and *Healthy Food Recipes* and co-edited *The Holistic Health Handbook* and *The Holistic Health Lifebook*. The vision of a rural healing community brought Edward to Heartwood College in 1983, where he initiated a nutritional consultant training program and directed the college's Wellness Clinic. In 1985, Edward and his wife, Chris Clay Bauman, will be settling in the Santa Fe, New Mexico, area, and opening a Center for Self Healing.

ARMAND IAN BRINT is the founder of the Berkeley Holistic Health Center, and co-editor of the *Holistic Health Handbook* and its companion volume, the *Holistic Health Lifebook*. Armand is a charter member of Iridologists International and has taught iri-

dology and related health practices throughout California. He currently is the administrator of a mental health clinic in Oakland, California.

PAMELA AMELIA WRIGHT is a holistic-health educator, lecturer, and administrator at the Berkeley Holistic Health Center, and has contributed greatly to the growth of the center. Currently she is helping to develop a holistic counseling and health evaluation program that will soon be available at the center. She is the mother of an eight-year-old son. She is a minister with the metaphysical Church of the Rising Star, and in her private practice specializes in psychic counseling, guided meditation, and relaxation techniques.

LORIN PIPER has served as an administrator with the Berkeley Holistic Health Center. A masseuse, flamenco dancer, and metaphysical practitioner, she is currently completing a program to become a professional prayer therapist through the Teaching of the Inner Christ, a nonsectarian metaphysical fellowship.